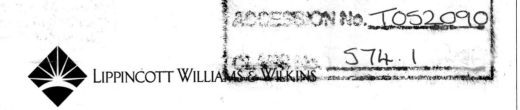

Memmler's
The Structure and Function
of the Human Body

Memmler's
The Structure and Function
of the Human Body

Eighth Edition

Barbara Janson Cohen

Jason James Taylor

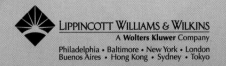

LIPPINCOTT WILLIAMS & WILKINS
A **Wolters Kluwer** Company

Philadelphia • Baltimore • New York • London
Buenos Aires • Hong Kong • Sydney • Tokyo

Senior Acquisitions Editor: *John Goucher*
Senior Development Editor: *Dana Knighten*
Associate Production Manager: *Kevin Johnson*
Associate Marketing Manager: *Hilary Henderson*
Cover and Interior Designer: *Armen Kojoyian*
Compositor: *Maryland Composition, Inc.*
Printer: *R.R. Donnelley & Sons-Willard*

351 West Camden Street
Baltimore, MD 21201

530 Walnut Street
Philadelphia, PA 19106

Printed in the United States of America

Library of Congress Cataloging-in-Publication Data

Cohen, Barbara J.
  Memmler's the structure and function of the human body.-- 8th ed. / Barbara Janson Cohen, Jason James Taylor.
      p. ; cm.
  Rev. ed. of: Memmler's the structure & function of the human body. 7th ed. / Barbara Janson Cohen, Dena Lion Wood. c2000.
  Includes bibliographical references and index.
  ISBN 0-7817-5184-5 (hardcover) -- ISBN 0-7817-4233-1 (softcover)
  1. Human physiology. 2. Human anatomy. I. Taylor, Jason J. II. Memmler, Ruth Lundeen. Structure & function of the human body. III. Cohen, Barbara J. Memmler's the structure & function of the human body. VI. Title. V. Title: Structure and function of the human body. [DNLM: 1. Anatomy. 2. Physiology. QS 4 C678m 2005]
  QP36.M54 2005
  612--dc22

                                    2004030916

To purchase additional copies of this book, call our customer service department at (800) 638-3030 or fax orders to (301) 824-7390. International customers should call (301) 714-2324.

Visit Lippincott Williams & Wilkins on the Internet: http://www.LWW.com. Lippincott Williams & Wilkins customer service representatives are available from 8:30 am to 6:00 pm, EST.

10 9 8 7 6 5 4 3 2 1

Reviewers

We gratefully acknowledge the generous contributions of the reviewers whose names appear in the list that follows. These instructors were kind enough to read the text thoroughly and make suggestions for improvement. Their comments determined many of the changes in content and direction for this revision, such as the increased number and types of learning aids, addition of new art and revisions to existing art, a stronger focus on teaching and learning anatomic and medical terminology, and an increased emphasis on physiology and the interrelatedness of structure and function. We hope they will be pleased with the results of their hard work in this 8th edition of *Memmler's The Structure and Function of the Human Body.*

LaVon Barrett, RN, BSN
Amarillo College
Amarillo, TX

Nina Beaman, MS, CMA, RNC
Allied Health Program Area
    Coordinator
Bryant and Stratton College
Richmond, VA

Mark Andrew Bloom, BS, MS
Instructor of Biology
Texas Christian University
Fort Worth, TX

Kathleen Bode, RN, MS
Chair, Division of Health
Flint Hills Technical College
Emporia, KS

William J. Burke, BA
Madison Area Technical College
Madison, WI
Blackhawk Area Technical College
Monroe, WI

Patti Calk, MEd, LOTR
University of Louisiana at Monroe
Monroe, LA

Kathy Carson, RPH
The Cleveland Institute of Dental-
    Medical Assistants, Inc.
Mentor, OH

Michelle Cleary, PhD
Florida International University
Miami, FL

Stephen M. Colarusso, BS, NCTMB,
    ACST
Director of Education
Charles of Italy School of Massage
    Therapy
Lake Havasu City, AZ

Zoe Hanson Cujak, BSN, MEd
Associate Dean, Service Occupations
Fox Valley Technical College
Appleton, WI

Glenn Grady, MEd, BSMT (ASCP),
    CMA
Allied Health Department Chair
Miller-Motte Technical College
Wilmington, NC

Kerry Hull, PhD
Associate Professor
Department of Biology
Bishop's University
Lennoxville, Quebec, Canada

Tammee Neuhaus, MLT
Minnesota School of Health Sciences
Apple Valley, MN

Debra J. Paul, BAM, CMA
Medical Assisting Program Instructor
IVY Tech State College
South Bend, IN

Lisa S. Reed, RN, MS, CNOR
Department Chairperson for Surgical
    Technology
New England Institute of Technology
Warwick, RI

Dyal N. P. Singh, BSc (Honors), MSc,
    PhD
Professor of Anatomy
Director of Neuroscience
Ross University School of Medicine
Dominica, West Indies

Rox Ann Sparks, RN, BSN, MICN
Vocational Nursing Instructor
Merced College
Merced, CA

Alan H. Stephenson, BS, MS, PhD
Chair, Science Department
Edgecombe Community College
Tarboro, NC

Jean A. Zorko, MS, BSMT (ASCP)
Assistant Professor, Science
Stark State College of Technology
Canton, OH

Preface

Memmler's The Structure and Function of the Human Body, 8th edition, is a textbook for introductory-level health professions and nursing students who need a basic understanding of anatomy and physiology and the interrelationships between structure and function.

Like preceding editions, the 8th edition remains true to Ruth Memmler's original vision. Designed for health professions and nursing students, the features and content specifically meet the needs of those who may be starting their health career preparation with little or no science background. This book's primary goals are:

- To provide the essential knowledge of human anatomy and physiology at an ideal level of detail, and in language that is clear and understandable.
- To illustrate the concepts discussed with anatomic art that depicts the appropriate level of detail with accuracy, simplicity, and elegance, and that is integrated seamlessly with the narrative.
- To incorporate the most recent scientific findings into the fundamental material on which Ruth Memmler's classic text is based.
- To include pedagogy designed to enhance interest in and understanding of the concepts presented.
- To teach the basic anatomic and medical terminology used in healthcare settings, preparing students to function efficiently in their chosen health career.
- To present an integrated teaching-learning package that includes all of the elements necessary for a successful learning experience.

This revision is the direct result of in-depth market feedback solicited to tell us what instructors and students at this level most need. We listened carefully to the feedback, and the results we obtained are integrated into every feature of this book. The text itself has been thoroughly revised and updated to reflect the latest accepted scientific thought in each area of the book. Because visual learning devices are so important to students at this level, this edition also features a completely revamped and expanded art program that includes revised versions of many of the figures from previous editions as well as numerous all-new, full-color anatomic line drawings and photographs. Last but not least, these features appear in an all-new design that makes the content more user-friendly and accessible than ever.

▶ Organization and Structure

Like previous editions, the 8th edition uses a body systems approach to the study of the normal human body.

The book is divided into six units, grouping related information and body systems together as follows:

- Unit I, The Body as a Whole (Chapters 1–5), focuses on the body's organization; basic chemistry needed to understand body functions; cells and their functions; tissues, glands, and membranes; and the skin.
- Unit II, Movement and Support (Chapters 6 and 7), includes the skeletal and muscular systems.
- Unit III, Coordination and Control (Chapters 8–11), focuses on the nervous system, the sensory system, and the endocrine system.
- Unit IV, Circulation and Body Defense (Chapters 12–15), includes the blood, the heart, blood vessels and ci factual recall.
- Unit V, Energy: Supply and Use (Chapters 16–19), includes the respiratory system; the digestive system; metabolism, nutrition, and temperature control; and the urinary system and body fluids.
- Unit VI, Perpetuating Life (Chapters 20 and 21), includes the male and female reproductive systems as well as development and heredity.

The main Glossary defines the chapters' boldfaced terms, and a Glossary of Word Parts is a reference tool that not only teaches basic medical and anatomic terminology but also helps students learn to recognize unfamiliar terms. Appendixes include a variety of supplementary information that students will find useful as they work with the text, as well as answers to the Chapter Checkpoint questions and Zooming In illustration questions (Appendix 4) that are found in every chapter.

▶ Pedagogic Features

Every chapter contains pedagogy that has been designed with the health professions and nursing student in mind (the User's Guide that follows the Preface provides a "guided tour" of these features and their pedagogic benefits).

- **Learning Outcomes:** Chapter objectives on the first page of every chapter help the student organize and prioritize learning.
- **Selected Key Terms:** List that accompanies the Learning Outcomes presents the most important terms covered in the chapter.
- **Chapter Checkpoints:** Brief questions at the end of main sections test and reinforce the student's recall of key information in that section.

▶ "Zooming In" questions (NEW to this edition): Questions with the figure legends test and reinforce the student's understanding of concepts depicted in the illustration. They are set in a red type to increase their visibility.

▶ Phonetic pronunciations: Easy-to-learn phonetic pronunciations are spelled out in the narrative, appearing in parentheses directly following many terms–no need for students to understand dictionary-style diacritical marks. (See the "Guide to Pronunciation" below.)

▶ Special interest boxes: Each chapter contains special interest boxes focusing on topics that augment chapter content. The book includes five types of boxes:

   ▶ A Closer Look: Provide additional in-depth scientific detail on topics in or related to the chapter.
   ▶ Clinical Perspective: Focus on what happens to the body when the normal structure-function relationship breaks down.
   ▶ Health Professions (NEW to this edition): Describe various careers in the health professions, highlighting the reasons why students need a thorough grounding in anatomy and physiology.
   ▶ Hot Topic (NEW to this edition): Focus on current trends and research, reinforcing the link between anatomy and physiology and related news coverage that students may have seen.
   ▶ Health Maintenance: Offer supplementary information on health and wellness issues.

▶ Figures: The greatly expanded and revised art program includes full-color anatomic line art, both new and revised, with a level of detail that matches that of the narrative. Also NEW to this edition are photomicrographs, radiographs, and other scans, included to give students a "preview" of what they might see in real-world healthcare settings.

▶ Tables: The numerous new and revised tables in this edition summarize key concepts and information in an easy-to-review form.

▶ Color figure and table numbers (NEW to this edition): Figure and table numbers appear in color in the narrative, helping students quickly find their place after stopping to look at an illustration or table. Figure callouts appear in blue type, and table callouts, in red.

▶ Word Anatomy: Organized by chapter headings, this chart groups various word parts used in terms found in the chapter. This learning tool helps students build vocabulary and promotes recognition of even unfamiliar terms based on a knowledge of common word parts.

▶ Summary: Outline-format summary provides a concise overview of chapter content, aiding in study and test preparation.

▶ Questions for Study and Review: Study questions have been thoroughly revised and organized hierarchically into three NEW levels in this edition (answers appear in the Instructor's Manual):

   ▶ Building Understanding: Includes fill-in-the-blanks, matching, and multiple choice questions that test factual recall.
   ▶ Understanding Concepts: Includes short-answer questions (define, describe, compare/contrast) that test and reinforce understanding of concepts.
   ▶ Conceptual Thinking: Includes short-essay questions that promote critical thinking skills.

▶ Guide to Pronunciation

The stressed syllable in each word is shown with capital letters. The vowel pronunciations are as follows:

Any vowel at the end of a syllable is given a long sound, as follows:

   a as in say
   e as in be
   i as in nice
   o as in go
   u as in true

A vowel followed by a consonant and the letter e (as in rate) also is given a long pronunciation.

Any vowel followed by a consonant receives a short pronunciation, as follows:

   a as in absent
   e as in end
   i as in bin
   o as in not
   u as in up

▶ Summary

In short, the 8th edition of *Memmler's The Structure and Function of the Human Body* builds on the successes of the previous seven editions by offering clear, concise narrative into which accurate, aesthetically pleasing anatomic art has been woven. We have made every effort to respond thoughtfully and thoroughly to reviewers' and instructors' comments, offering the ideal level of detail for students preparing for a career in the health professions and nursing, and the pedagogic features that best support it. We hope you will agree that the 8th edition of *Memmler's* is the best ever.

User's Guide

In today's health careers, a thorough understanding of human anatomy and physiology is more important than ever. Memmler's *The Structure and Function of the Human Body* not only provides the conceptual knowledge you'll need but also teaches you how to apply it. This User's Guide introduces you to the features and tools that will enhance your learning experience.

A unifying theme of this text is the relationship between structure and function. We've woven that theme into the book's design and approach. Take a few minutes to look through the text and get acquainted with its organization. The two tables of contents provide a framework for your learning: the Brief Contents gives a wide-angle view of the book's "skeleton"—the units and chapters–while the detailed Contents focuses in on the individual "bones," the topics themselves. As with the different body systems, specific topics build on each other from chapter to chapter, with each supporting the ones that follow.

Next, take a look at the chapters themselves. We've included some important tools to help you learn about anatomy and physiology and apply your new knowledge:

Outcomes and Selected Key Terms highlight important concepts—helping you organize and prioritize learning.

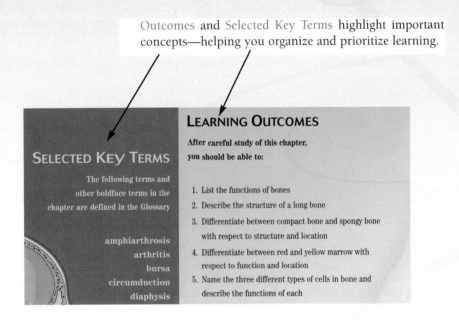

SELECTED KEY TERMS

The following terms and other boldface terms in the chapter are defined in the Glossary

amphiarthrosis
arthritis
bursa
circumduction
diaphysis

LEARNING OUTCOMES

After careful study of this chapter, you should be able to:

1. List the functions of bones

2. Describe the structure of a long bone

3. Differentiate between compact bone and spongy bone with respect to structure and location

4. Differentiate between red and yellow marrow with respect to function and location

5. Name the three different types of cells in bone and describe the functions of each

Health Professions boxes focus on a variety of health careers—showing how the knowledge of anatomy and physiology is applied in real-world jobs.

Box 1-3 · Health Professions

Health Information Technicians

Every time a patient receives medical treatment, information is added to the patient's medical record, which includes data about symptoms, medical history, test results, diagnoses, and treatment. **Health information technicians** organize and manage these records, working closely with physicians, nurses, and other health professionals to ensure that medical records provide a complete, accurate basis for quality patient care.

Accurate medical records are also essential for administrative purposes. Health information technicians assign a **code** to each diagnosis and procedure a patient receives, and this information is used for accurate patient billing. In addition, health information technicians analyze medical records to discover trends in health and disease. This research can be used to improve patient care, manage costs, and help establish new medical treatments.

Health information technicians need a strong clinical knowledge base. A thorough background in medical terminology is essential when reading and interpreting medical records. Anatomy and physiology are definitely required!

Most health information technologists work in hospitals and long-term care facilities. Others work in medical clinics, government agencies, insurance companies, and consulting firms. Job prospects are promising because of the growing need for healthcare. In fact, health information technology is projected to be one of the fastest growing careers in the United States. For more information about this profession, contact the American Health Information Management Association.

Hot Topic boxes provide cutting-edge content on trends and research—giving a view to what is happening in the larger scientific community.

Box 8-2   Hot Topics

Anabolic Steroids: Winning at All Costs?

Anabolic steroids mimic the effects of the male sex hormone testosterone by promoting metabolism and stimulating growth. These drugs are legally prescribed to promote muscle regeneration and prevent atrophy from disuse after surgery. However, athletes also purchase them illegally, using them to increase muscle size and strength and improve endurance.

When steroids are used illegally to enhance athletic performance, the doses needed are large enough to cause serious side effects. They increase blood cholesterol levels, which may lead to atherosclerosis, heart disease, kidney failure, and stroke. Steroids damage the liver, making it more susceptible to disease and cancer, and suppress the immune system, increasing the risk of infection and cancer. In men, steroids cause impotence, testicular atrophy, low sperm count, infertility, and the development of female sex characteristics such as breasts (gynecomastia). In women, steroids disrupt ovulation and menstruation and produce male sex characteristics such as breast atrophy, enlargement of the clitoris, increased body hair, and deepening of the voice. In both sexes steroids increase the risk for baldness and, especially in men, cause mood swings, depression and violence.

Clinical Perspective boxes focus on body processes as well as techniques used in clinical settings—providing additional content on the structure and function relationship.

Box 7-1   Clinical Perspectives

Landmarking: Seeing With Your Fingers

Most body structures lie beneath the skin, hidden from view except in dissection. A technique called landmarking allows health care providers to visualize hidden structures without cutting into the patient. Bony prominences, or landmarks, can be palpated (felt) beneath the skin to serve as reference points for locating other structures. Landmarking is used during physical examinations and surgeries, when giving injections, and for many other clinical procedures. The lower tip of the sternum, the xiphoid process, is a reference point in the administration of cardiopulmonary resuscitation (CPR).

Practice landmarking by feeling for some of the other bony prominences. You can feel the joint between the mandible and the temporal bone of the skull (the temporomandibular joint, or TMJ) anterior to the ear canal as you move your lower jaw up and down. Feel for the notch in the sternum (breast bone) between the clavicles (collar bones). Approximately 4 cm below this notch you will feel a bump called the sternal angle. This prominence is an important landmark because its location marks where the trachea splits to deliver air to both lungs. Move your fingers lateral to the sternal angle to palpate the second ribs, important landmarks for locating the heart and lungs. Feel for the most lateral bony prominence of the shoulder, the acromion process of the scapula (shoulder blade). Two to three fingerbreadths down from this point is the correct injection site into the deltoid muscle of the shoulder. Place your hands on your hips and palpate the iliac crest of the hip bone. Move your hands forward until you reach the anterior end of the crest, the anterior superior iliac spine (ASIS). Feel for the part of the bony pelvis that you sit on. This is the ischial tuberosity. It and the ASIS are important landmarks for locating safe injection sites in the gluteal region.

A Closer Look boxes provide additional detail on selected topics from the text—focusing in on the details of structure and function.

Box 13-1   A Closer Look

Hemoglobin: Door to Door Oxygen Delivery

The hemoglobin molecule is a protein made of four chains of amino acids (the globin part of the molecule), each of which holds an iron-containing heme group. Each of the four hemes can bind one molecule of oxygen.

Hemoglobin. This protein in red blood cells consists of four amino acid chains (globins), each with an oxygen-binding heme group.

Hemoglobin allows the blood to carry much more oxygen than it could were the oxygen simply dissolved in the plasma. A red blood cell contains about 250 million hemoglobins, each capable of binding four molecules of oxygen. So, a single red blood cell can carry about one billion oxygen molecules! Hemoglobin reversibly binds oxygen, picking it up in the lungs and releasing it in the body tissues. Active cells need more oxygen and also generate heat and acidity. These changing conditions promote the release of oxygen from hemoglobin into metabolically active tissues.

Immature red blood cells (erythroblasts) produce hemoglobin as they mature into erythrocytes in the red bone marrow. When the liver and spleen destroy old erythrocytes they break down the released hemoglobin. Some of its components are recycled, and the remainder leaves the body as a brown fecal pigment called stercobilin. In spite of some conservation, dietary protein and iron are still essential to maintain supplies.

Box 5-2 · Health Maintenance

The Cold Facts about the Common Cold

Every year, an estimated one billion Americans suffer from the symptoms of the common cold—runny nose, sneezing, coughing, and headache. Although most cases are mild and usually last a week, colds are the leading cause of doctor visits and missed days at work and school.

Colds are caused by a viral infection of the mucous membranes of the upper respiratory tract. More than 200 different viruses are known to cause cold symptoms. While most colds occur in winter, scientists have found that cold weather does not increase the risk of "catching" a cold; the incidence is probably higher in winter because people spend more time indoors, increasing the chances that the virus will spread from person to person.

Colds spread primarily from contact with a contaminated surface. When an infected person coughs or sneezes, small droplets of water filled with viral particles are propelled through the air. One unshielded sneeze may spread hundreds of thousands of viral particles several feet. Depending upon temperature and humidity, these particles may live as long as 3 to 6 hours, and others who touch the contaminated surface may pick up the particles on their hands.

To help prevent the transmission of cold viruses:

‣ Avoid close contact with someone who is sneezing or coughing.
‣ Wash hands frequently to remove any viral particles you may have picked up.
‣ Avoid touching or rubbing your eyes, nose, or mouth with contaminated hands.
‣ Clean contaminated surfaces with disinfectant.

There are currently no medically proven cures for the common cold, and treatments only ease the symptoms. Because viruses cause the common cold, antibiotics are of no benefit. Getting plenty of rest and drinking lots of fluids are the best ways to speed recovery.

The second type of bone tissue, called **spongy**, or **cancellous**, **bone** has more spaces than compact bone. It is made of a meshwork of small, bony plates filled with red marrow. Spongy bone is found at the epiphyses (ends) of the long bones and at the center of other bones. Figure 7-4 shows a photograph of both compact and spongy tissue in a bone section.

Checkpoint 7-1 A long bone has a long, narrow shaft and two irregular ends. What are the scientific names for the shaft and the ends of a long bone?

Checkpoint 7-2 What are the two types of osseous (bone) tissue and where is each type found

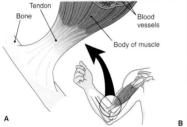

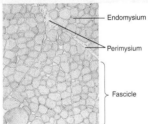

Figure 8-1 **Structure of a skeletal muscle.** Connective tissue coverings are shown. (B, Reprinted with permission from Gartner LP, Hiatt JL. Color Atlas of Histology. 3rd ed. Philadelphia: Lippincott Williams & Wilkins, 2000.) *ZOOMING IN ◆ What is the innermost layer of connective tissue in a muscle? What layer of connective tissue surrounds a fascicle of muscle fibers?*

head of the femur is the **greater trochanter** (tro-KAN-ter), used as a surface landmark. The **lesser trochanter**, a smaller elevation, is located on the medial side. On the posterior surface there is a long central ridge, the **linea aspera**, which is a point for attachment of hip muscles.

‣ The **patella** (pah-TEL-lah), or kneecap (see Fig. 7-1), is embedded in the tendon of the large anterior thigh muscle, the quadriceps femoris, where it crosses the

The Word Anatomy chart helps you learn to recognize new terms based on your knowledge of word parts—building vocabulary.

Word Anatomy

Medical terms are built from standardized word parts (prefixes, roots and suffixes). Learning the meanings of these parts can help you remember words and interpret unfamiliar terms.

WORD PART	MEANING	EXAMPLE
Bones		
dia-	through, between	The *diaphysis*, or shaft, of a long bone is between the two ends, or epiphyses.
oss, osse/o	bone, bone tissue	*Osseous* tissue is another name for bone tissue.
oste/o	bone, bone tissue	The *periosteum* is the fibrous membrane around a bone.
-clast	break	An *osteoclast* breaks down bone in the process of resorption.
Divisions of the Skeleton		
para-	near	The *paranasal* sinuses are near the nose.
pariet/o	wall	The *parietal* bones form the side walls of the skull.
cost/o	rib	*Intercostal* spaces are located between the ribs.
supra-	above, superior	The *supraspinous* fossa is a depression superior to the spine of the scapula
infra-	below, inferior	The *infraspinous* fossa is a depression inferior to the spine of the scapula.
meta-	near, beyond	The *metacarpal*

Summary

I. Types of muscle
A. Smooth muscle
  1. In walls of hollow organs, vessels, and respiratory passageways
  2. Cells tapered, single nucleus, nonstriated
  3. Involuntary; produces peristalsis; contracts and relaxes slowly
B. Cardiac muscle
  1. Muscle of heart wall
  2. Cells branch; single nucleus; lightly striated
  3. Involuntary; self-excitatory
C. Skeletal muscle
  1. Most attached to bones and move skeleton
  2. Cells long, cylindrical; multiple nuclei; heavily striated
  3. Voluntary; contracts and relaxes rapidly

II. Muscular system
  1. Functions
    a. Movement of skeleton
    b. Maintenance of posture
    c. Generation of heat

  3. Isometric contractions—tension increases, but muscle does not shorten

III. Mechanics of muscle movement
  1. Attachments of skeletal muscles
    a. Tendon—cord of connective tissue that attaches muscle to bone
      (1) Origin—attached to more fixed part
      (2) Insertion—attached to moving part
    b. Aponeurosis—broad band of connective tissue that attaches muscle to bone or other muscle
A. Muscles work together
  1. Prime mover—performs movement
  2. Antagonist—produces opposite movement
  3. Synergists—steady body parts and assist prime mover
B. Levers and body mechanics—muscles function with skeleton as lever systems
  1. Components
    a. Lever—bone
    b. Fulcrum—joint
    c. Force—muscle contraction

The Summary provides a quick review of key points in outline form—helping you prepare for exams.

Questions for Study and Review cover chapter content thoroughly—testing your recall of facts, reinforcing understanding of concepts, and teaching critical thinking.

Questions for Study and Review

Building Understanding

Fill in the blanks.
1. The shaft of a long bone is called the _____.
2. The structural unit of compact bone is the _____.
3. Red bone marrow manufactures _____.
4. Bones are covered by a connective tissue membrane called _____.
5. Bone matrix is produced by _____.

Matching
Match each numbered item with the most closely related lettered item.
___ 6. A rounded bony projection
___ 7. A sharp bony prominence
___ 8. A hole through bone
___ 9. A bony depression
___ 10. An air-filled bony cavity

a. condyle
b. foramen
c. fossa
d. sinus
e. spine

Multiple-choice
___ 11. On which of the following bones would the mastoid process be found?
  a. occipital bone
  b. femur

teoarthritis, rheumatoid arthritis, and gout?
b. hinge
c. pivot
d. ball-and-socket

The bonus CD contains a Human Body Review Atlas of electronic images and an Audio Pronunciations Glossary. The Altas, which contains the most important illustrations from the text, is a convenient study tool that lets you review and test your understanding of key body structures. The Glossary lets you hear the correct pronunciation of key terms from the text and practice saying them yourself, preparing you to communicate effectively in the healthcare setting.

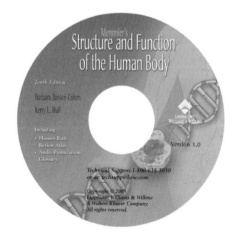

Ancillaries

A complete teaching and learning package is available for both faculty and students. For more information, please visit the text's companion website at http://connection. LWW.com/memmler, or contact your local LWW representative.

- Free Instructor's Manual packaged with Instructor's Resource CD, which includes a test generator, image bank, PowerPoint™ slides, and the Instructor's Manual files (0-7817-5392-9).
- Free transparency set (0-7817-6167-0).

- Free course preparation assistance for instructors and tutoring for students, powered by Smarthinking™, an online support service featuring access to live e-structors. To demo this service, please visit the website listed above.
- Online course materials and management powered by WebCT and Blackboard. To demo the online course, please visit the website listed above.
- Student Study Guide available for purchase either alone (0-7817-5172-1) or packaged with the text (0-7817-6207-3).

Acknowledgments

To prepare a textbook, an author needs the assistance of many skilled people. This is my opportunity to thank those who have helped with revisions for the 8th edition of *Memmler's The Structure and Function of the Human Body*. First and foremost, thanks go to my coauthor Jason Taylor, who had primary responsibility for reviewing and editing this manuscript, and who also wrote the special interest boxes and chapter summary questions. Senior Acquisitions Editor John Goucher has guided this project through from start to finish and showed great skills in putting out fires. Senior Development Editor Dana Knighten kept her eye on the big picture as well as the tiniest details—and everything in between. Kerry Hull's contribution as a reviewer landed her the job of writing all of the ancillary materials, assisted by Ancillary Editor Molly Ward. Elizabeth Connolly and Jennifer Clements kept the art program on track, managing all of the electronic art files.

My thanks to all the many reviewers, listed separately, who made such valuable and detailed comments on the text. Their insights and advice truly guided every aspect of this new edition.

Enormous thanks to Craig Durant and Dragonfly Media Group for their brilliant work on the art program. They understood our needs, often better than we did, and rendered art astonishing in its clarity, instructional value, and beauty of design.

And as always, thanks to my husband Matthew, currently an instructor in anatomy and physiology, for his advice on and contributions to the text.

—Barbara Janson Cohen

They say it takes a village to a raise a child. The same could be said about writing a textbook. As a first-time "parent" of a textbook, I especially appreciate the time and energy everybody at Lippincott invested into helping me navigate through the writing process. I am deeply indebted to Barbara Cohen and Senior Development Editor Dana Knighten, both of whom took me under their wings and taught me so much about being an author. They were always just an email or phone call away. Special thanks to Senior Acquisitions Editor John Goucher who showed so much faith in me throughout the project and made me feel like I had always been part of the team.

I am also deeply indebted to my wife Nicole, who gave birth to our daughter Emily while I helped birth this textbook. Without Nicole's love and support, I could not have finished this project, or much of anything else! Special thanks to my son Alek, who reminds me to always look at the world around and within me with the wide-eyed fascination of a child.

—Jason James Taylor

Brief Contents

Contents

Unit III ◖

COORDINATION AND CONTROL 135

Unit IV ◖

CIRCULATION AND BODY DEFENSE 211

Unit V ◖

ENERGY: SUPPLY AND USE 287

The Body as a Whole

This unit presents the basic levels of organization within the human body. Included is a description of the smallest units of life, called cells. Similar cells are grouped together as tissues, which are combined to form organs. Organs, in turn, work together in the various body systems, which together satisfy the needs of the entire organism. A short survey of chemistry, which deals with the composition of all matter and is important in understanding human anatomy and physiology is incorporated into this unit. These chapters prepare the student for the more detailed study of individual body systems in the units that follow. The final chapter in the unit illustrates some of these basic principles with a study of the skin and its associated structures.

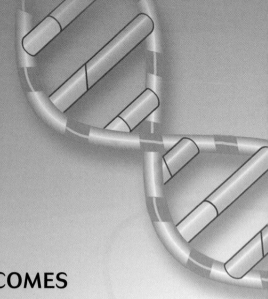

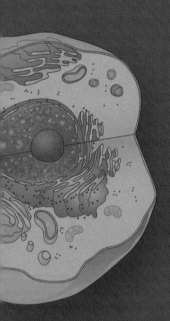

LEARNING OUTCOMES

After careful study of this chapter,
you should be able to:

1. Define the terms *anatomy* and *physiology*
2. Describe the organization of the body from chemicals to the whole organism
3. List 11 body systems and give the general function of each
4. Define *metabolism* and name the two phases of metabolism
5. Briefly explain the role of ATP in the body
6. Differentiate between extracellular and intracellular fluids
7. Define and give examples of homeostasis
8. Compare negative feedback and positive feedback
9. List and define the main directional terms for the body
10. List and define the three planes of division of the body
11. Name the subdivisions of the dorsal and ventral cavities
12. Name and locate subdivisions of the abdomen
13. Name the basic units of length, weight, and volume in the metric system
14. Define the metric prefixes kilo-, *centi-, milli-,*and *micro-*
15. Show how word parts are used to build words related to the body's organization (see Word Anatomy at the end of the chapter)

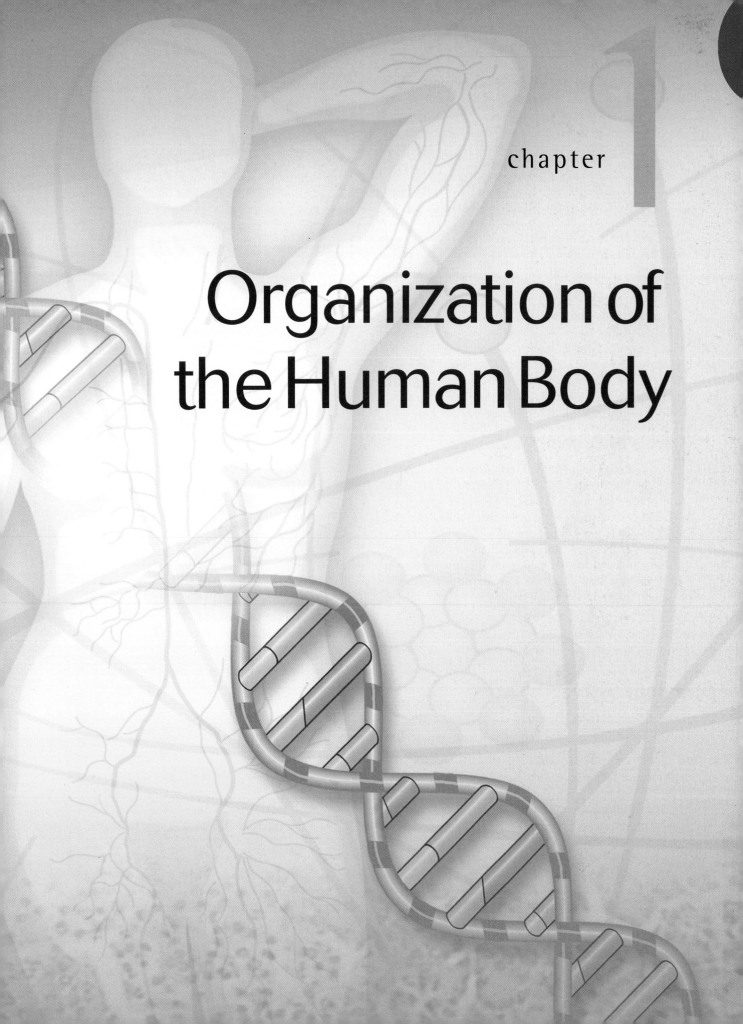

Organization of the Human Body

Studies of the normal structure and functions of the body are the basis for all medical sciences. It is only from understanding the normal that one can analyze what is going wrong in cases of disease. These studies give one an appreciation for the design and balance of the human body and for living organisms in general.

▶ Studies of the Human Body

The scientific term for the study of body structure is **anatomy** (ah-NAT-o-me). The *–tomy* part of this word in Latin means "cutting," because a fundamental way to learn about the human body is to cut it apart, or **dissect** (dis-sekt) it. **Physiology** (fiz-e-OL-o-je) is the term for the study of how the body functions, and is based on a Latin term meaning "nature." Anatomy and physiology are closely related—that is, form and function are intertwined. The stomach, for example, has a pouch-like shape because it stores food during digestion. The cells in the lining of the stomach are tightly packed to prevent strong digestive juices from harming underlying tissue.

Levels of Organization

All living things are organized from very simple levels to more complex levels (Fig. 1-1). Living matter is derived from simple chemicals. These chemicals are formed into the complex substances that make living **cells**—the basic units of all life. Specialized groups of cells form **tissues**, and tissues may function together as **organs**. Organs working together for the same general purpose make up the body **systems**. All of the systems work together to maintain the body as a whole organism.

> Checkpoint 1-1 In studying the human body, one may concentrate on its structure or its function. What are these two studies called?

▶ Body Systems

Most studies of the human body are organized according to the individual systems, as listed below, grouped according to their general functions.

▶ Protection, support, and movement
  ▶ The **integumentary** (in-teg-u-MEN-tar-e) **system**. The word *integument* (in-TEG-u-ment) means skin. The skin with its associated structures is considered a separate body system. The structures associated with the skin include the hair, the nails, and the sweat and oil glands.
  ▶ The **skeletal system**. The basic framework of the body is a system of 206 bones and the joints between them, collectively known as the **skeleton**.
  ▶ The **muscular system**. The muscles in this system are attached to the bones and produce movement of the skeleton. These skeletal muscles also give the body structure, protect organs, and maintain

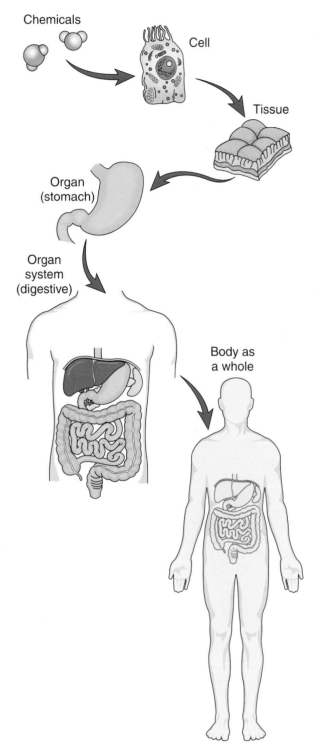

Figure 1-1 **Levels of organization.** The organ shown is the stomach, which is part of the digestive system.

posture. The two other types of muscles are smooth muscle, present in the walls of body organs, such as the stomach and intestine, and cardiac muscle, which makes up the wall of the heart.
▶ Coordination and control
  ▶ The **nervous system**. The brain, the spinal cord, and the nerves make up this complex system by which

the body is controlled and coordinated. The organs of special sense (the eyes, ears, taste buds, and organs of smell), together with the receptors for pain, touch, and other generalized senses, receive stimuli from the outside world. These stimuli are converted into impulses that are transmitted to the brain. The brain directs the body's responses to these outside stimuli and also to stimuli coming from within the body. Such higher functions as memory and reasoning also occur in the brain.

▶ The **endocrine** (EN-do-krin) **system.** The scattered organs known as endocrine glands are grouped together because they share a similar function. All produce special substances called hormones, which regulate such body activities as growth, food utilization within the cells, and reproduction. Examples of endocrine glands are the thyroid, pituitary, and adrenal glands.

▶ Circulation

▶ The **cardiovascular system.** The heart and blood vessels make up the system that pumps blood to all the body tissues, bringing with it nutrients, oxygen, and other needed substances. This system then carries waste materials away from the tissues to points where they can be eliminated.

▶ The **lymphatic system.** Lymphatic vessels assist in circulation by bringing fluids from the tissues back to the blood. Organs of the lymphatic system, such as the tonsils, thymus gland, and the spleen, play a role in immunity, protecting against disease. The lymphatic system also aids in the absorption of digested fats through special vessels in the intestine. The fluid that circulates in the lymphatic system is called lymph. The lymphatic and cardiovascular systems together make up the circulatory system.

▶ Nutrition and fluid balance

▶ The **respiratory system.** This system includes the lungs and the passages leading to and from the lungs. The purpose of this system is to take in air and conduct it to the areas designed for gas exchange. Oxygen passes from the air into the blood and is carried to all tissues by the cardiovascular system. In like manner, carbon dioxide, a gaseous waste product, is taken by the circulation from the tissues back to the lungs to be expelled.

▶ The **digestive system.** This system comprises all the organs that are involved with taking in nutrients (foods), converting them into a form that body cells can use, and absorbing these nutrients into the circulation. Organs of the digestive system include the mouth, esophagus, stomach, intestine, liver, and pancreas.

▶ The **urinary system.** The chief purpose of the urinary system is to rid the body of waste products and excess water. The main components of this system are the kidneys, the ureters, the bladder, and the urethra. (Note that some waste products are also eliminated by the digestive and respiratory systems and by the skin.)

▶ Production of offspring

▶ The **reproductive system.** This system includes the external sex organs and all related internal structures that are concerned with the production of offspring.

The number of systems may vary in different lists. Some, for example, show the sensory system as separate from the nervous system. Others have a separate entry for the immune system, which protects the body from foreign matter and invading organisms. The immune system is identified by its function rather than its structure and includes elements of both the cardiovascular and lymphatic systems. Bear in mind that even though the systems are studied as separate units, they are interrelated and must cooperate to maintain health.

▶ Metabolism and Its Regulation

All the life-sustaining reactions that go on within the body systems together make up **metabolism** (meh-TAB-o-lizm). Metabolism can be divided into two types of activities:

▶ In **catabolism** (kah-TAB-o-lizm), complex substances are broken down into simpler compounds (Fig. 1-2). The breakdown of the nutrients in food yields simple chemical building blocks and energy to power cell activities.

▶ In **anabolism** (ah-NAB-o-lizm), simple compounds are used to manufacture materials needed for growth, function, and repair of tissues. Anabolism is the building phase of metabolism.

The energy obtained from the breakdown of nutrients is used to form a compound often described as the "energy currency" of the cell. It has the long name of **adenosine triphosphate** (ah-DEN-o-sene tri-FOS-fate), but is commonly abbreviated **ATP.** Chapter 18 has more information on metabolism and ATP.

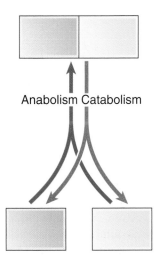

Anabolism Catabolism

Figure 1-2 Metabolism. In catabolism substances are broken down into their building blocks. In anabolism simple components are built into more complex substances.

Homeostatic Imbalance: When Feedback Fails

Each body structure contributes in some way to homeostasis, often through feedback mechanisms. The nervous and endocrine systems are particularly important in feedback. The nervous system's electrical signals react quickly to changes in homeostasis, while the endocrine system's chemical signals (hormones) react more slowly but over a longer time. Often both systems work together to maintain homeostasis.

As long as feedback keeps conditions within normal limits, the body remains healthy, but if feedback cannot maintain these conditions, the body enters a state of *homeostatic imbalance*. Moderate imbalance causes illness and disease, while severe imbalance causes death. At some level, all illnesses and diseases can be linked to homeostatic imbalance.

For example feedback mechanisms closely monitor and maintain normal blood pressure. When blood pressure rises, negative feedback mechanisms lower it to normal limits. If these mechanisms fail, *hypertension* (high blood pressure) develops. Hypertension further damages the cardiovascular system and, if untreated, may lead to death. With mild hypertension, lifestyle changes in diet, exercise, and stress management may lower blood pressure sufficiently, whereas severe hypertension often requires drug therapy. The various types of antihypertensive medication all help negative feedback mechanisms lower blood pressure.

Feedback mechanisms also regulate body temperature. When body temperature falls, negative feedback mechanisms raise it back to normal limits, but if these mechanisms fail and body temperature continues to drop, *hypothermia* develops. Its main effects are uncontrolled shivering, lack of coordination, decreased heart and respiratory rates, and, if left untreated, death. Cardiac surgeons use hypothermia to their advantage during open-heart surgery by cooling the body. This stops the heart and decreases its blood flow, creating a motionless and bloodless surgical field.

Homeostasis

Normal body function maintains a state of internal balance, an important characteristic of all living things. Such conditions as body temperature, the composition of body fluids, heart rate, respiration rate, and blood pressure must be kept within set limits to maintain health. (See Box 1-1, Homeostatic Imbalance: When Feedback Fails.) This steady state within the organism is called **homeostasis** (ho-me-o-STA-sis), which literally means "staying (stasis) the same (homeo)."

Fluid Balance Our bodies are composed of large amounts of fluids. The amount and composition of these fluids must be regulated at all times. One type of fluid bathes the cells, carries nutrient substances to and from the cells, and transports the nutrients into and out of the cells. This type is called **extracellular fluid** because it includes all body fluids outside the cells. Examples of extracellular fluids are blood, lymph, and the fluid between the cells in tissues. A second type of fluid, **intracellular fluid**, is contained within the cells. Extracellular and intracellular fluids account for about 60% of an adult's weight. Body fluids are discussed in more detail in Chapter 19.

Feedback The main method for maintaining homeostasis is **feedback**, a control system based on information returning to a source. We are all accustomed to getting feedback about the results of our actions and using that information to regulate our behavior. Grades on tests and assignments, for example, may inspire us to work harder if they're not so great or "keep up the good work" if they are good.

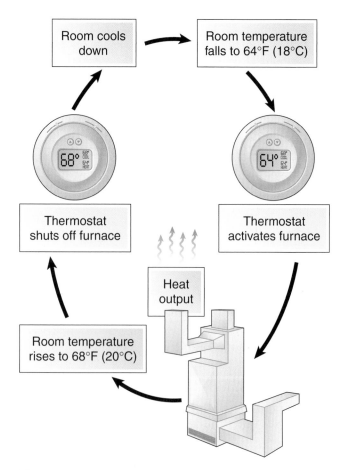

Figure 1-3 Negative feedback. A home thermostat illustrates how this type of feedback keeps temperature within a set range.

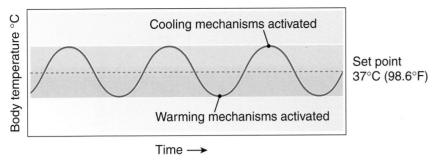

Figure 1-4 Negative feedback and body temperature. Body temperature is kept at a set point of 37° C by negative feedback acting on a center in the brain.

Most feedback systems keep body conditions within a set normal range by reversing any upward or downward shift. This form of feedback is called **negative feedback,** because actions are reversed. A familiar example of negative feedback is the thermostat in a house (Fig. 1-3). When the house temperature falls, the thermostat triggers the furnace to turn on and increase the temperature; when the house temperature reaches an upper limit, the furnace is shut off. In the body, a center in the brain detects changes in temperature and starts mechanisms for cooling or warming if the temperature is above or below the average set point of 37°C (98.6°F) (Fig. 1-4).

As another example, when glucose (a sugar) increases in the blood, the pancreas secretes insulin, which causes body cells to use more glucose. Increased uptake of glucose and the subsequent drop in blood sugar level serves as a signal to the pancreas to reduce insulin secretion (Fig. 1-5). As a result of insulin's action, the secretion of insulin is reversed. This type of self-regulating feedback loop is used in the endocrine system to maintain proper levels of hormones, as described in Chapter 11.

A few activities involve **positive feedback,** in which a given action promotes more of the same. The process of childbirth illustrates positive feedback. As the contractions of labor begin, the muscles of the uterus are stretched. The stretching sends nervous signals to the pituitary gland to release the hormone oxytocin into the blood. This hormone stimulates further contractions of the uterus. As contractions increase in force, the uterine muscles are stretched even more, causing further release of oxytocin. The escalating contractions and hormone release continue until the baby is born. In positive feedback, activity continues until the stimulus is removed or some outside force interrupts the activity. Positive and negative feedback are compared in Figure 1-6.

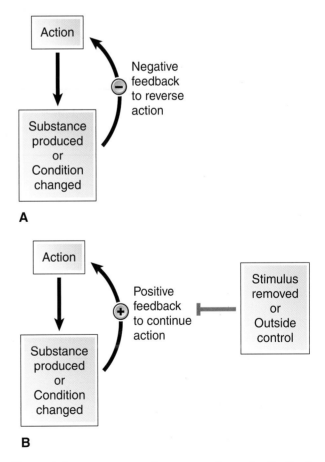

Figure 1-6 Comparison of positive and negative feedback. (A) In negative feedback, the result of an action reverses the action. **(B)** In positive feedback, the result of an action stimulates further action. Positive feedback continues until the stimulus is removed or an outside force stops the cycle.

Figure 1-5 Negative feedback in the endocrine system. Glucose utilization regulates insulin production by means of negative feedback.

The Effects of Aging

With age, changes occur gradually in all body systems. Some of these changes, such as wrinkles and gray hair, are obvious. Others, such as decreased kidney function, loss of bone mass, and formation of deposits within blood vessels, are not visible. However, they may make a person more subject to injury and disease. Changes due to aging will be described in chapters on the body systems.

> **Checkpoint 1-2** Metabolism is divided into a breakdown phase and a building phase. What are these two phases called?

> **Checkpoint 1-3** What type of system is used primarily to maintain homeostasis?

▶ Directions in the Body

Because it would be awkward and inaccurate to speak of bandaging the "southwest part" of the chest, a number of terms are used universally to designate position and directions in the body. For consistency, all descriptions assume that the body is in the **anatomical position**. In this posture, the subject is standing upright with face front, arms at the sides with palms forward, and feet parallel, as shown by the smaller illustration in Figure 1-7.

Directional Terms

The main terms for describing directions in the body are as follows (see Fig. 1-7):

▶ **Superior** is a term meaning above, or in a higher position. Its opposite, **inferior,** means below, or lower. The heart, for example, is superior to the intestine.
▶ **Ventral** and **anterior** have the same meaning in humans: located toward the belly surface or front of the body. Their corresponding opposites, **dorsal** and **posterior,** refer to locations nearer the back.
▶ **Cranial** means nearer to the head. **Caudal** means nearer to the sacral region of the spinal column (*i.e.,* where the tail is located in lower animals), or, in humans, in an inferior direction.
▶ **Medial** means nearer to an imaginary plane that passes through the midline of the body, dividing it into left and right portions. **Lateral,** its opposite, means farther away from the midline, toward the side.
▶ **Proximal** means nearer the origin of a structure; **distal,** farther from that point. For example, the part of your thumb where it joins your hand is its proximal region; the tip of the thumb is its distal region.

Planes of Division

To visualize the various internal structures in relation to each other, anatomists can divide the body along three planes, each of which is a cut through the body in a different direction (Fig. 1-8).

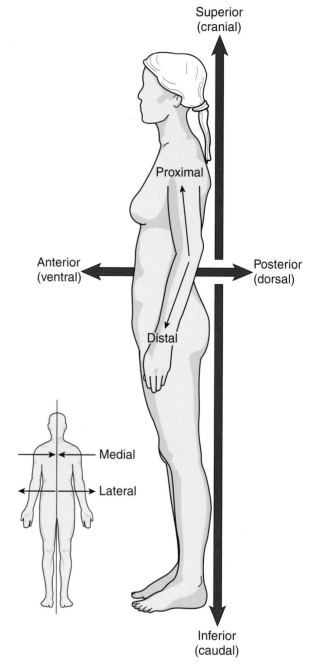

Figure 1-7 Directional terms. *ZOOMING IN ✦ What is the scientific name for the position in which the small figure is standing?*

▶ The **frontal plane.** If the cut were made in line with the ears and then down the middle of the body, you would see an anterior, or ventral (front), section and a posterior, or dorsal (back), section. Another name for this plane is *coronal plane.*
▶ The **sagittal** (SAJ-ih-tal) **plane.** If you were to cut the body in two from front to back, separating it into right and left portions, the sections you would see would be sagittal sections. A cut exactly down the midline of the body, separating it into equal right and left halves, is a **midsagittal** section.

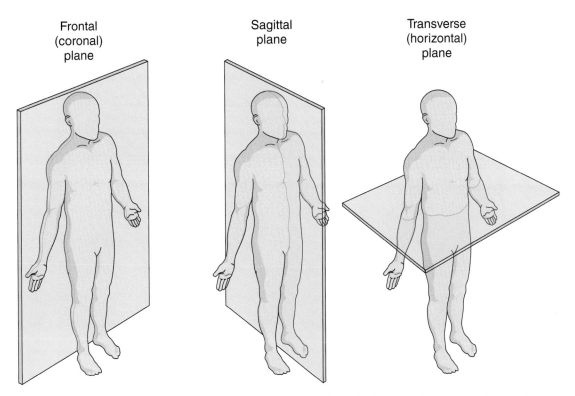

| Frontal (coronal) plane | Sagittal plane | Transverse (horizontal) plane |

Figure 1-8 Planes of division. *ZOOMING IN* ✦ *Which plane divides the body into superior and inferior parts? Which plane divides the body into anterior and posterior parts?*

▶ The **transverse plane.** If the cut were made horizontally, across the other two planes, it would divide the body into a superior (upper) part and an inferior (lower) part. There could be many such cross-sections, each of which would be on a transverse plane, also called a *horizontal plane.*

Tissue Sections Some additional terms are used to describe sections (cuts) of tissues, as used to prepare them for study under the microscope (Fig. 1-9). A cross section (see figure) is a cut made perpendicular to the long axis of an organ, such as a cut made across a banana to give a small round slice. A longitudinal section is made parallel to the long axis, as in cutting a banana from tip to tip to make a slice for a banana split. An oblique section is made at an angle. The type of section used will determine what is seen under the microscope, as shown with a blood vessel in Figure 1-9.

These same terms are used for images taken by techniques such as computed tomography (CT) or magnetic resonance imaging (MRI). (See Box 1-2, Medical Imaging: Seeing Without Making a Cut). In imaging studies, the term cross section is used more generally to mean any two-dimensional view of an internal structure obtained by imaging, as shown in Figure 1-10.

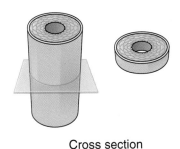

Cross section

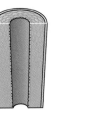

Longitudinal section

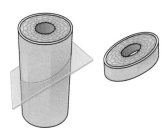

Oblique section

Figure 1-9 Tissue sections.

Box 1-2   Hot Topics

Medical Imaging: Seeing Without Making a Cut

Three imaging techniques that have revolutionized medicine are radiography, computed tomography, and magnetic resonance imaging. With them, physicians today can "see" inside the body without making a single cut. Each technique is so important that its inventor received a Nobel Prize.

The oldest is radiography (ra-de-OG-rah-fe), in which a machine beams x-rays (a form of radiation) through the body onto a piece of film. Like other forms of radiation, x-rays damage body tissues, but modern equipment uses extremely low doses. The resulting picture is called a radiograph. Dark areas indicate where the beam passed through the body and exposed the film, whereas light areas show where the beam did not pass through. Dense tissues (bone, teeth) absorb most of the x-rays, preventing them from exposing the film. For this reason, radiography is commonly used to visualize bone fractures and tooth decay as well as abnormally dense tissues like tumors. Radiography does not provide clear pictures of soft tissues because most of the beam passes through and exposes the film, but contrast media can help make structures like blood vessels and hollow organs more visible. For example, barium sulfate (which absorbs x-rays) coats the digestive tract when ingested.

Computed tomography (CT) is based on radiography and also uses very low doses of radiation. During a CT scan, a machine revolves around the patient, beaming x-rays through the body onto a detector. The detector takes numerous pictures of the beam and a computer assembles them into transverse sections, or "slices." Unlike conventional radiography, CT produces clear images of soft structures such as the brain, liver, and lungs. It is commonly used to visualize brain injuries and tumors, and even blood vessels when used with contrast media.

Magnetic resonance imaging uses a strong magnetic field and radiowaves. So far, there is no evidence to suggest that MRI causes tissue damage. The MRI patient lies inside a chamber within a very powerful magnet. The molecules in the patient's soft tissues align with the magnetic field inside the chamber. When radiowaves beamed at the region to be imaged hit the soft tissue, the aligned molecules emit energy that the MRI machine detects, and a computer converts these signals into a picture. MRI produces even clearer images of soft tissue than does computed tomography and can create detailed pictures of blood vessels without contrast media. MRI can visualize brain injuries and tumors that might be missed using CT.

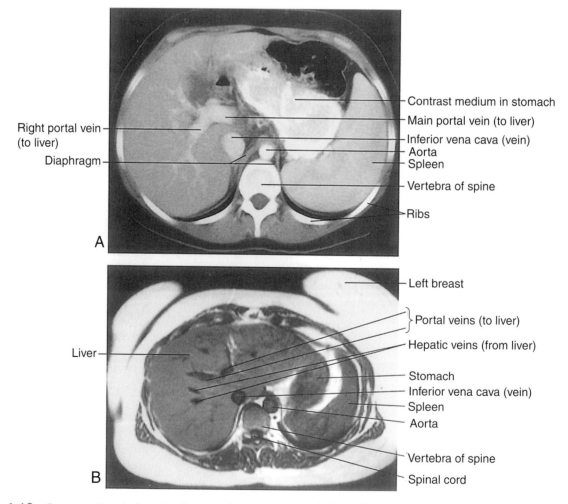

Figure 1-10   Cross-sections in imaging. Images taken across the body through the liver and spleen by **(A)** computed tomography (CT) and **(B)** magnetic resonance imaging (MRI). (Reprinted with permission from Erkonen WE. Radiology 101: Basics and Fundamentals of Imaging. Philadelphia: Lippincott Williams & Wilkins, 1998.)

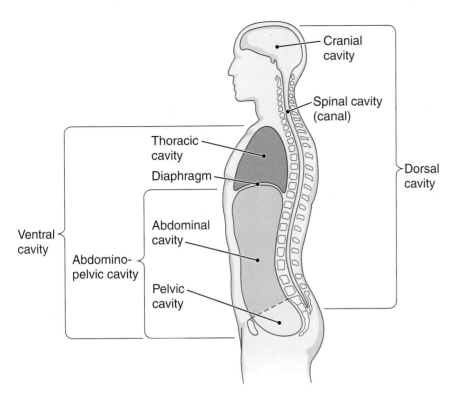

Figure 1-11 Body cavities, lateral view. Shown are the dorsal and ventral cavities with their subdivisions. *ZOOMING IN ✦ What cavity contains the diaphragm?*

heart, the lungs, and the large blood vessels that join the heart. The heart is contained in the pericardial cavity, formed by the pericardial sac; the lungs are in the pleural cavity, formed by the pleurae, the membranes that enclose the lungs (Fig. 1-12). The **mediastinum** (me-de-as-TI-num) is the space between the lungs, including the organs and vessels contained in that space.

The **abdominopelvic** (ab-dom-ih-no-PEL-vik) cavity (see Fig. 1-11) is located inferior to (below) the diaphragm. This space is further subdivided into two regions. The superior portion, the **abdominal cavity**, contains the stomach, most of the intestine, the liver, the gallbladder, the pancreas, and the spleen. The inferior portion, set off by an imaginary line across the top of the hip bones, is the **pelvic cavity**. This cavity contains the urinary bladder, the rectum, and the internal parts of the reproductive system.

Checkpoint 1-4 What are the three planes in which the body can be cut? What kind of a plane divides the body into two equal halves?

Checkpoint 1-5 There are two main body cavities, one posterior and one anterior. Name these two cavities.

Regions of the Abdomen It is helpful to divide the abdomen for examination and reference into nine regions (Fig. 1-13).

▶ Body Cavities

Internally, the body is divided into a few large spaces, or **cavities**, which contain the organs. The two main cavities are the **dorsal cavity** and **ventral cavity** (Fig. 1-11).

Dorsal Cavity

The dorsal body cavity has two subdivisions: the **cranial cavity**, containing the brain, and the **spinal cavity** (**canal**), enclosing the spinal cord. These two areas form one continuous space.

Ventral Cavity

The ventral cavity is much larger than the dorsal cavity. It has two main subdivisions, which are separated by the **diaphragm** (DI-ah-fram), a muscle used in breathing. The **thoracic** (tho-RAS-ik) **cavity** is located superior to (above) the diaphragm. Its contents include the

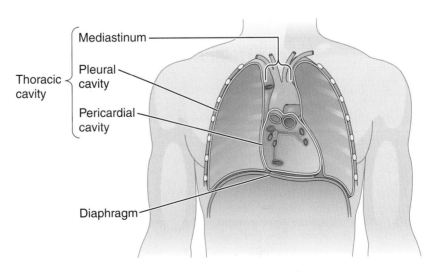

Figure 1-12 The thoracic cavity. Shown are the pericardial cavity, which contains the heart, and the pleural cavity, which contains the lungs.

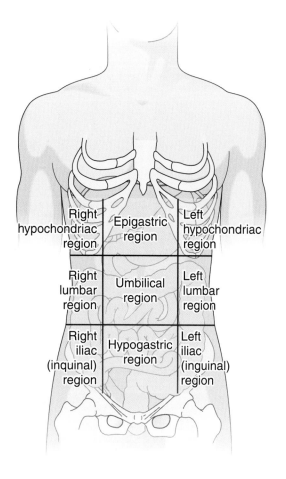

Figure 1-13   **The nine regions of the abdomen.**

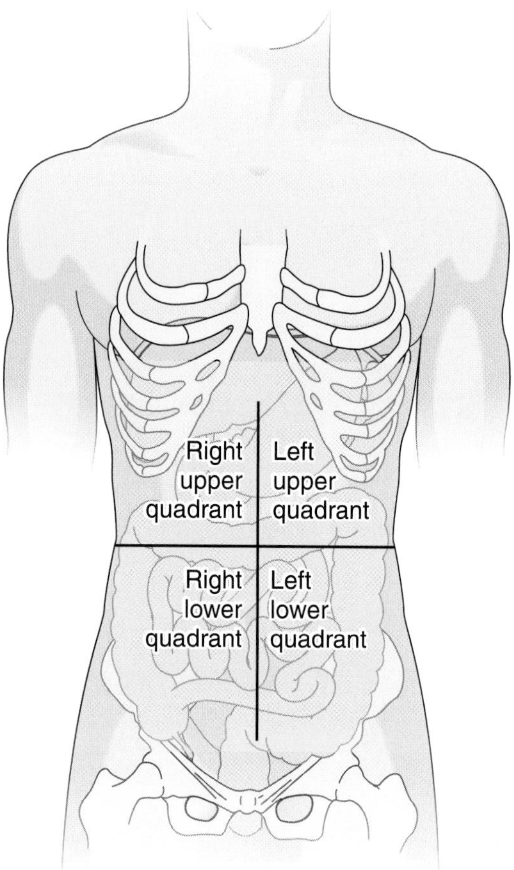

Figure 1-14   **Quadrants of the abdomen.** The organs within each quadrant are shown.

Box 1-3 · Health Professions

Health Information Technicians

Every time a patient receives medical treatment, information is added to the patient's medical record, which includes data about symptoms, medical history, test results, diagnoses, and treatment. **Health information technicians** organize and manage these records, working closely with physicians, nurses, and other health professionals to ensure that medical records provide a complete, accurate basis for quality patient care.

Accurate medical records are also essential for administrative purposes. Health information technicians assign a **code** to each diagnosis and procedure a patient receives, and this information is used for accurate patient billing. In addition, health information technicians analyze medical records to discover trends in health and disease. This research can be used to improve patient care, manage costs, and help establish new medical treatments.

Health information technicians need a strong clinical knowledge base. A thorough background in medical terminology is essential when reading and interpreting medical records. Anatomy and physiology are definitely required!

Most health information technologists work in hospitals and long-term care facilities. Others work in medical clinics, government agencies, insurance companies, and consulting firms. Job prospects are promising because of the growing need for healthcare. In fact, health information technology is projected to be one of the fastest growing careers in the United States. For more information about this profession, contact the American Health Information Management Association.

The three central regions, from superior to inferior are:

▶ the **epigastric** (ep-ih-GAS-trik) **region**, located just inferior to the breastbone
▶ the **umbilical** (um-BIL-ih-kal) **region** around the umbilicus (um-BIL-ih-kus), commonly called the *navel*
▶ the **hypogastric** (hi-po-GAS-trik) **region**, the most inferior of all the midline regions

The regions on the right and left, from superior to inferior, are:

▶ the **hypochondriac** (hi-po-KON-dre-ak) **regions**, just inferior to the ribs
▶ the **lumbar regions**, which are on a level with the lumbar regions of the spine
▶ the iliac, or **inguinal** (IN-gwih-nal), **regions**, named for the upper crest of the hipbone and the groin region, respectively

A simpler but less precise division into four quadrants is sometimes used. These regions are the right upper quadrant (RUQ), left upper quadrant (LUQ), right lower quadrant (RLQ), and left lower quadrant (LLQ) (Fig. 1-14). (See Box 1-3, Health Information Technicians, for description of a profession that uses anatomical, physiological, and medical terms)

Checkpoint 1-6 Name the three central regions and the three left and right lateral regions of the abdomen.

▶ The Metric System

Now that we have set the stage for further study of the body's structure and function, we should take a look at the metric system, because this system is used for all scientific measurements. The drug industry and the health- care industry already have converted to the metric system, so anyone who plans a career in healthcare should be acquainted with metrics.

The metric system is like the monetary system in the United States. Both are decimal systems based on multiples of the number 10. One hundred cents equal one dollar; one hundred centimeters equal one meter. Each multiple in the decimal system is indicated by a prefix:

kilo = 1000

centi = 1/100

milli = 1/1000

micro = 1/1,000,000

Units of Length

The basic unit of length in the metric system is the **meter** (m). Using the prefixes above, 1 kilometer is equal to 1000 meters. A centimeter is 1/100 of a meter; stated another way, there are 100 centimeters in 1 meter. The

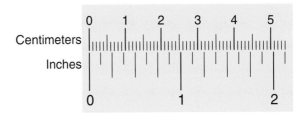

Figure 1-15 **Comparison of centimeters and inches.**

United States has not changed over to the metric system, as was once expected. Often, measurements on packages, bottles, and yard goods are now given according to both scales. In this text, equivalents in the more familiar units of inches and feet are included along with the metric units for comparison. There are 2.5 centimeters (cm) or 25 millimeters (mm) in 1 inch, as shown in Figure 1-15. Some equivalents that may help you to appreciate the size of various body parts are as follows:

1 mm = 0.04 inch, or 1 inch = 25 mm

1 cm = 0.4 inch, or 1 inch = 2.5 cm

1 m = 3.3 feet, or 1 foot = 30 cm

Units of Weight

The same prefixes used for linear measurements are used for weights and volumes. The **gram** (g) is the basic unit of weight. Thirty grams are about equal to 1 ounce, and 1 kilogram to 2.2 pounds. Drug dosages are usually stated in grams or milligrams. One thousand milligrams equal 1 gram; a 500-milligram (mg) dose would be the equivalent of 0.5 gram (g), and 250 mg is equal to 0.25 g.

Units of Volume

The dosages of liquid medications are given in units of volume. The basic metric measurement for volume is the **liter** (L) (LE-ter). There are 1000 milliliters (mL) in a liter. A liter is slightly greater than a quart, a liter being equal to 1.06 quarts. For smaller quantities, the milliliter is used most of the time. There are 5 ml in a teaspoon and 15 mL in a tablespoon. A fluid ounce contains 30 mL.

Temperature

The Celsius (centigrade) temperature scale, now in use by most countries and by scientists in this country, is discussed in Chapter 18.

A chart of all the common metric measurements and their equivalents is shown in Appendix 1. A Celsius-Fahrenheit temperature conversion scale appears in Appendix 2.

Checkpoint 1-7 Name the basic units of length, weight, and volume in the metric system.

Word Anatomy

Medical terms are built from standardized word parts (prefixes, roots, and suffixes). Learning the meanings of these parts can help you remember words and interpret unfamiliar terms.

WORD PART	MEANING	EXAMPLE
Studies of the Human Body		
-tomy	cutting, incision of	*Anatomy* can be revealed by making incisions in the body.
dis-	apart, away from	To *dissect* is to cut apart.
physi/o	nature, physical	*Physiology* is the study of how the body functions.
Body Processes		
cata-	down	*Catabolism* is the breakdown of complex substances into simpler ones.
ana-	upward, again, back	*Anabolism* is the building up of simple compounds into more complex substances.
home/o-	same	*Homeostasis* is the steady state (sameness) within an organism.
stat	stand, stoppage, constancy	In *homeostasis*, "-stasis" refers to constancy.

Summary

I. Studies of the human body
1. Anatomy—study of structure
2. Physiology—study of function

A. Levels of organization—chemicals, cell, tissue, organ, organ system, whole organism

II. Body systems
1. Integumentary system—skin and associated structures
2. Skeletal system—support
3. Muscular system—movement
4. Nervous system—reception of stimuli and control of responses
5. Endocrine system—production of hormones for regulation of growth, metabolism, reproduction
6. Cardiovascular system—movement of blood for transport
7. Lymphatic system—aids in circulation, immunity, and absorption of digested fats
8. Respiratory system—intake of oxygen and release of carbon dioxide
9. Digestive system—intake, breakdown, and absorption of nutrients
10. Urinary system—elimination of waste and water
11. Reproductive system—production of offspring

III. Metabolism and its regulation
1. Metabolism—all the chemical reactions needed to sustain life
   a. Catabolism—breakdown of complex substances into simpler substances; release of energy from nutrients
      (1) ATP (adenosine triphosphate)—energy compound of cells
   b. Anabolism—building of body materials

A. Homeostasis—steady state of body conditions

1. Fluid balance
   a. Extracellular fluid—outside the cells
   b. Intracellular fluid—inside the cells
2. Feedback—regulation by return of information within a system
   a. Negative feedback—reverses an action
   b. Positive feedback—promotes continued activity

B. Effects of aging—changes in all systems

IV. Directions in the body
1. Anatomical position—upright, palms forward, face front, feet parallel

A. Directional terms
1. Superior—above or higher; inferior—below or lower
2. Ventral (anterior)—toward belly or front surface; dorsal (posterior)—nearer to back surface
3. Cranial—nearer to head; caudal—nearer to sacrum
4. Medial—toward midline; lateral—toward side
5. Proximal—nearer to point of origin; distal—farther from point of origin

B. Planes of division
1. Body divisions
   a. Sagittal—from front to back, dividing the body into left and right parts
      (1) Midsagittal—exactly down the midline
   b Frontal (coronal)—from left to right, dividing the body into anterior and posterior parts
   c. Transverse—horizontally, dividing the body into superior and inferior parts
2. Tissue sections
   a. Cross section—perpendicular to long axis
   b. Transverse section—parallel to long axis
   c. Oblique section—at an angle

V. Body cavities

A. Dorsal cavity—contains cranial and spinal cavities for brain and spinal cord
B. Ventral cavity
  1. Thoracic—chest cavity
    a. Divided from abdominal cavity by diaphragm
    b. Contains heart and lungs
    c. Mediastinum—space between lungs and the organs contained in that space
  2. Abdominopelvic cavity
    a. Abdominal cavity—upper region containing stomach, most of intestine, pancreas, liver, spleen, and others
    b. Pelvic cavity—lower region containing reproductive organs, urinary bladder, rectum
  3. Nine regions of the abdomen
    a. Central—epigastric, umbilical, hypogastric
    b. Lateral (right and left)—hypochondriac, lumbar, iliac (inguinal)
  4. Quadrants—abdomen divided into four regions

VI. The metric system—based on multiples of 10

  1. Basic units
    a. Meter—length
    b. Gram—weight
    c. Liter—volume
  2. Prefixes—indicate multiples of 10
    a. Kilo—1000 times
    b. Centi—1/100th (0.01)
    c. Milli—1/1000th (0.001)
    d. Micro—1/1,000,000 (0.000001)
A. Units of length
B. Units of weight
C. Units of volume
D. Temperature—measured in Celsius (centigrade) scale

Questions for Study and Review

Building Understanding

Fill in the blanks
1. Tissues may function together as _____.
2. Glands that produce hormones belong to the _____ system.
3. The eyes are located _____ to the nose.
4. Normal body function maintains a state of internal balance called _____.
5. The basic unit of volume in the metric system is the _____.

Matching
Match each numbered item with the most closely related lettered item.
___ 6. One of two systems that control and coordinate other systems
___ 7. The system that brings needed substances to the body tissues
___ 8. The system that converts foods into a form that body cells can use
___ 9. The cavity that contains the liver
___ 10. The cavity that contains the urinary bladder

a. nervous system
b. abdominal cavity
c. cardiovascular system
d. pelvic cavity
e. digestive system

Multiple choice
___ 11. The study of normal body structure is
  a. homeostasis
  b. anatomy
  c. physiology
  d. metabolism
___ 12. Fluids contained within cells are described as
  a. intracellular
  b. ventral
  c. extracellular
  d. dorsal
___ 13. A type of feedback in which a given action promotes more of the same is called
  a. homeostasis
  b. biofeedback
  c. positive feedback
  d. negative feedback
___ 14. The cavity that contains the mediastinum is the
  a. dorsal
  b. ventral
  c. abdominal
  d. pelvic
___ 15. The foot is located _____ to the knee.
  a. superior
  b. inferior
  c. proximal
  d. distal

Understanding Concepts

16. Compare and contrast the studies of anatomy and physiology. Would it be wise to study one without the other?
17. List in sequence the levels of organization in the body from simplest to most complex. Give an example for each level.

18. Compare and contrast the anatomy and physiology of the nervous system with that of the endocrine system.

19. What is ATP? What type of metabolic activity releases the energy used to make ATP?

20. Compare and contrast intracellular and extracellular fluids.

21. Explain how an internal state of balance is maintained in the body.

22. List the subdivisions of the dorsal and ventral cavities. Name some organs found in each subdivision.

Conceptual Thinking

23. The human body is organized from very simple levels to more complex levels. With this in mind describe why a change at the chemical level can have an effect on organ system function.

24. When glucose levels in the blood drop below normal the pancreas releases a hormone called glucagon. Using your understanding of negative feedback, discuss the possible role of glucagon in blood glucose homeostasis.

25. Your patient's chart reads: "Patient reports pain in right lower quadrant of abdomen. X-ray reveals mass in right iliac region." Locate this region on yourself and explain why it is important for health professionals to use anatomical terminology when describing the human body.

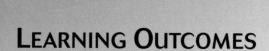

SELECTED KEY TERMS

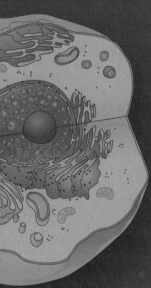

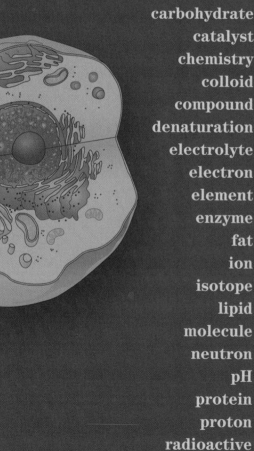

LEARNING OUTCOMES

After careful study of this chapter, you should be able to:

1. Define an element
2. Describe the structure of an atom
3. Differentiate between molecules and compounds
4. Explain why water is so important to the body
5. Define *mixture*; list the three types of mixtures and give two examples of each
6. Differentiate between ionic and covalent bonds
7. Define an electrolyte
8. Define the terms acid, *base*, and *salt*
9. Explain how the numbers on the pH scale relate to acidity and basicity (alkalinity)
10. Define *buffer* and explain why buffers are important in the body
11. Define *radioactivity* and cite several examples of how radioactive substances are used in medicine
12. List three characteristics of organic compounds
13. Name the three main types of organic compounds and the building blocks of each
14. Define *enzyme*; describe how enzymes work
15. Show how word parts are used to build words related to chemistry, matter, and life (see Word Anatomy at the end of the chapter)

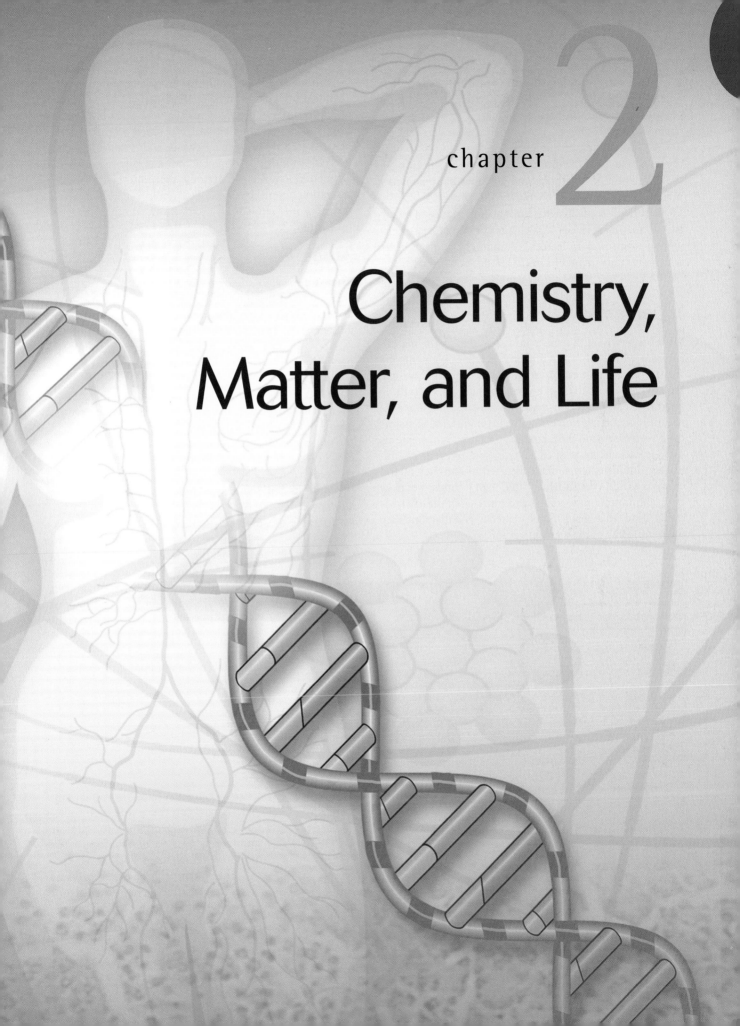

chapter 2

Chemistry, Matter, and Life

Greater understanding of living organisms has come to us through **chemistry**, the science that deals with the composition and properties of matter. Knowledge of chemistry and chemical changes helps us understand the normal functioning of the body. The digestion of food in the intestinal tract, the production of urine by the kidneys, the regulation of breathing, and all other body activities involve the principles of chemistry.

To provide some insights into the importance of chemistry in the life sciences, this chapter briefly describes elements, atoms and molecules, compounds, and mixtures, which are fundamental forms of matter.

▶ Elements

Matter is anything that takes up space, that is, the materials from which all of the universe is made. Elements are the substances that make up all matter. The food we eat, the atmosphere, water—everything around us, everything we can see and touch, is made of elements. There are 92 naturally occurring elements. (Twenty additional elements have been created in the laboratory.) Examples of elements include various gases, such as hydrogen, oxygen, and nitrogen; liquids, such as mercury used in barometers and other scientific instruments; and many solids, such as iron, aluminum, gold, silver, and zinc. Graphite (the so-called "lead" in a pencil), coal, charcoal, and diamonds are different forms of the element carbon.

Elements can be identified by their names or their chemical symbols, which are abbreviations of the modern or Latin names of the elements. Each element is also identified by its own number, which is based on the structure of its subunits, or atoms. The periodic table is a chart used by chemists to organize and describe the elements. Appendix 3 shows the periodic table and gives some information about how it is used. Table 2-1 lists some elements found in the human body along with their functions.

Atoms

The subunits of elements are **atoms**. These are the smallest complete units of matter. They cannot be broken down or changed into another form by ordinary chemical and physical means. These subunits are so small that millions of them could fit on the sharpened end of a pencil.

Atomic Structure Despite the fact that the atom is such a tiny particle, it has been carefully studied and has been found to have a definite structure. At the center of the atom is a nucleus, which contains positively charged electrical particles called **protons** (PRO-tonz) and noncharged particles called **neutrons** (NU-tronz). Together, the protons and neutrons contribute nearly all of the atom's weight.

In orbit outside the nucleus are **electrons** (e-LEK-tronz) (Fig. 2-1). These nearly weightless particles are negatively charged. It is the electrons that determine how the atom will react chemically. The protons and electrons of an atom always are equal in number, so that the atom as a whole is electrically neutral.

The **atomic number** of an element is equal to the number of protons that are present in the nucleus of each of its atoms. Because the number of protons is equal to the number of electrons, the atomic number also represents the number of electrons whirling around the nucleus. Each element has a specific atomic number. No two elements share the same number. In the Periodic Table of the Elements (see Appendix 3) the atomic number is located at the top of the box for each element.

The positively charged protons keep the negatively charged electrons in orbit around the nucleus by means of the opposite charges on the particles. Positively (+) charged protons attract negatively (−) charged electrons.

Table 2·1	Some Common Chemical Elements*		
NAME	**SYMBOL**	**FUNCTION**	
Oxygen	O	Part of water; needed to metabolize nutrients for energy	
Carbon	C	Basis of all organic compounds; in carbon dioxide, the waste gas of metabolism	
Hydrogen	H	Part of water; participates in energy metabolism, acid–base balance	
Nitrogen	N	Present in all proteins, ATP (the energy compound), and nucleic acids (DNA and RNA)	
Calcium	Ca	Builds bones and teeth; needed for muscle contraction, nerve impulse conduction, and blood clotting	
Phosphorus	P	Active ingredient in the energy-storing compound ATP; builds bones and teeth; in cell membranes and nucleic acids	
Potassium	K	Nerve impulse conduction; muscle contraction; water balance and acid–base balance	
Sulfur	S	Part of many proteins	
Sodium	Na	Active in water balance, nerve impulse conduction, and muscle contraction	
Chlorine	Cl	Active in water balance and acid–base balance; found in stomach acid	
Iron	Fe	Part of hemoglobin, the compound that carries oxygen in red blood cells	

The elements are listed in decreasing order by weight in the body.

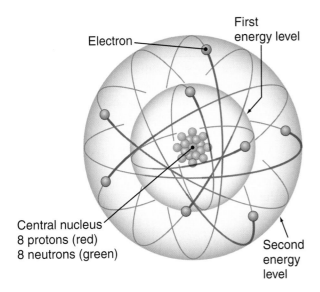

Figure 2-1 **Representation of the oxygen atom.** Eight protons and eight neutrons are tightly bound in the central nucleus. The eight electrons are in orbit around the nucleus, two at the first energy level and six at the second. *ZOOMING IN ✦ How does the number of protons in this atom compare with the number of electrons?*

Checkpoint 2-1 What are atoms?

Checkpoint 2-2 What are three types of particles found in atoms?

Energy Levels The electrons of an atom orbit at specific distances from the nucleus in regions called energy levels. The first energy level, the one closest to the nucleus, can hold only two electrons. The second energy level, the next in distance away from the nucleus, can hold eight electrons.

More distant energy levels can hold more than eight electrons, but they are stable (nonreactive) when they have eight.

The electrons in the energy level farthest away from the nucleus give the atom its chemical characteristics. If the outermost energy level has more than four electrons but less than its capacity of eight, the atom normally completes this level by gaining electrons. In the process, it becomes negatively charged, because it has more electrons than protons. The oxygen atom illustrated in Figure 2-1 has six electrons in its second, or outermost, level. When oxygen enters into chemical reactions, it gains two electrons, as when it reacts with hydrogen to form water (Fig. 2-2). The oxygen atom then has two more electrons than protons.

If the outermost energy level has fewer than four electrons, the atom normally loses those electrons. In so doing, it becomes positively charged, because it now has more protons than electrons.

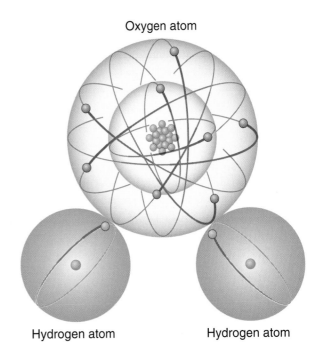

Figure 2-2 **Formation of water.** When oxygen reacts, two electrons are needed to complete the outermost energy level, as shown in this reaction with hydrogen to form water. *ZOOMING IN ✦ How many hydrogen atoms bond with an oxygen atom to form water?*

The number of electrons lost or gained by atoms of an element in chemical reactions is known as the **valence** of that element (from a Latin word that means "strength"). The outermost energy level, which determines the combining properties of the element, is the valence level. Valence is reported as a number with a + or – to indicate whether electrons are lost or gained in chemical reactions. Remember that electrons carry a negative charge, so when an atom gains electrons it becomes negatively charged and when an atom loses electrons it becomes positively charged. For example, the valence of oxygen, which gains two electrons in chemical reactions, is shown as O^{2-}.

❭ Molecules and Compounds

A **molecule** (MOL-eh-kule) is formed when two or more atoms unite on the basis of their electron structures. A molecule can be made of like atoms—the oxygen molecule is made of two identical atoms—but more often a molecule is made of atoms of two or more different elements. For example, a molecule of water (H_2O) contains one atom of oxygen (O) and two atoms of hydrogen (H) (see Fig. 2-2).

Substances composed of two or more different elements are called **compounds.** Molecules are the smallest subunits of a compound. Each molecule of a compound contains the elements that make up that compound in the proper ratio. Some compounds are made of a few elements in a simple combination. For example, the gas carbon monoxide (CO) contains 1 atom of carbon (C) and 1 atom of oxygen (O). Other compounds are very large and complex. Such complexity characterizes many of the compounds found in living organisms. Some proteins, for example, have thousands of atoms.

It is interesting to observe how different a compound is from any of its constituents. For example, a molecule of liquid water is formed from oxygen and hydrogen, both of which are gases. Another example is a crystal sugar, glucose ($C_6H_{12}O_6$). Its constituents include 12 atoms of the gas hydrogen, 6 atoms of the gas oxygen, and 6 atoms of the solid element carbon. The component gases and the solid carbon do not in any way resemble the glucose.

Checkpoint 2-3 What are molecules?

The Importance of Water

Water is the most abundant compound in the body. No plant or animal, including the human, can live very long without it. Water is of critical importance in all physiological processes in body tissues. Water carries substances to and from the cells and makes possible the essential processes of absorption, exchange, secretion, and excretion. What are some of the properties of water that make it such an ideal medium for living cells?

▶ Water can dissolve many different substances in large amounts. For this reason, it is called the **universal solvent**. Many of the materials needed by the body, such as gases, minerals, and nutrients, dissolve in water to be carried from place to place. Substances, such as salts, that mix with or dissolve in water are described as *hydrophilic* ("water-loving"); those, such as fats, that repel and do not dissolve in water are described as *hydrophobic* ("water-fearing").

▶ Water is stable as a liquid at ordinary temperatures. Water does not freeze until the temperature drops to 0°C (32° F) and does not boil until the temperature reaches 100° C (212° F). This stability provides a constant environment for body cells. Water can also be used to distribute heat throughout the body and to cool the body by evaporation of sweat from the body surface.

▶ Water participates in chemical reactions in the body. It is needed directly in the process of digestion and in many of the metabolic reactions that occur in the cells.

Checkpoint 2-4 What is the most abundant compound in the body?

Mixtures: Solutions and Suspensions

Not all elements or compounds combine chemically when brought together. The air we breathe every day is a mixture of gases, largely nitrogen, oxygen, and carbon dioxide, along with smaller percentages of other substances. The constituents in the air maintain their identity, although the proportions of each may vary. Blood plasma is also a mixture in which the various components maintain their identity. The many valuable compounds in the plasma remain separate entities with their own properties. Such combinations are called **mixtures**—blends of two or more substances (Table 2-2).

A mixture formed when one substance dissolves in another is called a **solution**. One example is salt water. In a solution, the component substances cannot be distinguished from each other and they remain evenly distributed throughout; that is, the mixture is homogeneous (ho-mo-JE-ne-us). The dissolving substance, which in the body is water, is the **solvent**. The substance dissolved, salt in the case of salt water, is the **solute**. An **aqueous** (A-kwe-us) **solution** is one in which water is the solvent. Aqueous solutions of glucose, salts, or both of these together are used for intravenous fluid treatments.

In some mixtures, the substance distributed in the background material is not dissolved and will settle out unless the mixture is constantly shaken. This type of non-uniform, or heterogeneous (het-er-o-JE-ne-us), mixture is called a **suspension**. The particles in a suspension are separate from the material in which they are dispersed, and they settle out because they are large and heavy. Examples of suspensions are milk of magnesia, finger paints, and, in the body, red blood cells suspended in blood plasma.

Table 2·2	Mixtures	
TYPE	**DEFINITION**	**EXAMPLE**
Solution	Homogeneous mixture formed when one substance (solute) dissolves in another (solvent)	Table salt (NaCl) dissolved in water; table sugar (sucrose) dissolved in water
Suspension	Heterogeneous mixture in which one substance is dispersed in another, but will settle out unless constantly mixed	Red blood cells in blood plasma; milk of magnesia
Colloid	Heterogeneous mixture in which the suspended material remains evenly distributed based on the small size and opposing charges of the particles	Blood plasma; cytosol

One other type of mixture is of importance in the body. Some organic compounds form **colloids**, in which the molecules do not dissolve yet remain evenly distributed in the suspending material. The particles have electrical charges that repel each other, and the molecules are small enough to stay in suspension. The fluid that fills the cells (cytosol) is a colloidal suspension, as is blood plasma.

Many mixtures are complex, with properties of solutions, suspensions, and colloidal suspensions. Blood plasma has dissolved compounds, making it a solution. The red blood cells and other formed elements give blood the property of a suspension. The proteins in the plasma give it the property of a colloidal suspension. Chocolate milk also has all three properties.

Checkpoint 2-5 Both solutions and suspensions are types of mixtures. What is the difference between them?

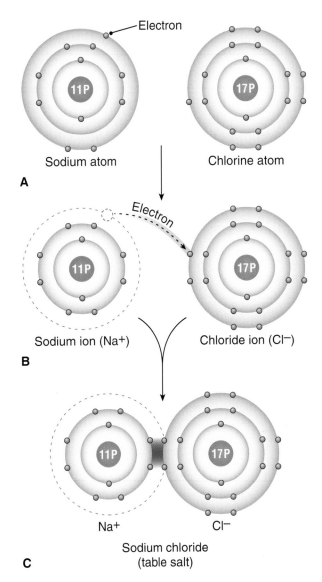

Figure 2-3 Ionic bonding. (A) A sodium atom has 11 protons and 11 electrons. A chlorine atom has 17 protons and 17 electrons. **(B)** A sodium atom gives up one electron to a chlorine atom in forming an ionic bond. The sodium atom now has 11 protons and 10 electrons, resulting in a positive charge of one. The chlorine becomes negatively charged by one, with 17 protons and 18 electrons. **(C)** The sodium ion (Na+) is attracted to the chloride ion (Cl-) in forming the compound sodium chloride (table salt).

▶ Chemical Bonds

When discussing the structure of the atom, we mentioned the positively charged (+) protons that are located in the nucleus and the equal number of orbiting negatively charged (−) electrons that neutralize the protons (Fig. 2-3 A). Atoms interact, however, to reach a stable number of electrons in the outermost energy level. These chemical interactions alter the neutrality of the atoms and also form a bond between them. In chemical reactions, electrons may be transferred from one atom to another or may be shared between atoms.

Ionic Bonds

When electrons are transferred from one atom to another, the type of bond formed is called an **ionic** (i-ON-ik) **bond**. The sodium atom, for example, tends to lose the single electron in its outermost shell (Fig. 2-3 B), leaving an outermost shell with a stable number of electrons (8). Removal of a single electron from the sodium atom leaves one more proton than electrons, and the atom then has a single net positive charge. The sodium atom in this form is symbolized as Na^+. An atom or group of atoms with a positive or negative charge is called an **ion** (I-on). Any ion that is positively charged is a **cation** (CAT-i-on).

Alternately, atoms can gain electrons so that there are more electrons than protons. Chlorine, which has seven electrons in its outermost energy level, tends to gain one electron to fill the level to its capacity. Such an atom of chlorine is negatively charged (Cl^-) (see Fig. 2-3 B). (Chemists refer to this charged form of chlorine as *chloride*.) Any negatively charged ion is an **anion** (AN-i-on).

Let us imagine a sodium atom coming in contact with a chlorine atom. The chlorine atom gains an electron from the sodium atom, forming an ionic bond. The two newly formed ions (Na^+ and Cl^-), because of their opposite charges, attract each other to produce the compound sodium chloride, ordinary table salt (see Fig. 2-3 C).

Electrolytes Ionically bonded substances, when they go into solution, separate into charged particles. Compounds formed by ionic bonds that release ions when they are in solution are called **electrolytes** (e-LEK-tro-lites). Note that in practice, the term *electrolytes* is also used to refer to the ions themselves in body fluids. Electrolytes include a variety of salts, such as sodium chloride and potassium chloride. They also include acids and bases, which are responsible for the acidity or alkalinity of body fluids, as described later in this chapter. Electrolytes must be present in exactly the right quantities in the fluid within the cell (intracellular fluid) and the fluid outside the cell (extracellular fluid), or very damaging effects will result, preventing the cells in the body from functioning properly.

Ions in the Body Many different ions are found in body fluids. Calcium ions (Ca^{2+}) are necessary for the clotting of blood, the contraction of muscle, and the health of bone tissue. Bicarbonate ions (HCO_3^-) are required for the regulation of acidity and alkalinity of body fluids. The stable condition of the normal organism, homeostasis, is influenced by ions.

Because ions are charged particles, electrolyte solutions can conduct an electric current. Records of electric currents in tissues are valuable indications of the functioning or malfunctioning of tissues and organs. The **electrocardiogram** (e-lek-tro-KAR-de-o-gram) and the **electroencephalogram** (e-lek-tro-en-SEF-ah-lo-gram) are graphic tracings of the electric currents generated by the heart muscle and the brain, respectively (see Chapters 9 and 13).

Checkpoint 2-6 What happens when an electrolyte goes into solution?

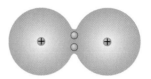

Hydrogen molecule (H₂)

Figure 2-4 A nonpolar covalent bond. The electrons involved in the bonding of a hydrogen molecule are equally shared between the two atoms of hydrogen. The electrons orbit evenly around the two. *ZOOMING IN ✦ How many electrons are needed to complete the energy level of each hydrogen atom?*

Covalent Bonds

Although ionic bonds form many chemical compounds, a much larger number of compounds are formed by another type of chemical bond. This bond involves not the exchange of electrons but a sharing of electrons between the atoms in the molecule and is called a **covalent bond**. This name comes from the prefix *co-*, meaning "together," and *valence*, referring to the electrons involved in chemical reactions between atoms. In a covalently bonded molecule, the valence electrons orbit around both of the atoms, making both of them stable. Covalent bonds may involve the sharing of one, two, or three pairs of electrons between atoms.

In some covalently bonded molecules, the electrons are equally shared, as in the case of a hydrogen molecule (H_2) and other molecules composed of atoms of the same element (Fig. 2-4). Electrons may also be shared equally in some

---

Box 2-1	A Closer Look

Hydrogen Bonds: Strength in Numbers

In contrast to ionic and covalent bonds, which hold atoms together, hydrogen bonds hold molecules together. Hydrogen bonds are much weaker than ionic or covalent bonds—in fact, they are more like "attractions" between molecules. While ionic and covalent bonds rely on electron transfer or sharing, hydrogen bonds form bridges between two molecules. A hydrogen bond forms when a slightly positive hydrogen atom in one molecule is attracted to a slightly negative atom in another molecule. Even though a single hydrogen bond is weak, many hydrogen bonds between two molecules can be strong.

Hydrogen bonds hold water molecules together, with the slightly positive hydrogen atom in one molecule attracted to a slightly negative oxygen atom in another. Many of water's unique properties come from its ability to form hydrogen bonds. For example, hydrogen bonds keep water liquid over a wide range of temperatures, which provides a constant environment for body cells.

Hydrogen bonds form not only between molecules but also within large molecules. Hydrogen bonds between regions of the same molecule cause it to fold and coil into a specific shape, as in the process that creates the precise three-dimensional structure of proteins. Because a protein's structure determines its function in the body, hydrogen bonds are essential to protein activity.

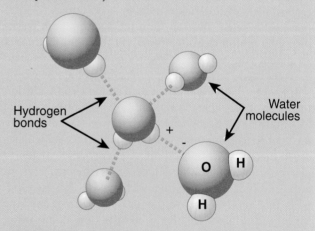

Hydrogen bonds. The bonds shown here are holding water molecules together.

molecules composed of different atoms, methane (CH_4), for example. If electrons are equally shared in forming a molecule, the electrical charges are evenly distributed around the atoms and the bond is described as a *nonpolar covalent bond.* That is, no part of the molecule is more negative or positive than any other part of the molecule. More commonly, the electrons are held closer to one atom than the other, as in the case of water (H_2O), shown in Figure 2-2. In a water molecule, the shared electrons are actually closer to the oxygen at any one time making that region of the molecule more negative. Such bonds are called *polar covalent bonds,* because one part of the molecule is more negative and one part is more positive at any one time. Anyone studying biological chemistry (biochemistry) is interested in covalent bonding because carbon, the element that is the basis of organic chemistry, forms covalent bonds with a wide variety of different elements. Thus, the compounds that are characteristic of living things are covalently bonded compounds. For a description of another type of bond, see Box 2-1, Hydrogen Bonds: Strength in Numbers.

Checkpoint 2-7 How is a covalent bond formed?

▶ Compounds: Acids, Bases, and Salts

An **acid** is a chemical substance capable of donating a hydrogen ion (H^+) to another substance. A common example is hydrochloric acid, the acid found in stomach juices:

$$HCl \rightarrow H^+ + Cl^-$$
(hydrochloric   (hydrogen ion)   (chloride ion)
acid)

A **base** is a chemical substance, usually containing a hydroxide ion (OH^-), that can accept a hydrogen ion. A base is also called an **alkali** (AL-kah-li). Sodium hydroxide, which releases hydroxide ion in solution, is an example of a base:

$$NaOH \rightarrow Na^+ + OH^-$$
(sodium   (sodium ion)   (hydroxide ion)
hydroxide)

A reaction between an acid and a base produces a **salt**, such as sodium chloride:

$$HCl + NaOH \rightarrow NaCl + H_2O$$

The pH Scale

The greater the concentration of hydrogen ions in a solution, the greater is the acidity of that solution. The greater the concentration of hydroxide ion (OH^-), the greater the basicity (alkalinity) of the solution. Based on changes in the balance of ions in solution, as the concentration of hydrogen ions increases, the concentration of hydroxide ions decreases. Conversely, as the concentration of hydroxide

ions increases, the concentration of hydrogen ions decreases. Acidity and alkalinity are indicated by **pH** units, which represent the relative concentrations of hydrogen and hydroxide ions in a solution. The pH units are listed on a scale from 0 to 14, with 0 being the most acidic and 14 being the most basic (Fig. 2-5). A pH of 7.0 is neutral. At pH 7.0 the solution has an equal number of hydrogen and hydroxide ions. Pure water has a pH of 7.0. Solutions that measure less than 7.0 are acidic; those that measure above 7.0 are alkaline (basic).

Because the pH scale is based on multiples of 10, each pH unit on the scale represents a 10-fold change in the number of hydrogen and hydroxide ions present. A solution registering 5.0 on the scale has 10 times the number of hydrogen ions as a solution that registers 6.0. The pH 5.0 solution also has one tenth the number of hydroxide ions as the solution of pH 6.0. A solution registering 9.0 has one tenth the number of hydrogen ions and 10 times the number of hydroxide ions as one registering 8.0. Thus, the lower the pH reading, the greater is the acidity, and the higher the pH, the greater is the alkalinity.

Blood and other body fluids are close to neutral but are slightly on the alkaline side, with a pH range of 7.35

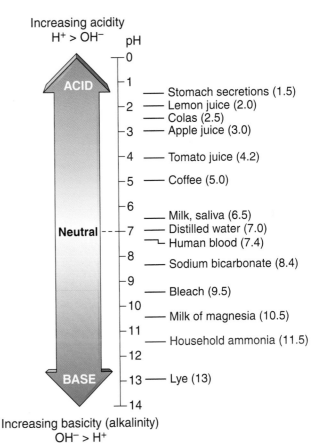

Figure 2-5 **The pH scale.** Degree of acidity or alkalinity is shown in pH units. This scale also shows the pH of some common substances. *ZOOMING IN ✦ What happens to the amount of hydroxide ion (OH^-) present in a solution when the amount of hydrogen ion (H^+) increases?*

to 7.45. Urine averages pH 6.0 but may range from 4.6 to 8.0 depending on body conditions and diet. Figure 2-5 shows the pH of some other common substances.

Because body fluids are on the alkaline side of neutral, the body may be considered to be in an acidic state even if the pH does not drop below 7.0. For example, if the pH falls below 7.35 but is still greater than 7.0, one is described as being in an acidic state known as *acidosis*. Thus, within a narrow range of the pH scale, physiologic acidity may differ from acidity from a chemical standpoint.

An increase in pH to readings greater than 7.45 is termed *alkalosis*. Any shifts in pH to readings above or below the normal range can be dangerous, even fatal.

Buffers

If a person is to remain healthy, a delicate balance must exist within the narrow limits of acidity and alkalinity of body fluids. This balanced chemical state is maintained in large part by **buffers**. Chemicals that serve as buffers form a system that prevents sharp changes in hydrogen ion concentration and thus maintains a relatively constant pH. Buffers are important in maintaining stability in the pH of body fluids. More information about body fluids, pH, and buffers can be found in Chapter 19.

Checkpoint 2-8 The pH scale is used to measure acidity and alkalinity of fluids. What number is neutral on the pH scale? What kind of compound measures lower than this number? Higher?

Checkpoint 2-9 What is a buffer?

▶ Isotopes and Radioactivity

Elements may exist in several forms, each of which is called an **isotope** (I-so-tope). These forms are alike in their numbers of protons and electrons, but differ in their atomic weights because of differing numbers of neutrons in the nucleus. The most common form of oxygen, for example, has eight protons and eight neutrons in the nucleus, giving the atom an atomic weight of 16 atomic mass units (amu). But there are some isotopes of oxygen with only 6 or 7 neutrons in the nucleus and others with 9 to 11 neutrons. The isotopes of oxygen thus range in weight from 14 to 19 amu.

Some isotopes are stable and maintain constant characteristics. Others disintegrate (fall apart) and give off rays of atomic particles. Such isotopes are said to be **radioactive**. Radioactive elements may occur naturally, as is the case with isotopes of the very heavy elements radium and uranium. Others may be produced artificially by placing the atoms of lighter, non-radioactive elements in accelerators that smash their nuclei together.

Use of Radioactive Isotopes

The rays given off by some radioactive elements, also called *radioisotopes*, have the ability to penetrate tissues, which has diagnostic value. X-rays penetrate tissues to produce an image of their interior on a photographic plate. Radioactive iodine and other "tracers" taken orally or injected into the bloodstream are used to image certain body organs, such as the thyroid gland. See Box 2-2, Radioactive Tracers: Medicine Goes Nuclear.

Box 2-2 | **Hot Topics**

Radioactive Tracers: Medicine Goes Nuclear

Like radiography, computed tomography, and MRI, **nuclear medicine imaging** (NMI) offers a noninvasive way to look inside the body. An excellent diagnostic tool, NMI shows not only structural details but also provides information about body function. NMI can diagnose cancer, stroke, and heart disease earlier than techniques that provide only structural information.

NMI uses **radiotracers**, radioactive substances that specific organs absorb. For example, radioactive iodine is used to image the thyroid gland, which absorbs more iodine than any other organ. After a patient ingests, inhales, or is injected with a radiotracer, a device called a gamma camera detects the radiotracer in the organ under study and produces a picture, which is used in making a diagnosis. Radiotracers are broken down and eliminated through urine or feces, so they leave the body quickly. A patient's exposure to radiation in NMI is usually considerably lower than with x-ray or CT scan.

Three NMI techniques are **positron emission tomography** (PET), **bone scanning**, and the **thallium stress test**. PET is often used to evaluate brain activity by measuring the brain's use of radioactive glucose. PET scans can reveal brain tumors because tumor cells are often more metabolically active than normal cells and thus absorb more radiotracer. Bone scanning detects radiation from a radiotracer absorbed by bone tissue with an abnormally high metabolic rate, such as a bone tumor. The thallium stress test is used to diagnose heart disease. A nuclear medicine technologist injects the patient with radioactive thallium, and a gamma camera images the heart during exercise and then rest. When compared, the two sets of images help to evaluate blood flow to the working, or "stressed," heart.

Radiation can also destroy tissue and is used to treat cancer. The sensitivity of the younger, dividing cells in a growing cancer allows selective destruction of these abnormal cells with minimal damage to normal tissues. Rigid precautions must be followed by health care personnel to protect themselves and the patient when using radiation in diagnosis or therapy because the rays can destroy both healthy and diseased tissues.

> **Checkpoint 2-10** Some isotopes are stable; others break down to give off atomic particles. What word is used to describe isotopes that give off radiation?

▶ Chemistry of Living Matter

Of the 92 elements that exist in nature, only 26 have been found in living organisms. Most of these are elements that are light in weight. Not all are present in large quantity. Hydrogen, oxygen, carbon, and nitrogen are the elements that make up about 96% of the body by weight (Fig. 2-6). Nine additional elements, calcium, sodium, potassium, phosphorus, sulfur, chlorine, magnesium, iron, and iodine make up most of the remaining 4% of the elements in the body. The remaining 13, including zinc, selenium, copper, cobalt, chromium, and others, are present in extremely small (trace) amounts totaling about 0.1% of body weight.

Organic Compounds

The chemical compounds that characterize living things are called **organic compounds.** All of these contain the element **carbon.** Because carbon can combine with a variety of different elements and can even bond to other carbon atoms to form long chains, most organic compounds consist of large, complex molecules. The starch found in potatoes, the fat in the tissue under the skin, hormones, and many drugs are examples of organic compounds. These large molecules are often formed from simpler molecules called *building blocks*, which bond together in long chains.

The main types of organic compounds are carbohydrates, lipids, and proteins. (Another category, the nucleic acids, which are important in cellular functions, are discussed in Chapter 3.) All of these organic compounds contain carbon, hydrogen, and oxygen as their main ingredients.

Carbohydrates, lipids, and proteins, in addition to minerals and vitamins, must be taken in as part of a normal diet. These compounds are discussed further in Chapters 17 and 18.

> **Checkpoint 2-11** Where are organic compounds found?

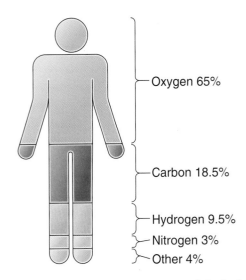

Figure 2-6 **Chemical composition of the body by weight.**

> **Checkpoint 2-12** What element is the basis of organic chemistry?

Carbohydrates The basic units of carbohydrates are simple sugars, or **monosaccharides** (mon-o-SAK-ah-rides) (Fig. 2-7 A). **Glucose** (GLU-kose), a simple sugar that circulates in the blood as a nutrient for cells, is an example of a monosaccharide. Two simple sugars may be linked together to form a **disaccharide** (Fig. 2-7 B), as represented by sucrose, table sugar. More complex carbohydrates, or **polysaccharides** (Fig. 2-7 C), consist of many simple sugars linked together with multiple side chains. Examples of polysaccharides are starch, which is manufactured in plant cells, and **glycogen** (GLI-ko-jen), a storage form of glucose found in liver cells and skeletal muscle cells. Carbohydrates in the form of sugars and starches are important sources of energy in the diet.

Lipids Lipids are a class of organic compounds mainly found in the body as **fat.** Fats provide insulation for the body and protection for organs. In addition, fats are the main form in which energy is stored.

Simple fats are made from a substance called **glycerol** (GLIS-er-ol), commonly known as glycerin, in combination with fatty acids (Fig. 2-8 A). One fatty acid is attached to each of the three carbon atoms in glycerol, so simple fats are described as **triglycerides** (tri-GLIS-er-ides). **Phospholipids** (fos-fo-LIP-ids) are complex lipids containing the element phosphorus. Among other functions, phospholipids make up a major part of the membrane around living cells. **Steroids** are lipids that contain

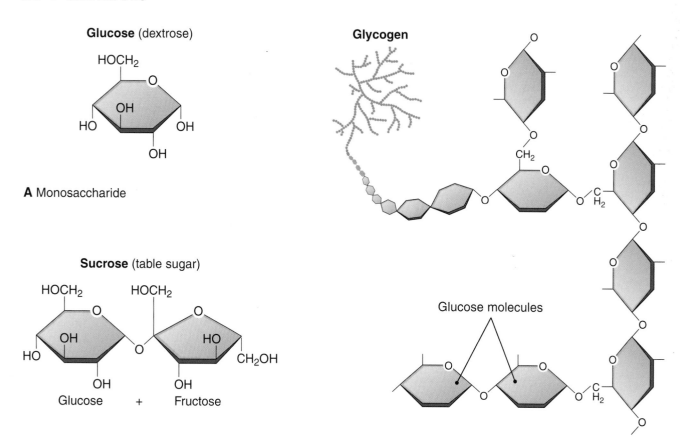

Glucose (dextrose)

A Monosaccharide

Sucrose (table sugar)

Glucose   +   Fructose

B Disaccharide

Glycogen

Glucose molecules

C Polysaccharide

Figure 2-7 **Examples of carbohydrates.** A monosaccharide (**A**) is a simple sugar. A disaccharide (**B**) consists of two simple sugars linked together, whereas a polysaccharide (**C**) consists of many simple sugars linked together in chains. *ZOOMING IN ♦ What are the building blocks of disaccharides and polysaccharides?*

rings of carbon atoms. They include **cholesterol** (ko-LES-ter-ol), another component of cell membranes (Fig. 2-8 B); the steroid hormones, such as cortisol, produced by the adrenal gland; the sex hormones, such as testosterone, produced by the testes; and estrogen and progesterone, produced by the ovaries.

Proteins All **proteins** (PRO-tenes) contain, in addition to carbon, hydrogen, and oxygen, the element **nitrogen** (NI-tro-jen). They may also contain sulfur or phosphorus. Proteins are the structural materials of the body, found in muscle, bone, and connective tissue. They also make up the pigments that give hair, eyes, and skin their color. It is protein that makes each individual physically distinct from others.

Proteins are composed of building blocks called **amino** (ah-ME-no) **acids** (Fig. 2-9 A). Although there are only about 20 different amino acids found in the body, a vast number of proteins can be made by linking them together in different sized molecules and in different combinations.

Each amino acid contains an acid group (COOH) and an amino group (NH_2), the part of the molecule that has the nitrogen. Many amino acids link together to form a polypeptide, which is then arranged into a particular shape. The polypeptide chain is coiled into a helix and may then be pleated or folded back on itself. Several chains also may be folded together (see Fig. 2-9 B). The overall shape of a protein is important to its function, as can be seen in the activity of enzymes.

Checkpoint 2-13 What are the three main categories of organic compounds?

Enzymes Enzymes (EN-zimes) are proteins that are essential for metabolism. They serve as **catalysts** in the hundreds of reactions that take place within cells. Without these catalysts, which speed the rate of chemical reactions, metabolism would not occur at a fast enough rate to sustain life. Because each enzyme works only on a spe-

Glycerol

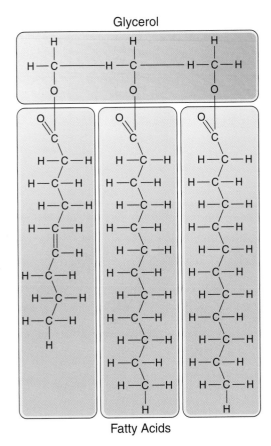

Fatty Acids

A   **Triglyceride (a simple fat)**

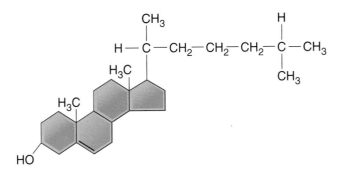

B   **Cholesterol (a steroid)**

Figure 2-8 **Lipids. (A)** A triglyceride, a simple fat, contains glycerol combined with three fatty acids. **(B)** Cholesterol is a type of steroid, a lipid that contains rings of carbon atoms. *ZOOMING IN ✦ How many carbon atoms are in glycerol?*

cific substance, or **substrate**, and does only one specific chemical job, many different enzymes are needed. Like all catalysts, enzymes take part in reactions only temporarily; they are not used up or changed by the reaction. Therefore, they are needed in very small amounts. Many of the vitamins and minerals required in the diet are parts of enzymes.

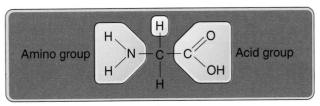

Simple amino acid

A

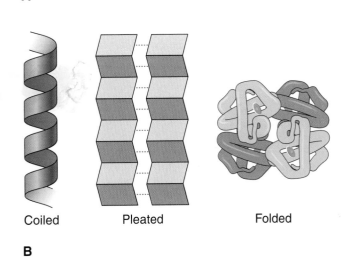

Coiled   Pleated   Folded

B

Figure 2-9 **Proteins. (A)** Amino acids are the building blocks of proteins. **(B)** Some shapes of proteins *ZOOMING IN ✦ What part of an amino acid contains nitrogen?*

The shape of the enzyme is important in its action. The enzyme's form must match the shape of the substrate or substrates the enzyme combines with in much the same way as a key fits a lock. This so-called "lock-and-key" mechanism is illustrated in Figure 2-10. Harsh conditions, such as extremes of temperature or pH, can alter the shape of an enzyme and stop its action. The alteration of any protein so that it can no longer function is termed **denaturation**. Such an event is always harmful to the cells.

You can usually recognize the names of enzymes because, with few exceptions, they end with the suffix *-ase*. Examples are lipase, protease, and oxidase. The first part of the name usually refers to the substance acted on or the type of reaction in which the enzyme is involved.

Checkpoint 2-14 Enzymes are proteins that act as catalysts. What is a catalyst?

For a description of professions that require knowledge of chemistry, see Box 2-3, Pharmacists and Pharmacy Technicians.

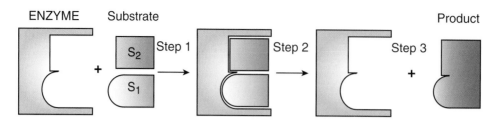

Figure 2-10 **Diagram of enzyme action.** The enzyme combines with substrate 1 (S_1) and substrate 2 (S_2). Once a new product is formed from the substrates, the enzyme is released unchanged. ZOOMING IN ✦ *How does the shape of the enzyme before the reaction compare with its shape after the reaction.*

Box 2-3 • Health Professions

Pharmacists and Pharmacy Technicians

Medications are chemicals designed to treat illness and improve quality of life. The role of pharmacists and pharmacy technicians is to ensure that patients receive the correct medication and the education they need to use it effectively and derive the intended health benefits.

As key members of the healthcare team, pharmacists need a strong clinical background with a thorough understanding of chemistry, anatomy, and physiology. Pharmacists not only dispense prescription medications and monitor patients' responses to them, they also educate patients about their appropriate use. They share their expertise with other health professionals and also participate in clinical research on drugs and their effects.

Pharmacy technicians also require a thorough understanding of chemistry, anatomy, and physiology to assist pharmacists with their duties. State rules and regulations vary, but pharmacy technicians may perform many of the tasks related to dispensing medications, such as preparing them and packaging them with appropriate labels and instructions for use.

Most pharmacists and pharmacy technicians work in retail pharmacies, whereas others work in hospitals and long-term care facilities. Job prospects are promising because of the growing need for healthcare. In fact, pharmacy is projected to be one of the fastest growing careers in the United States. For more information about careers in pharmacy, contact the American Association of Colleges of Pharmacy.

Word Anatomy

Medical terms are built from standardized word parts (prefixes, roots, and suffixes). Learning the meanings of these parts can help you to remember words and interpret unfamiliar terms.

WORD PART	MEANING	EXAMPLE
Molecules and Compounds		
hydr/o	water	*Dehydration* is a deficiency of water.
phil	to like	*Hydrophilic* substances "like" water—they mix with or dissolve in it.
-phobia	fear	*Hydrophobic* substances "fear" water—they repel and do *not* dissolve in it.
hom/o	same	*Homogeneous* mixtures are the same throughout.
heter/o-	different	*Heterogeneous* solutions are different (not uniform) throughout.
aqu/e	water	In an *aqueous* solution, water is the solvent.
Chemical Bonds		
co-	together	*Covalent* bonds form when atoms share electrons.
Chemistry of Living Matter		
sacchar/o	sugar	A *monosaccharide* consists of one simple sugar.
mon/o-	one	In *monosaccharide*, "mono-" refers to one.
di-	twice, double	A *disaccharide* consists of two simple sugars.
poly-	many	A *polysaccharide* consists of many simple sugars.
glyc/o	sugar, glucose, sweet	*Glycogen* is a storage form of glucose. It breaks down to release (generate) glucose.
tri-	three	*Triglycerides* have one fatty acid attached to each of three carbon atoms.

WORD PART	MEANING	EXAMPLE
Chemistry of Living Matter		
de-	remove	*Denaturation* of a protein removes its ability to function (changes its nature).
-ase	suffix used in naming enzymes	A *lipase* is an enzyme that acts on lipids.

Summary

I. Elements—substances from which all matter is made

A. Atoms—subunits of elements
  1. Atomic structure
     a. Protons—positively charged particles in the nucleus
     b. Neutrons—noncharged particles in the nucleus
     c. Electrons—negatively charged particles in energy levels around the nucleus
  2. Energy levels—orbits that hold electrons at specific distances from the nucleus
     a. Valence—number of electrons lost or gained in chemical reactions

II. Molecules and compounds

  1. Molecules—combinations of two or more atoms
  2. Compounds—substances composed of different elements
A. The importance of water—solvent; stable; essential for metabolism
B. Mixtures: solutions and suspensions
  1. Mixtures: blend of two or more substances
  2. Solution: substance (solute) remains evenly distributed in solvent (*e.g.*, salt in water); homogeneous
  3. Suspension—material settles out of mixture on standing (*e.g.*, red cells in blood plasma); heterogeneous
  4. Colloid—particles do not dissolve but remain suspended (*e.g.*, cytosol)

III. Chemical bonds

A. Ionic bonds—formed by transfer of electrons from one atom to another
  1. Electrolytes
     a. Ionically bonded substances
     b. Separate in solution into charged particles (ions); cation positive and anion negative
     c. Conduct electric current

  2. Ions in body fluids important for proper function
B. Covalent bonds—formed by sharing of electrons between atoms
  1. Nonpolar—equal sharing of electrons (*e.g.*, hydrogen gas, H_2)
  2. Polar—unequal sharing of electrons (*e.g.*, water, H_2O)

IV. Compounds: acids, bases and salts

  1. Acids—donate hydrogen ions
  2. Bases—accept hydrogen ions
  3. Salts—formed by reaction between acid and base
A. The pH scale
  1. Measure of acidity or alkalinity of a solution
  2. Scale goes from 0 to 14
     a. 7 is neutral; below 7 is acidic; above 7 is alkaline (basic)
B. Buffer—maintains constant pH of a solution

V. Isotopes and radioactivity

  1. Isotopes—forms of an element that differ in atomic weights (number of neutrons)
     a. Radioactive isotope gives off rays of atomic particles
A. Use of radioactive isotopes
  1. Diagnosis: tracers, x-rays
  2. Cancer therapy

VI. Chemistry of living matter

A. Organic compounds—all contain carbon
  1. Carbohydrates (*e.g.*, sugars, starches); made of simple sugars (monosaccharides)
  2. Lipids (*e.g.*, fats, steroids); fats made of glycerol and fatty acids
  3. Proteins (*e.g.*, structural materials, enzymes); made of amino acids
  4. Enzymes—organic catalysts

Questions for Study and Review

Building Understanding

Fill in the blanks
1. The basic units of matter are _____.
2. The atomic number is the number of_____ in an atom's nucleus.

3. A mixture of solute dissolved in solvent is called a(n) _____.
4. Blood has a pH of 7.35 to 7.45. Gastric juice has a pH of about 2.0. The more alkaline fluid is _____.
5. Proteins that catalyze metabolic reactions are called _____.

Matching

Match each numbered item with the most closely related lettered item.

___6. A simple carbohydrate such as glucose
___7. A complex carbohydrate such as glycogen
___8. An important component of cell membranes
___9. A hormone such as estrogen
___10. The basic building block of protein

a. polysaccharide
b. phospholipid
c. steroid
d. amino acid
e. monosaccharide

Multiple choice

___11. Red blood cells "floating" in plasma are an example of a mixture called a
  a. compound
  b. suspension
  c. colloid
  d. solution
___12. The most abundant compound in the body is
  a. carbohydrate
  b. protein
  c. lipid
  d. water
___13. A compound that releases ions when it is in solution is called a(n)
  a. solvent
  b. electrolyte
  c. anion
  d. colloid
___14. A chemical capable of donating hydrogen ions to other substances is called a(n)
  a. acid
  b. base
  c. salt
  d. catalyst
___15. Organic compounds always contain the element
  a. oxygen
  b. carbon
  c. nitrogen
  d. phosphorus

Understanding Concepts

16. Compare and contrast the following terms:
  a. element and atom
  b. molecule and compound
  c. proton, neutron, and electron
  d. anion and cation
  e. ionic bond and covalent bond
  f. acid and base
17. What are some of the properties of water that make it an ideal medium for living cells?
18. Explain the importance of ions in the structure and function of the human body.
19. What is pH? Discuss the role of buffers in maintaining pH homeostasis in the body.
20. Compare and contrast carbohydrates and proteins.
21. Describe three different types of lipid.
22. Define the term *enzyme* and discuss the relationship between enzyme structure and enzyme function.

Conceptual Thinking

23. Based on your understanding of strong acids and bases, why does the body have to be kept at a close-to-neutral pH?
24. Mrs. Alvarez has thyroid cancer and is undergoing radiation therapy. During one of her treatments she tells you that she had hoped her initial "thyroid scan" would have killed all of the cancer. Explain the difference between radiation therapy and nuclear medicine imaging.
25. Why do we need enzymes, when usually heat is used to speed up chemical reactions?

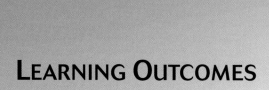

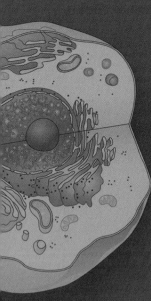
LEARNING OUTCOMES

After careful study of this chapter, you should be able to:

1. List three types of microscopes used to study cells
2. Describe the function and composition of the plasma membrane
3. Describe the cytoplasm of the cell, including the name and function of the main organelles
4. Describe the composition, location, and function of the DNA in the cell
5. Compare the function of three types of RNA in the cells
6. Explain briefly how cells make proteins
7. Name and briefly describe the stages in mitosis
8. Define eight methods by which substances enter and leave cells
9. Explain what will happen if cells are placed in solutions with concentrations the same as or different from those of the cell fluids
10. Show how word parts are used to build words related to cells and their functions (see Word Anatomy at the end of the chapter)

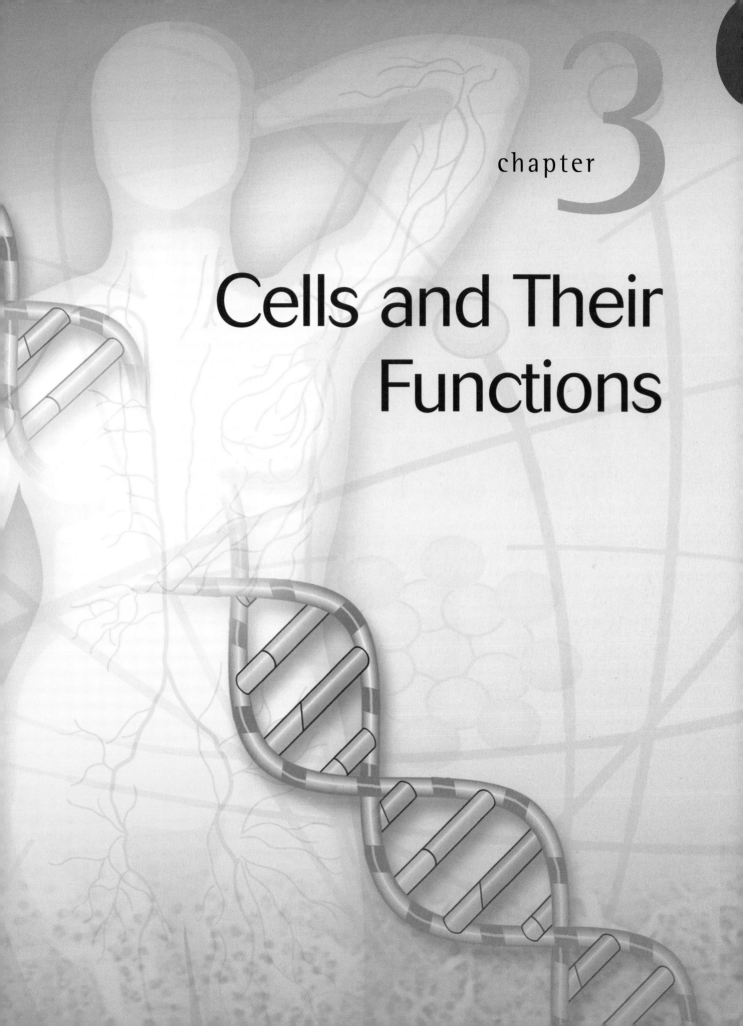

Cells and Their Functions

❱ The Role of Cells

The **cell** (sel) is the basic unit of all life. It is the simplest structure that shows all the characteristics of life, including organization, metabolism, responsiveness, homeostasis, growth, and reproduction. In fact, it is possible for a single cell to live independently of other cells. Examples of some free-living cells are microscopic organisms such as protozoa and bacteria, some of which produce disease. In a multicellular organism, cells make up all tissues. All the activities of the human body, which is composed of trillions of cells, result from the activities of individual cells. Cells produce all the materials manufactured within the body. The study of cells is **cytology** (si-TOL-o-je).

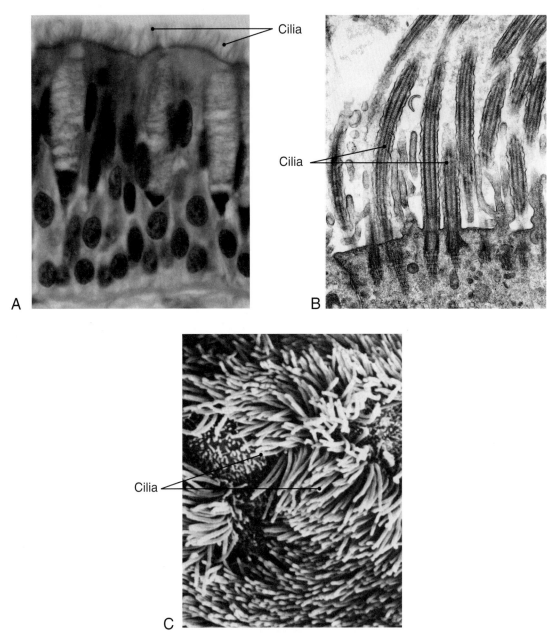

Figure 3-1 **Cilia photographed under three different microscopes. (A)** Cilia (hairlike projections) in cells lining the trachea under the highest magnification of a compound light microscope (1000×) **(B)** Cilia in the bronchial lining viewed with a transmission electron microscope (TEM). Internal components are visible at this much higher magnification. **(C)** Cilia on cells lining an oviduct as seen with a scanning electron microscope (SEM) (7000×). A three dimensional view can be seen. (A, Reprinted with permission from Cormack DH. Essential histology. 2nd ed. Philadelphia: Lippincott Williams & Wilkins, 2001. B, Reprinted with permission from Quinton P, Martinez R, eds. Fluid and electrolyte transport in exocrine glands in cystic fibrosis. San Francisco: San Francisco Press, 1982. C, Reprinted with permission from Hafez ESE, ed. Scanning electron microscopic atlas of mammalian reproduction. Tokyo: Igaku Shoin, 1975.) *ZOOMING IN ✦ Which microscope shows the most internal structure of the cilia? Which shows the cilia in three dimensions?*

▶ Microscopes

The outlines of cells were first seen in dried plant tissue almost 350 years ago. Study of their internal structure, however, depended on improvements in the design of the **microscope**, a magnifying instrument needed to examine structures not visible with the naked eye. The single-lens microscope used in the late 17th century was later replaced by the **compound light microscope** most commonly used in laboratories today. This instrument, which can magnify an object up to 1000 times, has two lenses and uses visible light for illumination. A much more powerful microscope, the **transmission electron microscope** (TEM), uses an electron beam in place of visible light and can magnify an image up to 1 million times. Another type of microscope, the **scanning electron microscope** (SEM), does not magnify as much (100,000×) and shows only surface features, but gives a three-dimensional view of an object. Figure 3-1 shows some cell structures viewed with each of these types of microscopes. The structures are cilia, short, hairlike projections from the cell that move nearby fluids. The metric unit used for microscopic measurements is the **micrometer** (MI-kro-me-ter), formerly called a micron. This unit is 1/1000 of a millimeter and is symbolized with the Greek letter mu (μ), as μm.

Before a scientist can examine cells and tissues under a microscope, he or she must usually color them with special dyes called **stains** to aid in viewing. These stains produce the variety of colors seen in pictures of cells and tissues taken under a microscope.

> **Checkpoint 3-1** The cell is the basic unit of life. What characteristics of life does it show?

> **Checkpoint 3-2** Name three types of microscopes.

▶ Cell Structure

Just as people may look different but still have certain features in common—two eyes, a nose, and a mouth, for example—all cells share certain characteristics. Refer to Figure 3-2 as we describe some of the parts that are common to most animal cells. Table 3-1 summarizes information about the main cell parts.

Plasma Membrane

The outer limit of the cell is the **plasma membrane**, formerly called the *cell membrane* (Fig. 3-3). The plasma membrane not only encloses the cell contents but also participates in many cellular activities, such as growth, reproduction, and interactions between cells, and is especially important in regulating what can enter and leave the cell. The main substance of this membrane is a double layer of lipid molecules, described as a bilayer. Because these lipids contain the element phosphorus, they are called **phospholipids**. Some molecules of cholesterol, another type of lipid, are located between the phospholipids. Cholesterol strengthens the membrane.

A variety of different proteins float within the lipid bilayer. Some of these proteins extend all the way through the membrane, and some are located near the inner or outer surfaces of the membrane. The importance of these proteins will be revealed in later chapters, but they are listed here along with their functions (Table 3-2):

▶ Channels—pores in the membrane that allow specific substances to enter or leave. Certain ions travel through channels in the membrane.

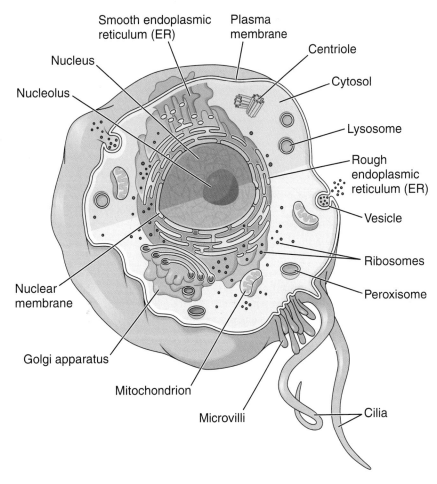

Figure 3-2 **A generalized animal cell, sectional view.** *ZOOMING IN ✦ What is attached to the ER to make it look rough? What is the liquid part of the cytoplasm called?*

Table 3•1 Cell Parts

NAME	DESCRIPTION	FUNCTION
Plasma membrane	Outer layer of the cell; composed mainly of lipids and proteins	Encloses the cell contents; regulates what enters and leaves the cell; participates in many activities, such as growth, reproduction, and interactions between cells
Microvilli	Short extensions of the cell membrane	Absorb materials into the cell
Nucleus	Large, dark-staining organelle near the center of the cell, composed of DNA and proteins	Contains the chromosomes, the hereditary units that direct all cellular activities
Nucleolus	Small body in the nucleus; composed of RNA, DNA, and protein	Makes ribosomes
Cytoplasm	Colloidal suspension that fills the cell from the nuclear membrane to the plasma membrane	Site of many cellular activities, consists of cytosol and organelles
Cytosol	The fluid portion of the cytoplasm	Surrounds the organelles
Endoplasmic reticulum (ER)	Network of membranes within the cytoplasm. Rough ER has ribosomes attached to it; smooth ER does not.	Rough ER sorts proteins and forms them into more complex compounds; smooth ER is involved with lipid synthesis.
Ribosomes	Small bodies free in the cytoplasm or attached to the ER; composed of RNA and protein	Manufacture proteins
Mitochondria	Large organelles with folded membranes inside	Convert energy from nutrients into ATP
Golgi apparatus	Layers of membranes	Makes compounds containing proteins; sorts and prepares these compounds for transport to other parts of the cell or out of the cell
Saclike bodies	Small, membrane-enclosed bodies	Store materials, transport materials through the plasma membrane, or destroy waste material
Lysosomes	Small sacs of digestive enzymes	Digest substances within the cell
Peroxisomes	Membrane-enclosed organelles containing enzymes	Break down harmful substances
Vesicles	Small membrane-bound bubbles in the cytoplasm	Store materials and move materials into or out of the cell in bulk
Centrioles	Rod-shaped bodies (usually two) near the nucleus	Help separate the chromosomes during cell division
Surface projections	Structures that extend from the cell	Move the cell or the fluids around the cell
Cilia	Short, hairlike projections from the cell	Move the fluids around the cell
Flagellum	Long, whiplike extension from the cell	Moves the cell

- Transporters—shuttle substances from one side of the membrane to the other. Glucose, for example, is carried into cells using transporters.
- Receptors—points of attachment for materials coming to the cell in the blood or tissue fluid. Some hormones, for example, must attach to receptors on the cell surface before they can act upon the cell, as described in Chapter 11 on the endocrine system.
- Enzymes—participate in reactions occurring at the plasma membrane.
- Linkers—give structure to the membrane and help attach cells to other cells.
- Cell identity markers—proteins unique to an individual's cells. These are important in the immune system and are also a factor in transplantation of tissue from one person to another.

Carbohydrates are present in small amounts in the plasma membrane, combined either with proteins (glycoproteins) or with lipids (glycolipids). These carbohydrates help cells to recognize each other and to stick together.

In some cells, the plasma membrane is folded out into multiple small projections called **microvilli** (mi-kro-VIL-li). Microvilli increase the surface area of the membrane, allowing for greater absorption of materials from the cell's environment, just as a sponge absorbs water. Microvilli are found on cells that line the small intestine, where they promote absorption of digested foods into the circulation. They are also found on kidney cells, where they reabsorb materials that have been filtered out of the blood.

Checkpoint 3-3 The outer limit of the cell is a complex membrane. What is the main substance of this membrane and what are three types of materials found within the membrane?

The Nucleus

Just as the body has different organs to carry out special functions, the cell contains specialized structures that perform different tasks. These structures are called

The Cytoplasm

The remaining organelles are part of the **cytoplasm** (SI-to-plazm), the material that fills the cell from the nuclear membrane to the plasma membrane. The liquid part of the cytoplasm is the **cytosol**, a suspension of nutrients, minerals, enzymes, and other specialized materials in water. The main organelles are described below (see Table 3-1).

The **endoplasmic reticulum** (en-do-PLAS-mik re-TIK-u-lum) is a network of membranes located between the nuclear membrane and the plasma membrane. Its name literally means "network" (reticulum) "within the cytoplasm" (endoplasmic), but for ease, it is almost always called simply the **ER**. In some areas, the ER appears to have an even surface, and is described as *smooth ER*. This type of ER is involved with the synthesis of lipids. In other areas, the ER has a gritty, uneven surface, causing it to be described as *rough ER*. The texture of rough ER comes from small bodies, called **ribosomes** (RI-bo-somz), attached to its surface. Ribosomes are necessary for the manufacture of proteins, as described later. They may be attached to the ER or be free in the cytoplasm.

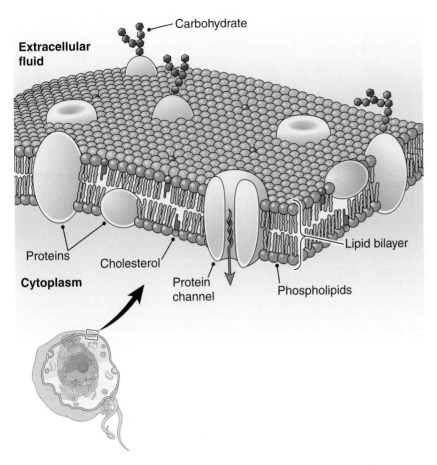

Figure 3-3 **The plasma membrane.** This drawing shows the current concept of its structure. *ZOOMING IN ✦ How many layers make up the main substance of the plasma membrane?*

organelles, which means "little organs." The largest of the organelles is the **nucleus** (NU-kle-us).

The nucleus is often called the *control center* of the cell because it contains the chromosomes, the threadlike units of heredity that are passed on from parents to their offspring. It is information contained in the **chromosomes** (KRO-mo-somes) that governs all cellular activities, as described later in this chapter. Most of the time, the chromosomes are loosely distributed throughout the nucleus, giving that organelle a uniform, dark appearance when stained and examined under a microscope (see Fig. 3-2). When the cell is dividing, however, the chromosomes tighten into their visible threadlike forms.

Within the nucleus is a smaller globule called the **nucleolus** (nu-KLE-o-lus), which means "little nucleus." The job of the nucleolus is to assemble ribosomes, small bodies outside the nucleus that are involved in the manufacture of proteins.

The **mitochondria** (mi-to-KON-dre-ah) are large organelles that are round or bean-shaped with folded membranes on the inside. Within the mitochondria, the energy from nutrients is converted to energy for the cell in the form of ATP. Mitochondria are the "power plants" of the cell. Active cells, such as muscle cells or sperm cells, need lots of energy and thus have large numbers of mitochondria.

Another organelle in a typical cell is the **Golgi** (GOL-je) **apparatus** (also called Golgi complex), a stack of membranous sacs involved in sorting and modifying proteins and then packaging them for export from the cell.

Several types of organelles appear as small sacs in the cytoplasm. These include **lysosomes** (LI-so-somz), which contain digestive enzymes. Lysosomes remove waste and foreign materials from the cell. They are also involved in destroying old and damaged cells as needed for repair and remodeling of tissue. **Peroxisomes** (per-OK-sih-somz) have enzymes that destroy harmful substances produced in metabolism (see Box 3-1, Lysosomes and Peroxisomes: Cellular Recycling). **Vesicles** (VES-ih-klz) are small, membrane-bound bubbles used for storage. They can be used to move materials into or out of the cell, as described later.

> **Checkpoint 3-4** What are cell organelles?

> **Checkpoint 3-5** Why is the nucleus called the control center of the cell?

Table 3·2 Proteins in the Plasma Membrane and Their Functions

TYPE OF PROTEIN	FUNCTION	ILLUSTRATION
Channels	Pores in the membrane that allow passage of specific substances, such as ions	
Transporters	Shuttle substances, such as glucose, across the membrane	
Receptors	Allow for attachment of substances, such as hormones, to the membrane	
Enzymes	Participate in reactions at the surface of the membrane	
Linkers	Give structure to the membrane and attach cells to other cells	
Cell identity markers	Proteins unique to a person's cells; important in the immune system and in transplantation of tissue from one person to another	

Box 3-1   Clinical Perspectives

Lysosomes and Peroxisomes: Cellular Recycling

Two organelles that play a vital role in cellular disposal and recycling are lysosomes and peroxisomes. **Lysosomes** contain enzymes that break down carbohydrates, lipids, proteins, and nucleic acids. These powerful enzymes must be kept within the lysosome because they would digest the cell if they escaped. In a process called **autophagy** (aw-TOF-ah-je), the cell uses lysosomes to safely recycle cellular structures, fusing with and digesting worn out organelles. The digested components then return to the cytoplasm for reuse. Lysosomes also break down foreign material, as when cells known as **phagocytes** (FAG-o-sites) engulf bacteria and then use lysosomes to destroy them. The cell may also use lysosomes to digest itself during **autolysis** (aw-TOL-ih-sis), a normal part of development. Cells that are no longer needed "self-destruct" by releasing lysosomal enzymes into their own cytoplasm.

Peroxisomes are small membranous sacs that resemble lysosomes but contain different kinds of enzymes. They break

down toxic substances that may enter the cell, such as drugs and alcohol, but their most important function is to break down free radicals. These substances are byproducts of normal metabolic reactions but can kill the cell if not neutralized by peroxisomes.

Disease may result if either lysosomes or peroxisomes are unable to function. In Tay-Sachs disease, nerve cells' lysosomes lack an enzyme that breaks down certain kinds of lipids. These lipids build up inside the cells, causing malfunction that leads to brain injury, blindness, and death. Disease may also result if lysosomes or peroxisomes function when they should not. Some investigators believe this is the case in autoimmune diseases, in which the body develops an immune response to its own cells. Phagocytes engulf the cells and lysosomes destroy them. In addition, body cells themselves may self-destruct through autolysis. The joint disease rheumatoid arthritis is one such example.

Centrioles (SEN-tre-olz) are rod-shaped bodies near the nucleus that function in cell division. They help to organize the cell and divide the cell contents during this process.

Surface Organelles

Some cells have structures projecting from their surface that are used for motion. **Cilia** (SIL-e-ah) are small, hairlike projections that wave, creating movement of the fluids around the cell. For example, cells that line the passageways of the respiratory tract have cilia that move impurities out of the system. Ciliated cells in the female reproductive tract move the egg cell along the oviduct toward the uterus.

A long, whiplike extension from the cell is a **flagellum** (flah-JEL-lum). The only type of cell in the human body that has a flagellum is the sperm cell of the male. Each human sperm cell has a flagellum that is used to propel the sperm cell toward the egg in the female reproductive tract.

Cellular Diversity

Although all body cells have some fundamental similarities, individual cells may vary widely in size, shape, and composition according to the function of each. The average cell size is 10 to 15 μm, but cells may range in size from the 7 μm of a red blood cell to the 200 μm or more in the length of a muscle cell.

Cell shape is related to cell function (Fig. 3-4). A neuron (nerve cell) has long fibers that transmit electrical energy from place to place in the nervous system. Cells in surface layers have a modified shape that covers and protects the tissue beneath. Red blood cells are small and round, which lets them slide through tiny blood vessels. They also have a thin outer membrane to allow for

passage of gases into and out of the cell. As red blood cells mature, they lose the nucleus and most of the other organelles, making the greatest possible amount of space available to carry oxygen.

Aside from cilia and flagella, most human cells have all the organelles described above. These may vary in number, however. For example, cells producing lipids have lots of smooth ER. Cells that secrete proteins have lots of ribosomes and a prominent Golgi apparatus. All active cells have lots of mitochondria to manufacture the ATP needed for energy.

Checkpoint 3-6 What are the two types of organelles used for movement, and what do they look like?

▶ Protein Synthesis

Because protein molecules play an indispensable part in the structure and function of the body, we need to identify the cellular substances that direct the production of proteins. As noted, the hereditary units that govern the cell are the chromosomes in the nucleus. Each chromosome in turn is divided into multiple subunits, called **genes** (Fig. 3-5). It is the genes that carry the messages for the development of particular inherited characteristics, such as brown eyes, curly hair, or blood type, and they do so by directing the manufacture of proteins in the cell.

Nucleic Acids: DNA and RNA

The genes are distinct segments of the complex organic chemical that makes up the chromosomes, a substance called **deoxyribonucleic** (de-ok-se-RI-bo-nu-kle-ik) **acid**, or **DNA**. DNA is composed of subunits called **nucleotides** (NU-kle-o-tides) (see Fig. 3-5). A related compound, **ribonucleic** (RI-bo-nu-kle-ik) **acid**, or **RNA**, which also

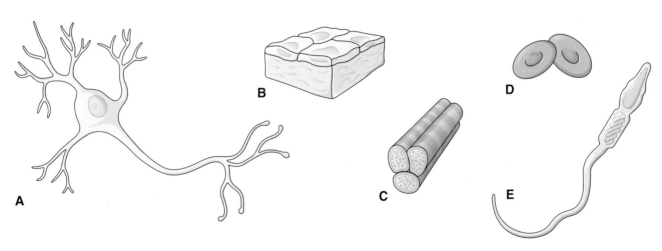

Figure 3-4 Cellular diversity. Cells vary in structure according to their functions. **(A)** A neuron has long extensions that pick up and transmit electrical impulses. **(B)** Epithelial cells cover and protect underlying tissue. **(C)** Muscle cells have fibers that produce contraction. **(D)** Red blood cells lose most organelles, which maximizes their oxygen-carrying capacity, and have a small, round shape that lets them slide through blood vessels. **(E)** A sperm cell is small and light and swims with a flagellum. *ZOOMING IN ✦ Which of the cells shown would best cover a large surface area?*

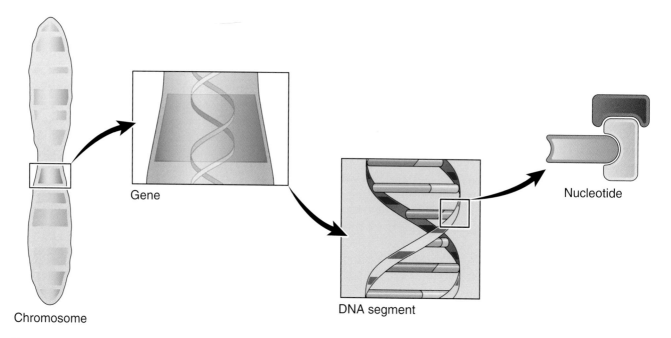

Figure 3-5 **Subdivisions of a chromosome.** A gene is a distinct region of a chromosome. The entire chromosome is made of DNA. Nucleotides are the building blocks of DNA.

participates in protein synthesis but is not part of the chromosomes, is also composed of nucleotides. There are four different nucleotides in DNA and four in RNA, but only three of these are common to both. Both DNA and RNA have the nucleotides adenine (A), guanine (G), and cytosine (C), but DNA has thymine (T), whereas RNA has uracil (U). Table 3-3 compares the structure and function of DNA and RNA.

Moving one step deeper into the structure of the nucleic acids, each nucleotide is composed of four units:

▶ A sugar, which in RNA is ribose and in DNA is a ribose that is missing one oxygen atom (that is, deoxyribose).
▶ A phosphorus-containing portion, or phosphate.
▶ A nitrogen-containing portion known as a nitrogen base.

The sugar and phosphate alternate to form a long chain to which the nitrogen bases are attached. It is variation in the nitrogen bases that accounts for the differences in the five different nucleotides.

DNA Most of the DNA in the cell is organized into chromosomes within the nucleus (a small amount of DNA is in the mitochondria located in the cytoplasm). Looking at Figure 3-6, which shows a section of a chromosome, you can see that the DNA exists as a double strand. Visualizing the complete molecule as a ladder, the sugar and phosphate units of the nucleotides make up the "side rails" of the ladder, and the nitrogen bases project from the side rails to make up the "steps" of the ladder. The two DNA strands are paired very specifically according to the identity of the nitrogen bases in the nucleotides. The adenine (A) nucleotide always pairs with the thymine (T) nucleotide; the guanine (G) nucleotide always pairs with the cytosine (C) nucleotide. The two strands of DNA are held together by weak bonds (hydrogen bonds; see Box 2-1).

Table 3·3	Comparison of DNA and RNA	
	DNA	**RNA**
Location	Almost entirely in the nucleus	Almost entirely in the cytoplasm
Composition	Nucleotides: adenine (A), guanine (G), cytosine (C), thymine (T)	Nucleotides: adenine (A), guanine (G), cytosine (C), uracil (U)
	Sugar: deoxyribose	Sugar: ribose
Structure	Double-stranded helix formed by nucleotide pairing A-T; G-C	Single strand
Function	Makes up the chromosomes, hereditary units that control all cell activities; divided into genes that carry the nucleotide codes for the manufacture of proteins	Manufacture proteins according to the nucleotide codes carried in the DNA; three types: messenger RNA (mRNA), ribosomal RNA (rRNA), and transfer RNA (tRNA)

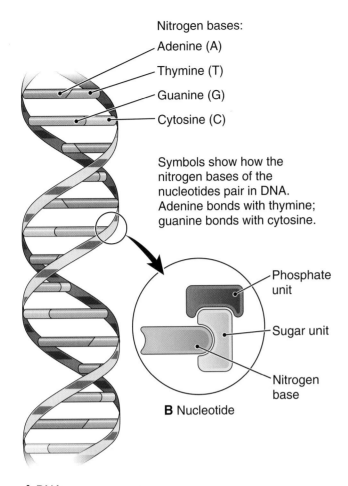

Nitrogen bases:
- Adenine (A)
- Thymine (T)
- Guanine (G)
- Cytosine (C)

Symbols show how the nitrogen bases of the nucleotides pair in DNA. Adenine bonds with thymine; guanine bonds with cytosine.

Phosphate unit

Sugar unit

Nitrogen base

B Nucleotide

A DNA

Figure 3-6 Structure of DNA. (A) This schematic representation of a chromosome segment shows the paired nucleic acid strands twisted into a double helix. **(B)** Each structural unit, or nucleotide, consists of a phosphate unit and a sugar unit attached to a nitrogen base. The sugar unit in DNA is deoxyribose. There are four different nucleotides in DNA. Their arrangement "spells out" the genetic instructions that control all activities of the cell. *ZOOMING IN ✦ Two of the DNA nucleotides (A and G) are larger in size than the other two (T and C). How do the nucleotides pair up with regard to size?*

The doubled strands then coil into a spiral, giving DNA the descriptive name *double helix.*

The message of the DNA that makes up the individual genes is actually contained in the varying pattern of the four nucleotides along the strand. The nucleotides are like four letters in an alphabet that can be combined in different ways to make a variety of words. The words represent the amino acids used to make proteins, and a long string of words makes up a gene. Each gene thus codes for the building of amino acids into a specific cellular protein. Remember that all enzymes are proteins, and enzymes are essential for all cellular reactions. DNA is thus the master blueprint for the cell.

In light of observations on cellular diversity, you may wonder how different cells in the body can vary in appearance and function if they all have the same amount and same kind of DNA. The answer to this question is that only portions of the DNA in a given cell are active at any one time. In some cells, regions of the DNA can be switched on and off, under the influence of hormones, for example. However, as cells differentiate during development and become more specialized, regions of the DNA are permanently shut down, leading to the variations in the different cell types. Scientists now realize that the control of DNA action throughout the life of the cell is a very complex matter involving not only the DNA itself but proteins as well.

Checkpoint 3-7 What are the building blocks of nucleic acids?

Checkpoint 3-8 What category of compounds does DNA code for in the cell?

The Role of RNA A blueprint is only a guide. The information it contains must be interpreted by appropriate actions, and RNA is the substance needed for these steps. RNA is much like DNA except that it exists as a single strand of nucleotides and has the nucleotide uracil (U) instead of thymine (T). Thus, when RNA pairs up with another molecule of nucleic acid to manufacture proteins, as explained below, adenine (A) bonds with uracil (U) in the RNA instead of thymine (T).

A detailed account of protein synthesis is beyond the scope of this book, but a highly simplified description and illustrations of the process are presented. The process begins with the transfer of information from DNA to RNA in the nucleus, a process known as *transcription* (Fig. 3-7). Before transcription begins, the DNA breaks its weak bonds and uncoils into single strands. Then a matching strand of RNA forms along one of the DNA strands by the process of nucleotide pairing. (For example, if the DNA strand reads CGAT, the corresponding mRNA will read GCUA. Recall that RNA uses the nucleotide U instead of A.) When complete, this messenger RNA (mRNA) leaves the nucleus and travels to a ribosome in the cytoplasm (Fig. 3-8). Recall that ribosomes are the site of protein synthesis in the cell.

Ribosomes are composed of a type of RNA called ribosomal RNA (rRNA) and also protein. At the ribosomes, the genetic message now contained within mRNA is decoded to build amino acids into the long chains that form proteins, a process termed *translation.* This final step requires a third type of RNA, transfer RNA (tRNA), small molecules present in the cytoplasm (see Fig. 3-8). Each transfer RNA carries a specific amino acid that can be added to a protein chain. A nucleotide code on each tRNA determines whether or not its amino acid will be added. After the amino acid chain is formed, it must be coiled and folded into the proper shape for that protein, as noted in Chapter 2. Table 3-4 summarizes information on the

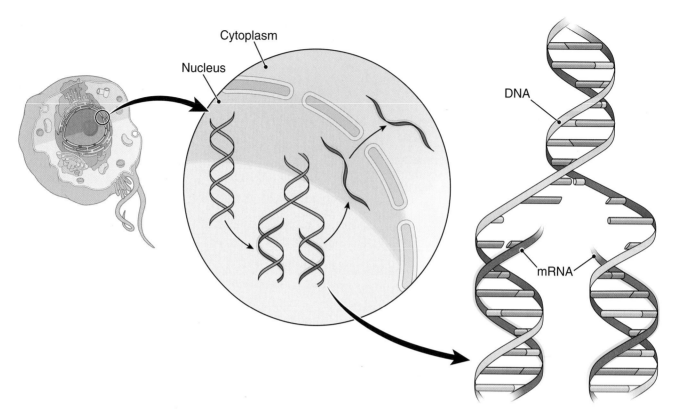

Figure 3-7   Transcription. In the first step of protein synthesis the DNA code is transcribed into messenger RNA (mRNA) by nucleotide base pairing. An enlarged view of the nucleic acids during transcription shows how mRNA forms according to the nucleotide pattern of the DNA. Note that adenine (A, red) in DNA bonds with uracil (U, brown) in RNA.

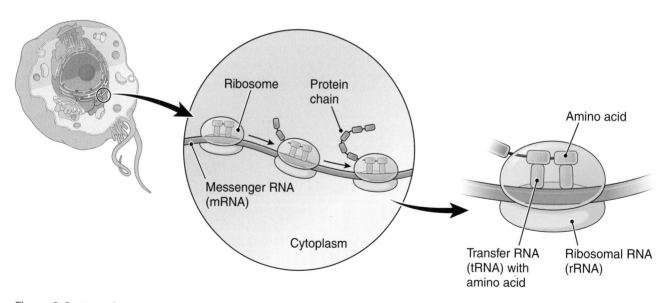

Figure 3-8   Translation. In protein synthesis, messenger RNA (mRNA) travels to the ribosomes in the cytoplasm. The information in the mRNA codes for the building of proteins from amino acids. Transfer RNA (tRNA) molecules bring amino acids to the ribosomes to build each protein.

Table 3·4	RNA
TYPES	**FUNCTION**
Messenger RNA (mRNA)	Is built on a strand of DNA in the nucleus and transcribes the nucleotide code; moves to cytoplasm and attaches to a ribosome
Ribosomal RNA (rRNA)	With protein makes up the ribosomes, the sites of protein synthesis in the cytoplasm; involved in the process of translating the genetic message into a protein
Transfer RNA (tRNA)	Works with other forms of RNA to translate the genetic code into protein; each molecule of tRNA carries an amino acid that can be used to build a protein at the ribosome

different types of RNA. Also see Box 3-2, Proteomics: So Many Proteins, So Few Genes.

Checkpoint 3-9 What three types of RNA are active in protein synthesis?

▶ Cell Division

For growth, repair, and reproduction, cells must multiply to increase their numbers. The cells that form the sex cells (egg and sperm) divide by the process of *meiosis* (mi-O-sis), which cuts the chromosome number in half to prepare for union of the egg and sperm in fertilization. If not for this preliminary reduction, the number of chromosomes in the offspring would constantly double. The process of meiosis is discussed in Chapter 21. All other body cells, known as *somatic cells*, divide by the process of **mitosis** (mi-TO-sis). In this process, described below, each original parent cell becomes two identical daughter cells.

Before mitosis can occur, the genetic information (DNA) in the parent cell must be doubled, so that each of the two new daughter cells will receive a complete set of chromosomes. For example, a cell that divides by mitosis in the human body must produce two cells with 46 chromosomes each, the same number of chromosomes that was present in the original parent cell. DNA duplicates during **interphase**, the stage in the life of a cell between one mitosis and the next. During this phase, DNA uncoils from its double-stranded form, and each strand takes on a matching strand of nucleotides according to the pattern of A-T, G-C pairing. There are now two strands, each identical to the original double helix. The strands are held together at a region called the *centromere* (SEN-tro-mere) until they separate during mitosis. A typical cell lives in interphase for most of its cycle and spends only a relatively short period in mitosis. For example, a cell reproducing every 20 hours spends only about 1 hour in mitosis and the rest of the time in interphase.

Checkpoint 3-10 What must happen to the DNA in a cell before mitosis can occur? During what stage in the life of a cell does this occur?

Stages of Mitosis

Although mitosis is a continuous process, distinct changes can be seen in the dividing cell at four stages (Fig. 3-9).

▶ In **prophase** (PRO-faze), the doubled strands of DNA return to their tightly wound spiral organization and

Box 3-2	Hot Topics

Proteomics: So Many Proteins, So Few Genes

To build the many different proteins that make up the body, cells rely on instructions encoded in genes on chromosomes. Collectively, all the different genes on all the chromosomes make up the **genome**. Genes contain the instructions for making proteins, while the proteins themselves perform the body's functions.

Scientists are now studying the human **proteome**—all the proteins that can be expressed in a cell—to help them understand the proteins' structure and function. Unlike the genome, the proteome changes as the cell's activities and needs change. In 2003, after a decade of intense scientific activity, investigators mapped the entire human genome and realized that it contained only 35,000 genes, far fewer than initially expected. How could this relatively small number of genes code for several million proteins? They concluded that genes were not the whole story.

Gene transcription is only the beginning of protein synthesis. In response to cell conditions, enzymes can snip newly transcribed mRNA into several pieces, each of which a ribosome can use to build a different protein. After each protein is built, enzymes can further modify the amino acid strands to produce several more different proteins. Other molecules help the newly formed proteins to fold into precise shapes and interact with each other, resulting in even more variations. Thus, while a gene may code for a specific protein, modifications after gene transcription can produce many more unique proteins. There is much left to discover about the proteome, but scientists hope that future research will lead to new techniques for detecting and treating disease.

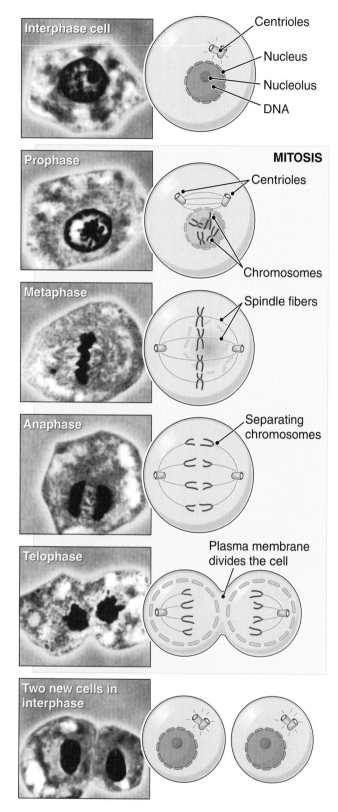

Figure 3-9 **The stages of mitosis.** When it is not dividing, the cell is in interphase. The cell shown is for illustration only. It is not a human cell, which has 46 chromosomes. (Photomicrographs reprinted with permission from Cormack DH. Essential Histology. 2nd ed. Philadelphia: Lippincott Williams & Wilkins, 2001.) *ZOOMING IN* ✦ *If the original cell shown has 46 chromosomes, how many chromosomes will each new daughter cell have?*

become visible under the microscope as dark, thread-like chromosomes. The nucleolus and the nuclear membrane begin to disappear. In the cytoplasm, the two centrioles move toward opposite ends of the cell and a spindle-shaped structure made of thin fibers begins to form between them.

‣ In **metaphase** (MET-ah-faze), the chromosomes line up across the center (equator) of the cell attached to the spindle fibers.

‣ In **anaphase** (AN-ah-faze), the centromere splits and the duplicated chromosomes separate and begin to move toward opposite ends of the cell.

‣ As mitosis continues into **telophase** (TEL-o-faze), a membrane appears around each group of separated chromosomes, forming two new nuclei.

Also during telophase, the plasma membrane pinches off to divide the cell. The midsection between the two areas becomes progressively smaller until, finally, the cell splits in two. There are now two new cells, or daughter cells, each with exactly the same kind and amount of DNA as was present in the parent cell. In just a few types of cells, skeletal muscle cells for example, the cell itself does not divide following nuclear division. The result, after multiple mitoses, is a giant single cell with multiple nuclei. This pattern is extremely rare in the human body.

During mitosis, all the organelles, except those needed for the division process, temporarily disappear. After the cell splits, these organelles reappear in each daughter cell. Also at this time, the centrioles usually duplicate in preparation for the next cell division.

Body cells differ in the rate at which they reproduce. Some, such as nerve cells and muscle cells, stop dividing at some point in development and are not replaced if they die. They remain in interphase. Others, such as blood cells, sperm cells, and skin cells, multiply rapidly to replace cells destroyed by injury, disease, or natural wear-and-tear. Cells that multiply slowly may be triggered to divide when tissue is injured, as in repair of a bone fracture.

Immature cells that retain the ability to divide and mature when necessary are known as **stem cells** (see Box 4-1 in Chapter 4). All blood cells, for example, are produced from stem cells in the red bone marrow. Research has been done on stimulating stem cells to divide into various cell types in the laboratory, but these studies have been controversial. Although it may be possible some day to use such cells to replace cells injured by disease, some people consider these studies to be unethical.

Checkpoint 3-11 What are the four stages of mitosis?

‣ Movement of Substances Across the Plasma Membrane

The plasma membrane serves as a barrier between the cell and its environment. Nevertheless, nutrients, oxygen, and many other substances needed by the cell must

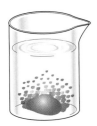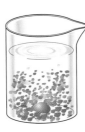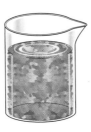

Figure 3-10 Diffusion of a solid in a liquid. The molecules of the solid tend to spread evenly throughout the liquid as they dissolve.

be taken in and waste products must be eliminated. Clearly, some substances can be exchanged between the cell and its environment through the plasma membrane. For this reason, the plasma membrane is described at a simple level as **semipermeable** (sem-e-PER-me-ah-bl). It is permeable, or passable, to some molecules but impassable to others. Some particles, proteins for example, are too large to travel through the membrane unaided.

The ability of a substance to travel through the membrane is based on several factors. Molecular size is the main factor that determines passage through the membrane, but solubility and electrical charge are also considerations. Water, a tiny molecule, is usually able to penetrate the membrane with ease. Nutrients, however, must be split into small molecules by the process of digestion so that they can travel through the plasma membrane. Sucrose (table sugar), for example, is converted to glucose and fructose, smaller molecules that enter the cell and serve as sources of energy.

Various physical processes are involved in exchanges through the plasma membrane. One way of grouping these processes is according to whether they do or do not require cellular energy.

Movement That Does Not Require Cellular Energy

The adjective *passive* describes movement through the plasma membrane that does not require energy output by the cell. Passive mechanisms depend on the internal energy of the moving particles or the application of some outside source of energy. The methods include:

▶ **Diffusion** is the constant movement of particles from a region of relatively higher concentration to one of lower concentration. Just as couples on a crowded dance floor spread out into all the available space to avoid hitting other dancers, diffusing substances spread throughout their available space until their concentration everywhere is the same—that is, they reach equilibrium (Fig. 3-10). This movement from higher to lower concentrations uses the internal energy of the particles and does not require cellular energy, just as a sled will move from the top to the bottom of a snowy hill. The particles are said to follow their *concentration gradient* from higher concentration to lower concentration.

▶ When substances diffuse through a membrane, such as the intact plasma membrane, passage is limited to those particles small enough to pass through spaces between molecules in the membrane, as shown with a large-scale example in Figure 3-11. In the body, soluble materials, such as nutrients, electrolytes, gases, and waste materials, are constantly moving into or out of the cells by diffusion.

▶ **Osmosis** (os-MO-sis) is a special type of diffusion. The term applies specifically to the diffusion of water through a semipermeable membrane. The water molecules move, as expected, from an area where there are more of them to an area where there are fewer of them. That is, the solvent (the water molecules) moves from an area of lower *solute* concentration to an area of higher *solute* concentration

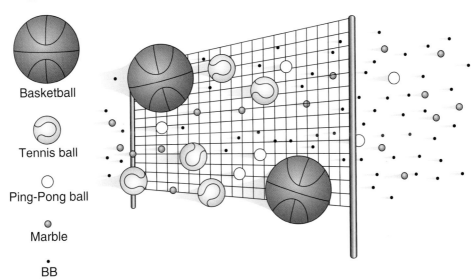

Basketball

Tennis ball

Ping-Pong ball

Marble

BB

Figure 3-11 Diffusion through a semipermeable membrane. In this example, large objects (basketballs, tennis balls) cannot pass through the net, whereas the smaller ones (ping-pong balls, marbles, BBs) can. In the human body, large particles in the blood, such as proteins and blood cells, cannot pass through the walls of the capillaries, whereas small particles, such as nutrients, electrolytes, and gases can. *ZOOMING IN ✦ If this picture represented diffusion in the body, what would the net be?*

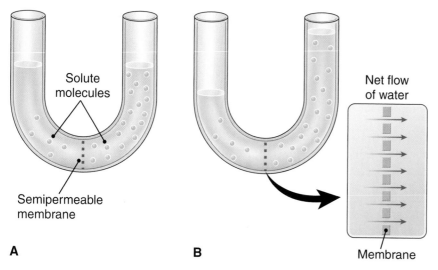

A   B

Figure 3-12 **A simple demonstration of osmosis.** Solute molecules are shown in yellow. All of the solvent (blue) is composed of water molecules. **(A)** Two solutions with different concentrations of solute are separated by a semipermeable membrane. Water can flow through the membrane, but the solute cannot. **(B)** Water flows into the more concentrated solution, raising the level of the liquid in that side. *ZOOMING IN* ✦ *What would happen in this system if the solute could pass through the membrane?*

(Fig. 3-12). For a physiologist studying the flow of water across membranes, as in exchange of fluids through capillaries in the circulation, it is helpful to know the direction in which water will flow and at what rate it will move. A measure of the force driving osmosis is called the *osmotic pressure*. This force can be measured, as illustrated in Figure 3-13, by applying enough pressure to the surface of a liquid to stop the inward flow of water by osmosis. The pressure needed to counteract osmosis is the osmotic pressure. In practice, the term osmotic pressure is used to describe the tendency of a solution to draw water into it. This force is directly related to concentration: the higher the concentration of a solution, the greater is its tendency to draw water in.

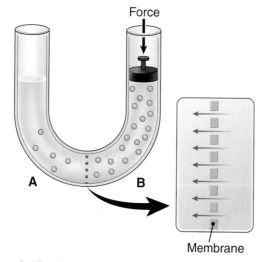

Figure 3-13 **Osmotic pressure.** Osmotic pressure is the force needed to stop the flow of water by osmosis. Pressure on the surface of the fluid in side B counteracts the osmotic flow of water from side A to side B. *ZOOMING IN* ✦ *What would happen to osmotic pressure if the concentration of solute were increased on side B of this system?*

▶ **Filtration** is the passage of water containing dissolved materials through a membrane as a result of a mechanical ("pushing") force on one side (Fig. 3-14). One example of filtration in the body is the movement of materials out of the capillaries and into the tissues under the force of blood pressure (see Chapter 14). Another example occurs in the kidneys as materials are filtered out of the blood in the first step of urine formation (see Chapter 19).

▶ **Facilitated diffusion** is the movement of materials across the plasma membrane in the direction of the concentration gradient (from higher to lower concentration) but using transporters to move the material at a faster rate (Fig. 3-15). Glucose, the sugar that is the main energy source for cells, moves through the plasma membrane by means of facilitated diffusion.

Movement That Requires Cellular Energy

Movement across the membrane that requires energy is describes as *active*. These methods include:

▶ **Active transport.** The plasma membrane has the ability to move small solute particles into or out of the cell opposite to the direction in which they would normally flow by diffusion. That is, the membrane moves them against the concentration gradient from an area where they are in relatively lower concentration to an area where they are in higher concentration. Because this movement goes against the natural flow of particles, it requires energy, just as getting a sled to the top of a hill requires energy. It also requires proteins in the cell membrane that act as **transporters** for the particles.

This process of active transport is one important function of the living cell membrane. The nervous system and muscular system, for example, depend on the active

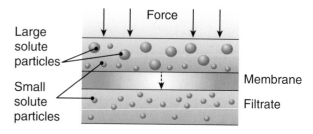

Figure 3-14 **Filtration.** A mechanical force pushes a substance through a membrane, although the membrane limits which particles can pass through based on size. The small particles go through the membrane and appear in the filtered solution (filtrate).

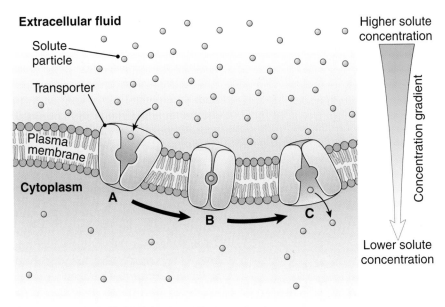

Figure 3-15 Facilitated diffusion. Transporters (proteins in the plasma membrane) move solute particles through a membrane from an area of higher concentration to an area of lower concentration. **(A)** A solute particle enters the transporter. **(B)** The transporter changes shape. **(C)** The transporter releases the solute particle on the other side of the membrane. *ZOOMING IN* ✦ *How would a change in the number of transporters affect the movement of a solute by facilitated diffusion?*

transport of sodium, potassium, and calcium ions for proper function. The kidneys also carry out active transport in regulating the composition of urine. By means of active transport, the cell can take in what it needs from the surrounding fluids and remove materials from the cell. Because the cell membrane can carry on active transport, the membrane is most accurately described, not as simply semipermeable, but as **selectively permeable.** It regulates

what can enter and leave based on the needs of the cell.

There are several active methods for moving large quantities of material into or out of the cell. These methods are grouped together as **bulk transport,** because of the amounts of material moved, or **vesicular transport,** because small bubbles, or vesicles, are needed for the processes.

▶ **Endocytosis** (en-do-si-TO-sis) is a term that describes the bulk movement of materials into the cell. There are two examples:

▶ In **phagocytosis** (fag-o-si-TO-sis), relatively large particles are engulfed by the plasma membrane and moved into the cell (Fig. 3-16). Certain white blood cells carry out phagocytosis to rid the body of foreign material and dead cells. Material taken into a cell by phagocytosis is first enclosed in a vesicle made from the plasma membrane and is later destroyed by lysosomes.

In **pinocytosis** (pi-no-si-TO-sis), the cell membrane engulfs droplets of fluid. This is a way for large protein molecules in suspension to travel into the cell. The word *pinocytosis* means "cell drinking."

▶ In **exocytosis,** the cell moves materials out in vesicles (Fig. 3-17). One example of exocytosis is the export of neurotransmitters from neurons (neurotransmitters are chemicals that control the activity of the nervous system).

The transport methods described above are summarized in Table 3-5.

> **Checkpoint 3-12** Substances are constantly moving into and out of cells through the plasma membrane. What types of movement do not require cellular energy and what types of movement do require cellular energy?

How Osmosis Affects Cells

As stated earlier, water usually moves easily through the cell membrane. Therefore, for a normal fluid balance to be maintained, the fluid outside all cells must have the same concentration of dissolved substances (solutes) as the fluids inside the cells (Fig. 3-18). If not, water will move rapidly into or out of the cell by osmosis. Solutions with concentrations equal to the concentration of the cytoplasm are described as **isotonic** (i-so-TON-ik). Tissue fluids and blood plasma are isotonic for body cells. Manufactured solutions that are isotonic for the cells and can thus be used to replace body fluids include 0.9% salt, or **normal saline,** and 5% dextrose (glucose).

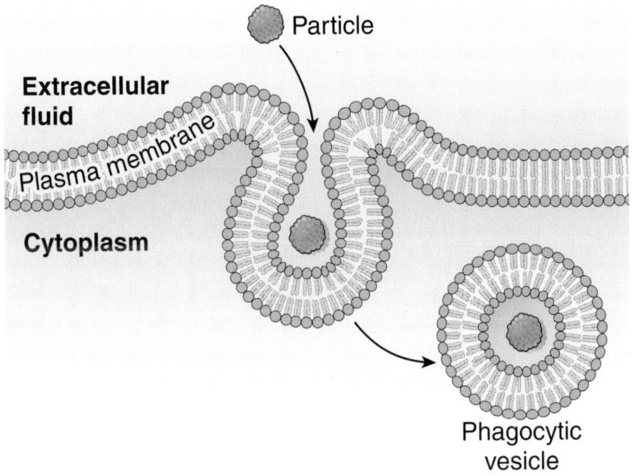

Figure 3-16 Phagocytosis. The plasma membrane encloses a particle from the extracellular fluid. The membrane then pinches off, forming a vesicle that carries the particle into the cytoplasm. *ZOOMING IN* ✦ *What organelle would likely help to destroy a particle taken in by phagocytosis?*

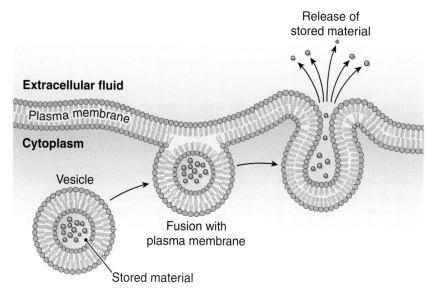

Figure 3-17 **Exocytosis.** A vesicle fuses with the plasma membrane then ruptures and releases its contents.

When a red blood cell draws in water and bursts in this way, the cell is said to undergo **hemolysis** (he-MOL-ih-sis). If a cell is placed in a **hypertonic** solution, which is more concentrated than the cellular fluid, it loses water to the surrounding fluids and shrinks, a process termed **crenation** (kre-NA-shun) (see Fig. 3-18).

Fluid balance is an important facet of homeostasis and must be properly regulated for health. You can figure out in which direction water will move through the plasma membrane if you remember the saying "water follows salt," salt meaning any dissolved material (solute). The total amount and distribution of body fluids is discussed in Chapter 19. Table 3-6 summarizes the effects of different solution concentrations on cells.

A solution that is less concentrated than the intracellular fluid is described as **hypotonic**. Based on the principles of osmosis already explained, a cell placed in a hypotonic solution draws water in, swells, and may burst.

Checkpoint 3-13 The concentration of fluids in and around the cell is important in homeostasis. What term describes a fluid that is the same concentration as the fluid within the cell (intracellular fluid)? What type of fluid is less concentrated? More concentrated?

Table 3·5	Membrane Transport	
PROCESS	**DEFINITION**	**EXAMPLE**
Do not require cellular energy (passive)		
Diffusion	Random movement of particles with the concentration gradient (from higher concentration to lower concentration) until they reach equilibrium	Movement of nutrients, electrolytes, gases, wastes, and other soluble materials into and out of the cell
Osmosis	Diffusion of water through a semipermeable membrane	Movement of water across the plasma membrane
Filtration	Movement of materials through a membrane under mechanical force	Movement of materials out of the blood under the force of blood pressure
Facilitated diffusion	Movement of materials across the plasma membrane along the concentration gradient using transporters to speed the process	Movement of glucose into the cells
Require cellular energy		
Active transport	Movement of materials through the plasma membrane against the concentration gradient using transporters	Transport of ions (*e.g.*, Na^+, K^+, Ca^{2+}) in the nervous system and muscular system
Endocytosis	Transport of bulk amounts of materials into the cell using vesicles	Phagocytosis, intake of large particles, as when white blood cells take in waste materials; also pinocytosis—intake of fluid
Exocytosis	Transport of bulk amounts of materials out of the cell using vesicles	Release of neurotransmitters from neurons

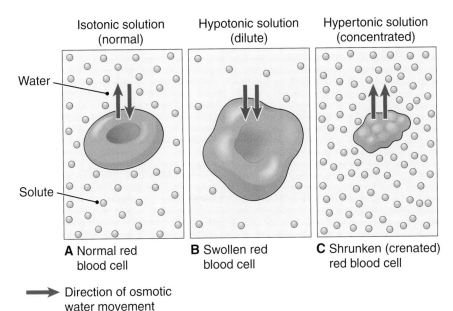

Water

Solute

A Normal red blood cell

B Swollen red blood cell

C Shrunken (crenated) red blood cell

➡ Direction of osmotic water movement

Figure 3-18 **The effect of osmosis on cells.** Water moves through a red blood cell membrane in solutions with three different concentrations of solute. **(A)** The isotonic (normal) solution has the same concentration as the cell fluid, and water moves into and out of the cell at the same rate. **(B)** A cell placed in a hypotonic (more dilute) solution draws water in, causing the cell to swell and perhaps undergo hemolysis (bursting). **(C)** The hypertonic (more concentrated) solution draws water out of the cell, causing it to shrink, an effect known as crenation. *ZOOMING IN* ✦ *What would happen to red blood cells if blood lost through injury were replaced with pure water?*

▶ Cell Aging

As cells multiply throughout life, changes occur that may lead to their damage and death. Harmful substances known as *free radicals*, produced in the course of normal metabolism, can injure cells unless these materials are destroyed. Chapter 18 covers free radicals in more detail. Lysosomes may deteriorate as they age, releasing enzymes that can harm the cell. Alteration of the genes, or **mutations**, are a natural occurrence in the process of cell division and are increased by exposure to harmful substances and radiation in the environment. Mutations usually harm cells and may lead to cancer.

As a person ages, the overall activity of the body cells slows. One example of this change is the slowing down of repair processes. A bone fracture, for example, takes considerably longer to heal in an old person than in a young person.

One theory on aging holds that cells are preprogrammed to divide only a certain number of times before they die. Support for this idea comes from the fact that cells taken from a young person divide more times when grown in the laboratory than similar cells taken from an older individual. This programmed cell death, known as *apoptosis* (ah-pop-TO-sis), is a natural part of growth and remodeling before birth in the developing embryo and in repair and remodeling of tissue throughout life (see Box 3-3, Necrosis and Apoptosis: Cellular Homicide and Suicide).

Table 3·6	Solutions and Their Effects on Cells		
TYPE OF SOLUTION	**DESCRIPTION**	**EXAMPLES**	**EFFECT ON CELLS**
Isotonic	Has the same concentration of dissolved substances as the fluid in the cell	0.9% salt (normal saline); 5% dextrose (glucose)	None; cell in equilibrium with its environment
Hypotonic	Has a lower concentration of dissolved substances than the fluid in the cell	Less than 0.9% salt or 5% dextrose	Cell takes in water, swells, and may burst; red blood cell undergoes hemolysis
Hypertonic	Has a higher concentration of dissolved substances than the fluid in the cell	Higher than 0.9% salt or 5% dextrose	Cell will lose water and shrink; cell undergoes crenation

Box 3-3	A Closer Look

Necrosis and Apoptosis: Cellular Homicide and Suicide

Cell death happens in two ways: by necrosis, because the cell is injured; or by apoptosis, because the cell is programmed to die. One way of remembering the difference is to think of necrosis as "cellular homicide" and apoptosis as "cellular suicide."

Necrosis disrupts the cell's normal water-balancing mechanisms and stimulates autolysis (see Box 3-1). As a result, the cell swells and its organelles break down. Finally, the cell ruptures, releasing its contents into the surrounding tissue. These contents contain digestive enzymes that damage adjacent cells, producing more injury and necrosis.

Apoptosis is an orderly, genetically programmed cell death triggered by the cell's own genes. Under the right circumstances, these "suicide genes" produce enzymes called capsases that destroy the cell swiftly and neatly. The cell shrinks, and phagocytes quickly digest it. In contrast to necrosis, apoptotic cells do not cause further chaos when they die.

Apoptosis is a normal bodily process. It is especially important during embryonic development because it removes unneeded cells, such as those from limb buds to form fingers and toes. Apoptosis also occurs after birth, as when cells subject to extreme wear and tear regularly undergo apoptosis and are replaced. For example, the cells lining the digestive tract are removed and replaced every 2 to 3 days.

Word Anatomy

Medical terms are built from standardized word parts (prefixes, roots, and suffixes). Learning the meanings of these parts can help you remember words and interpret unfamiliar terms.

WORD PART	MEANING	EXAMPLE
The Role of Cells		
cyt/o	cell	*Cytology* is the study of cells.
Microscopes		
micr/o	small	*Microscopes* are used to view structures too small to see with the naked eye.
Cell Structure		
bi-	two	The lipid *bilayer* is a double layer of lipid molecules.
-some	body	*Ribosomes* are small bodies outside the cell's nucleus that help make proteins.
chrom/o-	color	*Chromosomes* are small, threadlike bodies that stain darkly with basic dyes.
Cell Structure		
end/o-	in, within	The *endoplasmic* reticulum is a network of membranes within the cytoplasm.
lys/o	loosening, dissolving, separating	*Lysosomes* are small bodies (organelles) with enzymes that dissolve materials (see also *hemolysis* below).
Cell Functions		
inter-	between	*Interphase* is the stage between one cell division (mitosis) and the next.
pro-	before, in front of	*Prophase* is the first stage of mitosis.
meta-	change	*Metaphase* is the second stage of mitosis when the chromosomes change position and line up across the equator.
ana-	upward, back, again	In the *anaphase* stage of mitosis, chromosomes move to opposite sides of the cell.
tel/o-	end	*Telophase* is the last stage of mitosis.
semi-	partial, half	A *semipermeable* membrane lets some molecules pass through but not others.
phag/o	to eat, ingest	In *phagocytosis* the cell membrane engulfs large particles and moves them into the cell.
pino	to drink	In *pinocytosis* the cell membrane "drinks" (engulfs) droplets of fluid.
ex/o-	outside, out of, away from	In *exocytosis* the cell moves material out in vesicles.
iso-	same, equal	An *isotonic* solution has the same concentration as that of the cytoplasm.
hypo-	deficient, below, beneath	A *hypotonic* solution's concentration is lower than that of the cytoplasm.
hem/o	blood	*Hemolysis* is the destruction of red blood cells.
hyper-	above, over, excessive	A *hypertonic* solution's concentration is higher than that of the cytoplasm.

Summary

I. The Role of Cells
1. Basic unit of life
2. Show all characteristics of life—organization, metabolism, responsiveness, homeostasis, growth, reproduction

II. Microscopes
1. Types
   a. Compound light microscope
   b. Transmission electron microscope—magnifies up to 1 million times
   c. Scanning electron microscope—gives three-dimensional image
2. Micrometer—metric unit commonly used for microscopic measurements
3. Stains—dyes used to aid in viewing cells under the microscope

III. Cell Structure
A. Plasma membrane—regulates what enters and leaves cell
1. Phospholipid bilayer with proteins, carbohydrates, cholesterol
   a. Proteins—channels, transporters, receptors, enzymes, linkers, cell identity markers
B. Nucleus
1. Control center of the cell
2. Contains the chromosomes (units of heredity)
3. Contains the nucleolus, which manufactures ribosomes
C. Cytoplasm—colloidal suspension that holds organelles
1. Cytosol—liquid portion
2. Organelles—structures that carry out special functions
   a. ER (endoplasmic reticulum), ribosomes, mitochondria, Golgi apparatus, lysosomes, peroxisomes, vesicles, centrioles
D. Surface organelles
1. Cilia, flagellum—used for movement
E. Cellular diversity

IV. Protein synthesis
A. Nucleic acids—DNA and RNA
1. Composed of nucleotides
   a. Each nucleotide has sugar, phosphate, nitrogen base
   b. Nitrogen bases vary, giving five nucleotides
2. DNA
   a. Carries the genetic message
   b. Located almost entirely in the nucleus
   c. Composed of nucleotides adenine (A), guanine (G), cytosine (C), thymine (T)
   d. Double stranded by pairing of A-T, G-C, and wound into helix
3. The role of RNA
   a. Single strand of nucleotides—A, G, C, and uracil (U)
   b. Located in the cytoplasm
   c. Translates DNA message into proteins
   d. Three types
      (1) Messenger RNA (mRNA)—transcribes the message of the DNA
      (2) Ribosomal RNA (rRNA)—makes up the ribosomes, the site of protein synthesis
      (3) Transfer RNA (tRNA)—brings amino acids to be made into proteins

V. Cell division
1. Meiosis—forms the sex cells (egg and sperm)
   a. Divides the chromosome number in half
2. Mitosis—division of somatic (body) cells
   a. Chromosomes first duplicate during interphase
   b. Division of cell into two identical daughter cells
A. Stages of mitosis—prophase, metaphase, anaphase, telophase

VI. Movement of substances across plasma membrane
A. Movement that does not require cellular energy (passive)
1. Diffusion—molecules move from area of higher concentration to area of lower concentration
2. Osmosis—diffusion of water through semipermeable membrane
   a. Osmotic pressure—measure of tendency of a solution to draw in water
3. Filtration—movement of materials through plasma membrane under mechanical force
4. Facilitated diffusion—movement of materials with aid of transporters in plasma membrane
B. Movement that requires cellular energy (active)
1. Active transport
   a. Movement of solute particles from area of lower concentration to area of higher concentration
   b. Requires transporters
2. Endocytosis—movement of bulk amounts of material into the cell in vesicles
   a. Phagocytosis—engulfing of large particles
   b. Pinocytosis—intake of droplets of fluid
3. Exocytosis—movement of bulk amounts of materials out of the cell in vesicles
C. How osmosis affects cells
1. Isotonic solution—same concentration as cell fluids; cell remains the same
2. Hypotonic solution—lower concentration than cell fluids; cell swells and may undergo hemolysis (bursting)
3. Hypertonic solution—higher concentration than cell fluids; cell undergoes crenation (shrinking)

VII. Cell aging
A. Mutations (changes) occur in genes
B. Slowing of cellular activity
C. Apoptosis—programmed cell death

Questions for Study and Review

Building Understanding

Fill in the blanks

1. The part of the cell that regulates what can enter or leave is the _____.
2. Distinct segments of DNA that code for specific proteins are called _____.
3. The cytosol and organelles make up the _____.
4. If Solution A has more solute and less water than Solution B, then Solution A is _____ to Solution B.
5. Mechanisms that require energy to move substances across the plasma membrane are called _____ transport mechanisms.

Matching

Match each numbered item with the most closely related lettered item.

___6. DNA duplication takes place
___7. DNA is tightly wound into chromosomes
___8. Chromosomes line up along the cell's equator
___9. Chromosomes separate and move toward opposite ends of the cell
___10. Cell membrane pinches off, dividing the cell into two new daughter cells

a. metaphase
b. anaphase
c. telophase
d. interphase
e. prophase

Multiple choice

___ 11. The main component of the plasma membrane is
   a. phospholipid
   b. cholesterol
   c. carbohydrate
   d. protein
___ 12. ATP is synthesized in the
   a. nucleus
   b. Golgi apparatus
   c. endoplasmic reticulum
   d. mitochondria
___ 13. Transcription of the DNA strand TGAAC would produce an mRNA strand with the sequence
   a. CAGGU
   b. ACTTG
   c. CAGGT
   d. ACUUG
___ 14. Somatic cells divide by the process called
   a. mitosis
   b. meiosis
   c. crenation
   d. hemolysis
___ 15. Movement of solute from a region of high concentration to one of lower concentration is called
   a. exocytosis
   b. diffusion
   c. endocytosis
   d. osmosis

Understanding Concepts

16. List the components of the plasma membrane and state a function for each.
17. Compare and contrast the following cellular components:

a. microvilli and cilia
b. nucleus and nucleolus
c. rough ER and smooth ER
d. lysosome and peroxisome
e. DNA and RNA
f. chromosome and gene

18. Describe the role of each of the following in protein synthesis: DNA, nucleotide, RNA, ribosomes, rough ER, and Golgi apparatus.
19. List and define six methods by which materials cross the cell membrane. Which of these requires cellular energy?
20. Why is the cell membrane described as selectively permeable?
21. What will happen to a red blood cell placed in a 5.0% salt solution? In distilled water?

Conceptual Thinking

22. Cigarette smoke paralyzes the cilia of cells lining the respiratory tract. Explain the effects of this on respiratory system function.
23. A particular type of cell manufactures a protein needed elsewhere in the body. Beginning with events in the nucleus, describe the process of making that protein and exporting it out of the cell.
24. Kidney failure causes a buildup of waste and water in the blood. A procedure called hemodialysis removes these substances from the blood. During this procedure, the patient's blood passes by a semipermeable membrane within the dialysis machine. Waste and water from the blood diffuses across the membrane into dialysis fluid on the other side. Based on this information, compare the osmotic concentration of the blood with that of the dialysis fluid.

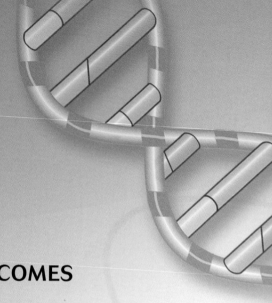

SELECTED KEY TERMS

The following terms and
other boldface terms in the
chapter are defined in the Glossary

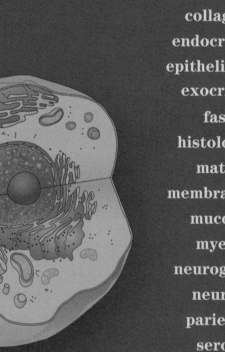

adipose

areolar

cartilage

collagen

endocrine

epithelium

exocrine

fascia

histology

matrix

membrane

mucosa

myelin

neuroglia

neuron

parietal

serosa

visceral

LEARNING OUTCOMES

After careful study of this chapter,
you should be able to:

1. Name the four main groups of tissues and give the location and
   general characteristics of each
2. Describe the difference between exocrine and endocrine glands
   and give examples of each
3. Give examples of liquid, soft, fibrous, and hard
   connective tissues
4. Describe three types of epithelial membranes
5. List several types of connective tissue membranes
6. Show how word parts are used to build words related to
   tissues, glands, and membranes (see Word Anatomy
   at the end of the chapter)

chapter 4

Tissues, Glands, and Membranes

Tissues are groups of cells similar in structure, arranged in a characteristic pattern, and specialized for the performance of specific tasks. The study of tissues is known as **histology** (his-TOL-o-je). This study shows that the form, arrangement, and composition of cells in different tissues account for their properties. For a description of the health professional who prepares tissues for study, see Box 4-1, Histotechnologist.

The tissues in our bodies might be compared with the different materials used to construct a building. Think for a moment of the great variety of building materials used according to need—wood, stone, steel, plaster, insulation, and others. Each of these has different properties, but together they contribute to the building as a whole. The same may be said of tissues.

◗ Tissue Classification

The four main groups of tissue are the following:

◗ **Epithelial** (ep-ih-THE-le-al) **tissue** covers surfaces, lines cavities, and forms glands.
◗ **Connective tissue** supports and forms the framework of all parts of the body.
◗ **Muscle tissue** contracts and produces movement.
◗ **Nervous tissue** conducts nerve impulses.

This chapter concentrates mainly on epithelial and connective tissues; muscle and nervous tissues receive more attention in later chapters.

◗ Epithelial Tissue

Epithelial tissue, or **epithelium** (ep-ih-THE-le-um), forms a protective covering for the body. It is the main tissue of the skin's outer layer. It also forms membranes, ducts, and the lining of body cavities and hollow organs, such as the organs of the digestive, respiratory, and urinary tracts.

Structure of Epithelial Tissue

Epithelial cells are tightly packed to better protect underlying tissue or form barriers between systems. The cells vary in shape and arrangement according to their function. Epithelial tissue is classified on the basis of these characteristics. In shape, the cells may be described as follows:

◗ **Squamous** (SKWA-mus)—flat and irregular.
◗ **Cuboidal**—square.
◗ **Columnar**—long and narrow.

The cells may be arranged in a single layer, in which case it is described as **simple** (Fig. 4-1). Simple epithelium functions as a thin barrier through which materials can pass fairly easily. For example, simple epithelium allows for absorption of materials from the lining of the digestive tract into the blood and allows for passage of oxygen from the blood to body tissues. Areas subject to wear-and-tear that require protection are covered with epithelial cells in multiple layers, an arrangement described as **stratified** (Fig. 4-2). If the cells are staggered so that they appear to be in multiple layers but really are not, they are termed *pseudostratified*. Terms for both shape and arrangement are used to describe epithelial tissue. Thus, a single layer of flat, irregular cells would be described as *simple squamous epithelium*, whereas tissue with many layers of these same cells would be described as *stratified squamous epithelium*.

Some organs, such as the urinary bladder, must vary a great deal in size as they work. These organs are lined with **transitional epithelium**, which is capable of great expansion but returns to its original form once tension is relaxed—as when, in this case, the bladder is emptied.

Box 4-1 · Health Professions

Histotechnologist

In the clinical laboratory, the histotechnologist is the health-care professional who prepares tissue samples for microscopic examination. When a tissue sample arrives at the laboratory, the histotechnologist cuts it into very thin slices, called sections, mounts the sections on glass slides, and treats them with various chemicals to preserve and prepare them for staining. The histotechnologist then stains the preserved sections with specific dyes to emphasize cellular details that a pathologist might look for. To perform these tasks, histotechnologists require a strong clinical background and a thorough understanding of chemistry, anatomy, and physiology.

Most histotechnologists work in hospital and medical clinic laboratories, although some find employment in research laboratories, pharmaceutical companies, and government agencies. Job prospects are promising because of the growing need for health-care and the development of new laboratory tests and technologies. For more information about careers in histotechnology, contact the American Society for Clinical Laboratory Science.

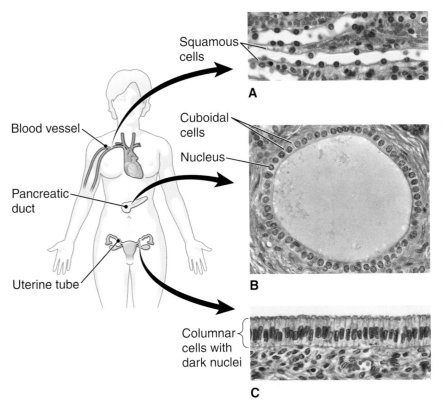

Figure 4-1   **Simple epithelial tissues.** **(A)** Simple squamous has flat, irregular cells. **(B)** Cuboidal cells are square in shape with darkly staining round nuclei. **(C)** Columnar cells are long and narrow with darkly staining nuclei. (A and C, Reprinted with permission from Cormack DH. Essential Histology. 2nd ed. Philadelphia: Lippincott Williams & Wilkins, 2001; B, reprinted with permission from Ross MH, Kaye GI, Pawlina W. Histology. 4th ed. Philadelphia: Lippincott Williams & Wilkins, 2003.) *ZOOMING IN ✦ In how many layers are these epithelial cells?*

Special Functions of Epithelial Tissue

The cells of some epithelium produce secretions, including **mucus** (MU-kus) (a clear, sticky fluid), digestive juices, sweat, and other substances. The air that we breathe passes over epithelium that lines the passageways of the respiratory (breathing) system. Mucus-secreting **goblet cells**, named for their shape, are scattered among the pseudostratified epithelial cells (Fig. 4-3 A). The epithelial cells also have tiny hairlike projections called **cilia**. Together, the mucus and the cilia help trap bits of dust and other foreign particles that could otherwise reach the lungs and damage them. The digestive tract is lined with simple columnar epithelium that also contains goblet cells. They secrete mucus that protects the lining of the digestive organs (Fig. 4-3 B).

Epithelium repairs itself quickly after it is injured. In areas of the body subject to normal wear and tear, such as the skin, the inside of the mouth, and the lining of the intestinal tract, epithelial cells reproduce frequently, replacing damaged tissue. Certain areas of the epithelium that form the outer layer of the skin are capable of modifying themselves for greater strength whenever they are subjected to unusual wear and tear; the growth of calluses is a good example of this response.

Checkpoint 4-1 Epithelium is classified according to cell shape. What are the three basic shapes?

Glands

The active cells of many glands are epithelial cells. A gland is an organ specialized to produce a substance that is sent out to other parts of the body. The gland manufactures these secretions from materials removed from the blood. Glands are divided into two categories based on how they release their secretions:

▸ **Exocrine** (EK-so-krin) **glands** have ducts or tubes to carry secretions away from the gland. The secretions may be

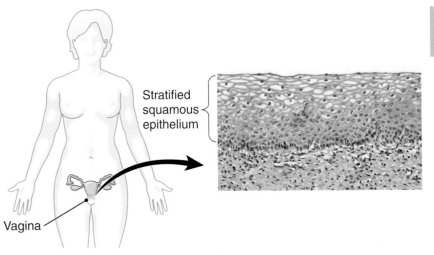

Figure 4-2   **Stratified squamous epithelium.** Cells are arranged in multiple layers. (Reprinted with permission from Cormack DH. Essential Histology. 2nd ed. Philadelphia: Lippincott Williams & Wilkins, 2001.)

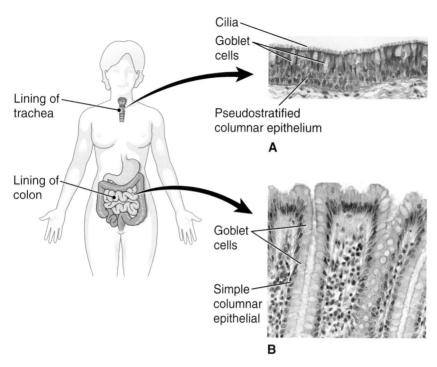

Figure 4-3 Special features of epithelial tissues. (A) The lining of the trachea showing cilia and goblet cells that secrete mucus. **(B)** The lining of the intestine showing goblet cells. (A, Reprinted with permission from Ross MH, Kaye GI, Pawlina W. Histology. 4th ed. Philadelphia: Lippincott Williams & Wilkins, 2003; B, reprinted with permission from Cormack DH. Essential Histology. 2nd ed. Philadelphia: Lippincott Williams & Wilkins, 2001.)

carried to another organ, to a body cavity, or to the body surface. They are effective in a limited area near their source. Examples of exocrine glands include the glands in the gastrointestinal tract that secrete digestive juices, the sebaceous (oil) glands of the skin, and the lacrimal glands that produce tears. These and other exocrine glands are discussed in the chapters on specific systems.

In structure, an exocrine gland may consist of a single cell, such as the cells that secrete mucus into the digestive tract. Most, however, are composed of multiple cells in various arrangements (Fig. 4-4). They may be tubular, in a simple straight form or in a branched formation, as are found in the digestive tract. They may also be coiled, as are the sweat glands of the skin. They may be saclike, as are the sebaceous (oil) glands of the skin, or compound formations of tubes and sacs, as are the salivary glands in the mouth.

- **Endocrine** (EN-do-krin) **glands** secrete directly into the blood, which then carries their secretions to another area of the body. These secretions, called **hormones,** have effects on specific tissues known as the *target tissues.* Endocrine glands have an extensive network of blood vessels. These so-called *ductless glands* include the pituitary, thyroid, adrenal glands, and others described in greater detail in Chapter 11.

Checkpoint 4-2 Glands are classified according to whether they secrete through ducts or secrete directly into the bloodstream. What are these two categories of glands?

Connective Tissue

The supporting fabric of all parts of the body is connective tissue. This is so extensive and widely distributed that if we were able to dissolve all the tissues except connective tissue, we would still be able to recognize the contours of the entire body. Connective tissue has large amounts of nonliving material between the cells. This intercellular background material or **matrix** (MA-trix) contains varying amounts of water, fibers, and hard minerals.

There are several ways of classifying connective tissue. Some is considered more generalized because it occurs throughout the body wherever structure and protection are needed. Others, such as bone and blood, have a more specialized function. Based on the composition of the matrix, the various connective tissues also differ in their degree of hardness. For simplicity, we will categorize them according to these physical properties:

- Liquid connective tissue—blood and lymph (the fluid that circulates in the lymphatic system) are examples of liquid connective tissues (Fig. 4-5). The cells in liquid connective tissue are suspended in a fluid environment. Chapters 12 and 15 have more information on the liquid connective tissues.
- Soft connective tissue—loosely held together with semi-liquid material between the cells; includes adipose (fat) tissue and areolar (loose) connective tissue.
- Fibrous connective tissue—most connective tissue contains some fibers, but this type is densely packed with them. Cells called *fibroblasts* produce the fibers in connective tissue. (The word ending *-blast* refers to a young and active cell.) Examples of structures composed of fibrous connective tissue are ligaments, tendons, and the capsules (coverings) around certain organs.
- Hard connective tissue—has a very firm consistency, as in cartilage, or is hardened by minerals in the matrix, as in bone.

Checkpoint 4-3 Connective tissue varies according to the composition of the material that is between the cells. What is the general name for this intercellular material?

Soft Connective Tissue

The **areolar** (ah-RE-o-lar), or loose, form of connective tissue (see Fig. 4-5) is found in membranes around vessels and organs, between muscles, and under the skin. It

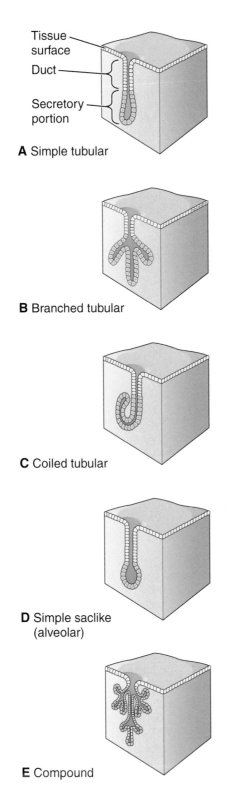

Tissue surface

Duct

Secretory portion

A Simple tubular

B Branched tubular

C Coiled tubular

D Simple saclike (alveolar)

E Compound

Figure 4-4 **Some structural types of exocrine glands. (A)** Simple tubular, as found in the intestine. **(B)** Branched tubular, as found in the stomach. **(C)** Coiled tubular, such as the sweat glands of the skin. **(D)** Simple saclike (alveolar), such as the oil glands of the skin. **(E)** Compound, with tubes and sacs, such as the salivary glands.

is the most common type of connective tissue in the body. It contains cells and fibers in a very loose, jellylike background material.

Adipose (AD-ih-pose) **tissue** (see Fig. 4-5) contains cells that are able to store large amounts of fat. The fat in this tissue is used as a reserve energy supply for the body. Adipose tissue also serves as a heat insulator and as protective padding for organs and joints.

Fibrous Connective Tissue

Fibrous connective tissue (Fig. 4-6 A) is very dense and has large numbers of fibers that give it strength and flexibility. The main type of fiber in this and other connective tissues is **collagen** (KOL-ah-jen), a flexible white protein. (See Box 4-2, Collagen: The Body's Scaffolding.)

Some fibrous connective tissue contains large amounts of elastic fibers that allow the tissue to stretch and then return to its original length. This type of elastic connective tissue appears in the vocal cords, the passageways of the respiratory tract, and the walls of the large arteries (blood vessels).

Fibrous connective tissue makes up the fibrous membranes that cover various organs, as described later in this chapter. Particularly strong forms make up the tough **capsules** around certain organs, such as the kidneys, the liver, and some glands. If the fibers in the connective tissue are all arranged in the same direction, like the strands of a cable, the tissue can pull in one direction. Examples are the cordlike **tendons,** which connect muscles to bones, and the **ligaments,** which connect bones to other bones.

Hard Connective Tissue

The hard connective tissues, cartilage and bone, are more solid than the other groups.

Cartilage Because of its strength and flexibility, cartilage is used as a structural material and as reinforcement. It is also used as a shock absorber and as a bearing surface that reduces friction between moving parts, as at joints. A common form of cartilage known as **hyaline** (HI-ah-lin) **cartilage** forms the tough, translucent material, popularly called *gristle*, seen over the ends of the long bones (see Fig. 4-6 B). Hyaline cartilage is also found at the tip of the nose and in parts of the larynx ("voicebox") and the trachea ("windpipe").

Another form of cartilage, **fibrocartilage** (fi-bro-KAR-tih-laj), is found between segments of the spine, at the anterior joint between the pubic bones of the hip, and in the knee joint. **Elastic cartilage** can spring back into shape after it is bent. An easy place to observe the properties of elastic cartilage is in the outer portion of the ear. It is also located in the larynx.

The cells that produce cartilage are **chondrocytes** (KON-dro-sites), a name derived from the word root

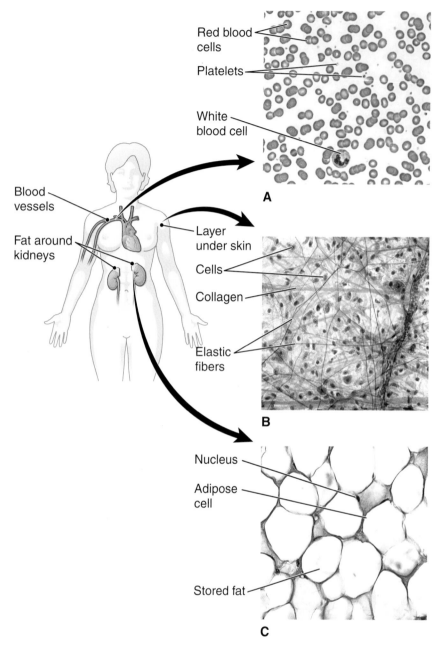

Red blood cells

Platelets

White blood cell

A

Blood vessels

Fat around kidneys

Layer under skin

Cells

Collagen

Elastic fibers

B

Nucleus

Adipose cell

Stored fat

C

Figure 4-5 Liquid and soft connective tissue. (A) Blood smear showing various blood cells in a liquid matrix. **(B)** Areolar (loose) connective tissue, a mixture of cells and fibers in a jellylike matrix. **(C)** Adipose tissue showing stored fat. The nuclei are at the edges of the cells. (Reprinted with permission from Ross MH, Kaye GI, Pawlina W. Histology. 4th ed. Philadelphia: Lippincott Williams & Wilkins, 2003.) *ZOOMING IN* ✦ *Which of these tissues has the most fibers? Which of these tissues is modified for storage?*

chondro, meaning "cartilage" and the root *cyto,* meaning "cell."

Bone The tissue of which bones are made, called **os-seous** (OS-e-us) **tissue,** is much like cartilage in its cellu-lar structure (see Fig. 4-6 C). In fact, the skeleton of the fetus in the early stages of development is made almost entirely of cartilage. This tissue gradually becomes im-pregnated with salts of calcium and phosphorus that

make bone characteristically solid and hard. The cells that form bone are called **osteoblasts** (OS-te-o-blasts), a name that combines the root for bone (*osteo*) with a root (*blast*) that means an immature cell. As these cells ma-ture, they are referred to as **osteocytes** (OS-te-o-sites). Within the osseous tissue are nerves and blood vessels. Enclosed within bones is a specialized type of tissue, the bone marrow. The red bone marrow contained in certain bone regions produces blood cells. Chapter 6 has more information on bones.

Checkpoint 4-4 Connective tissue is the supportive and protective material found throughout the body. What are some ex-amples of liquid, soft, fibrous, and hard connective tissue?

▶ Muscle Tissue

Muscle tissue is designed to produce movement by contraction of its cells, which are called **muscle fibers** because most of them are long and threadlike. If a piece of well-cooked meat is pulled apart, small groups of these muscle fibers may be seen. Muscle tissue is usually classified as follows:

▶ **Skeletal muscle,** which works with tendons and bones to move the body (Fig. 4-7 A). This type of tissue is de-scribed as **voluntary muscle** because it can be made to contract by con-scious thought. The cells in skeletal muscle are very large and are re-markable in having multiple nuclei and a pattern of dark and light band-ing described as **striations.** This type of muscle is also called striated mus-cle. Chapter 7 has more details on skeletal muscles.

▶ **Cardiac muscle,** which forms the bulk of the heart wall and is known also as **myocardium** (mi-o-KAR-de-um) (see Fig. 4-7 B). This is the muscle that produces the reg-ular contractions known as *heartbeats.* Cardiac muscle is described as **involuntary muscle** because it typically con-tracts independently of thought. Most of the time we are not aware of its actions at all. Cardiac muscle has branch-ing cells and specialized membranes between the cells that appear as dark lines under the microscope. Their technical name is *intercalated* (in-TER-cal-a-ted) *disks.*

Box 4-2   A Closer Look

Collagen: The Body's Scaffolding

The most abundant protein in the body, making up about 25% of total protein, is collagen. Its name, derived from a Greek word meaning "glue," reveals its role as the main structural protein in connective tissue.

Fibroblasts secrete collagen molecules into the surrounding matrix, where the molecules are then assembled into fibers. These fibers give the matrix its strength and its flexibility. Collagen fibers' high tensile strength makes them stronger than steel fibers of the same size, and their flexibility confers resilience on the tissues that contain them. For example, collagen in skin, bone, tendons, and ligaments resists pulling forces, whereas collagen found in joint cartilage and between vertebrae resists compression. Based on amino acid structure, there are at least 19 types of collagen, each of which imparts a different property to the connective tissue containing it.

The arrangement of collagen fibers in the matrix reveals much about the tissue's function. In the skin and membranes covering muscles and organs, collagen fibers are arranged irregularly, with fibers running in all directions. The result is a tissue that can resist stretching forces in many different directions. In tendons and ligaments, collagen fibers have a parallel arrangement, forming strong ropelike cords that can resist longitudinal pulling forces. In bone tissue, collagen fibers' meshlike arrangement promotes deposition of calcium salts into the tissue, which gives bone strength while also providing flexibility.

Collagen's varied properties are also evident in the preparation of a gelatin dessert. Gelatin is a collagen extract made by boiling animal bones and other connective tissue. It is a viscous liquid in hot water but forms a semisolid gel on cooling.

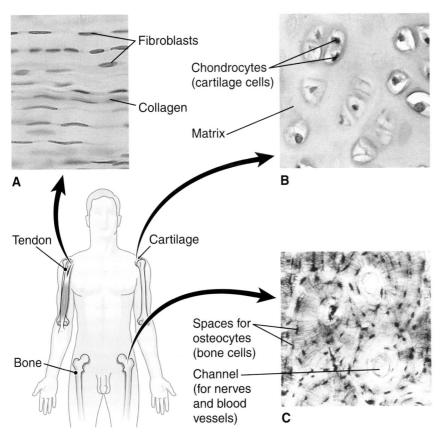

A Fibroblasts
Collagen

B Chondrocytes (cartilage cells)
Matrix

Tendon
Cartilage
Bone

C Spaces for osteocytes (bone cells)
Channel (for nerves and blood vessels)

Figure 4-6 Fibrous and hard connective tissue. (A) Fibrous connective tissue. In tendons and ligaments, the fibers are arranged in the same direction. **(B)** In cartilage, the cells (chondrocytes) are enclosed in a firm matrix. **(C)** Bone is the hardest connective tissue. The cells (osteocytes) are within the hard matrix. (Reprinted with permission from Ross MH, Kaye GI, Pawlina W.. Histology. 4th ed. Philadelphia: Lippincott Williams & Wilkins, 2003.)

The heart and cardiac muscle are discussed in Chapter 13.

▶ **Smooth muscle** is also involuntary muscle (see Fig. 4-7 C). It forms the walls of the hollow organs in the ventral body cavities, including the stomach, intestines, gallbladder, and urinary bladder. Together these organs are known as viscera (VIS-eh-rah), so smooth muscle is sometimes referred to as *visceral muscle*. Smooth muscle is also found in the walls of many tubular structures, such as the blood vessels and the tubes that carry urine from the kidneys. A smooth muscle is attached to the base of each body hair. Contraction of these muscles causes the condition of the skin that we call *gooseflesh*. Smooth muscle cells are of a typical size and taper at each end. They are not striated and have only one nucleus per cell. Structures containing smooth muscle are discussed in the chapters on the various body systems.

Muscle tissue, like nervous tissue, repairs itself only with difficulty or not at all once an injury has been sustained. When injured, muscle tissue is frequently replaced with connective tissue.

Checkpoint 4-5 What are the three types of muscle tissue?

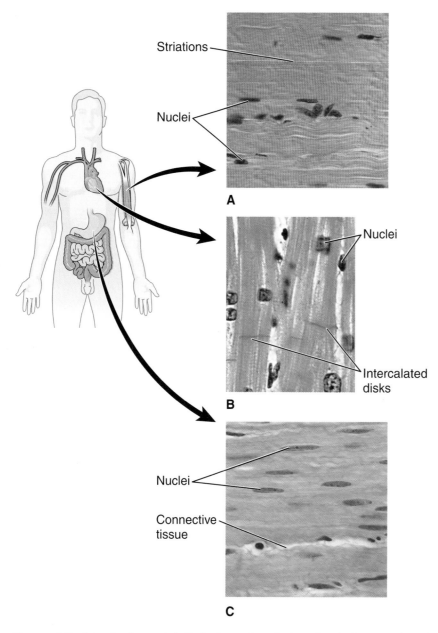

Figure 4-7 Muscle tissue. (A) Skeletal muscle cells have bands (striations) and multiple nuclei. **(B)** Cardiac muscle makes up the wall of the heart. **(C)** Smooth muscle is found in soft body organs and in vessels. (A and B, Reprinted with permission from Ross MH, Kaye GI, Pawlina W. Histology. 4th ed. Philadelphia: Lippincott Williams & Wilkins, 2003; C, reprinted with permission from Cormack DH. Essential Histology. 2nd ed. Philadelphia: Lippincott Williams & Wilkins, 2001.)

▶ Nervous Tissue

The human body is made up of countless structures, both large and small, each of which contributes something to the action of the whole organism. This aggregation of structures might be compared to a large corporation. For all the workers in the corporation to coordinate their efforts, there must be some central control, such as the president or CEO. In the body, this central agent is the **brain.** Each structure of the body is in direct communica-

tion with the brain by means of its own set of "wires," called **nerves.** Nerves from even the most remote parts of the body come together and form a great trunk cable called the **spinal cord,** which in turn leads into the central switchboard of the brain. Here, messages come in and orders go out 24 hours a day. Some nerves, the cranial nerves, connect directly with the brain and do not form part of the spinal cord. This entire communication system, including the brain, is made of nervous tissue.

The Neuron

The basic unit of nervous tissue is the **neuron** (NU-ron), or nerve cell (Fig. 4-8 A). A neuron consists of a nerve cell body plus small branches from the cell called *fibers.* One type of fiber, the **dendrite** (DEN-drite), is generally short and forms tree-like branches. This type of fiber carries messages in the form of nerve impulses to the nerve cell body. A single fiber, the **axon** (AK-son), carries impulses away from the nerve cell body. Neurons may be quite long; their fibers can extend for several feet. A **nerve** is a bundle of such nerve cell fibers held together with connective tissue (see Fig. 4-8 B).

Just as wires are insulated to keep them from being short-circuited, some axons are insulated and protected by a coating of material called **myelin** (MI-eh-lin). Groups of myelinated fibers form "white matter," so called because of the color of the myelin, which is much like fat in appearance and consistency.

Not all neurons have myelin, however; some axons are unmyelinated, as are all dendrites and all cell bodies. These areas appear gray in color. Because the outer layer of the brain has large collections of cell bodies and unmyelinated fibers, the brain is popularly termed *gray matter,* even though its interior is composed of white matter (see Fig. 4-8 C).

Neuroglia

Nervous tissue is supported by specialized cells known as **neuroglia** (nu-ROG-le-ah) or *glial* (GLI-al) *cells,* which are named from the Greek word *glia* meaning "glue." Some of these cells protect the brain from harmful substances; oth-

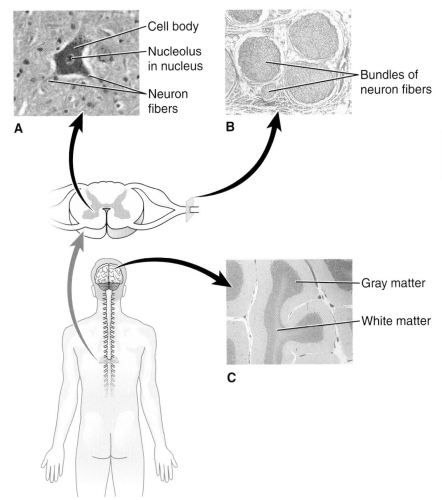

Figure 4-8 Nervous tissue. (A) A neuron, or nerve cell. **(B)** Cross-section of a nerve. **(C)** Brain tissue. (Reprinted with permission from Cormack DH. Essential Histology. 2nd ed. Philadelphia: Lippincott Williams & Wilkins, 2001.)

ers get rid of foreign organisms and cellular debris; still others form the myelin sheath around axons. They do not, however, transmit nerve impulses.

A more detailed discussion of nervous tissue and the nervous system can be found in Chapters 8 and 9.

> **Checkpoint 4-6** What is the basic cellular unit of the nervous system and what is its function?

> **Checkpoint 4-7** What are the nonconducting support cells of the nervous system called?

All of the various tissues discussed previously develop from primitive cells. Read about these cells in Box 4-3, Stem Cells: So Much Potential.

▶ Membranes

Membranes are thin sheets of tissue. Their properties vary: some are fragile, others tough; some are transparent, others opaque (*i.e.*, they cannot be seen through). Membranes may cover a surface, may serve as a dividing partition, may line a hollow organ or body cavity, or may anchor an organ. They may contain cells that secrete lubricants to ease the movement of organs, such as the heart and lung, and the movement of joints. Epithelial membranes and connective tissue membranes are described below.

Box 4-3   Hot Topics

Stem Cells: So Much Potential

At least 200 different types of cells are found in the human body, each with its own unique structure and function. All originate from unspecialized precursors called **stem cells**, which exhibit two important characteristics: they can divide repeatedly and have the potential to become specialized cells.

Stem cells come in two types. **Embryonic stem cells**, found in early embryos, are the source of all body cells and potentially can differentiate into any type of cell. **Adult stem cells**, found in babies and children as well as adults, are stem cells that remain in the body after birth and can differentiate into only a few cell types. They assist with tissue growth and repair. For example, in red bone marrow, these cells differentiate into blood cells, whereas in the skin, they differentiate into new skin cells after a cut or scrape.

The potential healthcare applications of stem cell research are numerous. In the near future, stem cell trans-plants may be used to repair damaged tissues in treating illnesses such as diabetes, cancer, heart disease, Parkinson disease, and spinal cord injury. This research may also help explain how cells develop and why some cells develop abnormally, causing birth defects and cancer. Stem cells may also be used to test drugs before trying them on animals and humans.

But stem cell research is controversial. Some argue that it is unethical to use embryonic stem cells because they are obtained from aborted fetuses or fertilized eggs left over from in vitro fertilization. Others argue that these cells would be discarded anyway and have the potential to improve lives. A possible solution is the use of adult stem cells. However, adult stem cells are less abundant and lack embryonic stem cells' potential to differentiate, so more research is needed to make this a viable option.

Epithelial Membranes

An **epithelial membrane** is so named because its outer surface is made of epithelium. Underneath, however, there is a layer of connective tissue that strengthens the membrane, and in some cases, there is a thin layer of smooth muscle under that. Epithelial membranes are made of closely packed active cells that manufacture lubricants and protect the deeper tissues from invasion by microorganisms. Epithelial membranes are of several types:

▸ **Serous** (SE-rus), **membranes** line the walls of body cavities and are folded back onto the surface of internal organs, forming their outermost layer.

Air (equivalent to serous fluid)

Outer balloon wall (equivalent to parietal membrane)

Inner balloon wall (equivalent to visceral membrane)

A

Lung
Heart

Myocardium (heart muscle)

Visceral layer
Serous pericardium { Parietal layer
Pericardial cavity

Parietal pleura

Visceral pleura

Fibrous pericardium

Lung

B

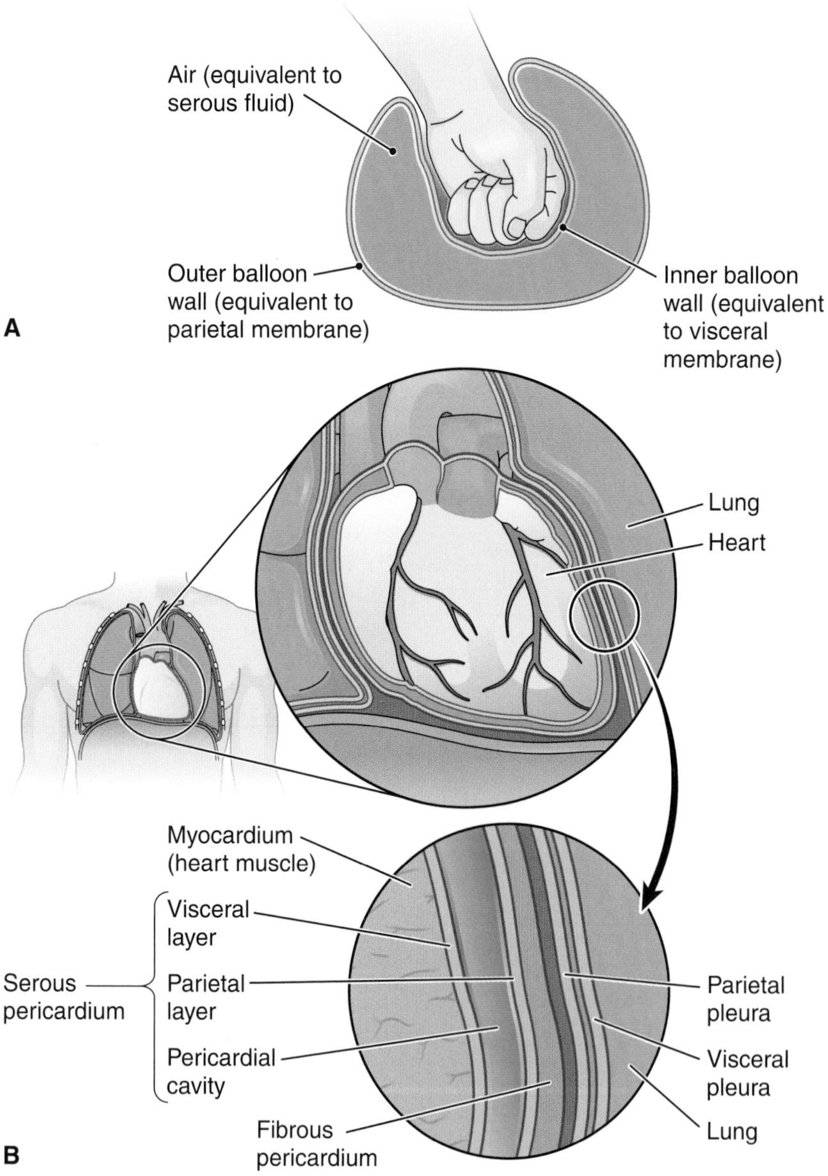

Figure 4-9   Organization of serous membranes. (A) An organ fits into a serous membrane like a fist punching into a soft balloon. **(B)** The outer layer of a serous membrane is the parietal layer. The inner layer is the visceral layer. The fibrous pericardium reinforces the parietal pericardium.

▸ **Mucous** (MU-kus) **membranes** line tubes and other spaces that open to the outside of the body.
▸ The **cutaneous** (ku-TA-ne-us) **membrane,** commonly known as the *skin,* has an outer layer of epithelium. This membrane is complex and is discussed in detail in Chapter 5 on the integumentary system.

Serous Membranes Serous membranes line the closed ventral body cavities and do not connect with the outside of the body. They secrete a thin, watery lubricant, known as serous fluid, that allows organs to move with a minimum of friction. The thin epithelium of serous membranes is a smooth, glistening kind of tissue called **mesothelium** (mes-o-THE-le-um). The membrane itself may be referred to as the **serosa** (se-RO-sah).

There are three serous membranes:

▸ The **pleurae** (PLU-re), or **pleuras** (PLU-rahs), line the thoracic cavity and cover each lung.
▸ The **serous pericardium** (per-ih-KAR-de-um) forms part of a sac that encloses the heart, which is located in the chest between the lungs.
▸ The **peritoneum** (per-ih-to-NE-um) is the largest serous membrane. It lines the walls of the abdominal cavity, covers the organs of the abdomen, and forms supporting and protective structures within the abdomen (see Fig. 17-3 in Chapter 17).

Serous membranes are arranged so that one portion forms the lining of a closed cavity, while another part folds back to cover the surface of the organ contained in that cavity. The relationship between an organ and the serous membrane around it can be visualized by imagining your fist punching into a large, soft balloon (Fig. 4-9). Your fist is the organ and the serous membrane around it is in two layers, one against your fist and one folded back to form an outer layer. Although in two layers, each serous membrane is continuous.

The portion of the serous membrane attached to the wall of a cavity or sac is known as the **parietal** (pah-RI-eh-tal) **layer;** the word *parietal* refers to a wall. In the example above, the parietal layer is represented by the outermost layer of the balloon. Parietal pleura lines the thoracic (chest) cavity, and parietal pericardium lines the fibrous sac (the fibrous pericardium) that encloses the heart (see Fig. 4-9).

Because internal organs are called *viscera,* the portion of the serous membrane attached to an organ is the **visceral layer.** Visceral pericardium is on the surface of the heart, and each lung surface is covered by visceral pleura. Portions of the peritoneum that cover organs in the abdomen are named according to the particular organ involved. The visceral layer in our balloon example is in direct contact with your fist.

The visceral and parietal layers of a serous membrane normally are in direct contact with a minimal amount of lubricant between them. The area between the two layers of the membrane forms a **potential space.** That is, it is *possible* for a space to exist there, although normally one does not. Only if substances accumulate between the layers, as when inflammation causes the production of excessive amounts of fluid, is there an actual space.

Mucous Membranes Mucous membranes are so named because they produce a thick and sticky substance called **mucus** (MU-kus). (Note that the adjective *mucous* contains an "o," whereas the noun *mucus* does not.) These membranes form extensive continuous linings in the digestive, respiratory, urinary, and reproductive systems, all of which are connected with the outside of the body. These membranes vary somewhat in both structure and function. The cells that line the nasal cavities and the passageways of the respiratory tract are supplied with tiny, hairlike extensions called *cilia,* described in Chapter 3. The microscopic cilia move in waves that force secretions outward. In this way, foreign particles, such as bacteria, dust, and other impurities trapped in the sticky mucus, are prevented from entering the lungs and causing harm. Ciliated epithelium is also found in certain tubes of both the male and the female reproductive systems.

The mucous membranes that line the digestive tract have special functions. For example, the mucous membrane of the stomach serves to protect the deeper tissues from the action of powerful digestive juices. If for some reason a portion of this membrane is injured, these juices begin to digest a part of the stomach itself—as happens in cases of peptic ulcers. Mucous membranes located farther along in the digestive system are designed to absorb nutrients, which the blood then transports to all body cells.

The noun **mucosa** (mu-KO-sah) is used in referring to the mucous membrane of an organ.

Checkpoint 4-8 Epithelial membranes have an outer layer of epithelium. Which are the three type of epithelial membranes?

Connective Tissue Membranes

The following list is an overview of membranes that consist of connective tissue with no epithelium. These membranes are described in greater detail in later chapters.

▸ **Synovial** (sin-O-ve-al) **membranes** are thin connective tissue membranes that line the joint cavities. They secrete a lubricating fluid that reduces friction between the ends of bones, thus permitting free movement of the joints. Synovial membranes also line small cushioning sacs near the joints called **bursae** (BUR-se).
▸ The **meninges** (men-IN-jeze) are several layers of membranes covering the brain and the spinal cord.

Fascia (FASH-e-ah) refers to fibrous bands or sheets that support organs and hold them in place. Fascia is found in two regions:

▸ **Superficial fascia** is the continuous sheet of tissue that underlies the skin and contains adipose (fat) tissue that insulates the body and protects the skin. This tissue is also called *subcutaneous fascia,* because it is located beneath the skin.
▸ **Deep fascia** covers, separates, and protects skeletal muscles.

Finally, there are membranes whose names all start with the prefix *peri-* because they are around organs:

▸ The **fibrous pericardium** (per-e-KAR-de-um) forms the cavity that encloses the heart, the pericardial cavity. This fibrous sac and the serous pericardial membranes described above are often referred to together as the pericardium (see Fig. 4-9 B).
▸ The **periosteum** (per-e-OS-te-um) is the membrane around a bone.
▸ The **perichondrium** (per-e-KON-dre-um) is the membrane around cartilage.

▸ Tissues and Aging

With aging, tissues lose elasticity and collagen becomes less flexible. These changes affect the skin most noticeably, but internal changes occur as well. The blood vessels, for example, have a reduced capacity to expand. Less blood supply and lower metabolism slow the healing process. Tendons and ligaments stretch, causing a stooped posture and joint instability. Bones may lose calcium salts, becoming brittle and prone to fracture. With age, muscles and other tissues waste from loss of cells, a process termed *atrophy* (AT-ro-fe) (Fig. 4-10). Changes that apply to specific organs and systems are described in later chapters.

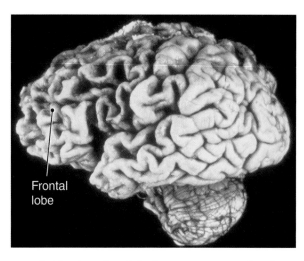

Figure 4-10 Atrophy of the brain. Brain tissue has thinned and larger spaces appear between sections of tissue, especially in the frontal lobe. (Reprinted with permission from Okazaki H, Scheithauer BW. Atlas of neuropathology. New York: Gower Medical Publishing, 1988. By permission of the author.)

Word Anatomy

Medical terms are built from standardized word parts (prefixes, roots, and suffixes). Learning the meanings of these parts can help you remember words and interpret unfamiliar terms.

WORD PART	MEANING	EXAMPLE
hist/o	tissue	*Histology* is the study of tissues.
Epithelial Tissue		
epi-	on, upon	*Epithelial* tissue covers body surfaces.
pseud/o-	false	*Pseudostratified* epithelium appears to be in multiple layers, but is not.
Connective Tissue		
-blast	immature cell, early stage of cell	A *fibroblast* is a cell that produces fibers.
chondr/o	cartilage	A *chondrocyte* is a cartilage cell.
oss, osse/o	bone, bone tissue	*Osseous* tissue is bone tissue.
oste/o	bone, bone tissue	An *osteocyte* is a mature bone cell.
Muscle Tissue		
my/o	muscle	The *myocardium* is the heart muscle.
cardi/o	heart	
Nervous Tissue		
neur/o	nerve, nervous system	A *neuron* is a nerve cell.
Membranes		
pleur/o	side, rib	The *pleurae* are membranes that line the chest cavity.
peri-	around	The *peritoneum* wraps around the abdominal organs.

Summary

I. Tissue classification—epithelial tissue, connective tissue, muscle tissue, nervous tissue

II. Epithelial tissue—covers surfaces; lines cavities, organs, and ducts
A. Structure of epithelial tissue
   1. Cells—squamous, cuboidal, columnar
   2. Arrangement—simple or stratified
B. Special functions
   1. Produces secretions, *e.g.*, mucus, digestive juices, sweat
   2. Filters impurities using cilia
C. Glands—active cells are epithelial cells
   1. Exocrine
      a. Secrete through ducts
      b. Examples: digestive glands, tear glands, sweat and oil glands of skin
   2. Endocrine
      a. Secrete into bloodstream
      b. Produce hormones

III. Connective tissue—supports, binds, forms framework of body
A. Liquid
   1. Blood
   2. Lymph
B. Soft—jellylike intercellular material (matrix)
   1. Areolar (loose)
   2. Adipose—stores fat
C. Fibrous—dense tissue with collagenous or elastic fibers between cells
   1. Examples
      a. Tendons—attach muscle to bone
      b. Ligaments—connect bones
      c. Capsules—around organs
      d. Fascia—bands or sheets that support organs
D. Hard—firm and solid
   1. Cartilage—found at joints and ends of bones, nose, outer ear, trachea, etc.
      a. Types—hyaline, elastic, fibrocartilage
      b. Cells—chondrocytes
   2. Bone
      a. Contains mineral salts
      b. Cells
         (1) Osteoblasts—produce bone
         (2) Osteocytes—mature cells

IV. Muscle tissue—contracts to produce movement
   1. Skeletal muscle—voluntary; moves skeleton
   2. Cardiac muscle—forms main part of the heart
   3. Smooth muscle—involuntary; forms visceral organs

V. Nervous tissue
A. Neuron—nerve cell
   1. Cell body—contains nucleus
   2. Dendrite—fiber carrying impulses toward cell body
   3. Axon—fiber carrying impulses away from cell body
      a. Myelin—fatty material that insulates some axons
         (1) Myelinated fibers—make up white matter
         (2) Unmyelinated cells and fibers—make up gray matter
B. Neuroglia—support and protect nervous tissue

VI. Membranes—thin sheets of tissue
A. Epithelial membranes—outer layer epithelium
   1. Serous membrane—secretes watery fluid
      a. Parietal layer—lines body cavity
      b. Visceral layer—covers internal organs
      c. Examples—pleurae, pericardium, peritoneum
   2. Mucous membrane
      a. Secretes mucus
      b. Lines tube or space that opens to the outside (*e.g.*, respiratory, digestive, reproductive tracts)
   3. Cutaneous membrane—skin
B. Connective tissue membranes
   1. Synovial membrane—lines joint cavity
   2. Meninges—around brain and spinal cord
   3. Fascia—under skin and around muscles
   4. Pericardium—around heart; periosteum—around bone; perichondrium—around cartilage

VII. Tissues and aging—atrophy

Questions for Study and Review

Building Understanding

Fill in the blanks

1. A group of similar cells arranged in a characteristic pattern is called a(n) _____.

2. Glands that secrete their products directly into the blood are called _____ glands.

3. Tissue that supports and forms the framework of the body is called _____ tissue.

4. Skeletal muscle is also described as _____ muscle.

5. Nervous tissue is supported by specialized cells known as _____.

Matching

Match each numbered item with the most closely related lettered item.

___6. Membrane around the heart
___7. Membrane around each lung
___8. Membrane around bone
___9. Membrane around cartilage
___10. Membrane around abdominal organs

a. perichondrium
b. pericardium
c. peritoneum
d. periosteum
e. pleura

Multiple choice

___11. Epithelium composed of a single layer of long and narrow cells is called
    a. simple cuboidal epithelium
    b. simple columnar epithelium
    c. stratified cuboidal epithelium
    d. stratified columnar epithelium

___12. Tendons and ligaments are examples of
    a. liquid connective tissue
    b. soft connective tissue
    c. fibrous connective tissue
    d. hard connective tissue

___13. A tissue composed of long striated cells with multiple nuclei is
    a. smooth muscle tissue
    b. cardiac muscle tissue
    c. skeletal muscle tissue
    d. nervous tissue

___14. A bundle of nerve cell fibers held together with connective tissue is called a(n)
    a. dendrite
    b. axon
    c. nerve
    d. myelin

___15. All of the following are types of epithelial membranes except
    a. cutaneous membrane
    b. mucous membrane
    c. serous membrane
    d. synovial membrane

Understanding Concepts

16. Explain how epithelium is classified and discuss at least three functions of this tissue type.

17. Compare the structure and function of exocrine and endocrine glands and give two examples of each type.

18. Describe the functions of connective tissue. Name two kinds of fibers found in connective tissue and discuss how their presence affects tissue function.

19. Compare and contrast the three different types of muscle tissue.

20. Compare serous and mucous membranes.

Conceptual Thinking

21. Prolonged exposure to cigarette smoke causes damage to ciliated epithelium that lines portions of the respiratory tract. Discuss the implications of this damage.

22. The middle ear is connected to the throat by a tube called the eustachian (auditory) tube. All are lined by a continuous mucous membrane. Using this information, describe why a throat infection (pharyngitis) may lead to an ear infection (otitis media).

23. Osteogenesis imperfecta is a connective tissue disease characterized by abnormal collagen fiber synthesis. Based on the fact that collagen is the predominant fiber type in connective tissue, list some possible symptoms of this disease.

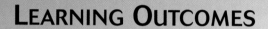

SELECTED KEY TERMS

The following terms and
other boldface terms in the
chapter are defined in the Glossary

arrector pili
dermis
epidermis
integument
keratin
melanin
sebaceous
sebum
stratum
subcutaneous
sudoriferous

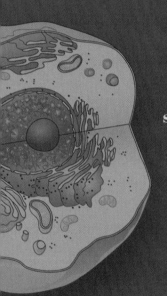

LEARNING OUTCOMES

After careful study of this chapter,
you should be able to:

1. Name and describe the layers of the skin
2. Describe the subcutaneous tissue
3. Give the location and function of the accessory
   structures of the skin
4. List the main functions of the skin
5. Discuss the factors that contribute to skin color
6. Show how word parts are used to build words related to
   the skin (see Word Anatomy at the end of the chapter)

The Integumentary System

The skin is the one system that can be inspected in its entirety without requiring specialized medical imaging techniques. The skin not only gives clues to its own health but also reflects the health of other body systems. Although the skin may be viewed simply as a membrane enveloping the body, it is far more complex than the other epithelial membranes described in Chapter 4.

The skin is associated with accessory structures, also known as appendages, which include glands, hair, and nails. Together with blood vessels, nerves, and sensory organs, the skin and its associated structures form the **integumentary** (in-teg-u-MEN-tar-e) **system**. This name is from the word integument (in-TEG-u-ment), which means "covering." The term cutaneous (ku-TA-ne-us) also refers to the skin. The functions of this system are discussed later in the chapter after a description of its structure.

▶ Structure of the Skin

The skin consists of two layers (Fig. 5-1):

▶ The **epidermis** (ep-ih-DER-mis), the outermost portion, which itself is subdivided into thin layers called **strata** (STRA-tah) (sing. stratum). The epidermis is composed entirely of epithelial cells and contains no blood vessels.

▶ The **dermis**, or true skin, which has a framework of connective tissue and contains many blood vessels, nerve endings, and glands.

Figure 5-2 is a photograph of the skin as seen through a microscope showing the layers and some accessory structures.

Epidermis

The epidermis is the surface portion of the skin, the outermost cells of which are constantly lost through wear and tear. Because there are no blood vessels in the epidermis, the cells must be nourished by capillaries in the underlying dermis. New epidermal cells are produced in the deepest layer, which is closest to the dermis. The cells in this layer, the **stratum basale** (bas-A-le), or **stratum germinativum** (jer-min-a-TI-vum), are constantly dividing and producing daughter cells, which are then pushed upward toward the surface of the skin. As the epidermal cells die from the gradual loss of nourishment, they undergo changes. Mainly, their cytoplasm is replaced by

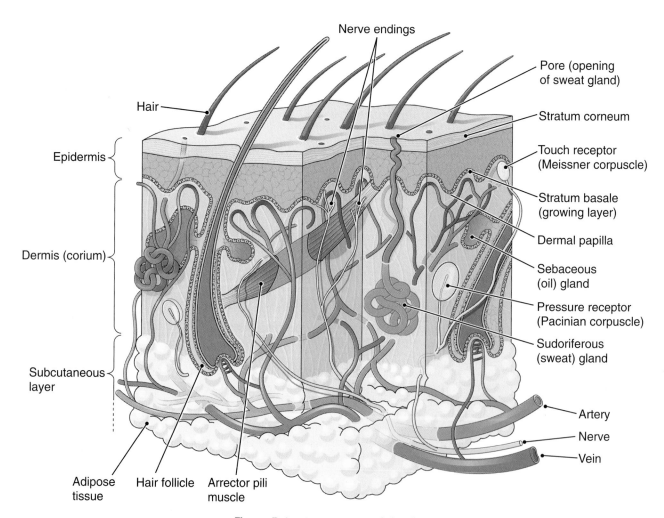

Figure 5-1 Cross-section of the skin.

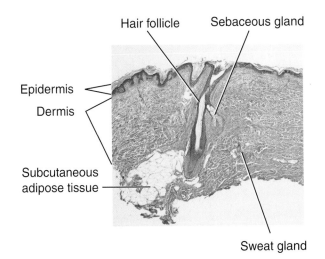

Figure 5-2 Microscopic view of thin skin. Tissue layers and some accessory structures are labeled. (Reprinted with permission from Cormack DH. Essential Histology. 2nd ed. Philadelphia: Lippincott Williams & Wilkins, 2001.)

large amounts of a protein called **keratin** (KER-ah-tin), which serves to thicken and protect the skin (Fig. 5-3).

By the time epidermal cells approach the surface, they have become flat, filled with keratin, and horny, forming the uppermost layer of the epidermis, the **stratum corneum** (KOR-ne-um). The stratum corneum is a protective layer and is deeper in thick skin than in thin skin. Cells at the surface are constantly being lost and replaced from below, especially in areas of the skin that are subject to wear and tear, as on the scalp, face, soles of the feet, and palms of the hands. Although this process of **exfoliation** (eks-fo-le-A-shun) occurs naturally at all times, many cosmetics companies sell products to promote exfoliation, presumably to "enliven" and "refresh" the skin.

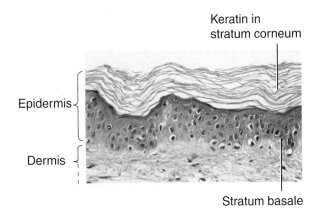

Figure 5-3 Upper portion of the skin. Layers of keratin in the stratum corneum are visible at the surface. Below are layers of stratified squamous epithelium making up the remainder of the epidermis. (Reprinted with permission from Cormack DH. Essential Histology. 2nd ed. Philadelphia: Lippincott Williams & Wilkins, 2001.)

Between the stratum basale and the stratum corneum there are additional layers of stratified epithelium that vary in number and quantity depending on the thickness of the skin.

Cells in the deepest layer of the epidermis produce **melanin** (MEL-ah-nin), a dark pigment that colors the skin and protects it from the harmful rays of sunlight. The cells that produce this pigment are the **melanocytes** (MEL-ah-no-sites). Irregular patches of melanin are called freckles.

Dermis

The **dermis**, the so-called "true skin," has a framework of elastic connective tissue and is well supplied with blood vessels and nerves. Because of its elasticity, the skin can stretch, even dramatically as in pregnancy, with little damage. Most of the accessory structures of the skin, including the sweat glands, the oil glands, and the hair, are located in the dermis and may extend into the subcutaneous layer under the skin.

The thickness of the dermis also varies in different areas. Some places, such as the soles of the feet and the palms of the hands, are covered with very thick layers of skin, whereas others, such as the eyelids, are covered with very thin and delicate layers. (See Box 5-1, Thick and Thin Skin: Getting a Grip on Their Differences.)

Portions of the dermis extend upward into the epidermis, allowing blood vessels to get closer to the surface cells (see Figs. 5-1 and 5-2). These extensions, or **dermal papillae**, can be seen on the surface of thick skin, such as at the tips of the fingers and toes. Here they form a distinct pattern of ridges that help to prevent slipping, such as when grasping an object. The unchanging patterns of the ridges are determined by heredity. Because they are unique to each person, fingerprints and footprints can be used for identification.

Checkpoint 5-1 The skin and all its associated structures comprise a body system. What is the name of this system?

Checkpoint 5-2 The skin itself is composed of two layers. Moving from the superficial to the deeper layer, what are the names of these two layers?

Subcutaneous Layer

The dermis rests on the **subcutaneous** (sub-ku-TA-ne-us) **layer**, sometimes referred to as the hypodermis or the superficial fascia (see Fig. 5-1). This layer connects the skin to the surface muscles. It consists of loose connective tissue and large amounts of adipose (fat) tissue. The fat serves as insulation and as a reserve supply for energy. Continuous bundles of elastic fibers connect the subcutaneous tissue with the dermis, so there is no clear boundary between the two.

| Box 5-1 | A Closer Look |

Thick and Thin Skin: Getting a Grip on Their Differences

The skin is the largest organ in the body, weighing about 4 kg. Though it appears uniform in structure and function, its thickness in fact varies, from less than 1 mm covering the eyelids to more than 5 mm on the upper back. Many of the functional differences between skin regions reflect the thickness of the epidermis and not the skin's overall thickness. Based on epidermal thickness, skin can be categorized as **thick** (about 1 mm deep) or **thin** (about 0.1 mm deep).

Areas of the body exposed to significant wear and tear (the palms, fingertips, and bottoms of the feet and toes) are covered with thick skin. It is composed of a thick stratum corneum and an extra layer not found in thin skin, the stratum lucidum, both of which make thick skin resistant to abrasion. Thick skin is also characterized by epidermal ridges (*e.g.,* fingerprints) and numerous sweat glands, but lacks hair and

sebaceous (oil) glands. These adaptations make the thick skin covering the hands and feet effective for grasping or gripping. Thick skin's dermis also contains many sensory receptors, giving the hands and feet a superior sense of touch.

Thin skin covers areas of the body not exposed to much wear and tear. It has a very thin stratum corneum and lacks a distinct stratum lucidum. Though thin skin lacks epidermal ridges and has fewer sensory receptors than thick skin, it has several specializations that thick skin does not. Thin skin is covered with hair, which may help prevent heat loss from the body. In fact, hair is most densely distributed in skin that covers regions of great heat loss—the head, axillae (armpits), and groin. Thin skin also contains numerous sebaceous glands, making it supple and free of cracks that may let infectious organisms enter.

The blood vessels that supply the skin with nutrients and oxygen and help to regulate body temperature run through the subcutaneous layer. This tissue is also rich in nerves and nerve endings, including those that supply nerve impulses to and from the dermis and epidermis. The thickness of the subcutaneous layer varies in different parts of the body; it is thinnest on the eyelids and thickest on the abdomen.

Checkpoint 5-3 What is the composition of the subcutaneous layer?

▶ Accessory Structures of the Skin

The integumentary system includes some structures associated with the skin—glands, hair, and nails—that not only protect the skin itself but have some more generalized functions as well.

Sebaceous (Oil) Glands

The **sebaceous** (se-BA-shus) **glands** are saclike in structure, and their oily secretion, **sebum** (SE-bum), lubricates the skin and hair and prevents drying. The ducts of the sebaceous glands open into the hair follicles (Fig. 5-4 A).

Babies are born with a covering produced by these glands that resembles cream cheese; this secretion is called the **vernix caseosa** (VER-niks ka-se-O-sah), which literally means "cheesy varnish." Modified sebaceous glands, **meibomian** (mi-BO-me-an) **glands**, are associated with the eyelashes and produce a secretion that lubricates the eyes.

Blackheads consist of a mixture of dried sebum and keratin that may collect at the openings of the sebaceous glands. If these glands become infected, pimples result. If a sebaceous gland becomes blocked, a sac of accumulated sebum may form and gradually increase in size. Such a

sac is referred to as a **sebaceous cyst.** Usually, it is not difficult to remove such tumorlike cysts by surgery.

Sudoriferous (Sweat) Glands

The **sudoriferous** (su-do-RIF-er-us) **glands,** or sweat glands, are coiled, tubelike structures located in the dermis and the subcutaneous tissue (see Fig. 5-4 B). Most of the sudoriferous glands function to cool the body. They release sweat, or perspiration, that draws heat from the skin as the moisture evaporates at the surface. These **eccrine** (EK-rin) type sweat glands are distributed throughout the skin. Each gland has a secretory portion and an excretory tube that extends directly to the surface and opens at a pore (see also Fig. 5-2). Because sweat contains small amounts of dissolved salts and other wastes in addition to water, these glands also serve a minor excretory function.

Present in smaller number, the **apocrine** (AP-o-krin) sweat glands are located mainly in the armpits (axillae) and groin area. These glands become active at puberty and release their secretions through the hair follicles in response to emotional stress and sexual stimulation. The apocrine glands release some cellular material in their secretions. Body odor develops from the action of bacteria in breaking down these organic cellular materials.

Several types of glands associated with the skin are modified sweat glands. These are the **ceruminous** (seh-RU-min-us) **glands** in the ear canal that produce ear wax, or **cerumen;** the **ciliary** (SIL-e-er-e) **glands** at the edges of the eyelids; and the **mammary glands.**

Checkpoint 5-4 Some skin glands produce an oily secretion called sebum. What is the name of these glands?

Checkpoint 5-5 What is the scientific name for the sweat glands?

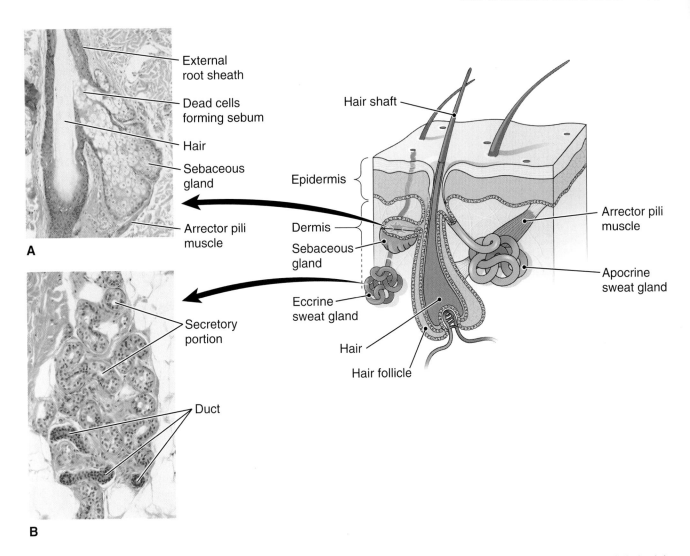

Figure 5-4 **Portion of skin showing associated glands and hair.** **(A)** A sebaceous (oil) gland and its associated hair follicle. **(B)** An eccrine (temperature-regulating) sweat gland. (A and B, Reprinted with permission from Cormack DH. Essential Histology. 2nd ed. Philadelphia: Lippincott Williams & Wilkins, 2001.) *ZOOMING IN ✦ How do the sebaceous glands and apocrine sweat glands secrete to the outside? What kind of epithelium makes up the sweat glands?*

Hair

Almost all of the body is covered with hair, which in most areas is soft and fine. Hairless regions are the palms of the hands, soles of the feet, lips, nipples, and parts of the external genital areas. Hair is composed mainly of keratin and is not living. Each hair develops, however, from living cells located in a bulb at the base of the **hair follicle**, a sheath of epithelial and connective tissue that encloses the hair (see Fig. 5-4). Melanocytes in this growth region add pigment to the developing hair. Different shades of melanin produce the various hair colors we see in the population. The part of the hair that projects above the skin is the **shaft**; the portion below the skin is the **root** of the hair.

Attached to most hair follicles is a thin band of involuntary muscle (see Fig. 5-1). When this muscle contracts, the hair is raised, forming "goose bumps" on the skin.

The name of this muscle is **arrector pili** (ah-REK-tor PI-li), which literally means "hair raiser." This response is of no importance to humans but helps animals with furry coats to conserve heat. As the arrector pili contracts, it presses on the sebaceous gland associated with the hair follicle, causing the release of sebum to lubricate the skin.

Checkpoint 5-6 Each hair develops within a sheath. What is this sheath called?

Nails

Nails protect the fingers and toes and also help in grasping small objects with the hands. They are made of hard keratin produced by cells that originate in the outer layer of the epidermis (stratum corneum) (Fig. 5-5). New cells form continuously in a growth region (nail matrix) located under the proximal end of the nail, a portion called

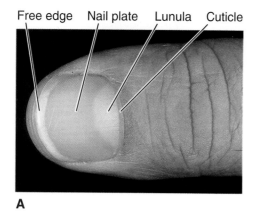

Free edge   Nail plate   Lunula   Cuticle

A

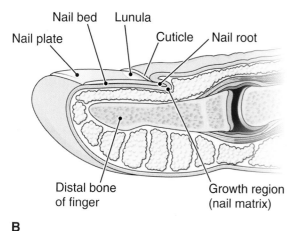

Nail bed   Lunula
Nail plate   Cuticle   Nail root

Distal bone
of finger   Growth region
                   (nail matrix)

B

Figure 5-5   Nail structure. (A) Photograph of a nail, superior view. **(B)** Midsagittal section of a fingertip. (A, Reprinted with permission from Bickley LS. Bates' Guide to Physical Examination and History Taking. 8th ed. Philadelphia: Lippincott Williams & Wilkins, 2003.)

the **nail root.** The remainder of the **nail plate** rests on a **nail bed** of epithelial tissue. The color of the dermis below the nail bed can be seen through the clear nail. The pale **lunula** (LU-nu-lah), literally "little moon," at the proximal end of the nail appears lighter because it lies over the thicker growing region of the nail. The **cuticle,** an extension of the stratum corneum, seals the space between the nail plate and the skin above the root.

Nails of both the toes and the fingers are affected by general health. Changes in nails, including abnormal color, thickness, shape, or texture (*e.g.*, grooves or splitting), occur in chronic diseases such as heart disease, peripheral vascular disease, malnutrition, and anemia.

▶ Functions of the Skin

Although the skin has many functions, the following are its four major functions:

▶ Protection against infection.
▶ Protection against dehydration (drying).
▶ Regulation of body temperature.
▶ Collection of sensory information.

Protection Against Infection

Intact skin forms a primary barrier against invasion of pathogens. The cells of the stratum corneum form a tight interlocking pattern that is resistant to penetration. The surface cells are constantly being shed, causing the mechanical removal of pathogens. Rupture of this barrier, as in cases of wounds or burns, invites infection of deep tissues. The skin also protects against bacterial toxins (poisons) and some harmful chemicals in the environment.

Protection Against Dehydration

Both keratin in the epidermis and the oily sebum released to the surface of the skin from the sebaceous glands help to waterproof the skin and prevent water loss by evaporation from the surface.

Regulation of Body Temperature

Both the loss of excess heat and protection from cold are important functions of the skin. Indeed, most of the blood supply to the skin is concerned with temperature regulation. In cold conditions, vessels in the skin constrict (become narrower) to reduce the flow of blood to the surface and diminish heat loss. The skin may become visibly pale under these conditions. Special vessels that directly connect arteries and veins in the skin of the ears, nose, and other exposed locations provide the volume of blood flow needed to prevent freezing.

To cool the body, the skin forms a large surface for radiating body heat to the surrounding air. When the blood vessels dilate (widen), more blood is brought to the surface so that heat can be dissipated.

The other mechanism for cooling the body involves the sweat glands, as noted above. The evaporation of perspiration draws heat from the skin. A person feels uncomfortable on a hot and humid day because water does not evaporate as readily from the skin into the surrounding air. A dehumidifier makes one more comfortable even when the temperature remains high.

As is the case with so many body functions, temperature regulation is complex and involves several parts of the body, including certain centers in the brain.

Collection of Sensory Information

Because of its many nerve endings and other special receptors, the skin may be regarded as one of the chief sensory organs of the body. Free nerve endings detect pain and moderate changes in temperature. Other types of sensory receptors in the skin respond to light touch and deep pressure. Figure 5-1 shows some free nerve endings, a touch receptor (Meissner corpuscle), and a deep pressure receptor (Pacinian corpuscle) in a section of skin.

Many of the reflexes that make it possible for humans to adjust themselves to the environment begin as sensory impulses from the skin. As elsewhere in the body, the skin works with the brain and the spinal cord to accomplish these important functions.

Other Activities of the Skin

Substances can be absorbed through the skin in limited amounts. Some drugs, for example, estrogens, other steroids, anesthetics, and medications to control motion sickness, can be absorbed from patches placed on the skin. (See Box 5-2, Medication Patches: No Bitter Pill to Swallow.) Most medicated ointments used on the skin, however, are for the treatment of local conditions only. Even medication injected into the subcutaneous tissues is absorbed very slowly.

There is also a minimal amount of excretion through the skin. Water and electrolytes (salts) are excreted in sweat (perspiration). Some nitrogen-containing wastes are eliminated through the skin, but even in disease, the amount of waste products excreted by the skin is small.

Vitamin D needed for the development and maintenance of bone tissue is manufactured in the skin under the effects of ultraviolet radiation in sunlight.

Note that the human skin does not "breathe." The pores of the epidermis serve only as outlets for perspiration from the sweat glands and sebum (oil) from the sebaceous glands. They are not used for exchange of gases.

Checkpoint 5-7 What two mechanisms are used to regulate temperature through the skin?

▶ Skin Color

The color of the skin depends on a number of factors, including the following:

▶ Amount of pigment in the epidermis.
▶ Quantity of blood circulating in the surface blood vessels.
▶ Composition of the circulating blood, including:
  ▶ Quantity of oxygen.
  ▶ Concentration of hemoglobin.
  ▶ Presence of bile, silver compounds, or other chemicals.

Pigment

The main pigment of the skin, as we have noted, is called **melanin.** This pigment is also found in the hair, the middle coat of the eyeball, the iris of the eye, and certain tumors. Melanin is common to all races, but darker people have a much larger quantity in their tissues. The melanin in the skin helps to protect against damaging ultraviolet radiation from the sun. Thus, skin that is exposed to the sun shows a normal increase in this pigment, a response we call tanning.

Sometimes, there are abnormal increases in the quantity of melanin, which may occur either in localized areas or over the entire body surface. For example, diffuse

---

Box 5-2	**Clinical Perspectives**

Medication Patches: No Bitter Pill to Swallow

For most people, pills are a convenient way to take medication, but for others, they have drawbacks. Pills must be taken at regular intervals to ensure consistent dosing, and they must be digested and absorbed into the bloodstream before they can begin to work. For those who have difficulty swallowing or digesting pills, **transdermal (TD) patches** offer an effective alternative to oral medications.

TD patches deliver a consistent dose of medication that diffuses at a constant rate through the skin into the bloodstream. There is no daily schedule to follow, nothing to swallow, and no stomach upset. TD patches can also deliver medication to unconscious patients, who would otherwise require intravenous drug delivery. TD patches are used in hormone replacement therapy, to treat heart disease, to manage pain, and to suppress motion sickness. Nicotine patches are also used as part of programs to quit smoking.

TD patches must be used carefully. Drug diffusion through the skin takes time, so it is important to know how long the patch must be in place before it is effective. It is also important to know how long the medication's effects take to disappear after the patch is removed. Because the body continues to absorb what has already diffused into the skin, removing the patch does not entirely remove the medicine.

A recent advance in TD drug delivery is **iontophoresis.** Based on the principle that like charges repel each other, this method uses a mild electrical current to move ionic drugs through the skin. A small electrical device attached to the patch uses positive current to "push" positively charged drug molecules through the skin, and a negative current to push negatively charged ones. Even though very low levels of electricity are used, people with pacemakers should not use iontophoretic patches. Another disadvantage is that they can move only ionic drugs through the skin.

spots of pigmentation may be characteristic of some endocrine disorders. In **albinism** (AL-bih-nizm), a hereditary disorder that affects melanin production, there is lack of pigment in the skin, hair, and eyes.

Another pigment that imparts color to the skin is carotene, a pigment obtained from carrots and other orange and yellow vegetables. Carotene is stored in fatty tissue and skin. Also visible is hemoglobin, the pigment that gives blood its color, which can be seen through the vessels in the dermis.

Checkpoint 5-8 What are some pigments that impart color to the skin?

▶ Effects of Aging on the Integumentary System

As people age, wrinkles, or crow's feet, develop around the eyes and mouth owing to the loss of fat and collagen in the underlying tissues. The dermis becomes thinner, and the skin may become transparent and lose its elasticity, the effect of which is sometimes called "parchment skin." The formation of pigment decreases with age. However, there may be localized areas of extra pigmentation in the skin with the formation of brown spots ("liver spots"), especially on areas exposed to the sun (*e.g.*, the back of the hands). Circulation to the dermis decreases, so white skin looks paler.

The hair does not replace itself as rapidly as before and thus becomes thinner on the scalp and elsewhere on the body. Decreased melanin production leads to gray or white hair. The texture of the hair changes as the hair shaft becomes less dense, and hair, like the skin, becomes drier with a decrease in sebum production.

The sweat glands decrease in number, so there is less output of perspiration and lowered ability to withstand heat. The elderly are also more sensitive to cold because of less fat in the skin and poor circulation. The fingernails may flake, become brittle, or develop ridges, and toenails may become discolored or abnormally thickened.

▶ Care of the Skin

The most important factors in caring for the skin are those that ensure good general health. Proper nutrition and adequate circulation are vital to the maintenance of the skin. Regular cleansing removes dirt and dead skin debris and sustains the slightly acid environment that inhibits bacterial growth on the skin. Careful hand washing with soap and water, with attention to the undernail areas, is a simple measure that reduces the spread of disease.

The skin needs protection from continued exposure to sunlight to prevent premature aging and cancerous changes. Appropriate applications of sunscreens before and during time spent in the sun can prevent skin damage. (See Box 5–3, The Dark Side of the Sun.)

Box 5-3 · Health Maintenance

The Dark Side of the Sun

The three most common forms of skin cancer—basal cell carcinoma, squamous cell carcinoma, and malignant melanoma—share a common risk factor: excessive exposure to the ultraviolet radiation (UV) found in sunlight. UV rays also cause premature aging of the skin, including wrinkling, discoloration ("age spots" or "liver spots"), and a change in texture most often referred to as "leathery skin." Excessive sun exposure is also a risk factor for cataracts and other eye problems.

The damaging radiation found in sunlight occurs in two different forms, ultraviolet-A (UVA) and ultraviolet-B (UVB). UVA damages the skin's deeper layers, resulting in a loss of elasticity and a general decrease in blood flow to the skin. UVB damages the skin's outermost layers, causing the erythema (redness), inflammation, and peeling common to the average "sunburn." Excessive UV exposure causes genetic mutations in skin cells that make them unable to repair themselves and possibly cancerous. Tanning booths also produce UVA and UVB rays and are no safer than sun tanning.

You can reduce the damage caused by UVA and UVB by the following:

▶ Limit exposure during midday when the level of UV radiation is highest.
▶ Cover up with a hat, long pants, and a long-sleeved shirt when outdoors.
▶ Wear sunglasses that block UV rays.
▶ Apply a sunscreen with an SPF (sun protection factor) of 15 or higher 30 minutes before going outdoors. Reapply during exposure, especially after swimming.
▶ Stay in the shade, where exposure to UVA and UVB is significantly decreased.
▶ Avoid tanning booths.

Word Anatomy

Medical terms are built from standardized word parts (prefixes, roots, and suffixes). Learning the meanings of these parts can help you remember words and interpret unfamiliar terms.

WORD PART	MEANING	EXAMPLE
Structure of the Skin		
derm/o	skin	The *epidermis* is the outermost layer of the skin.
corne/o	horny	The stratum *corneum* is the outermost thickened, horny layer of the skin.
melan/o	dark, black	A *melanocyte* is a cell that produces the dark pigment melanin.
sub-	under, below	The *subcutaneous* layer is under the skin.
Accessory Structures of the Skin		
ap/o-	separation from, derivation from	The *apocrine* sweat glands release some cellular material in their secretions.
pil/o	hair	The arrector *pili* muscle raises the hair to produce "goose bumps."
Skin Color		
alb/i	white	*Albinism* is a condition associated with a lack of pigment, so the skin appears white.

Summary

I. Structure of the skin
A. Epidermis—surface layer of the skin
    1. Stratum basale (stratum germinativum)
        a. Produces new cells
        b. Melanocytes produce melanin—dark pigment
    2. Stratum corneum
        a. Surface layer of dead cells
        b. Contain keratin
B. Dermis (true skin)
    1. Deeper layer of the skin
    2. Has blood vessels and accessory structures
C. Subcutaneous layer
    1. Under the skin
    2. Made of connective tissue and adipose (fat) tissue

II. Accessory structures of the skin
A. Sebaceous (oil) glands
    1. Release sebum—lubricates skin and hair
B. Sudoriferous (sweat) glands
    1. Eccrine type
        a. Control body temperature
        b. Widely distributed
        c. Vent directly to surface
    2. Apocrine type
        a. Respond to stress
        b. In armpit and groin
        c. Excrete through hair follicle

C. Hair
    1. Develop in hair follicle (sheath)
    2. Active cells at base of follicle
D. Nails
    1. Grow from nail matrix at proximal end

III. Functions of the skin
A. Protection against infection—barrier
B. Protection against dehydration—keratin and sebum waterproof skin
C. Regulation of body temperature—blood supply and sweat glands
D. Collection of sensory information—receptors in skin
E. Other activities of the skin—absorption, excretion, manufacture of vitamin D

IV. Skin Color
A. Pigment
    1. Mainly melanin, also carotene, hemoglobin

V. Effects of aging on the integumentary system

VI. Care of the skin—good nutrition, cleansing, sun protection

Questions for Study and Review

Building Understanding

Fill in the blanks

1. The skin and its associated structures form the _____ system.

2. Cells of the stratum corneum contain large amounts of a protein called _____.

3. Sweat glands located in the axillae and groin are called _____ sweat glands.

4. The name of the muscle that raises the hair is _____.

5. A dark-colored pigment that protects the skin from ultraviolet light is called _____.

Matching

Match each numbered item with the most closely related lettered item.

____ 6. The uppermost protective epithelial layer of skin

____ 7. The lowermost dividing epithelial layer of skin

____ 8. Accessory structure of skin that senses deep touch

____ 9. A modified sweat gland that produces ear wax

____ 10. Accessory structure of skin that lubricates the eye

a. Pacinian corpuscle
b. stratum basale
c. ceruminous gland
d. stratum corneum
e. meibomian gland

Multiple choice

____ 11. The epidermis is _____ to the dermis.
    a. superficial
    b. deep
    c. lateral
    d. medial

____ 12. The layer of skin that has its own blood supply is called
    a. epidermis
    b. dermis
    c. hypodermis
    d. subcutaneous layer

____ 13. Fingerprints and footprints are formed by
    a. melanocytes
    b. Meissner corpuscles
    c. Pacinian corpuscles
    d. dermal papillae

____ 14. The _____ glands are responsible for temperature regulation
    a. apocrine
    b. eccrine
    c. ciliary
    d. ceruminous

____ 15. Nails grow from the
    a. lunula
    b. cuticle
    c. nail bed
    d. nail root

Understanding Concepts

16. Compare and contrast the epidermis, dermis, and hypodermis. How are the outermost cells of the epidermis replaced?

17. What are the four most important functions of the skin?

18. Describe the location and function of the two types of skin glands.

19. What changes may occur in the skin with age?

Conceptual Thinking

20. Skin is the largest organ in your body. Explain why it is an organ.

21. Ross Baker sustained full-thickness burns to his legs while lighting a fire with gasoline. After Mr. Baker is informed that he will require skin grafting, he asks you why his own skin won't heal by itself. How would you answer his question?

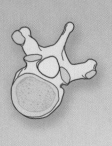

Movement and Support

$\mathcal{T}$his unit deals with the skeletal and muscular systems, which work together to execute movement and to support and protect vital organs. It covers the additional functions of the skeletal system in housing the blood-forming tissue and storing some minerals. The chapter on muscles describes the characteristics of all types of muscles and then concentrates on the muscles that are attached to the skeleton and how they function. The main skeletal muscles are named and located and their actions are described.

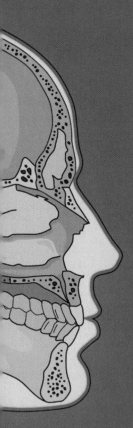

SELECTED KEY TERMS

The following terms and other boldface terms in the chapter are defined in the Glossary

amphiarthrosis

bursa

circumduction

diaphysis

diarthrosis

endosteum

epiphysis

fontanel

joint

osteoblast

osteoclast

osteocyte

osteon

periosteum

resorption

skeleton

synarthrosis

synovial

LEARNING OUTCOMES

After careful study of this chapter, you should be able to:

1. List the functions of bones
2. Describe the structure of a long bone
3. Differentiate between compact bone and spongy bone with respect to structure and location
4. Differentiate between red and yellow marrow with respect to function and location
5. Name the three different types of cells in bone and describe the functions of each
6. Explain how a long bone grows
7. Name and describe various markings found on bones
8. List the bones in the axial skeleton
9. Explain the purpose of the infant fontanels
10. Describe the normal curves of the spine and explain their purpose
11. List the bones in the appendicular skeleton
12. Compare the structure of the female pelvis and the male pelvis
13. Describe how the skeleton changes with age
14. Describe the three types of joints
15. Describe the structure of a synovial joint and give six examples of synovial joints
16. Demonstrate six types of movement that occur at synovial joints
17. Show how word parts are used to build words related to the skeleton (see Word Anatomy at the end of the chapter)

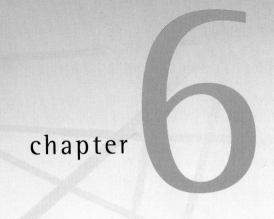

chapter 6

The Skeleton: Bones and Joints

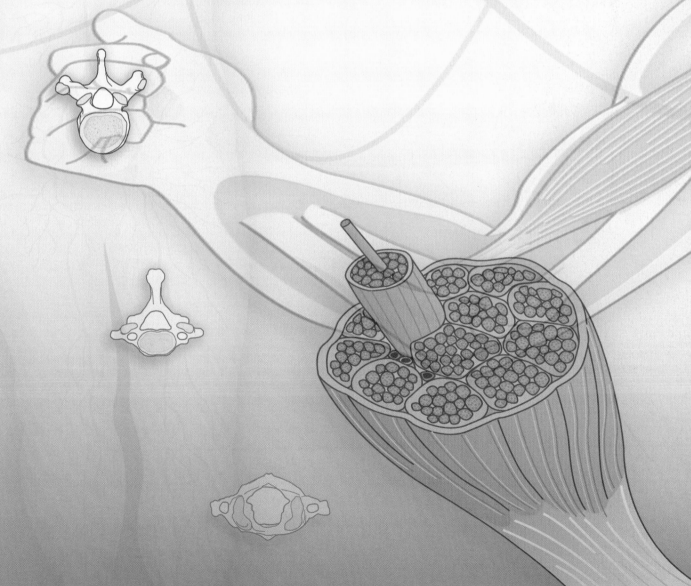

The skeleton is the strong framework on which the body is constructed. Much like the frame of a building, the skeleton must be strong enough to support and protect all the body structures. Bone tissue is the most dense form of the connective tissues described in Chapter 4. Bones work with muscles to produce movement at the joints. The bones and joints, together with supporting connective tissue, form the skeletal system.

▶ Bones

Bones have a number of functions, several of which are not evident in looking at the skeleton:

▶ To serve as a firm framework for the entire body
▶ To protect such delicate structures as the brain and the spinal cord
▶ To serve as levers, working with attached muscles to produce movement
▶ To serve as a storehouse for calcium salts, which may be resorbed into the blood if there is not enough calcium in the diet
▶ To produce blood cells (in the red marrow)

Bone Structure

The complete bony framework of the body, known as the **skeleton** (Fig. 6-1), consists of 206 bones. It is divided into a central portion, the axial skeleton, and the extremities, which make up the appendicular skeleton. The individual bones in these two divisions will be described in detail later in this chapter. The bones of the skeleton can be of several different shapes. They may be flat (ribs, cranium), short (carpals of wrist, tarsals of ankle), or irregular (vertebrae, facial bones). The most familiar shape, however, is the **long bone**, the type of bone that makes up almost all of the skeleton of the arms and legs. The long narrow shaft of this type of bone is called the **diaphysis** (di-AF-ih-sis). At the center of the diaphysis is a **medullary** (MED-u-lar-e) **cavity**, which contains bone marrow. The long bone also has two irregular ends, a proximal and a distal **epiphysis** (eh-PIF-ih-sis) (Fig. 6-2).

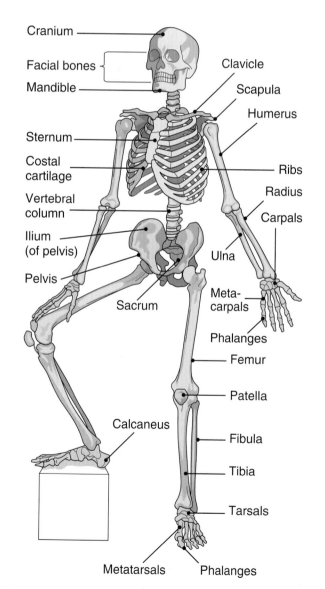

Figure 6-1   **The skeleton.** The axial skeleton is shown in yellow; the appendicular, in blue.

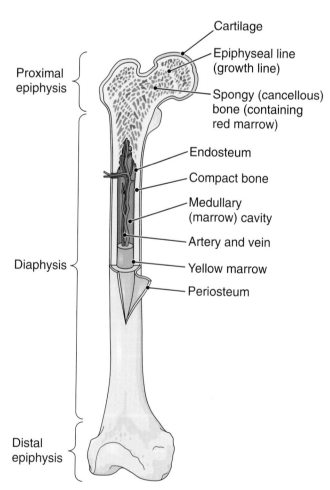

Figure 6-2   **The structure of a long bone.**

Bone Tissue Bones are not lifeless. Even though the spaces between the cells of bone tissue are permeated with stony deposits of calcium salts, the bone cells themselves are very much alive. Bones are organs, with their own system of blood vessels, lymphatic vessels, and nerves.

There are two types of bone tissue, also known as **osseous** (OS-e-us) **tissue**. One type is **compact bone**, which is hard and dense (Fig. 6-3). This tissue makes up the main shaft of a long bone and the outer layer of other bones. The cells in this type of bone are located in rings of bone tissue around a central **haversian** (ha-VER-shan) **canal** containing nerves and blood vessels. The bone cells live in spaces (lacunae) between the rings and extend out into many small radiating channels so that they can be in contact with nearby cells. Each ringlike unit with its central canal makes up a **haversian system**, also known as an **osteon** (OS-te-on) (see Fig. 6-3 B). Forming a channel across the bone, from one side of the shaft to the other, are many **perforating** (Volkmann) **canals**, which also house blood vessels and nerves.

The second type of bone tissue, called **spongy**, or **cancellous**, **bone**, has more spaces than compact bone. It is made of a meshwork of small, bony plates filled with red marrow. Spongy bone is found at the epiphyses (ends) of the long bones and at the center of other bones. Figure 6-4 shows a photograph of both compact and spongy tissue in a bone section.

> **Checkpoint 6-1** A long bone has a long, narrow shaft and two irregular ends. What are the scientific names for the shaft and the ends of a long bone?

> **Checkpoint 6-2** What are the two types of osseous (bone) tissue and where is each type found?

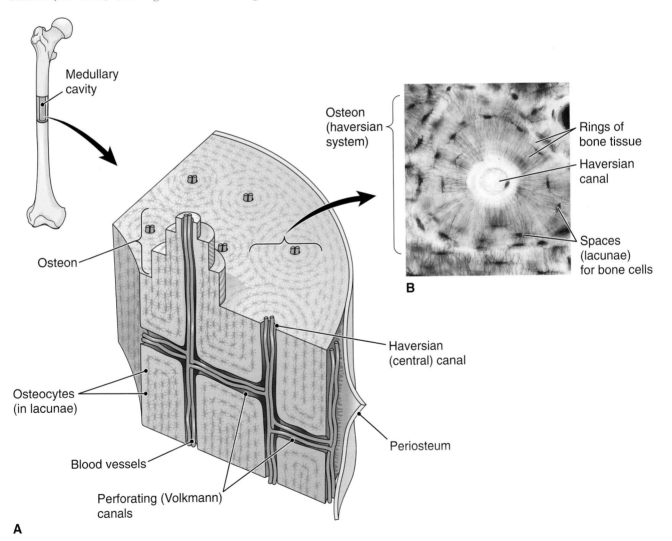

Medullary cavity

Osteon

Osteocytes (in lacunae)

Blood vessels

Perforating (Volkmann) canals

A

Osteon (haversian system)

Rings of bone tissue

Haversian canal

Spaces (lacunae) for bone cells

B

Haversian (central) canal

Periosteum

Figure 6-3   Compact bone tissue. (A) This section shows osteocytes (bone cells) within osteons (haversian systems). It also shows the canals that penetrate the tissue. **(B)** Microscopic view of compact bone in cross section (×300) showing a complete osteon. In living tissue, osteocytes (bone cells) reside in spaces (lacunae) and extend out into channels that radiate from these spaces. (B, Reprinted with permission from Ross MH, Kaye GI, Pawlina, W. Histology. 4th ed. Philadelphia: Lippincott Williams & Wilkins, 2003.)

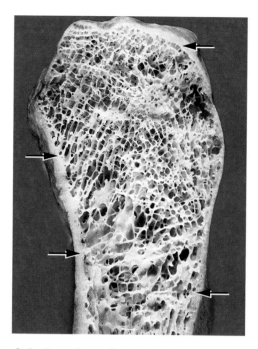

Figure 6-4 Bone tissue, longitudinal section. Spongy (cancellous) bone makes up most of the epiphysis (end) of this long bone, shown by the arrows. (Reprinted with permission from Ross MH, Kaye GI, Pawlina, W. Histology. 4th ed. Philadelphia: Lippincott Williams & Wilkins, 2003.)

Bone Marrow Bones contain two kinds of marrow. **Red marrow** is found at the ends of the long bones and at the center of other bones (see Fig. 6-2). Red bone marrow manufactures blood cells. **Yellow marrow** is found chiefly in the central cavities of the long bones. Yellow marrow is composed largely of fat.

Bone Membranes Bones are covered on the outside (except at the joint region) by a membrane called the **periosteum** (per-e-OS-te-um) (see Fig. 6-2). The inner layer of this membrane contains cells (osteoblasts) that are essential in bone formation, not only during growth but also in the repair of injuries. Blood vessels and lymphatic vessels in the periosteum play an important role in the nourishment of bone tissue. Nerve fibers in the periosteum make their presence known when one suffers a fracture, or when one receives a blow, such as on the shinbone. A thinner membrane, the **endosteum** (en-DOS-te-um), lines the marrow cavity of a bone; it too contains cells that aid in the growth and repair of bone tissue.

Bone Growth and Repair

During early development, the embryonic skeleton is at first composed almost entirely of cartilage. (Portions of the skull develop from fibrous connective tissue.) The conversion of cartilage to bone, a process known as **ossification**, begins during the second and third months of embryonic life. At this time, bone-building cells, called

osteoblasts (OS-te-o-blasts), become active. First, they begin to manufacture the **matrix**, which is the material located between the cells. This intercellular substance contains large quantities of **collagen**, a fibrous protein that gives strength and resilience to the tissue. Then, with the help of enzymes, calcium compounds are deposited within the matrix.

Once this intercellular material has hardened, the cells remain enclosed within the lacunae (small spaces) in the matrix. These cells, now known as **osteocytes** (OS-te-o-sites), are still living and continue to maintain the existing bone matrix, but they do not produce new bone tissue. When bone has to be remodeled or repaired later in life, new osteoblasts develop from stem cells in the endosteum and periosteum.

One other type of cell found in bone develops from a type of white blood cell (monocyte). These large, multinucleated **osteoclasts** (OS-te-o-klasts) are responsible for the process of **resorption**, which is the breakdown of bone tissue. Resorption is necessary for remodeling and repair of bone, as occurs during growth and after injury. Bone tissue is also resorbed when its stored minerals are needed by the body.

The formation and resorption of bone tissue are regulated by several hormones. Vitamin D promotes the absorption of calcium from the intestine. Other hormones involved in these processes are produced by glands in the neck. Calcitonin from the thyroid gland promotes the uptake of calcium by bone tissue. Parathyroid hormone (PTH) from the parathyroid glands at the posterior of the thyroid causes bone resorption and release of calcium into the blood. These hormones are discussed more fully in Chapter 11.

Checkpoint 6-3 What are the three types of cells found in bone and what is the role of each?

Formation of a Long Bone In a long bone, the transformation of cartilage into bone begins at the center of the shaft during fetal development. Around the time of birth, secondary bone-forming centers, or **epiphyseal** (ep-ih-FIZ-e-al) **plates**, develop across the ends of the bones. The long bones continue to grow in length at these centers by calcification of new cartilage through childhood and into the late teens. Finally, by the late teens or early 20s, the bones stop growing in length. Each epiphyseal plate hardens and can be seen in x-ray films as a thin line, the epiphyseal line, across the end of the bone. Physicians can judge the future growth of a bone by the appearance of these lines on x-ray films.

As a bone grows in length, the shaft is remodeled so that it grows wider as the central marrow cavity increases in size. Thus, alterations in the shape of the bone are a result of the addition of bone tissue to some surfaces and its resorption from others.

The processes of bone resorption and bone formation continue throughout life, more actively in some places than in others, as bones are subjected to "wear and tear" or injuries. The bones of small children are relatively pliable because they contain a larger proportion of cartilage and are undergoing active bone formation. In elderly people, there is a slowing of the processes that continually renew bone tissue. As a result, the bones are weaker and more fragile. Elderly people also have a decreased ability to form the protein framework on which calcium salts are deposited. Fractures in elderly people heal more slowly because of these decreases in bone metabolism.

> **Checkpoint 6-4** As the embryonic skeleton is converted from cartilage to bone, the intercellular matrix becomes hardened. What compounds are deposited in the matrix to harden it?

> **Checkpoint 6-5** After birth, long bones continue to grow in length at secondary centers. What are these centers called?

Bone Markings

In addition to their general shape, bones have other distinguishing features, or **bone markings**. These markings include raised areas and depressions that help to form joints or serve as points for muscle attachments and various holes that allow the passage of nerves and blood vessels. Some of these identifying features are described next.

Projections

- **Head**—a rounded, knoblike end separated from the rest of the bone by a slender region, the neck.
- **Process**—a large projection of a bone, such as the upper part of the ulna in the forearm that creates the elbow.
- **Condyle** (KON-dile)—a rounded projection; a small projection above a condyle is an epicondyle.

- **Crest**—a distinct border or ridge, often rough, such as over the top of the hip bone.
- **Spine**—a sharp projection from the surface of a bone, such as the spine of the scapula (shoulder blade).

Depressions or Holes

- **Foramen** (fo-RA-men)—a hole that allows a vessel or a nerve to pass through or between bones. The plural is foramina (fo-RAM-ih-nah).
- **Sinus** (SI-nus)—an air space found in some skull bones.
- **Fossa** (FOS-sah)—a depression on a bone surface. The plural is fossae (FOS-se).
- **Meatus** (me-A-tus)—a short channel or passageway, such as the channel in the temporal bone of the skull that leads to the inner ear.

Examples of these and other markings can be seen on the bones illustrated in this chapter. To find out how these markings can be used in healthcare, see Box 6-1, Landmarking: Seeing With Your Fingers.

> **Checkpoint 6-6** Bones have a number of projections, depressions, and holes. What are some functions of these markings?

▶ Bones of the Axial Skeleton

The skeleton may be divided into two main groups of bones (see Fig. 6-1):

- The **axial** (AK-se-al) **skeleton** consists of 80 bones and includes the bony framework of the head and the trunk.
- The **appendicular** (ap-en-DIK-u-lar) **skeleton** consists of 126 bones and forms the framework for the **extremities** (limbs) and for the shoulders and hips.

Box 6-1	*Clinical Perspectives*

Landmarking: Seeing With Your Fingers

Most body structures lie beneath the skin, hidden from view except in dissection. A technique called **landmarking** allows healthcare providers to visualize hidden structures without cutting into the patient. Bony prominences, or landmarks, can be palpated (felt) beneath the skin to serve as reference points for locating other structures. Landmarking is used during physical examinations and surgeries, when giving injections, and for many other clinical procedures. The lower tip of the sternum, the xiphoid process, is a reference point in the administration of cardiopulmonary resuscitation (CPR).

Practice landmarking by feeling for some of the other bony prominences. You can feel the joint between the mandible and the temporal bone of the skull (the temporomandibular joint, or TMJ) anterior to the ear canal as you move your lower jaw up and down. Feel for the notch in the sternum (breast bone) between the clavicles (collar bones). Approximately 4 cm below this notch you will feel a bump called the sternal angle. This prominence is an important landmark because its location marks where the trachea splits to deliver air to both lungs. Move your fingers lateral to the sternal angle to palpate the second ribs, important landmarks for locating the heart and lungs. Feel for the most lateral bony prominence of the shoulder, the acromion process of the scapula (shoulder blade). Two to three fingerbreadths down from this point is the correct injection site into the deltoid muscle of the shoulder. Place your hands on your hips and palpate the iliac crest of the hip bone. Move your hands forward until you reach the anterior end of the crest, the anterior superior iliac spine (ASIS). Feel for the part of the bony pelvis that you sit on. This is the ischial tuberosity. It and the ASIS are important landmarks for locating safe injection sites in the gluteal region.

Table 6·1	Bones of the Skeleton	
REGION	**BONES**	**DESCRIPTION**
Axial Skeleton		
Skull		
Cranium	Cranial bones (8)	Chamber enclosing the brain; houses the ear and forms part of the eye socket
Facial portion	Facial bones (14)	Form the face and chambers for sensory organs
Hyoid		U-shaped bone under lower jaw; used for muscle attachments
Ossicles	Ear bones (3)	Transmit sound waves in inner ear
Trunk		
Vertebral column	Vertebrae (26)	Encloses the spinal cord
Thorax	Sternum	Anterior bone of the thorax
	Ribs (12 pair)	Enclose the organs of the thorax
Appendicular Skeleton		
Upper division		
Shoulder girdle	Clavicle	Anterior; between sternum and scapula
	Scapula	Posterior, anchors muscles that move arm
Upper extremity	Humerus	Proximal arm bone
	Ulna	Medial bone of forearm
	Radius	Lateral bone of forearm
	Carpals (8)	Wrist bones
	Metacarpals (5)	Bones of palm
	Phalanges (14)	Bones of fingers
Lower division		
Pelvis	Os coxae (2)	Join sacrum and coccyx of vertebral column to form the bony pelvis
Lower extremity	Femur	Thigh bone
	Patella	Kneecap
	Tibia	Medial bone of leg
	Fibula	Lateral bone of leg
	Tarsal bones (7)	Ankle bones
	Metatarsals (5)	Bones of instep
	Phalanges (14)	Bones of toes

We describe the axial skeleton first and then proceed to the appendicular skeleton. Table 6-1 provides an outline of all the bones included in this discussion.

Framework of the Skull

The bony framework of the head, called the **skull**, is subdivided into two parts: the cranium and the facial portion. Refer to Figures 6-5 through 6-8, which show different views of the skull, as you study the following descriptions. Color-coding of the bones will aid in identification as the skull is seen from different positions.

Cranium This rounded chamber that encloses the brain is composed of eight distinct cranial bones.

▶ The **frontal bone** forms the forehead, the anterior of the skull's roof, and the roof of the eye orbit (socket). The frontal sinuses (air spaces) communicate with the nasal cavities (see Figs. 6-7 and 6-8). These sinuses and others near the nose are described as **paranasal sinuses**.

▶ The two **parietal** (pah-RI-eh-tal) bones form most of the top and the side walls of the cranium.

▶ The two **temporal bones** form part of the sides and some of the base of the skull. Each one contains **mastoid sinuses** as well as the ear canal, the eardrum, and the entire middle and internal portions of the ear. The **mastoid process** of the temporal bone projects downward immediately behind the external part of the ear. It contains the mastoid air cells and serves as a place for muscle attachment.

▶ The **ethmoid** (ETH-moyd) **bone** is a light, fragile bone located between the eyes (see Fig. 6-7). It forms a part of the medial wall of the eye orbit, a small portion of the cranial floor, and most of the nasal cavity roof. It contains several air spaces, comprising some of the paranasal sinuses. A thin, platelike, downward extension of this bone (the perpendicular plate) forms much of the nasal septum, a midline partition in the nose (see Fig. 6-5 A).

▶ The **sphenoid** (SFE-noyd) **bone**, when seen from a superior view, resembles a bat with its wings extended. It lies at the base of the skull anterior to the temporal bones and forms part of the eye socket. The sphenoid contains a saddlelike depression, the **sella turcica** (SEL-ah TUR-sih-ka), that holds and protects the pituitary gland (see Fig. 6-7).

▶ The **occipital** (ok-SIP-ih-tal) **bone** forms the posterior and a part of the base of the skull. The **foramen magnum**, located at the base of the occipital bone, is a large opening through which the spinal cord communicates with the brain (see Figs. 6-6 and 6-7).

Uniting the bones of the skull is a type of flat, immovable joint known as a **suture** (SU-chur) (see Fig. 6-5). Some of the most prominent cranial sutures are the:

▶ Coronal (ko-RO-nal) suture, which joins the frontal bone with the two parietal bones along the coronal plane.

▶ Squamous (SKWA-mus) suture, which joins the temporal bone to the parietal bone on the lateral surface of the cranium (named because it is in a flat portion of the skull).

▶ Lambdoid (LAM-doyd) suture, which joins the occipital bone with the parietal bones in the posterior cranium (named because it resembles the Greek letter lambda).

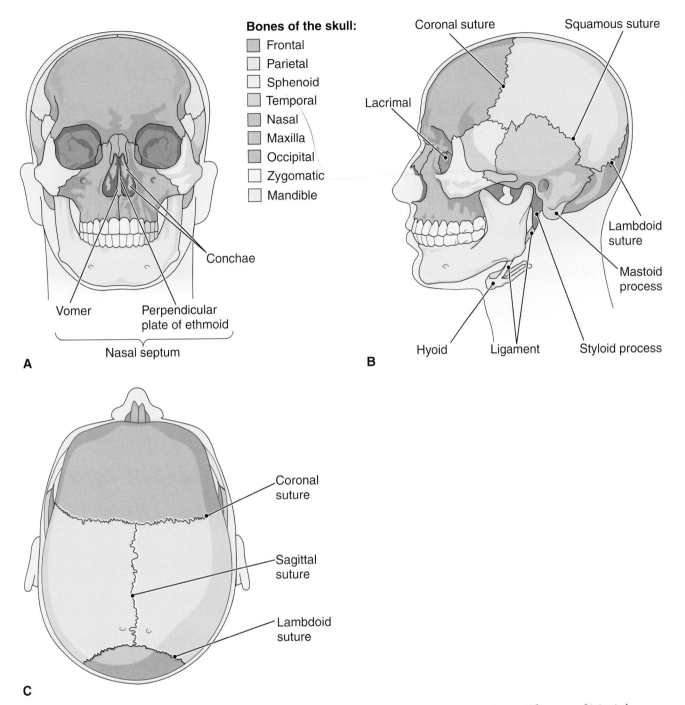

Figure 6-5 **The skull. (A)** Anterior view. **(B)** Left lateral view. **(C)** Superior view.   *ZOOMING IN ✦ What type of joint is between bones of the skull?*

▶ Sagittal (SAJ-ih-tal) suture, which joins the two parietal bones along the superior midline of the cranium, along the sagittal plane.

Facial Bones The facial portion of the skull is composed of 14 bones (see Fig. 6-5):

▶ The **mandible** (MAN-dih-bl), or lower jaw bone, is the only movable bone of the skull.
▶ The two **maxillae** (mak-SIL-e) fuse in the midline to form the upper jaw bone, including the front part of the

hard palate (roof of the mouth). Each maxilla contains a large air space, called the **maxillary sinus**, that communicates with the nasal cavity.
▶ The two **zygomatic** (zi-go-MAT-ik) **bones**, one on each side, form the prominences of the cheeks.
▶ Two slender **nasal bones** lie side by side, forming the bridge of the nose.
▶ The two **lacrimal** (LAK-rih-mal) **bones**, each about the size of a fingernail, lie near the inside corner of the eye in the front part of the medial wall of the orbital cavity.

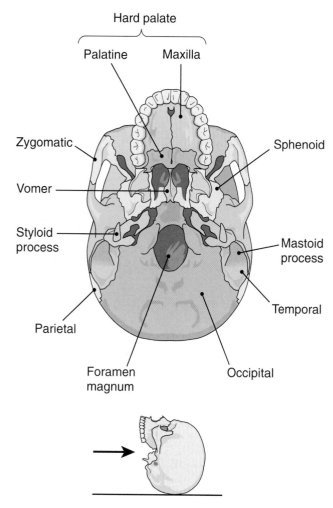

Hard palate

Palatine   Maxilla

Zygomatic

Vomer

Sphenoid

Styloid process

Mastoid process

Parietal

Temporal

Foramen magnum

Occipital

Figure 6-6 The skull, inferior view. The mandible (lower jaw) has been removed. *ZOOMING IN ✦ What two bones make up each side of the hard palate?*

▶ The **vomer** (VO-mer), shaped like the blade of a plow, forms the lower part of the nasal septum (see Fig. 6-5 A).
▶ The paired **palatine** (PAL-ah-tine) **bones** form the back part of the hard palate (see Figs. 6-6 and 6-8).
▶ The two **inferior nasal conchae** (KON-ke) extend horizontally along the lateral wall (sides) of the nasal cavities. The paired superior and middle conchae are part of the ethmoid bone (see Figs. 6-5 A and 6-8).

In addition to the bones of the cranium and the facial bones, there are three tiny bones, or **ossicles** (OS-sik-ls), in each middle ear (see Chapter 10) and a single horseshoe, or **U**-shaped, bone just below the skull proper, called the **hyoid** (HI-oyd) **bone**, to which the tongue and other muscles are attached (see Fig. 6-5 B).

Openings in the base of the skull provide spaces for the entrance and exit of many blood vessels, nerves, and other structures. Projections and slightly elevated portions of the bones provide for the attachment of muscles. Some portions protect delicate structures, such as the eye orbit and the part of the temporal bone that encloses the inner portions of the ear. The sinuses provide lightness and serve as resonating chambers for the voice (which is why your voice sounds better to you as you are speaking than it sounds when you hear it played back as a recording).

Infant Skull The skull of the infant has areas in which the bone formation is incomplete, leaving so-called soft spots, properly called **fontanels** (fon-tah-NELS) (Fig. 6-9). These flexible regions allow the skull to compress and change shape during the birth process. They also allow for rapid growth of the brain during infancy. Although there are a number of fontanels, the largest and most recognizable is near the front of the skull at the junction of the two parietal bones and the frontal bone. This **anterior fontanel** usually does not close until the child is about 18 months old.

Framework of the Trunk

The bones of the trunk include the spine, or **vertebral** (VER-teh-bral), **column**, and the bones of the chest, or **thorax** (THO-raks).

Vertebral Column This bony sheath for the spinal cord is made of a series of irregularly shaped bones. These number 33 or 34 in the child, but because of fusions that occur later in the lower part of the spine, there usually are just 26 separate bones in the adult spinal column. Figures 6-10 and 6-11 show the vertebral column from lateral and anterior views.

The **vertebrae** (VER-teh-bre) have a drum-shaped **body** (centrum) lo-

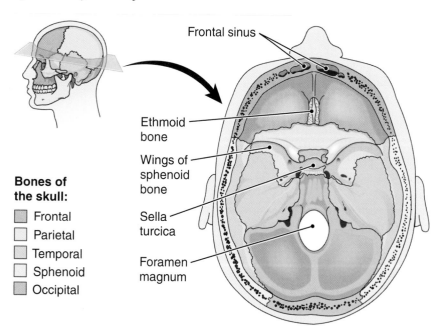

Frontal sinus

Bones of the skull:
- ☐ Frontal
- ☐ Parietal
- ☐ Temporal
- ☐ Sphenoid
- ☐ Occipital

Ethmoid bone

Wings of sphenoid bone

Sella turcica

Foramen magnum

Figure 6-7 Floor of cranium, superior view. The internal surfaces of some of the cranial bones are visible. *ZOOMING IN ✦ What is a foramen?*

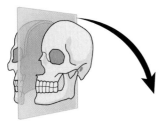

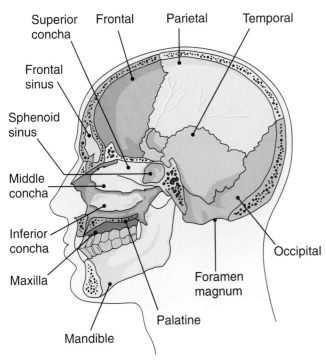

Figure 6-8 The skull, sagittal section.

Labels on figure: Superior concha, Frontal, Parietal, Temporal, Frontal sinus, Sphenoid sinus, Middle concha, Inferior concha, Maxilla, Mandible, Palatine, Foramen magnum, Occipital

cated anteriorly (toward the front) that serves as the weight-bearing part; disks of cartilage between the vertebral bodies act as shock absorbers and provide flexibility (see Fig. 6-11). In the center of each vertebra is a large hole, or foramen. When all the vertebrae are linked in series by strong connective tissue bands (ligaments), these spaces form the spinal canal, a bony cylinder that protects the spinal cord. Projecting dorsally (toward the back) from the bony arch that encircles the spinal cord is the **spinous process**, which usually can be felt just under the skin of the back. Projecting laterally is a **transverse process** on each side. These processes are attachment points for muscles. When viewed from a lateral aspect, the vertebral column can be seen to have a series of **intervertebral foramina**, formed between the vertebrae as they join together, through which spinal nerves emerge as they leave the spinal cord (see Fig. 6-10).

The bones of the vertebral column are named and numbered from above downward, on the basis of location. There are five regions:

▶ The **cervical** (SER-vih-kal) **vertebrae**, seven in number (C1 to C7), are located in the neck (see Fig. 6-11). The

first vertebra, called the **atlas**, supports the head (Fig. 6-12). (This vertebra is named for the mythologic character who was able to support the world in his hands.) When one nods the head, the skull rocks on the atlas at the occipital bone. The second cervical vertebra, the **axis** (see Fig. 6-12), serves as a pivot when the head is turned from side to side. It has an upright toothlike part, the **dens**, that projects into the atlas and serves as a pivot point. The absence of a body in these vertebrae allows for the extra movement. Only the cervical vertebrae have a hole in the tranverse process on each side (see Fig. 6-11). These **transverse foramina** accommodate blood vessels and nerves that supply the neck and head.

▶ The **thoracic vertebrae**, 12 in number (T1 to T12), are located in the chest. They are larger and stronger than the cervical vertebrae and each has a longer spinous process that points downward (see Fig. 6-11). The posterior ends of the 12 pairs of ribs are attached to these vertebrae.

▶ The **lumbar vertebrae**, five in number (L1 to L5), are located in the small of the back. They are larger and heavier than the vertebrae superior to them and can support more weight (see Fig. 6-11). All of their processes are shorter and thicker.

▶ The **sacral** (SA-kral) **vertebrae** are five separate bones in the child. They eventually fuse to form a single bone,

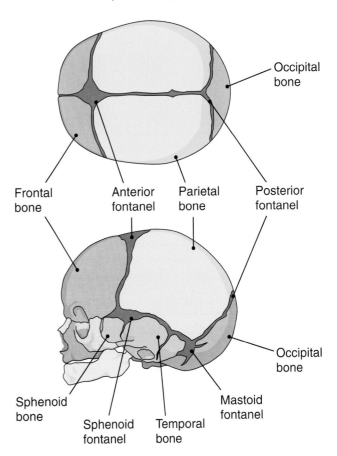

Labels on figure: Occipital bone, Frontal bone, Anterior fontanel, Parietal bone, Posterior fontanel, Sphenoid bone, Sphenoid fontanel, Temporal bone, Mastoid fontanel, Occipital bone

Figure 6-9 Infant skull, showing fontanels. *ZOOMING IN ✦ Which is the largest fontanel?*

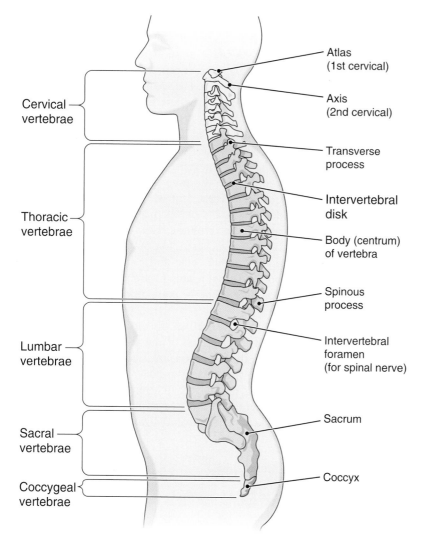

Atlas
(1st cervical)

Axis
(2nd cervical)

Transverse
process

Intervertebral
disk

Body (centrum)
of vertebra

Spinous
process

Intervertebral
foramen
(for spinal nerve)

Sacrum

Coccyx

Cervical
vertebrae

Thoracic
vertebrae

Lumbar
vertebrae

Sacral
vertebrae

Coccygeal
vertebrae

Figure 6-10 Vertebral column, left lateral view. *ZOOMING IN ✦ From an anterior view, which group(s) of vertebrae form a convex curve? Which group(s) form a concave curve?*

called the **sacrum** (SA-krum), in the adult. Wedged between the two hip bones, the sacrum completes the posterior part of the bony pelvis.

▶ The **coccygeal** (kok-SIJ-e-al) **vertebrae** consist of four or five tiny bones in the child. These later fuse to form a single bone, the **coccyx** (KOK-siks), or tail bone, in the adult.

Curves of the Spine When viewed from the side, the vertebral column can be seen to have four curves, corresponding to the four groups of vertebrae (see Fig. 6-10). In the fetus, the entire column is concave forward (curves away from a viewer facing the fetus), as seen in Figure 6-13. This is the primary curve.

When an infant begins to assume an erect posture, secondary curves develop. These curves are convex (curve toward the viewer). The cervical curve appears when the head is held up at about 3 months of age; the lumbar curve appears when the child begins to walk. The thoracic and sacral curves remain the two primary curves.

These curves of the vertebral column provide some of the resilience and spring so essential in balance and movement.

Thorax The bones of the **thorax** form a cone-shaped cage (Fig. 6-14). Twelve pairs of **ribs** form the bars of this cage, completed by the **sternum** (STER-num), or breastbone, anteriorly. These bones enclose and protect the heart, lungs, and other organs contained in the thorax.

The superior portion of the sternum is the broadly T-shaped **manubrium** (mah-NU-bre-um) that joins laterally on the right and left with the clavicle (collarbone) (see Fig. 6-1). The point on the manubrium where the clavicle joins can be seen on Figure 6-14 as the clavicular notch. Laterally, the manubrium joins with the anterior ends of the first pair of ribs. The **body** of the sternum is long and bladelike. It joins along each side with ribs two through seven. Where the manubrium joins the body of the sternum, there is a slight elevation, the **sternal angle**, which easily can be felt as a surface landmark.

The lower end of the sternum consists of a small tip that is made of cartilage in youth but becomes bone in the adult. This is the **xiphoid** (ZIF-oyd) **process**. It is used as a landmark for CPR (cardiopulmonary resuscitation) to locate the region for chest compression.

All 12 of the ribs on each side are attached to the vertebral column posteriorly. However, variations in the anterior attachment of these slender, curved bones have led to the following classification:

▶ **True ribs,** the first seven pairs, are those that attach directly to the sternum by means of individual extensions called **costal** (KOS-tal) **cartilages.**
▶ **False ribs** are the remaining five pairs. Of these, the 8th, 9th, and 10th pairs attach to the cartilage of the rib above. The last two pairs have no anterior attachment at all and are known as **floating ribs.**

The spaces between the ribs, called **intercostal spaces,** contain muscles, blood vessels, and nerves.

Checkpoint 6-7 The axial skeleton consists of the bones of the skull and the trunk. What bones make up the skeleton of the trunk?

Checkpoint 6-8 What are the five regions of the vertebral column?

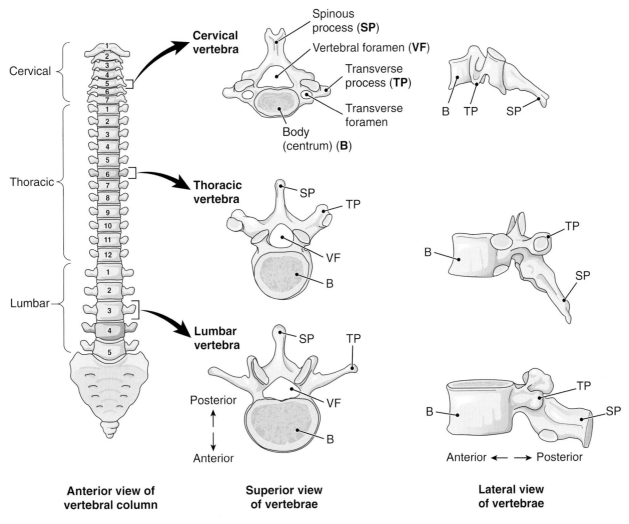

Figure 6-11   The vertebral column and vertebrae.

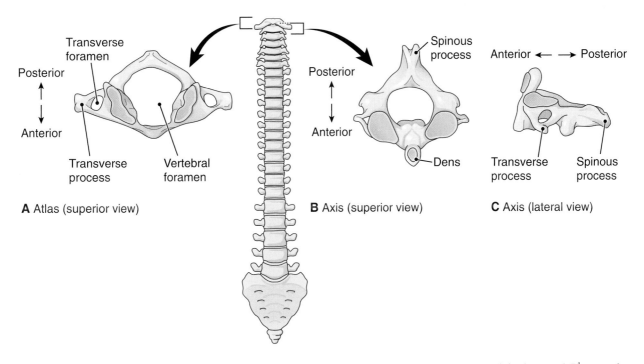

Figure 6-12   The first two cervical vertebrae. (A) The atlas (1st cervical vertebra), superior view. **(B)** The axis (2nd cervical vertebra), superior view. **(C)** The axis, lateral view.

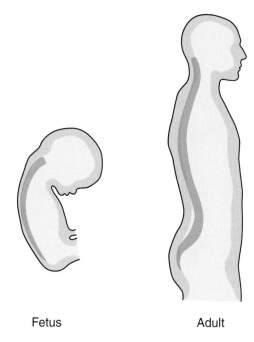

Fetus   Adult

Figure 6-13 **Curves of the spine.** Compare the fetus (*left*) with the adult (*right*).

▶ Bones of the Appendicular Skeleton

The appendicular skeleton may be considered in two divisions: upper and lower. The upper division on each side includes the shoulder, the arm (between the shoulder and the elbow), the forearm (between the elbow and the wrist), the wrist, the hand, and the fingers. The lower division includes the hip (part of the pelvic girdle), the thigh (between the hip and the knee), the leg (between the knee and the ankle), the ankle, the foot, and the toes.

The Upper Division of the Appendicular Skeleton

The bones of the upper division may be divided into two groups, the shoulder girdle and the upper extremity.

The Shoulder Girdle The shoulder girdle consists of two bones (Fig. 6-15):

▶ The **clavicle** (KLAV-ih-kl), or collarbone, is a slender bone with two shallow curves. It joins the sternum anteriorly and the scapula laterally and helps to support the shoulder. Because it often receives the full force of falls on outstretched arms or of blows to the shoulder, it is the most frequently broken bone.

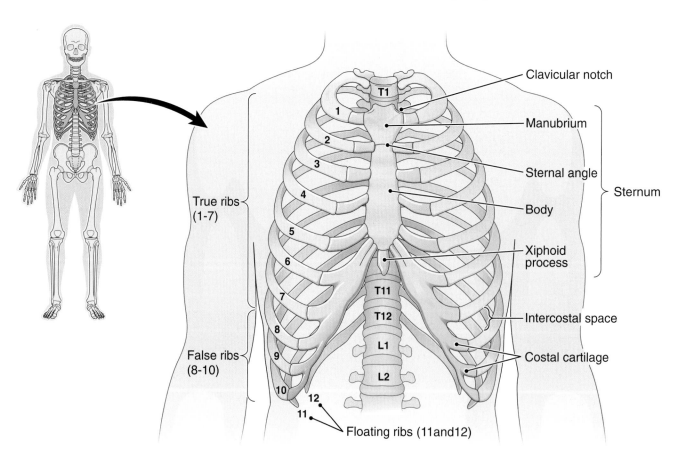

Figure 6-14 **Bones of the thorax, anterior view.** The first seven pairs of ribs are the true ribs; pairs 8 through 12 are the false ribs, of which the last two pairs are also called floating ribs. *ZOOMING IN ✦ To what bones do the costal cartilages attach?*

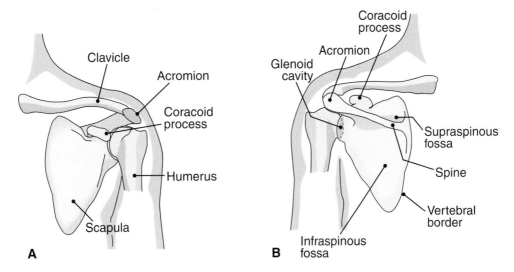

Figure 6-15 **The shoulder girdle and scapula. (A)** Bones of the shoulder girdle, left anterior view. **(B)** Left scapula, posterior view. *ZOOMING IN ✦ What does the prefix* supra *mean? What does the prefix* infra *mean?*

▶ The **scapula** (SKAP-u-lah), or shoulder blade, is shown from anterior and posterior views in Figure 6-15. The **spine** of the scapula is the posterior raised ridge that can be felt behind the shoulder in the upper portion of the back. Muscles that move the arm attach to fossae (depressions), known as the **supraspinous fossa** and the **infraspinous fossa**, superior and inferior to the scapular spine. The **acromion** (ah-KRO-me-on) is the process that joins the clavicle. This can be felt as the highest point of the shoulder. Below the acromion there is a shallow socket, the **glenoid cavity**, that forms a ball-and-socket joint with the arm bone (humerus). Medial to the glenoid cavity is the **coracoid** (KOR-ah-koyd) **process**, to which muscles attach.

The Upper Extremity The upper extremity is also referred to as the upper limb, or simply the arm, although technically, the arm is only the region between the shoulder and the elbow. The region between the elbow and wrist is the forearm. The upper extremity consists of the following bones:

▶ The proximal bone is the **humerus** (HU-mer-us), or arm bone (Fig. 6-16). The head of the humerus forms a joint with the glenoid cavity of the scapula. The distal end has a projection on each side, the medial and lateral epicondyles (ep-ih-KON-diles), to which tendons attach, and a pulley-shaped midportion, the **trochlea** (TROK-le-ah), that forms a joint with the ulna of the forearm.

▶ The forearm bones are the **ulna** (UL-nah) and the **radius** (RA-de-us). In the anatomic position, the ulna lies on the medial side of the forearm in line with the little finger, and the radius lies laterally, above the thumb (Fig. 6-17). When the forearm is supine, with the palm up or forward, the two bones are parallel; when the forearm is prone, with the palm down or back, the distal end of the radius rotates around the ulna so that the shafts of the two bones are crossed (Fig. 6-18). In this

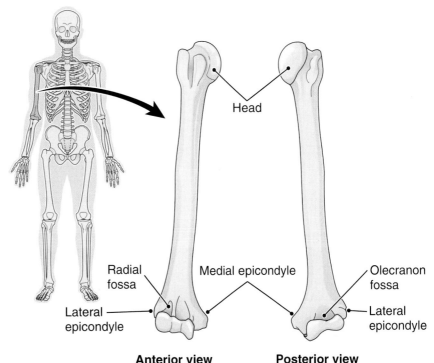

Figure 6-16 **The right humerus.**

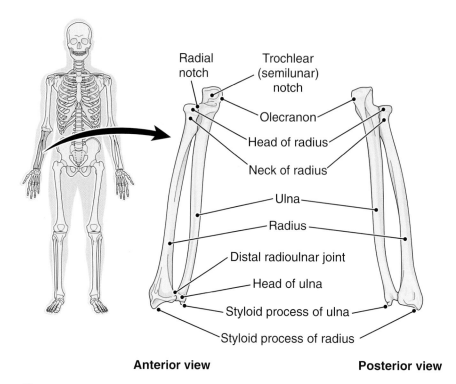

Figure 6-17 **Radius and ulna of the right forearm.** *ZOOMING IN ✦ What is the lateral bone of the forearm?*

position, a distal projection (styloid process) of the ulna pops up at the outside of the wrist.

▶ The proximal end of the ulna has the large **olecranon** (o-LEK-rah-non) that forms the point of the elbow (see Fig. 6-17). The trochlea of the distal humerus fits into the deep **trochlear notch** of the ulna, allowing a hinge action at the elbow joint. This ulnar depression, because of its deep half-moon shape, is also known as the semilunar notch (Fig. 6-19).

▶ The wrist contains eight small **carpal** (KAR-pal) **bones** arranged in two rows of four each. The names of these eight different bones are given in Figure 6-20.

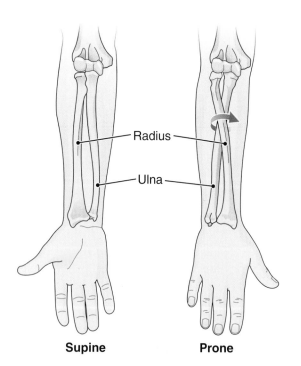

Figure 6-18 **Movements of the forearm.** When the palm is supine (facing up or forward), the radius and ulna are parallel. When the palm is prone (facing down or to the rear), the radius crosses over the ulna.

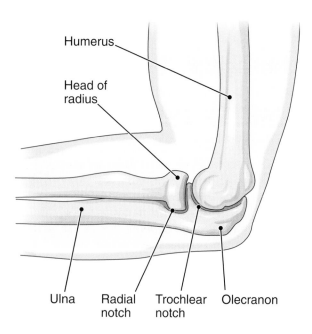

Figure 6-19 **Left elbow, lateral view.** *ZOOMING IN ✦ What part of what bone forms the bony prominence of the elbow?*

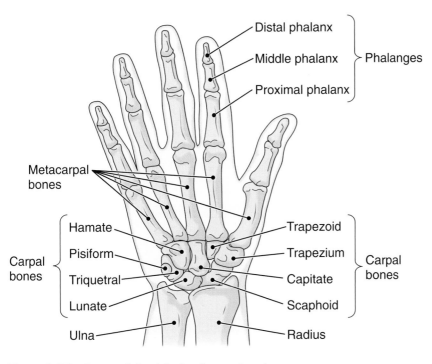

Figure 6-20 Bones of the right hand, anterior view.

▸ Five **metacarpal bones** are the framework for the palm of each hand. Their rounded distal ends form the knuckles.

▸ There are 14 **phalanges** (fah-LAN-jeze), or finger bones, in each hand, two for the thumb and three for each finger. Each of these bones is called a **phalanx** (FA-lanx). They are identified as the first, or proximal, which is attached to a metacarpal; the second, or middle; and the third, or distal. Note that the thumb has only two phalanges, a proximal and a distal (see Fig. 6-20).

The Lower Division of the Appendicular Skeleton

The bones of the lower division also fall into two groups, the pelvis and the lower extremity.

The Pelvic Bones The hip bone, or **os coxae**, begins its development as three separate bones that later fuse (Fig. 6-21). These individual bones are:

▸ The **ilium** (IL-e-um), which forms the upper, flared portion. The **iliac** (IL-e-ak) **crest** is the curved rim along the superior border of the ilium. It can be felt just below the waist. At either end of the crest are two bony projections. The most prominent of these is the **anterior superior iliac spine**, which is often used as a surface landmark in diagnosis and treatment.

▸ The **ischium** (IS-ke-um), which is the lowest and strongest part. The **ischial** (IS-ke-al) **spine** at the posterior of the pelvic outlet is used as a point of reference during childbirth to indicate the progress of the presenting part (usually the baby's head) down the birth canal. Just inferior to this spine is the large **ischial tuberosity**, which helps support the weight of the trunk when one sits down. One is sometimes aware of this projection of the ischium when sitting on a hard surface for a while.

▸ The **pubis** (PU-bis), which forms the anterior part. The joint formed by the union of the two hip bones anteriorly is called the **pubic symphysis** (SIM-fih-sis). This joint becomes more flexible late in pregnancy to allow for passage of the baby's head during childbirth.

Portions of all three pelvic bones contribute to the formation of the **acetabulum** (as-eh-TAB-u-lum), the deep socket that holds the head of the femur (thigh bone) to form the hip joint.

The largest foramina in the entire body are found near the front of each hip bone, one on each side of the pubic symphysis. Each opening is partially covered by a membrane and is called an **obturator** (OB-tu-ra-tor) **foramen** (see Fig. 6-21).

The two ossa coxae join in forming the pelvis, a strong bony girdle completed by the sacrum and coccyx of the spine posteriorly. The pelvis supports the trunk and the organs in the lower abdomen, or pelvic cavity, including the urinary bladder, the internal reproductive organs, and parts of the intestine.

The female pelvis is adapted for pregnancy and childbirth (Fig. 6-22). Some of the ways in which the female pelvis differs from that of the male are:

▸ It is lighter in weight.
▸ The ilia are wider and more flared.
▸ The pubic arch, the anterior angle between the pubic bones, is wider.
▸ The pelvic opening is wider and more rounded.
▸ The lower diameter, the pelvic outlet, is larger.
▸ The sacrum and coccyx are shorter and less curved.

The Lower Extremity The lower extremity is also referred to as the lower limb, or simply the leg, although technically the leg is only the region between the knee and the ankle. The portion of the extremity between the hip and the knee is the thigh. The lower extremity consists of the following bones:

▸ The **femur** (FE-mer), the bone of the thigh, is the longest and strongest bone in the body. Proximally, it has a large ball-shaped head that joins the os coxae (Fig. 6-23). The large lateral projection near the head of the femur is the **greater trochanter** (tro-KAN-ter), used as a surface landmark. The **lesser trochanter**, a smaller elevation, is located on the medial side. On the posterior surface there is a long central ridge, the **linea aspera**, which is a point for attachment of hip muscles.

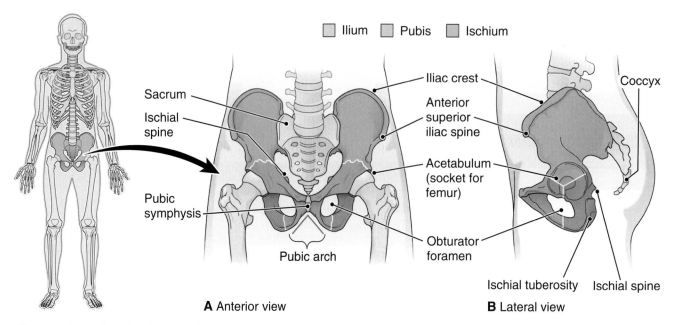

☐ Ilium ☐ Pubis ☐ Ischium

A Anterior view

B Lateral view

Figure 6-21   **The pelvic bones. (A)** Anterior view. **(B)** Lateral view; shows joining of the three pelvic bones to form the acetabulum.   *ZOOMING IN ✦ What bone is nicknamed the "sit bone"?*

▶ The **patella** (pah-TEL-lah), or kneecap (see Fig. 6-1), is embedded in the tendon of the large anterior thigh muscle, the quadriceps femoris, where it crosses the knee joint. It is an example of a **sesamoid** (SES-ahmoyd) **bone**, a type of bone that develops within a tendon or a joint capsule.

▶ There are two bones in the leg (Fig. 6-24). Medially (on the great toe side), the **tibia**, or shin bone, is the longer, weight-bearing bone. It has a sharp anterior crest that can be felt at the surface of the leg. Laterally, the slender **fibula** (FIB-u-lah) does not reach the knee joint; thus, it is not a weight-bearing bone. The **medial malleolus** (mal-LE-o-lus) is a downward projection at the distal end of the tibia; it forms the prominence on the inner aspect of the ankle. The lat-

eral **malleolus,** at the distal end of the fibula, forms the prominence on the outer aspect of the ankle. Most people think of these projections as their "ankle bones," whereas, in truth, they are features of the tibia and fibula.

▶ The structure of the foot is similar to that of the hand. However, the foot supports the weight of the body, so it is stronger and less mobile than the hand. There are seven **tarsal bones** associated with the ankle and foot. These are named and illustrated in Figure 6-25. The largest of these is the **calcaneus** (kal-KA-ne-us), or heel bone.

▶ Five **metatarsal bones** form the framework of the instep, and the heads of these bones form the ball of the foot (see Fig. 6-25).

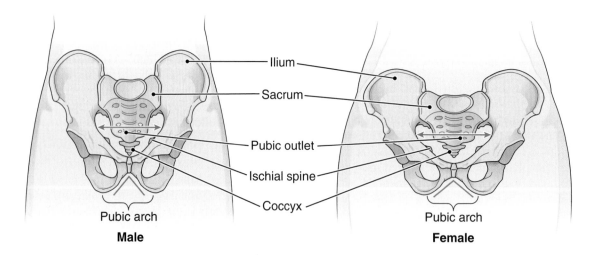

Male

Female

Figure 6-22   **Comparison of male and female pelvis, anterior view.** Note the broader angle of the pubic arch and the wider pelvic outlet in the female. Also, the ilia are wider and more flared; the sacrum and coccyx are shorter and less curved.

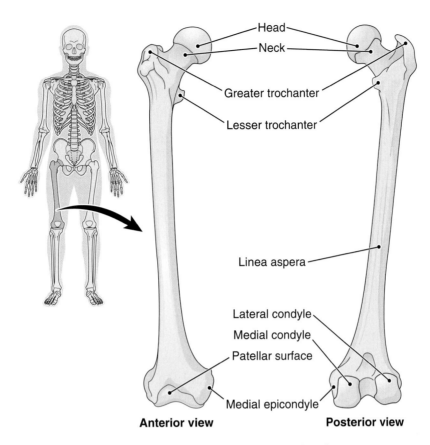

Figure 6-23 **The right femur (thigh bone).**

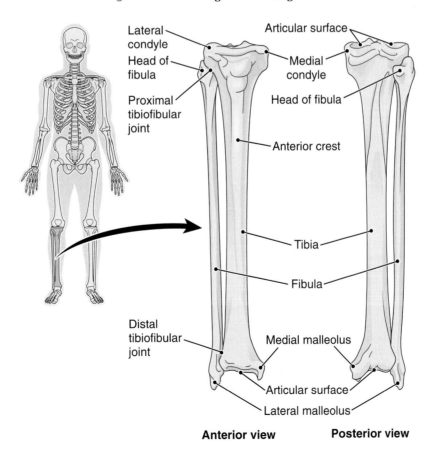

Figure 6-24 **Tibia and fibula of the right leg.** *ZOOMING IN ✦ What is the medial bone of the leg?*

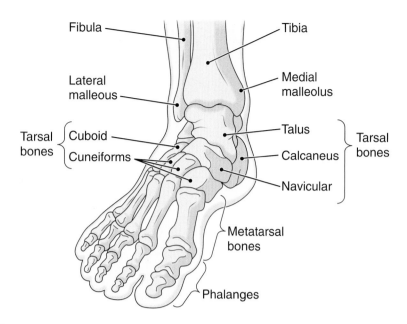

Figure 6-25 **Bones of the right foot.** *ZOOMING IN* ✦ *Which tarsal bone is the heel bone?*

▶ The **phalanges** of the toes are counterparts of those in the fingers. There are three of these in each toe except for the great toe, which has only two.

Checkpoint 6-9 What division of the skeleton consists of the bones of the shoulder girdle, hip, and extremities?

▶ Skeletal Changes in the Aging

The aging process includes significant changes in all connective tissues, including bone. There is a loss of calcium salts and a decrease in the amount of protein formed in bone tissue. The reduction of collagen in bone and in tendons, ligaments, and skin contributes to the stiffness so often found in older people. Muscle tissue is also lost throughout adult life. Thus, there is a tendency to decrease the exercise that is so important to the maintenance of bone tissue. To learn about ways to slow bone degeneration, see Box 6-2, Three Steps Toward a Strong and Healthy Skeleton.

Changes in the vertebral column with age lead to a loss in height. Approximately 1.2 cm (about 0.5 inches) are lost each 20 years beginning at 40 years of age, owing primarily to a thinning of the intervertebral disks (between the bodies of the vertebrae). Even the vertebral bodies themselves may lose height in later years. The costal (rib) cartilages become calcified and less flexible, and the chest may decrease in diameter by 2 to 3 cm (about 1 inch), mostly in the lower part.

▶ The Joints

An **articulation**, or **joint**, is an area of junction or union between two or more bones. Joints are classified into three main types on the basis of the material between the adjoining bones. They may also be classified according to the degree of movement permitted (Table 6-2):

Box 6-2 • Health Maintenance

Three Steps Toward a Strong and Healthy Skeleton

The skeleton is the body's framework. It supports and protects internal organs, helps to produce movement, and manufactures blood cells. Bone also stores nearly all of the body's calcium, releasing it into the blood when needed for processes such as nerve transmission, muscle contraction, and blood clotting. Proper nutrition, exercise, and a healthy lifestyle can help the skeleton perform all these essential roles.

A well-balanced diet supplies the nutrients and energy needed for strong, healthy bones. Calcium and phosphorus confer strength and rigidity. Protein supplies the amino acids needed to make collagen, which gives bone tissue flexibility, and vitamin C helps stimulate collagen synthesis. Foods rich in both calcium and phosphorus include dairy products, fish, beans, and leafy green vegetables. Meat is an excellent source of protein, whereas citrus fruits are rich in vitamin C. Vitamin D helps the digestive system absorb calcium into the bloodstream, making it available for bone. Foods rich in vitamin D include fish, liver, and eggs.

When body fluids become too acidic, bone releases calcium and phosphate and is weakened. Both magnesium and potassium help regulate the pH of body fluids, with magnesium also helping bone absorb calcium. Foods rich in magnesium and potassium include beans, potatoes, and leafy green vegetables. Bananas and dairy products are high in potassium.

Like muscle, bone becomes weakened with disuse. Consistent exercise promotes a stronger, denser skeleton by stimulating bone to absorb more calcium and phosphate from the blood, reducing the risk of osteoporosis. A healthy lifestyle also includes avoiding smoking and excessive alcohol consumption, both of which decrease bone calcium and inhibit bone growth. High levels of caffeine in the diet may also rob the skeleton of calcium.

Table 6·2 Joints

TYPE	MOVEMENT	MATERIAL BETWEEN THE BONES	EXAMPLES
Fibrous	Immovable (synarthrosis)	No joint cavity; fibrous connective tissue between bones	Sutures between bones of skull
Cartilaginous	Slightly movable (amphiarthrosis)	No joint cavity; cartilage between bones	Pubic symphysis; joints between bodies of vertebrae
Synovial	Freely movable (diarthrosis)	Joint cavity containing synovial fluid	Gliding, hinge, pivot, condyloid, saddle, ball-and-socket joints

▶ **Fibrous joint.** The bones in this type of joint are held together by fibrous connective tissue. An example is a **suture** (SU-chur) between bones of the skull. This type of joint is immovable and is termed a **synarthrosis** (sin-ar-THRO-sis).

▶ **Cartilaginous joint.** The bones in this type of joint are connected by cartilage. Examples are the joint between the pubic bones of the pelvis—the pubic symphysis—and the joints between the bodies of the vertebrae. This type of joint is slightly movable and is termed an **amphiarthrosis** (am-fe-ar-THRO-sis).

▶ **Synovial** (sin-O-ve-al) **joint.** The bones in this type of joint have a potential space between them called the **joint cavity**, which contains a small amount of thick, colorless fluid. This lubricant, **synovial fluid**, resembles uncooked egg white (ov is the root, meaning "egg") and is secreted by the membrane that lines the joint cavity. The synovial joint is freely movable and is termed a **diarthrosis** (di-ar-THRO-sis). Most joints are synovial joints; they are described in more detail next.

Checkpoint 6-10 What are the three types of joints classified according to the type of material between the adjoining bones?

More About Synovial Joints

The bones in freely movable joints are held together by **ligaments**, bands of fibrous connective tissue. Additional ligaments reinforce and help stabilize the joints at various points (Fig. 6-26 A). Also, for strength and protection, there is a **joint capsule** of connective tissue that encloses each joint and is continuous with the periosteum of the bones. The bone surfaces in freely movable joints are protected by a smooth layer of hyaline cartilage called the **articular** (ar-TIK-u-lar) **cartilage** (see Fig. 6-26 B). Some complex joints may have cartilage between the bones that acts as a cushion, such as the crescent-shaped medial **meniscus** (meh-NIS-kus) and lateral meniscus in the knee joint (Fig. 6-27). Fat may also appear as padding around a joint.

Near some joints are small sacs called **bursae** (BER-se), which are filled with synovial fluid (see Fig. 6-27). These lie in areas subject to stress and help ease movement over and around the joints. Inflammation of a bursa, as a result of injury or irritation, is called **bursitis**. Joint injury may require medical attention. For more information see Box 6-3, Arthroplasty: Bionic Parts for a Better Life.

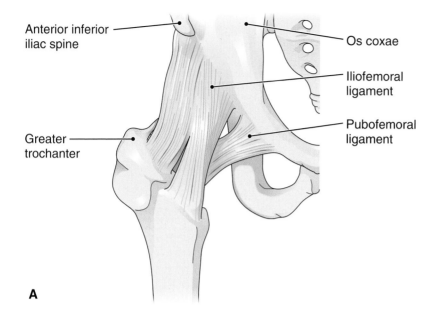

A

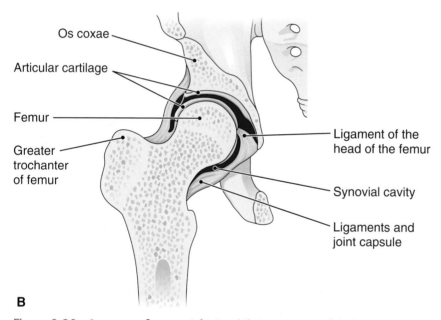

B

Figure 6-26 Structure of a synovial joint. (A) Anterior view of the hip joint showing ligaments that reinforce and stabilize the joint. **(B)** Frontal section through right hip joint showing protective structures.

Types of Synovial Joints Synovial joints are classified according to the types of movement they allow, as described and illustrated in Table 6-3. Listed in order of increasing range of motion, they are:

▶ Gliding joint
▶ Hinge joint
▶ Pivot joint
▶ Condyloid joint
▶ Saddle joint
▶ Ball-and-socket joint

Movement at Synovial Joints The chief function of the freely movable joints is to allow for changes of posi-

tion and so provide for motion. These movements are named to describe changes in the positions of body parts (Fig. 6-28). For example, there are four kinds of angular movement, or movement that changes the angle between bones, as listed below:

▶ **Flexion** (FLEK-shun) is a bending motion that decreases the angle between bones, as in bending the fingers to close the hand.
▶ **Extension** is a straightening motion that increases the angle between bones, as in straightening the fingers to open the hand.
▶ **Abduction** (ab-DUK-shun) is movement away from the midline of the body, as in moving the arms straight out to the sides.
▶ **Adduction** is movement toward the midline of the body, as in bringing the arms back to their original position beside the body.

A combination of these angular movements enables one to execute a movement referred to as **circumduction** (ser-kum-DUK-shun). To perform this movement, stand with your arm outstretched and draw a large imaginary circle in the air. Note the smooth combination of flexion, abduction, extension, and adduction that makes circumduction possible.

Rotation refers to a twisting or turning of a bone on its own axis, as in turning the head from side to side to say "no," or rotating the forearm to turn the palm up and down.

There are special movements that are characteristic of the forearm and the ankle:

▶ **Supination** (su-pin-A-shun) is the act of turning the palm up or forward; **pronation** (pro-NA-shun) turns the palm down or backward.
▶ **Inversion** (in-VER-zhun) is the act of turning the sole inward, so that it faces the opposite foot; **eversion** (e-VER-zhun) turns the sole outward, away from the body.
▶ In **dorsiflexion** (dor-sih-FLEK-shun), the foot is bent upward at the ankle, narrowing the angle between the leg and the top of the foot; in **plantar flexion**, the toes point downward, as in toe dancing, flexing the arch of the foot.

Checkpoint 6-11 What is the most freely movable type of joint?

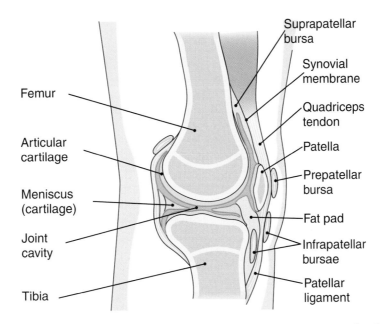

Femur

Articular
cartilage

Meniscus
(cartilage)

Joint
cavity

Tibia

Suprapatellar
bursa

Synovial
membrane

Quadriceps
tendon

Patella

Prepatellar
bursa

Fat pad

Infrapatellar
bursae

Patellar
ligament

Figure 6-27 **The knee joint, sagittal section.** Protective structures are also shown.

Box 6-3	Hot Topics

Arthroplasty: Bionic Parts for a Better Life

Since the first total hip replacement in the early 1960s, millions of joint replacements, called **arthroplasties,** have been performed successfully. Most are done to decrease joint pain in older people with arthritis and other chronic degenerative bone diseases after other treatments such as weight loss, physical therapy, and medication have been tried. Hips and knees are most commonly restored, with 300,000 hip arthroplasties and an equal number of knee replacements performed each year in the United States. Orthopedic surgeons can also replace shoulder, elbow, wrist, hand, ankle, and foot joints.

Artificial, or **prosthetic,** joints are engineered to be strong, nontoxic, corrosion-resistant, and firmly bondable to the patient. Computer-controlled machines now produce individualized joints in less time and at less cost than before. Ball-and-socket joint prostheses, like those used in total hip replacement, consist of a cup, ball, and stem. The cup replaces the hip socket (acetabulum) and is bonded to the pelvis using screws or glue. The cup is usually plastic but may also be made of longer-lasting ceramic or metal. The ball, made of metal or ceramic, replaces the femoral head and is attached to the stem, which is implanted into the femoral shaft. Stems are made of various metal alloys such as cobalt and titanium and are often glued into place. Stems designed to promote bone growth into them are usually used in younger, more active patients because it is believed that they will remain firmly attached longer.

Until recently, arthroplasty was rarely performed on young people because prosthetics had a short lifespan of about 10 years. Today's materials and surgical techniques could increase the lifespan to 20 years or more, and young people who undergo arthroplasty will require fewer future replacements. This is especially important because sports-related joint injuries in young adults are increasing.

Table 6·3 Synovial Joints

TYPE OF JOINT	TYPE OF MOVEMENT	EXAMPLES
Gliding joint	Bone surfaces slide over one another	Joints in the wrist and ankles (Figs. 6-20, 6-25)
Hinge joint	Allows movement in one direction, changing the angle of the bones at the joint	Elbow joint; joints between phalanges of fingers and toes (Figs. 6-19, 6-20, 6-25)
Pivot joint	Allows rotation around the length of the bone	Joint between the first and second cervical vertebrae; joint at proximal ends of the radius and ulna (Figs. 6-10, 6-19)
Condyloid joint	Allows movement in two directions	Joint between the metacarpal and the first phalanx of the finger (knuckle) (Fig. 6-20); joint between the occipital bone of the skull and the first cervical vertebra (atlas) (Fig. 6-10)
Saddle joint	Like a condyloid joint, but with deeper articulating surfaces	Joint between the wrist and the metacarpal bone of the thumb (Fig. 6-20)
Ball-and-socket joint	Allows movement in many directions around a central point. Gives the greatest freedom of movement	Shoulder joint and hip joint (Figs. 6-15, 6-26)

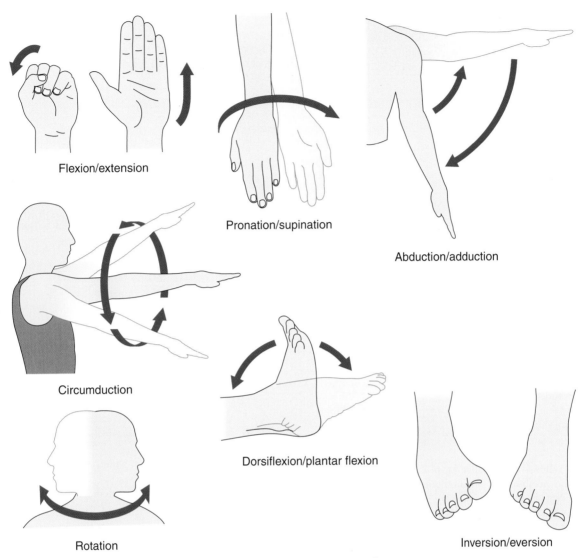

Flexion/extension

Pronation/supination

Abduction/adduction

Circumduction

Dorsiflexion/plantar flexion

Rotation

Inversion/eversion

Figure 6-28 Movements at synovial joints.

Word Anatomy

Medical terms are built from standardized word parts (prefixes, roots and suffixes). Learning the meanings of these parts can help you remember words and interpret unfamiliar terms.

WORD PART	MEANING	EXAMPLE
Bones		
dia-	through, between	The *diaphysis*, or shaft, of a long bone is between the two ends, or epiphyses.
oss, osse/o	bone, bone tissue	*Osseous* tissue is another name for bone tissue.
oste/o	bone, bone tissue	The *periosteum* is the fibrous membrane around a bone.
-clast	break	An *osteoclast* breaks down bone in the process of resorption.
Divisions of the Skeleton		
para-	near	The *paranasal* sinuses are near the nose.
pariet/o	wall	The *parietal* bones form the side walls of the skull.
cost/o	rib	*Intercostal* spaces are located between the ribs.
supra-	above, superior	The *supraspinous* fossa is a depression superior to the spine of the scapula.
infra-	below, inferior	The *infraspinous* fossa is a depression inferior to the spine of the scapula.
meta-	near, beyond	The *metacarpal* bones of the palm are near and distal to the carpal bones of the wrist.

WORD PART	MEANING	EXAMPLE
The Joints		
arthr/o	joint, articulation	A *synarthrosis* is an immovable joint, such as a suture.
amphi-	on both sides, around, double	An *amphiarthrosis* is a slightly movable joint.
ab-	away from	*Abduction* is movement away from the midline of the body.
ad-	toward, added to	*Adduction* is movement toward the midline of the body.
circum-	around	*Circumduction* is movement around a joint in a circle.

Summary

I. Bones

1. Main functions of bones—serve as body framework; protect organs; serve as levers for movement; store calcium salts; form blood cells
A. Bone structure
   1. Long bone
      a. Diaphysis—shaft
      b. Epiphysis—end
   2. Bone tissue
      a. Compact—in shaft of long bones; outside of other bones
      b. Spongy (cancellous)—in end of long bones; center of other bones
   3. Bone marrow
      a. Red—in spongy bone
      b. Yellow—in central cavity of long bones
   4. Bone membranes—contain bone-forming cells
      a. Periosteum—covers bone
      b. Endosteum—lines marrow cavity
B. Bone growth and repair
   1. Bone cells
      a. Osteoblasts—bone-forming cells
      b. Osteocytes—mature bone cells that maintain bone
      c. Osteoclasts—cells that break down (resorb) bone; derived from monocytes, types of white blood cells
   2. Formation of a long bone—begins in center of shaft and continues at epiphyseal plate
C. Bone markings
   1. Projections—head, process, condyle, crest, spine
   2. Depressions and holes—foramen, sinus, fossa, meatus

II. Bones of the axial skeleton

A. Framework of the skull
   1. Cranium—frontal, parietal, temporal, ethmoid, sphenoid, occipital
   2. Facial bones—mandible, maxilla, zygomatic, nasal, lacrimal, vomer, palatine, inferior nasal conchae
   3. Other—ossicles (of ear), hyoid
   4. Infant skull—fontanels (soft spots)
B. Framework of the trunk
   1. Vertebral column—divisions: cervical, thoracic, lumbar, sacral, coccygeal
      a. Curves
         (1) Thoracic and sacral—concave, primary
         (2) Cervical and lumbar—convex, secondary

2. Thorax
   a. Sternum—manubrium, body, xiphoid process
   b. Ribs
      (1) True—first seven pairs
      (2) False—remaining five pairs, including two floating ribs

III. Bones of the appendicular skeleton

A. Upper division
   1. Shoulder girdle—clavicle, scapula
   2. Upper extremity—humerus, ulna, radius, carpals, metacarpals, phalanges
B. Lower division
   1. Pelvic bones—os coxae (hip bone): ilium, ischium, pubis
      a. Female pelvis lighter, wider, more rounded than male
   2. Lower extremity—femur, patella, tibia, fibula, tarsals, metatarsals, phalanges

IV. Skeletal changes in aging— Loss of calcium salts, decreased production of collagen, thinning of intervertebral disks, loss of flexibility

V. Joints (articulations)

1. Kinds of joints
   a. Fibrous—immovable (synarthrosis)
   b. Cartilaginous—slightly movable (amphiarthrosis)
   c. Synovial—freely movable (diarthrosis)
A. More about synovial joints
   1. Structure of synovial joints
      a. Joint cavity—contains synovial fluid
      b. Ligaments—hold joint together
      c. Joint capsule—strengthens and protects joint
      d. Articular cartilage—covers ends of bones
      e. Bursae—fluid-filled sacs near joints; cushion and protect joints and surrounding tissue
   2. Types of synovial joints—gliding, hinge, pivot, condyloid, saddle, ball-and-socket
   3. Movement at synovial joints
      a. Angular—flexion, extension, abduction, adduction
      b. Circular—circumduction, rotation
      c. Special at forearm—supination, pronation,
      d. Special at ankle—inversion, eversion, dorsiflexion, plantar flexion

Questions for Study and Review

Building Understanding

Fill in the blanks
1. The shaft of a long bone is called the _____.
2. The structural unit of compact bone is the _____.
3. Red bone marrow manufactures _____.
4. Bones are covered by a connective tissue membrane called _____.
5. Bone matrix is produced by _____.

Matching
Match each numbered item with the most closely related lettered item.
___ 6. A rounded bony projection
___ 7. A sharp bony prominence
___ 8. A hole through bone
___ 9. A bony depression
___ 10. An air-filled bony cavity

a. condyle
b. foramen
c. fossa
d. sinus
e. spine

Multiple choice
___ 11. The cells responsible for bone resorption are called
    a. osteoblasts
    b. osteoclasts
    c. osteocytes
    d. osteons
___ 12. On which of the following bones would the mastoid process be found?
    a. occipital bone
    b. femur
    c. temporal bone
    d. humerus
___ 13. On which of the following bones would the greater trochanter be found?
    a. humerus
    b. ulna
    c. femur
    d. tibia
___ 14. A joint that is freely moveable is called a(n) _____ joint.
    a. arthrotic
    b. amphiarthrotic
    c. diarthrotic
    d. synarthrotic
___ 15. Which of the following synovial joints describes the hip?
    a. gliding
    b. hinge
    c. pivot
    d. ball-and-socket

Understanding Concepts

16. List five functions of bone and describe how a long bone's structure enables it to carry out each of these functions.

17. Explain the differences between the terms in each of the following pairs:
    a. osteoblast and osteocyte
    b. periosteum and endosteum
    c. compact bone and spongy bone
    d. epiphysis and diaphysis
    e. axial skeleton and appendicular skeleton
18. Discuss the process of long bone formation during fetal development and childhood. What role does resorption play in bone formation?
19. Name the bones of the:
    a. cranium and face
    b. thoracic cavity, vertebral column, and pelvis
    c. upper and lower limbs
20. List the structural differences between the male and female pelvis.
21. Name three effects of aging on the skeletal system.
22. Differentiate between the terms in each of the following pairs:
    a. flexion and extension
    b. abduction and adduction
    c. supination and pronation
    d. inversion and eversion
    e. circumduction and rotation
    f. dorsiflexion and plantar flexion

Conceptual Thinking

23. The vertebral bodies are much larger in the lower back than the neck. What is the functional significance of this structural difference?
24. Nine-year-old Alek is admitted into Emergency with a closed fracture of the right femur. Radiography reveals that the fracture crosses the distal epiphyseal plate. What concerns should Alek's healthcare team have about the location of his injury?

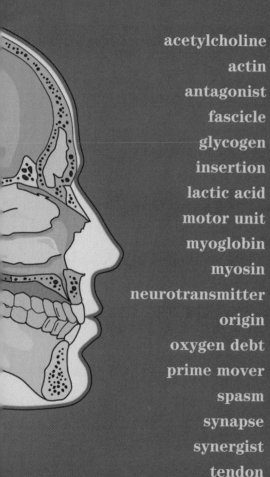

LEARNING OUTCOMES

After careful study of this chapter, you should be able to:

1. Compare the three types of muscle tissue

2. Describe three functions of skeletal muscle

3. Briefly describe how skeletal muscles contract

4. List the substances needed in muscle contraction and describe the function of each

5. Define the term oxygen debt

6. Describe three compounds stored in muscle that are used to generate energy in highly active muscle cells

7. Cite the effects of exercise on muscles

8. Compare isotonic and isometric contractions

9. Explain how muscles work in pairs to produce movement

10. Compare the workings of muscles and bones to lever systems

11. Explain how muscles are named

12. Name some of the major muscles in each muscle group and describe the main function of each

13. Describe how muscles change with age

14. Show how word parts are used to build words related to the muscular system (see Word Anatomy at the end of the chapter)

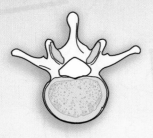

chapter 7

The Muscular System

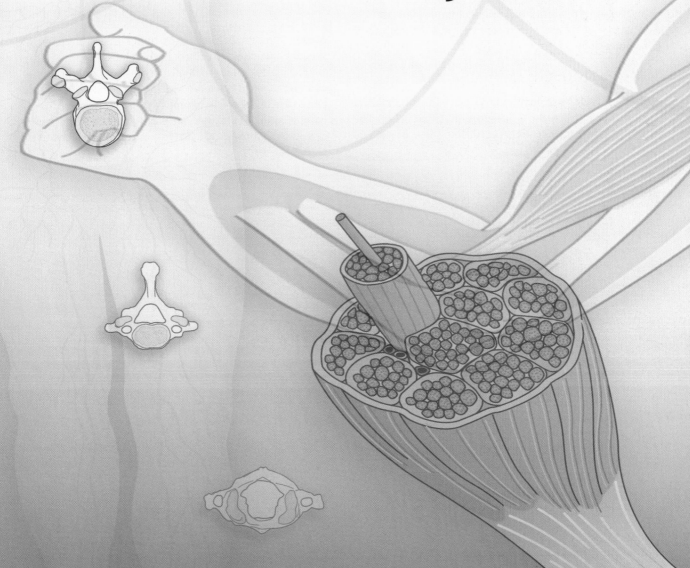

▶ Types of Muscle

There are three kinds of muscle tissue: smooth, cardiac, and skeletal muscle, as introduced in Chapter 4. After a brief description of all three types (Table 7-1), this chapter concentrates on skeletal muscle, which has been studied the most.

Smooth Muscle

Smooth muscle makes up the walls of the hollow body organs as well as those of the blood vessels and respiratory passageways. It moves involuntarily and produces the wavelike motions of peristalsis that move substances through a system. Smooth muscle can also regulate the diameter of an opening, such as the central opening of blood vessels, or produce contractions of hollow organs, such as the uterus. Smooth muscle fibers (cells) are tapered at each end and have a single, central nucleus. The cells appear smooth under the microscope because they do not contain the visible bands, or **striations**, that are seen in the other types of muscle cells. Smooth muscle may contract in response to a nerve impulse, hormonal stimulation, stretching, and other stimuli. The muscle contracts and relaxes slowly and can remain contracted for a long time.

Cardiac Muscle

Cardiac muscle, also involuntary, makes up the wall of the heart and creates the pulsing action of that organ. The cells of cardiac muscle are striated, like those of skeletal muscle. They differ in having one nucleus per cell and branching interconnections. The membranes between the cells are specialized to allow electrical impulses to travel rapidly through them, so that contractions can be better coordinated. These membranes appear as dark lines between the cells (see Table 7-1) and are called intercalated (in-TER-kah-la-ted) disks, because they are "inserted between" the cells. The electrical impulses that produce contractions of cardiac muscle are generated within the muscle itself but can be modified by nervous stimuli and hormones.

Skeletal Muscle

When viewed under the microscope, skeletal muscle cells appear heavily striated. The arrangement of protein threads within the cell that produces these striations is described later. The cells are very long and cylindrical and have multiple nuclei per cell. During development, the nuclei of these cells divide repeatedly by mitosis without division of the cell contents, resulting in a large, multinucleated cell. Such cells can contract as a large unit when stimulated. The nervous system stimulates skeletal muscle to contract, and the tissue usually contracts and relaxes rapidly. Because it is under conscious control, skeletal muscle is described as voluntary.

Skeletal muscle is so named because most of these muscles are attached to bones and produce movement at the joints. There are a few exceptions. The muscles of the abdominal wall, for example, are partly attached to other muscles, and the muscles of facial expression are attached to the

Table 7·1	Comparison of the Different Types of Muscle		
	SMOOTH	**CARDIAC**	**SKELETAL**
Location	Wall of hollow organs, vessels, respiratory passageways	Wall of heart	Attached to bones
Cell characteristics	Tapered at each end, branching networks, nonstriated	Branching networks; special membranes (intercalated disks) between cells; single nucleus; lightly striated	Long and cylindrical; multinucleated; heavily striated
Control	Involuntary	Involuntary	Voluntary
Action	Produces peristalsis; contracts and relaxes slowly; may sustain contraction	Pumps blood out of heart; self-excitatory but influenced by nervous system and hormones	Produces movement at joints; stimulated by nervous system; contracts and relaxes rapidly

skin. Skeletal muscles constitute the largest amount of the body's muscle tissue, making up about 40% of the total body weight. This muscular system is composed of more than 600 individual skeletal muscles. Although each one is a distinct structure, muscles usually act in groups to execute body movements.

Table 7·2	Connective Tissue Layers in Skeletal Muscle	
NAME OF LAYER	**LOCATION**	
Endomysium	Around each individual muscle fiber.	
Perimysium	Around fascicles (bundles) of muscle fibers.	
Epimysium	Around entire muscle; forms the innermost layer of the deep fascia.	

Checkpoint 7-1 What are the three types of muscle?

The Muscular System

The three primary functions of skeletal muscles are:

▶ Movement of the skeleton. Muscles are attached to bones and contract to change the position of the bones at a joint.
▶ Maintenance of posture. A steady partial contraction of muscle, known as **muscle tone**, keeps the body in position. Some of the muscles involved in maintaining posture are the large muscles of the thighs, back, neck, and shoulders as well as the abdominal muscles.
▶ Generation of heat. Muscles generate most of the heat needed to keep the body at 37°C (98.6°F). Heat is a natural byproduct of muscle cell metabolism. When we are cold, muscles can boost their heat output by the rapid small contractions we know of as shivering.

Checkpoint 7-2 What are the three main functions of skeletal muscle?

Structure of a Muscle

In forming whole muscles, individual muscle fibers are arranged in bundles, or **fascicles** (FAS-ih-kls), held together by fibrous connective tissue (Fig. 7-1, Table 7-2). The deepest layer of this connective tissue, the **endomysium** (en-do-MIS-e-um) surrounds the individual fibers in the fascicles. Around each fascicle is a connective tissue layer known as the **perimysium** (per-ih-MIS-e-um). The entire muscle is then encased in a tough connective tissue sheath, the **epimysium** (ep-ih-MIS-e-um), which forms the innermost layer of the **deep fascia**, the tough, fibrous sheath that encloses a muscle. (Note that all these layers are named with prefixes that describe their position added to the root *my/o*, meaning "muscle.") All of these supporting tissues merge to form the **tendon**, the band of connective tissue that attaches a muscle to a bone (see Fig. 7-1).

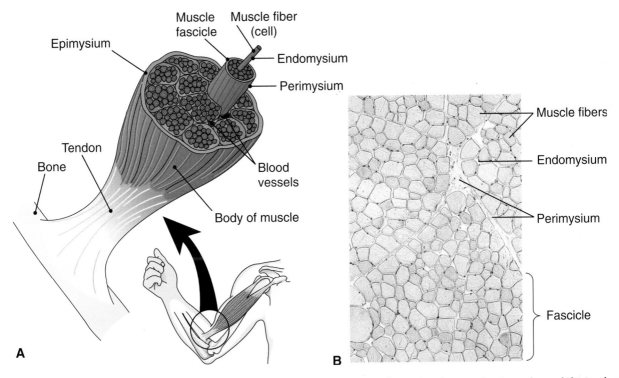

Figure 7-1 **Structure of a skeletal muscle. (A)** Structure of a muscle showing the tendon that attaches it to a bone. **(B)** Muscle tissue seen under a microscope. Portions of several fascicles are shown with connective tissue coverings. (B, Reprinted with permission from Gartner LP, Hiatt JL. Color Atlas of Histology. 3rd ed. Philadelphia: Lippincott Williams & Wilkins, 2000.) *ZOOMING IN ✦ What is the innermost layer of connective tissue in a muscle? What layer of connective tissue surrounds a fascicle of muscle fibers?*

Muscle Cells in Action

Nerve impulses coming from the brain and the spinal cord stimulate skeletal muscle fibers (see Chap. 8). Because these impulses are traveling away from the central nervous system (CNS), they are described as **motor** impulses (as contrasted to sensory impulses traveling toward the CNS), and the neurons (nerve cells) that carry these impulses are described as motor neurons. As the neuron contacts the muscle, its axon (fiber) branches to supply from a few to hundreds of individual muscle cells, or in some cases more than 1000 (Fig. 7-2).

A single neuron and all the muscle fibers it stimulates comprise a **motor unit**. Small motor units are used in fine coordination, as in movements of the eye. Larger motor units are used for maintaining posture or for broad movements, such as walking or swinging a tennis racquet.

The Neuromuscular Junction The point at which a nerve fiber contacts a muscle cell is called the **neuromuscular junction** (NMJ) (Fig. 7-3). It is here that a chemical classified as a **neurotransmitter** is released from the neuron to stimulate the muscle fiber. The specific neurotransmitter released here is **acetylcholine** (as-e-til-KO-lene), abbreviated ACh, which is found elsewhere in the body as well. A great deal is known about the events that occur at this junction, and this information is important in understanding muscle action.

The neuromuscular junction is an example of a **synapse** (SIN-aps), a point of communication between cells. Between the cells there is a tiny space, the **synaptic cleft**, across which the neurotransmitter must travel. Until its release, the neurotransmitter is stored in tiny membranous sacs, called vesicles, in the endings of the nerve fiber. Once released, the neurotransmitter crosses the synaptic cleft and attaches to receptors, which are proteins embedded in the muscle cell membrane. The membrane forms multiple folds at this point that increase surface area and hold a maximum number of receptors. The receiving membrane of the muscle cell is known as the **motor end plate**.

Muscle fibers, like nerve cells, show the property of **excitability**; that is, they are able to transmit electrical current along the plasma membrane. When the muscle is stimulated at the neuromuscular junction, an electrical impulse is generated that spreads rapidly along the muscle cell membrane. This spreading wave of electrical current is called the **action potential** because it calls the muscle cell into action. Chapter 8 provides more information on synapses and the action potential.

> **Checkpoint 7-3** Muscles are activated by the nervous system. What is the name of the special synapse where a nerve cell makes contact with a muscle cell?

> **Checkpoint 7-4** What neurotransmitter is involved in the stimulation of skeletal muscle cells?

Contraction Another important property of muscle tissue is **contractility**. This is the capacity of a muscle fiber to undergo shortening and to change its shape, becoming thicker. Studies of muscle chemistry and observation of cells under the powerful electron microscope have given a concept of how muscle cells work.

These studies reveal that each skeletal muscle fiber contains many threads, or filaments, made of two kinds of proteins, called **actin** (AK-tin) and **myosin** (MI-o-sin). Filaments made of actin are thin and light; those made of myosin are thick and dark. The filaments are present in alternating bundles within the muscle cell (Fig. 7-4). It is the alternating bands of light actin and heavy myosin filaments that give skeletal muscle its striated appearance. They also give a view of what occurs when muscles contract.

Note that the actin and myosin filaments overlap where they meet, just as your fingers overlap when you fold your hands together. A contracting subunit of skeletal muscle is called a **sarcomere** (SAR-ko-mere). It consists of a band of myosin filaments and the actin filaments on each side of them (see Fig. 7-4). In movement, the myosin filaments "latch on" to the actin filaments in their overlapping region by means of many paddlelike extensions called myosin heads. In this way, the myosin heads form attachments between the actin and myosin filaments that are described as cross-bridges. Using the energy of ATP for repeated movements, the myosin heads, like the oars of a boat moving water, pull all the actin strands closer together within each sarcomere. As the overlapping filaments slide together, the

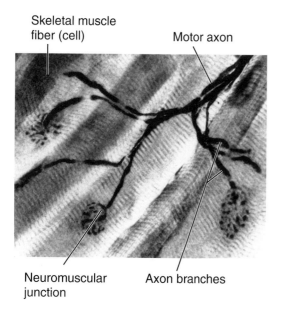

Skeletal muscle fiber (cell)

Motor axon

Neuromuscular junction

Axon branches

Figure 7-2 Nervous stimulation of skeletal muscle. A motor axon branches to stimulate multiple muscle fibers (cells). The point of contact between the neuron and the muscle cell is the neuromuscular junction. (Reprinted with permission from Cormack DH. Essential Histology. 2nd ed. Philadelphia: Lippincott Williams & Wilkins, 2001.)

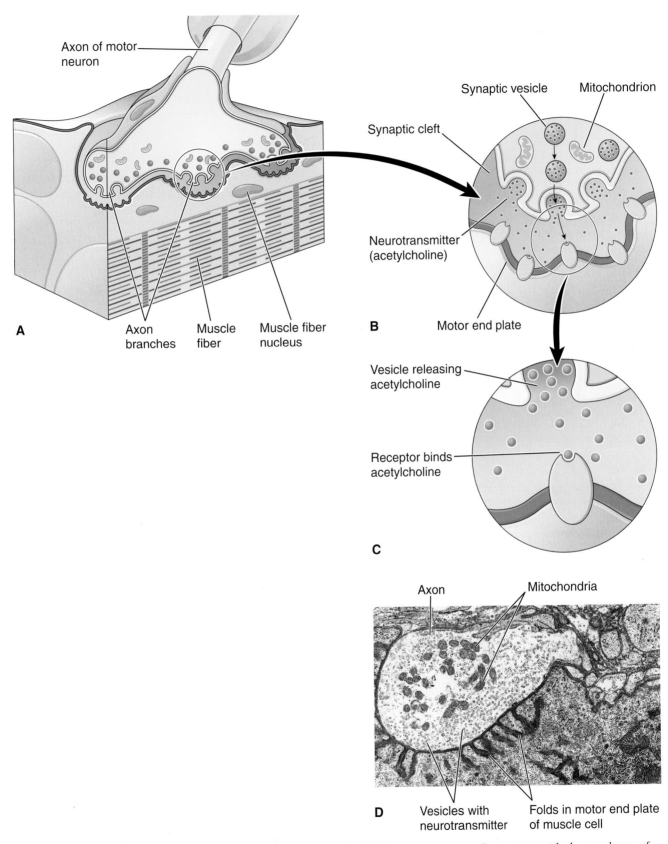

Figure 7-3 Neuromuscular junction (NMJ). (A) The branched end of a motor neuron makes contact with the membrane of a muscle fiber (cell). **(B)** Enlarged view of the NMJ showing release of neurotransmitter (acetylcholine) into the synaptic cleft. **(C)** Acetylcholine attaches to receptors in the motor end plate, whose folds increase surface area. **(D)** Electron microscope photograph of the neuromuscular junction. (D, Courtesy of A. Sima.)

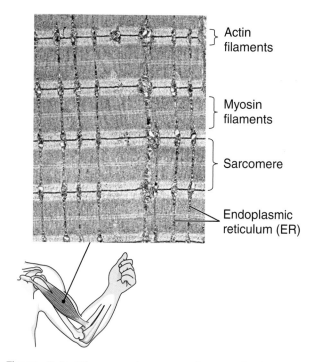

Actin filaments

Myosin filaments

Sarcomere

Endoplasmic reticulum (ER)

Figure 7-4 **Electron microscope photograph of skeletal muscle cell (×6500).** Actin makes up the light band and myosin makes up the dark band. The dark line in the actin band marks points where actin filaments are held together. A sarcomere is a contracting subunit of skeletal muscle. (Photomicrograph reprinted with permission from Ross MH, Kaye GI, Pawlina W. Histology. 4th ed. Philadelphia: Lippincott Williams & Wilkins, 2003.)

muscle fiber contracts, becoming shorter and thicker. Figure 7-5 shows a section of muscle as it contracts. Once the cross-bridges form, the myosin heads move the actin filaments forward, then they detach and move back to position for another "power stroke." Note that the filaments overlap increasingly as the cell contracts. (In reality, not all the myosin heads are moving at the same time. About one half are forward at any time, and the rest are preparing for another swing.) During contraction, each sarcomere becomes shorter, but the individual filaments do not change in length. As in shuffling a deck of cards, as you push the cards together, the deck becomes smaller, but the cards do not change in length.

Checkpoint 7-5 What are two properties of muscle cells that are needed for response to a stimulus?

Checkpoint 7-6 What are the filaments that interact to produce muscle contraction?

The Role of Calcium In additional to actin, myosin, and ATP, calcium is needed for muscle contraction. It enables cross-bridges to form between actin and myosin so the sliding filament action can begin. When muscles are at rest, two additional proteins called **troponin** (tro-PO-nin) and **tropomyosin** (tro-po-MI-o-sin) block the sites on actin filaments where cross-bridges can form (Fig. 7-6). When calcium attaches to these proteins, they

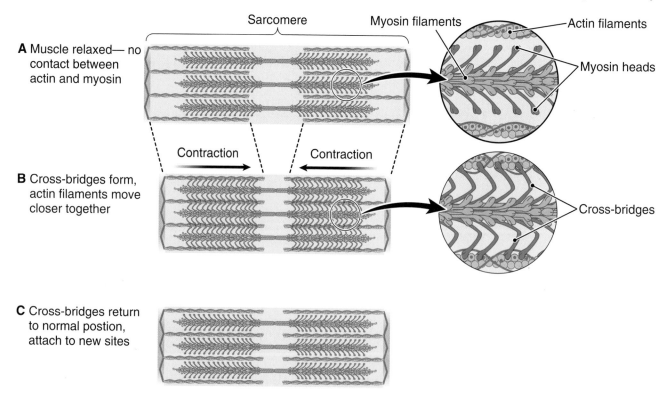

Sarcomere

Myosin filaments

Actin filaments

A Muscle relaxed— no contact between actin and myosin

Myosin heads

B Cross-bridges form, actin filaments move closer together

Contraction   Contraction

Cross-bridges

C Cross-bridges return to normal postion, attach to new sites

Figure 7-5 **Sliding filament mechanism of skeletal muscle contraction. (A)** Muscle is relaxed and there is no contact between the actin and myosin filaments. **(B)** Cross-bridges form and the actin filaments are moved closer together as the muscle fiber contracts. **(C)** The cross-bridges return to their original position and attach to new sites to prepare for another pull on the actin filaments and further contraction. *ZOOMING IN ✦ Do the actin or myosin filaments change in length as contraction proceeds?*

move aside, uncovering the binding sites. In resting muscles, the calcium is not available because it is stored within the endoplasmic reticulum (ER) of the muscle cell. It is released into the cytoplasm only when the cell is stimulated by a nerve fiber. Muscles relax when nervous stimulation stops and the calcium is then pumped back into the ER, ready for the next contraction.

A summary of the events in a muscle contraction is as follows:

1. Acetylcholine (ACh) is released from a neuron ending into the synaptic cleft at the neuromuscular junction.
2. ACh binds to the motor end plate of the muscle and produces an action potential.
3. The action potential travels to the endoplasmic reticulum (ER).
4. The endoplasmic reticulum releases calcium into the cytoplasm.
5. Calcium shifts troponin and tropomyosin so that binding sites on actin are exposed.
6. Myosin heads bind to actin, forming cross-bridges.
7. Myosin heads pull actin filaments together within the sarcomeres and cell shortens.
8. ATP is used to detach myosin heads and move them back to position for another "power stroke."
9. Muscle relaxes when stimulation ends and the calcium is pumped back into the ER.

Box 7-1, Muscle Contraction and Energy, has additional details on skeletal muscle contraction.

Energy Sources

As noted earlier, all muscle contraction requires energy in the form of ATP. The source of this energy is the oxidation (commonly called "burning") of nutrients within the cells.

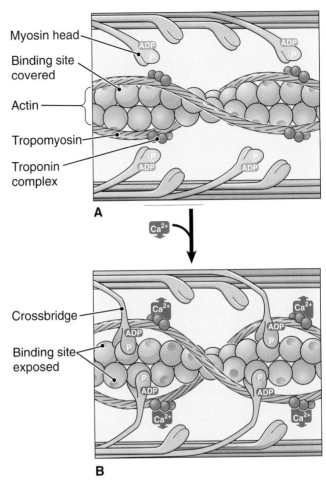

Figure 7-6 **Role of calcium in muscle contraction. (A)** Troponin and tropomyosin cover the binding sites where cross-bridges can form between actin and myosin. **(B)** Calcium shifts troponin and tropomyosin away from binding sites so cross-bridges can form.

Box 7-1 | **A Closer Look**

Muscle Contraction and Energy

When we think of muscle contraction, we might imagine a runner's rippling muscles. But muscle contraction actually occurs at a microscopic level within the sarcomere's working parts: the thick and thin filaments.

Thick filaments are composed of many myosin molecules, each shaped like two golf clubs twisted together with the myosin heads projecting away from the sarcomere's center (see Fig. 7-6). Each myosin head can bind ATP and convert it into ADP and a phosphate molecule, which remain bound. The chemical energy released during this reaction charges the myosin head, enabling it to do work.

Thin filaments' actin molecules are twisted together like two strands of beads. Each "bead" has a myosin-binding site, but the two regulatory proteins, troponin and tropomyosin, cover the binding sites when the muscle is at rest. When calcium shifts these proteins away from the binding sites, the following cycle of events occurs:

1. The charged myosin heads attach to the actin molecules and form cross-bridges between the thick and thin filaments.
2. Using their stored energy, the myosin heads pull the thin filaments to the center of the sarcomere, releasing the ADP and phosphate molecules.
3. New ATP molecules bind to the myosin heads, causing them to detach from actin and breaking the cross-bridges.
4. The myosin heads convert ATP into ADP and phosphate, which recharges them.

After death, muscles enter a stage of rigidity known as rigor mortis. This phenomenon illustrates ATP's crucial role in muscle contraction. Shortly after death, muscle cells begin to degrade. Calcium escapes into the cytoplasm, and the muscle filaments slide together. Metabolism has ceased, however, and there is no ATP to disengage the filaments, so they remain locked in a contracted state. Rigor mortis lasts about 24 hours, gradually fading as enzymes break down the muscle filaments.

To produce ATP, muscle cells must have an adequate supply of oxygen and glucose or other usable nutrient. The circulating blood constantly brings these substances to the cells, but muscle cells also store a small reserve supply of each to be used when needed, during vigorous exercise, for example. The following are compounds that store oxygen, energy, or nutrients in muscle cells:

- **Myoglobin** (mi-o-GLO-bin) stores additional oxygen. This compound is similar to the blood's hemoglobin but is located specifically in muscle cells, as indicated by the prefix *myo-* in its name.
- **Glycogen** (GLI-ko-jen) stores additional glucose. It is a polysaccharide made of multiple glucose molecules and it can be broken down into glucose when needed by the muscle cells.
- **Creatine** (KRE-ah-tin) **phosphate** stores energy. It is a compound similar to ATP, in that it has a high energy bond that releases energy when it is broken. This energy is used to make ATP for muscle contraction when the muscle cell has used up its ATP.

Checkpoint 7-7 What mineral is needed to allow actin and myosin to interact?

Checkpoint 7-8 Muscle cells obtain energy for contraction from the oxidation of nutrients. What compound is formed in oxidation that supplies the energy for contraction?

Oxygen Consumption During most activities of daily life, the tissues receive adequate oxygen, and muscles can function aerobically. During strenuous activity, however, a person may not be able to breathe in oxygen rapidly enough to meet the needs of the hard-working muscles. At first, the myoglobin, glycogen, and creatine phosphate stored in the tissues meet the increased demands, but continual exercise depletes these stores.

For a short time, glucose may be used anaerobically, that is, without the benefit of oxygen. This anaerobic process generates ATP rapidly and permits greater magnitude of activity than would otherwise be possible, as, for example, allowing sprinting instead of jogging. However, anaerobic metabolism is inefficient; it does not produce as much ATP as does metabolism in the presence of oxygen. Also, an organic acid called **lactic acid** accumulates in the cells when this alternate pathway of metabolism is used. Anaerobic metabolism can continue only until the buildup of lactic acid causes the muscles to fatigue.

Muscles operating anaerobically are in a state of **oxygen debt**. After stopping exercise, a person must continue to take in extra oxygen by continued rapid breathing (panting) until the debt is paid in full. That is, enough oxygen must be taken in to convert the lactic acid to other substances that can be metabolized further. In addition, the glycogen, myoglobin, and creatine phosphate that are stored in the cells must be replenished. The time after strenuous exercise during which extra oxygen is needed is known as the period of recovery oxygen consumption.

Checkpoint 7-9 When muscles work without oxygen, a compound is produced that causes muscle fatigue. What is the name of this compound?

Effects of Exercise

Regular exercise results in a number of changes in muscle tissue. These changes correspond to the three components of exercise: stretching, aerobics, and resistance training. When muscles are stretched, they contract more forcefully, as the internal filaments can interact over a greater length. Stretching also helps with balance and promotes flexibility at the joints. Aerobic exercise, that is, exercise that increases oxygen consumption, such as running, biking, or swimming, leads to improved endurance. Resistance training, such as weight lifting, causes muscle cells to increase in size, a condition known as hypertrophy (hi-PER-tro-fe). This change can be seen in the enlarged muscles of body-builders. Some of the changes in muscle tissue that lead to improved endurance and strength include:

- Increase in the number of capillaries in the muscle tissue, which brings more blood to the cells.
- Increase in the number of mitochondria to increase production of ATP.
- Increase in reserves of myoglobin, glycogen, and creatine phosphate to promote endurance.

An exercise program should include all three methods—stretching, aerobic exercise, and resistance training—with periods of warm-up and cool-down before and after working out. This type of varied program is described as cross-training or interval training.

In addition to affecting muscle tissue itself, exercise causes some systemic changes. The **vasodilation** (vas-o-di-LA-shun), or widening of blood vessel diameter, that occurs during exercise allows blood to flow more easily to muscle tissue. With continued work, more blood is pumped back to the heart. The temporarily increased load on the heart strengthens the heart muscle and improves its circulation. With exercise training, the chambers of the heart gradually enlarge to accommodate more blood. The resting heart rate of a trained athlete is lower than the average rate because the heart can function more efficiently.

Regular exercise also improves breathing and respiratory efficiency. Circulation in the capillaries surrounding the alveoli (air sacs) is increased, and this brings about enhanced gas exchange. The more efficient distribution and use of oxygen delays the onset of oxygen debt. Even moderate regular exercise has the additional benefits of weight control, strengthening of the bones, decreased blood pressure, and decreased risk of heart attacks. The effects of exercise on the body are studied in the fields of

Anabolic Steroids: Winning at All Costs?

Anabolic steroids mimic the effects of the male sex hormone testosterone by promoting metabolism and stimulating growth. These drugs are legally prescribed to promote muscle regeneration and prevent atrophy from disuse after surgery. However, athletes also purchase them illegally, using them to increase muscle size and strength and improve endurance.

When steroids are used illegally to enhance athletic performance, the doses needed are large enough to cause serious side effects. They increase blood cholesterol levels, which may lead to atherosclerosis, heart disease, kidney failure, and stroke. Steroids damage the liver, making it more susceptible to disease and cancer, and suppress the immune system, increasing the risk of infection and cancer. In men, steroids cause impotence, testicular atrophy, low sperm count, infertility, and the development of female sex characteristics such as breasts (gynecomastia). In women, steroids disrupt ovulation and menstruation and produce male sex characteristics such as breast atrophy, enlargement of the clitoris, increased body hair, and deepening of the voice. In both sexes steroids increase the risk for baldness and, especially in men, cause mood swings, depression, and violence.

---

sports medicine and exercise physiology. Box 7-2, Anabolic Steroids: Winning at all Costs?, has information on how steroids affect muscles.

Types of Muscle Contractions

Muscle **tone** refers to a partially contracted state of the muscles that is normal even when the muscles are not in use. The maintenance of this tone, or **tonus** (TO-nus), is due to the action of the nervous system in keeping the muscles in a constant state of readiness for action. Muscles that are little used soon become flabby, weak, and lacking in tone.

In addition to the partial contractions that are responsible for muscle tone, there are two other types of contractions on which the body depends:

▸ **Isotonic** (i-so-TON-ik) **contractions** are those in which the tone or tension within the muscle remains the same but the muscle as a whole shortens, producing movement; that is, work is accomplished. Lifting weights, walking, running, or any other activity in which the muscles become shorter and thicker (forming bulges) are isotonic contractions.

▸ **Isometric** (i-so-MET-rik) **contractions** are those in which there is no change in muscle length but there is a great increase in muscle tension. Pushing against an immovable force produces an isometric contraction. For example, if you push the palms of your hands hard against each other, there is no movement, but you can feel the increased tension in your arm muscles.

Most movements of the body involve a combination of both isotonic and isometric contractions. When walking, for example, some muscles contract isotonically to propel the body forward, but at the same time, other muscles are contracting isometrically to keep your body in position.

▸ The Mechanics of Muscle Movement

Most muscles have two or more points of attachment to the skeleton. The muscle is attached to a bone at each end by means of a cordlike extension called a **tendon** (Fig. 7-7). All of the connective tissue within and around the muscle merges to form the tendon, which then attaches directly to the periosteum of the bone (see Fig. 7-1). In some instances, a broad sheet called an **aponeurosis** (ap-o-nu-RO-sis) may attach muscles to bones or to other muscles.

In moving the bones, one end of a muscle is attached to a more freely movable part of the skeleton, and the other end is attached to a relatively stable part. The less movable (more fixed) attachment is called the **origin**; the attachment to the part of the body that the muscle puts into action is called the **insertion**. When a muscle contracts, it pulls on both points of attachment, bringing the more movable insertion closer to the origin and thereby causing movement

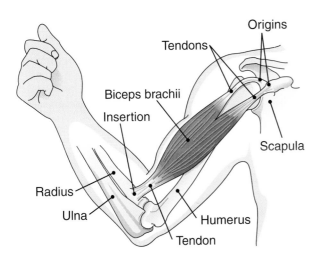

Figure 7-7 Muscle attachments to bones. Three attachments are shown—two origins and one insertion. *ZOOMING IN ✦ Does contraction of the biceps brachii produce flexion or extension at the elbow?*

of the body part. Figure 7-7 shows the action of the biceps brachii (in the upper arm) in flexing the arm at the elbow. The insertion on the radius of the forearm is brought toward the origin at the scapula of the shoulder girdle.

> **Checkpoint 7-10** Muscles are attached to bones by means of tendons: one attached to a less movable part of the skeleton, and one attached to a movable part. What are the names of these two attachment points?

Muscles Work Together

Many of the skeletal muscles function in pairs. A movement is performed by a muscle called the **prime mover**; the muscle that produces an opposite movement to that of the prime mover is known as the **antagonist**. Clearly, for any given movement, the antagonist must relax when the prime mover contracts. For example, when the biceps brachii at the front of the arm contracts to flex the arm, the triceps brachii at the back must relax; when the triceps brachii contracts to extend the arm, the biceps brachii must relax. In addition to prime movers and antagonists, there are also muscles that serve to steady body parts or to assist prime movers. These "helping" muscles are called **synergists** (SIN-er-jists), because they work with the prime movers to accomplish a movement.

As the muscles work together, body movements are coordinated, and a large number of complicated movements can be carried out. At first, however, the nervous system must learn to coordinate any new, complicated movement. Think of a child learning to walk or to write, and consider the number of muscles she or he uses unnecessarily or forgets to use when the situation calls for them.

> **Checkpoint 7-11** Muscles work together to produce movement. What is the name of the muscle that produces a movement as compared with the muscle that produces an opposite movement?

Levers and Body Mechanics

Proper body mechanics help conserve energy and ensure freedom from strain and fatigue; conversely, such ailments as lower back pain—a common complaint—can be traced to poor body mechanics. Body mechanics have special significance to healthcare workers, who are frequently called on to move patients and handle cumbersome equipment. Maintaining the body segments in correct relation to one another has a direct effect on the working capacity of the vital organs that are supported by the skeleton.

If you have had a course in physics, recall your study of levers. A lever is simply a rigid bar that moves about a fixed pivot point, the fulcrum. There are three classes of levers, which differ only in the location of the fulcrum (F), the effort (E), or force, and the resistance (R), the weight or load. In a first-class lever, the fulcrum is located between the resistance and the effort; a see-saw or a scissors is an example of this class (Fig. 7-8 A). The second-class lever has the resistance located between the fulcrum and the effort; a wheelbarrow or a mattress lifted at one end is an illustration of this class (Fig. 7-8 B). In the third-class lever, the effort is between the resistance and the fulcrum. A forceps or a tweezers is an example of this type of lever. The effort is applied in the center of the tool, between the fulcrum, where the pieces join, and the resistance at the tip.

The musculoskeletal system can be considered a system of levers, in which the bone is the lever, the joint is the fulcrum, and the force is applied by a muscle. An example of a first-class lever in the body is using the muscles at the back of the neck to lift the head at the joint between the occipital bone of the skull and the first cervical vertebra (atlas) (see Fig. 7-8). A second-class lever is exemplified by raising your weight to the ball of your foot (the fulcrum) using muscles of the calf.

However, there are very few examples of first- and second-class levers in the body. Most lever systems in the body are of the third-class type. A muscle usually inserts over a joint and exerts force between the fulcrum and the resistance. That is, the fulcrum is behind both the point of effort and the weight. As shown in Figure 7-8 C, when the biceps brachii flexes the forearm at the elbow, the muscle exerts its force at its insertion on the radius. The weight of the hand and forearm creates the resistance, and the fulcrum is the elbow joint, which is behind the point of effort.

By understanding and applying knowledge of levers to body mechanics, the healthcare worker can improve his or her skill in carrying out numerous clinical maneuvers and procedures.

> **Checkpoint 7-12** Muscles and bones work together as lever systems. Of the three classes of levers, which one represents the action of most muscles?

▶ Skeletal Muscle Groups

The study of muscles is made simpler by grouping them according to body regions. Knowing how muscles are named can also help in remembering them. A number of different characteristics are used in naming muscles, including the following:

- Location, named for a nearby bone, for example, or for position, such as lateral, medial, internal, or external.
- Size, using terms such as maximus, major, minor, longus, brevis.
- Shape, such as circular (orbicularis), triangular (deltoid), trapezoid (trapezius).
- Direction of fibers, including straight (rectus) or angled (oblique).
- Number of heads (attachment points) as indicated by the suffix -ceps, as in biceps, triceps, quadriceps.
- Action, as in flexor, extensor, adductor, abductor, levator.

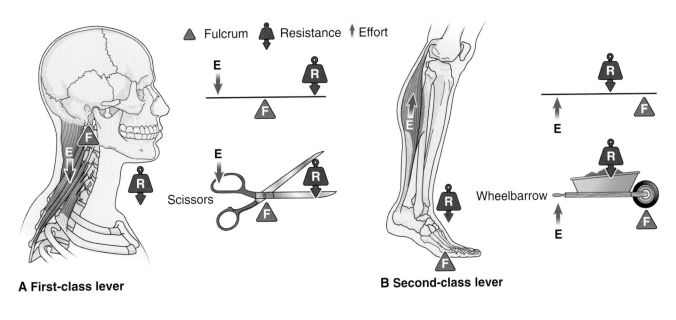

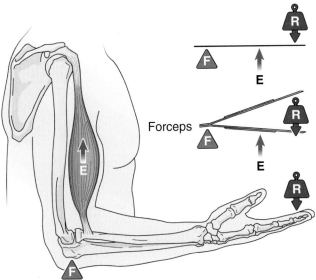

A First-class lever

B Second-class lever

C Third-class lever

Figure 7-8   Levers. Three classes of levers are shown along with tools and anatomic examples that illustrate each type. R = resistance (weight); E = effort (force); F = fulcrum (pivot point).

Often, more than one feature is used in naming. Refer to Figures 7-9 and 7-10 as you study the locations and functions of some of the skeletal muscles and try to figure out why each has the name that it does. Although they are described in the singular, most of the muscles are present on both sides of the body.

Muscles of the Head

The principal muscles of the head are those of facial expression and of mastication (chewing) (Fig. 7-11, Table 7-3).

The muscles of facial expression include ring-shaped ones around the eyes and the lips, called the **orbicularis** (or-bik-u-LAH-ris) **muscles** because of their shape (think

of "orbit"). The muscle surrounding each eye is called the **orbicularis oculi** (OK-u-li), whereas the muscle of the lips is the **orbicularis oris.** These muscles, of course, all have antagonists. For example, the **levator palpebrae** (PAL-pe-bre) **superioris,** or lifter of the upper eyelid, is the antagonist for the orbicularis oculi.

One of the largest muscles of expression forms the fleshy part of the cheek and is called the **buccinator** (BUK-se-na-tor). Used in whistling or blowing, it is sometimes referred to as the trumpeter's muscle. You can readily think of other muscles of facial expression: for instance, the antagonists of the orbicularis oris can produce a smile, a sneer, or a grimace. There are a number of scalp muscles by means of which the eyebrows are lifted or drawn together into a frown.

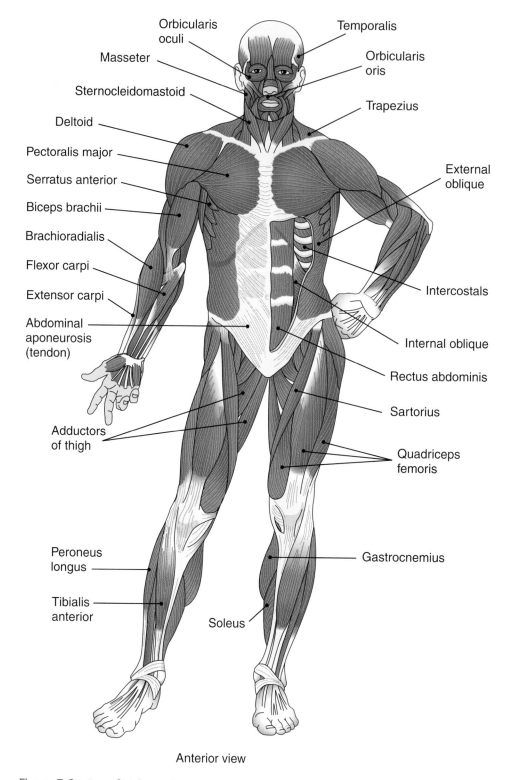

Orbicularis oculi

Temporalis

Masseter

Orbicularis oris

Sternocleidomastoid

Trapezius

Deltoid

Pectoralis major

External oblique

Serratus anterior

Biceps brachii

Brachioradialis

Flexor carpi

Extensor carpi

Intercostals

Abdominal aponeurosis (tendon)

Internal oblique

Rectus abdominis

Sartorius

Adductors of thigh

Quadriceps femoris

Peroneus longus

Gastrocnemius

Tibialis anterior

Soleus

Anterior view

Figure 7-9 Superficial muscles, anterior view. Associated structure is labeled in parentheses.

There are four pairs of muscles of mastication, all of which insert on and move the mandible. The largest are the **temporalis** (TEM-po-ral-is), which is superior to the ear, and the **masseter** (mas-SE-ter) at the angle of the jaw.

The tongue has two groups of muscles. The first group, called the **intrinsic muscles**, is located entirely within the tongue. The second group, the **extrinsic muscles**, originates outside the tongue. It is because of these many muscles that the tongue has such remarkable flexibility and can perform so many different functions. Consider the intricate tongue motions involved in speaking, chewing, and swallowing.

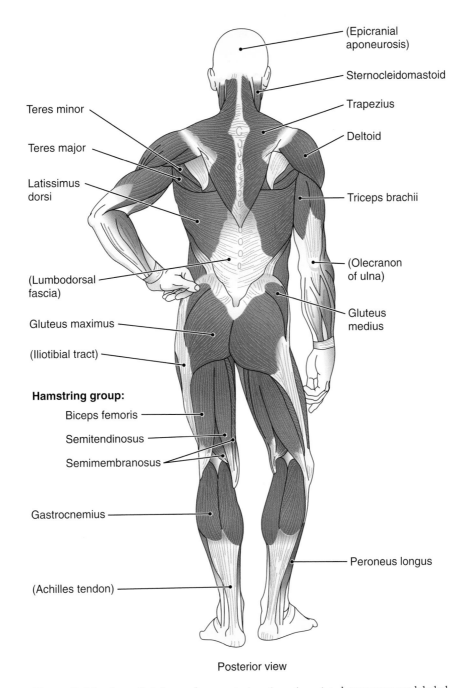

Teres minor

Teres major

Latissimus dorsi

(Lumbodorsal fascia)

Gluteus maximus

(Iliotibial tract)

Hamstring group:

Biceps femoris

Semitendinosus

Semimembranosus

Gastrocnemius

(Achilles tendon)

(Epicranial aponeurosis)

Sternocleidomastoid

Trapezius

Deltoid

Triceps brachii

(Olecranon of ulna)

Gluteus medius

Peroneus longus

Posterior view

Figure 7-10 Superficial muscles, posterior view. Associated structures are labeled in parentheses.

Figure 7-11 shows some additional muscles of the face.

Muscles of the Neck

The neck muscles tend to be ribbonlike and extend up and down or obliquely in several layers and in a complex manner (Fig. 7-11, Table 7-3). The one you will hear of most frequently is the **sternocleidomastoid** (ster-no-kli-do-MAS-toyd), sometimes referred to simply as the ster-nomastoid. This strong muscle extends superiorly from the sternum across the side of the neck to the mastoid process. When the left and right muscles work together, they bring the head forward on the chest (flexion). Working alone, each muscle tilts and rotates the head so as to orient the face toward the side opposite that muscle. If the head is abnormally fixed in this position, the person is said to have **torticollis** (tor-tih-KOL-is), or wryneck; this condition may be due to injury or spasm of the muscle.

A portion of the trapezius muscle (described later) is located at the posterior of the neck, where it helps hold

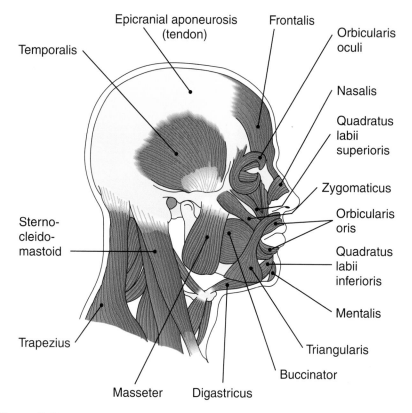

Temporalis

Epicranial aponeurosis (tendon)

Frontalis

Orbicularis oculi

Nasalis

Quadratus labii superioris

Zygomaticus

Orbicularis oris

Quadratus labii inferioris

Mentalis

Triangularis

Buccinator

Digastricus

Masseter

Trapezius

Sterno-cleido-mastoid

Figure 7-11 Muscles of the head. Associated structure is labeled in parentheses. *ZOOMING IN ✦ Which of the muscles in this illustration is named for a bone it is near?*

Muscles That Move the Shoulder and Arm

The position of the shoulder depends to a large extent on the degree of contraction of the **trapezius** (trah-PE-ze-us), a triangular muscle that covers the posterior neck and extends across the posterior shoulder to insert on the clavicle and scapula (Fig. 7-10, Table 7-4). The trapezius muscles enable one to raise the shoulders and pull them back. The upper portion of each trapezius can also extend the head and turn it from side to side.

The **latissimus** (lah-TIS-ih-mus) **dorsi** is the wide muscle of the back and lateral trunk. It originates from the vertebral spine in the middle and lower back and covers the lower half of the thoracic region, forming the posterior portion of the axilla (armpit). The fibers of each muscle converge to a tendon that inserts on the humerus. The latissimus dorsi powerfully extends the arm, bringing it down forcibly as, for example, in swimming.

A large **pectoralis** (pek-to-RAL-is) **major** is located on either side of the superior part of the chest (see Fig. 7-9). This muscle arises from the sternum, the upper ribs, and the clavicle and forms the anterior "wall" of the armpit, or axilla; it inserts on the superior part of the humerus. The pectoralis major flexes and adducts the arm, pulling it across the chest.

The **serratus** (ser-RA-tus) **anterior** is below the axilla, on the lateral part of the chest. It originates on the upper eight or nine ribs on the lateral and anterior thorax and inserts in the scapula on the side toward the vertebrae. The serratus anterior moves the scapula forward when, for example, one is pushing something. It also aids in raising the arm above the horizontal level.

The **deltoid** covers the shoulder joint and is responsible for the roundness of the upper part of the arm just inferior to the shoulder (see Figs. 7-9 and 7-10). This muscle is named for its triangular shape, which resembles the Greek letter delta. The deltoid is often used as an injection site. Arising from the shoulder girdle (clavicle and scapula), the deltoid fibers converge to insert on the lateral surface of the humerus. Contraction of this muscle abducts the arm, raising it laterally to the horizontal position.

The shoulder joint allows for a very wide range of movement. This freedom

the head up (extension). Other larger deep muscles are the chief extensors of the head and neck.

Muscles of the Upper Extremities

Muscles of the upper extremities include the muscles that determine the position of the shoulder, the anterior and posterior muscles that move the arm, and the muscles that move the forearm and hand.

Table 7·3	Muscles of the Head and Neck*	
NAME	**LOCATION**	**FUNCTION**
Orbicularis oculi	Encircles eyelid	Closes eye
Levator palpebrae superioris (deep muscle; not shown)	Back of orbit to upper eyelid	Opens eye
Orbicularis oris	Encircles mouth	Closes lips
Buccinator	Fleshy part of cheek	Flattens cheek; helps in eating, whistling, and blowing wind instruments
Temporalis	Above and near ear	Closes jaw
Masseter	At angle of jaw	Closes jaw
Sternocleidomastoid	Along side of neck, to mastoid process	Flexes head; rotates head toward opposite side from muscle

These and other muscles of the face are shown in Fig. 7–11.

Table 7·4	Muscles of the Upper Extremities*	
NAME	**LOCATION**	**FUNCTION**
Trapezius	Posterior of neck and upper back, to clavicle and scapula	Raises shoulder and pulls it back; extends head
Latissimus dorsi	Middle and lower back, to humerus	Extends and adducts arm behind back
Pectoralis major	Superior, anterior chest, to humerus	Flexes and adducts arm across chest; pulls shoulder forward and downward
Serratus anterior	Below axilla on lateral chest to scapula	Moves scapula forward; aids in raising arm, punching, or reaching forward
Deltoid	Covers shoulder joint, to lateral humerus	Abducts arm
Biceps brachii	Anterior arm along humerus, to radius	Flexes forearm at the elbow and supinates hand
Brachioradialis	Lateral forearm from distal end of humerus to distal end of radius	Flexes forearm at the elbow
Triceps brachii	Posterior arm, to ulna	Extends forearm to straighten upper extremity
Flexor carpi groups	Anterior forearm, to hand	Flex hand
Extensor carpi groups	Posterior forearm, to hand	Extend hand
Flexor digitorum groups	Anterior forearm, to fingers	Flex fingers
Extensor digitorum groups	Posterior forearm, to fingers	Extend fingers

These and other muscles of the upper extremities are shown in Figs. 7–9, 7–10, and 7–12.

of movement is possible because the humerus fits into a shallow socket, the glenoid cavity of the scapula. This joint requires the support of four deep muscles and their tendons, which compose the **rotator cuff**. The four muscles are the supraspinatus, infraspinatus, teres minor, and subscapularis, known together as SITS, based on the first letters of their names. In certain activities, such as swinging a golf club, playing tennis, or pitching a baseball, the muscles of the rotator cuff may be injured, even torn, and may require surgery for repair.

Muscles That Move the Forearm and Hand

The **biceps brachii** (BRA-ke-i), located at the anterior arm along the humerus, is the muscle you usually display when you want to "flex your muscles" to show your strength (Fig. 7-12 A). It inserts on the radius and flexes the forearm. It is a supinator of the hand.

Another flexor of the forearm at the elbow is the **brachioradialis** (bra-ke-o-ra-de-A-lis), a prominent muscle of the forearm that originates at the distal end of the humerus and inserts on the distal radius.

The **triceps brachii**, located on the posterior of the arm, inserts on the olecranon of the ulna (Fig. 7-12 B). It is used to straighten the arm, as in lowering a weight from an arm curl. It is also important in pushing because it converts the arm and forearm into a sturdy rod.

Most of the muscles that move the hand and fingers originate from the radius and the ulna (see Fig. 7-12). Some of them insert on the carpal bones of the wrist, whereas others have long tendons that cross the wrist and insert on bones of the hand and the fingers.

The **flexor carpi** and the **extensor carpi muscles** are responsible for many movements of the hand. Muscles that produce finger movements are the several **flexor digitorum** (dij-e-TO-rum) and the **extensor digitorum muscles**. The names of these muscles may include bones they are near, their action, or their length, for example, longus for long and brevis for short.

Special groups of muscles in the fleshy parts of the hand are responsible for the intricate movements that can be performed with the thumb and the fingers. The thumb's freedom of movement has been one of the most useful capacities of humans.

Muscles of the Trunk

The muscles of the trunk include the muscles involved in breathing, the thin muscle layers of the abdomen, and the muscles of the pelvic floor. The following discussion also includes the deep muscles of the back that support and move the vertebral column.

Muscles of Respiration

The most important muscle involved in the act of breathing is the **diaphragm**. This dome-shaped muscle forms the partition between the thoracic cavity superiorly and the abdominal cavity inferiorly (Fig. 7-13). When the diaphragm contracts, the central dome-shaped portion is pulled downward, thus enlarging the thoracic cavity from top to bottom.

The **intercostal muscles** are attached to and fill the spaces between the ribs. The external and internal intercostals run at angles in opposite directions. Contraction of the intercostal muscles serves to elevate the ribs, thus enlarging the thoracic cavity from side to side and from anterior to posterior. The mechanics of breathing are described in Chapter 16.

Checkpoint 7-13 What muscle is most important in breathing?

Muscles of the Abdomen and Pelvis

The wall of the abdomen has three layers of muscle that extend from the back (dorsally) and around the sides (laterally) to the front (ventrally) (Fig. 7-14, Table 7-5). They are the **ex-**

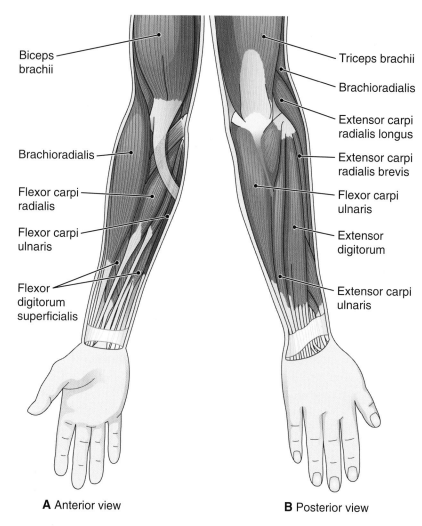

Biceps brachii

Brachioradialis

Flexor carpi radialis

Flexor carpi ulnaris

Flexor digitorum superficialis

Triceps brachii

Brachioradialis

Extensor carpi radialis longus

Extensor carpi radialis brevis

Flexor carpi ulnaris

Extensor digitorum

Extensor carpi ulnaris

A Anterior view   **B** Posterior view

Figure 7-12   **Muscles that move the forearm and hand.**

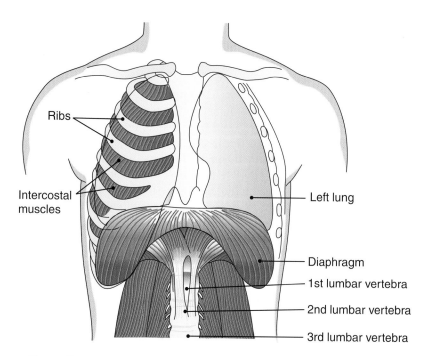

Ribs

Intercostal muscles

Left lung

Diaphragm

1st lumbar vertebra

2nd lumbar vertebra

3rd lumbar vertebra

Figure 7-13   **Muscles of respiration.** Associated structures are also shown.

ternal **oblique** on the outside, the **internal oblique** in the middle, and the **transversus abdominis**, the innermost. The connective tissue from these muscles extends forward and encloses the vertical **rectus abdominis** of the anterior abdominal wall. The fibers of these muscles, as well as their connective tissue extensions (aponeuroses), run in different directions, resembling the layers in plywood and resulting in a strong abdominal wall. The midline meeting of the aponeuroses forms a whitish area called the **linea alba** (LIN-e-ah AL-ba), which is an important landmark on the abdomen. It extends from the tip of the sternum to the pubic joint.

These four pairs of abdominal muscles act together to protect the internal organs and compress the abdominal cavity, as in coughing, emptying the bladder (urination) and bowel (defecation), sneezing, vomiting, and childbirth (labor). The two oblique muscles and the rectus abdominis help bend the trunk forward and sideways.

The pelvic floor, or **perineum** (per-ih-NE-um), has its own form of diaphragm, shaped somewhat like a shallow dish. One of the principal muscles of this pelvic diaphragm is the **levator ani** (le-VA-tor A-ni), which acts on the rectum and thus aids in defecation. The superficial and deep muscles of the female perineum are shown in Figure 7-15 along with some associated structures.

Checkpoint 7-14 What structural feature gives strength to the muscles of the abdominal wall?

Deep Muscles of the Back The deep muscles of the back, which act on the vertebral column itself, are thick vertical masses that lie under the trapezius and latissimus dorsi. The **erector spinae** muscles make up a large group located between the sacrum and the skull. These muscles extend the spine and maintain the vertebral column in an erect posture. The muscles can be strained in lifting heavy objects if the spine is flexed while lifting. One should bend at the hip and knee in-

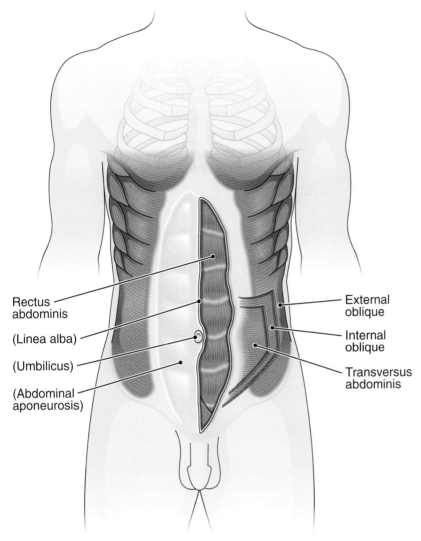

Rectus abdominis

(Linea alba)

(Umbilicus)

(Abdominal aponeurosis)

External oblique

Internal oblique

Transversus abdominis

Figure 7-14 **Muscles of the abdominal wall.** Surface tissue is removed on the right side to show deeper muscles. Associated structures are labeled in parentheses.

Table 7·5	Muscles of the Trunk*	
NAME	**LOCATION**	**FUNCTION**
Diaphragm	Dome-shaped partition between thoracic and abdominal cavities	Dome descends to enlarge thoracic cavity from top to bottom
Intercostals	Between ribs	Elevate ribs and enlarge thoracic cavity
Muscles of abdominal wall: External oblique Internal oblique Transversus abdominis Rectus abdominis	Anterolateral abdominal wall	Compress abdominal cavity and expel substances from body; flex spinal column
Levator ani	Pelvic floor	Aids defecation
Erector spinae (deep; not shown)	Group of deep vertical muscles betweeen the sacrum and skull	Extends vertebral column to produce erect posture

These and other muscles of the trunk are shown in Figs. 7–13, 7–14 and 7–15.

stead and use the thigh and buttock muscles to help in lifting.

Deeper muscles in the lumbar area extend the vertebral column in that region. These deep muscles of the back are not shown in the illustrations.

Muscles of the Lower Extremities

The muscles in the lower extremities, among the longest and strongest muscles in the body, are specialized for locomotion and balance. They include the muscles that move the thigh and leg and those that control movement of the foot.

Muscles that Move the Thigh and Leg The **gluteus maximus** (GLU-te-us MAK-sim-us), which forms much of the fleshy part of the buttock, is relatively large in humans because of its support function when a person is standing in the erect position (Fig. 7-10, Table 7-6). This muscle extends the thigh and is important in walking and running. The **gluteus medius**, which is partially covered by the gluteus maximus, abducts the thigh. It is one of the sites used for intramuscular injections.

The **iliopsoas** (il-e-o-SO-as) arises from the ilium and the bodies of the lumbar vertebrae; it crosses the anterior of the hip joint to insert on the femur (Fig. 7-16 A). It is a powerful flexor of the thigh and helps keep the trunk from falling backward when one is standing erect.

The **adductor muscles** are located on the medial part of the thigh. They arise from the pubis and ischium and insert on the femur. These strong muscles press the thighs together, as in grasping a saddle between the knees when riding a horse. They include the **adductor longus** and **adductor magnus**.

The **sartorius** (sar-TO-re-us) is a long, narrow muscle that begins at the iliac spine, winds downward and inward across the entire thigh, and ends on the upper medial surface of the tibia. It is called the tailor's muscle because it is used in crossing the legs in

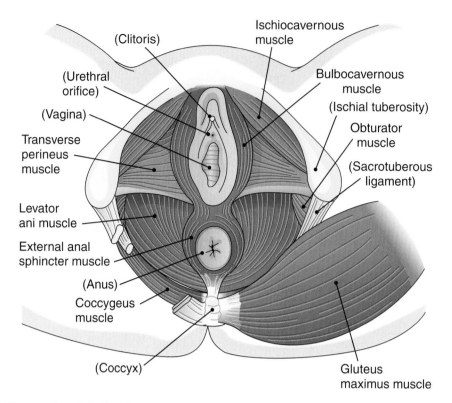

Figure 7-15 **Muscles of the female perineum (pelvic floor).** Associated structures are labeled in parentheses.

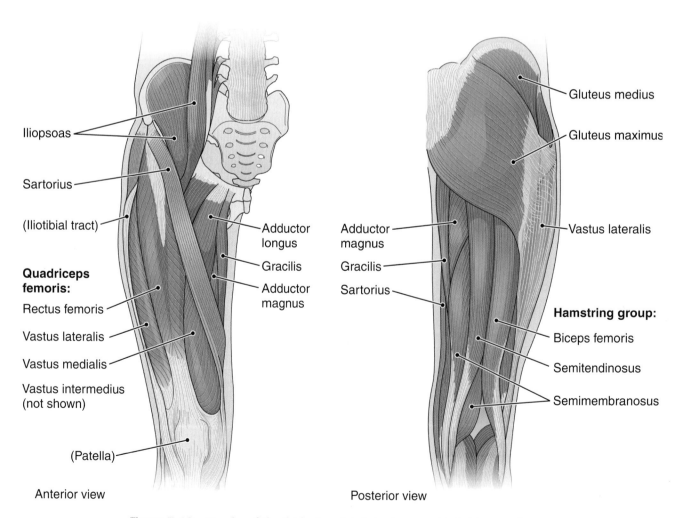

Anterior view

Posterior view

Figure 7-16 **Muscles of the thigh.** Associated structures are labeled in parentheses.

Table 7·6 Muscles of the Lower Extremities*

NAME	LOCATION	FUNCTION
Gluteus maximus	Superficial buttock, to femur	Extends thigh
Gluteus medius	Deep buttock, to femur	Abducts thigh
Iliopsoas	Crosses front of hip joint, to femur	Flexes thigh
Adductor group (e.g., adductor longus, adductor magnus)	Medial thigh, to femur	Adducts thigh
Sartorius	Winds down thigh, ilium to tibia	Flexes thigh and leg (to sit cross-legged)
Gracilis	Pubic bone to medial surface of tibia	Adducts thigh at hip; flexes leg at knee
Quadriceps femoris: Rectus femoris Vastus medialis Vastus lateralis Vastus intermedius (deep; not shown)	Anterior thigh, to tibia	Extends leg
Hamstring group: Biceps femoris Semimembranosus Semitendinosus	Posterior thigh, to tibia and fibula	Flexes leg
Gastrocnemius	Calf of leg, to calcaneus, inserting by the Achilles tendon	Plantar flexes foot at ankle (as in tiptoeing)
Soleus	Posterior leg deep to gastrocnemius	Plantar flexes foot at ankle
Tibialis anterior	Anterior and lateral shin, to foot	Dorsiflexes foot (as in walking on heels); inverts foot (sole inward)
Peroneus longus	Lateral leg, to foot	Everts foot (sole outward)
Flexor digitorum groups	Posterior leg and foot to inferior surface of toe bones	Flex toes
Extensor digitorum groups	Anterior surface of leg bones to superior surface of toe bones	Extend toes

These and other muscles of the lower extremities are shown in Figs. 7–16 and 7–17.

the manner of tailors, who in days gone by sat cross-legged on the floor. The **gracilis** (grah-SIL-is) extends from the pubic bone to the medial surface of the tibia. It adducts the thigh at the hip and flexes the leg at the knee.

The anterior and lateral femur are covered by the **quadriceps femoris** (KWOD-re-seps FEM-or-is), a large muscle that has four heads of origin. The individual parts are as follows: in the center, covering the anterior thigh, the **rectus femoris**; on either side, the **vastus medialis** and **vastus lateralis**; deeper in the center, the **vastus intermedius.** One of these muscles (rectus femoris) originates from the ilium, and the other three are from the femur, but all four have a common tendon of insertion on the tibia. You may remember that this is the tendon that encloses the knee cap, or patella. This muscle extends the

leg, as in kicking a ball. The vastus lateralis is also a site for intramuscular injections.

The **hamstring muscles** are located in the posterior part of the thigh (see Fig. 7-16 B). Their tendons can be felt behind the knee as they descend to insert on the tibia and fibula. The hamstrings flex the leg on the thigh, as in kneeling. Individually, moving from lateral to medial position, they are the **biceps femoris**, the **semimembranosus**, and the **semitendinosus.** The name of this muscle group refers to the tendons at the back of the knee by which these muscles insert on the leg.

Muscles That Move the Foot

The **gastrocnemius** (gas-trok-NE-me-us) is the chief muscle of the calf of the leg (its name means "belly of the leg") (Fig. 7-17). It has been called the toe dancer's muscle because it is used in standing on tiptoe. It ends near the heel in a prominent cord called the **Achilles tendon** (see Fig. 7-17 B), which attaches to the calcaneus (heel bone). The Achilles tendon is the largest tendon in the body. According to Greek mythology, the region above the heel was the only place that Achilles was vulnerable, and if the Achilles tendon is cut, it is impossible to walk. The **soleus** (SO-le-us) is a flat muscle deep to the gastrocnemius. It also inserts by means of the Achilles tendon and, like the gastrocnemius, flexes the foot at the ankle.

Another leg muscle that acts on the foot is the **tibialis** (tib-e-A-lis) **anterior,** located on the anterior region of the leg (see Fig. 7-17 A). This muscle performs the opposite function of the gastrocnemius. Walking on the heels uses the tibialis anterior to raise the rest of the foot off the ground (dorsiflexion). This muscle is also responsible for inversion of the foot. The muscle for eversion of the foot is the **peroneus** (per-o-NE-us) **longus,** located on the lateral part of the leg. The long tendon of this muscle crosses under the foot, forming a sling that supports the transverse (metatarsal) arch.

The toes, like the fingers, are provided with flexor and extensor muscles. The tendons of the extensor muscles are located in superior part of the foot and insert on the superior surface of the phalanges (toe bones). The flexor digitorum tendons cross the sole of the foot and insert on the undersurface of the phalanges.

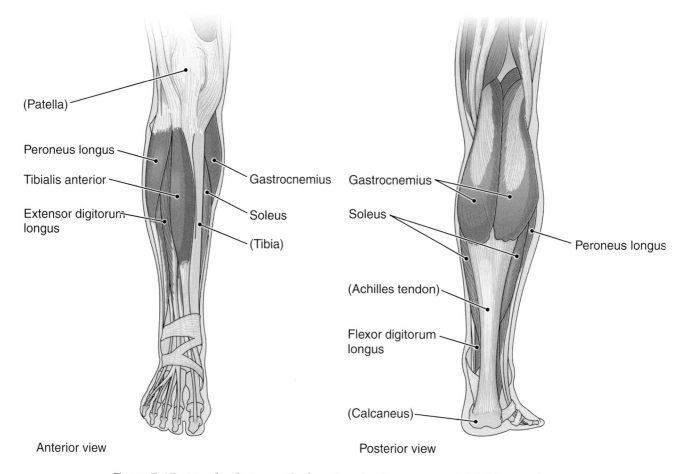

(Patella)

Peroneus longus

Tibialis anterior

Extensor digitorum longus

Gastrocnemius

Soleus

(Tibia)

Gastrocnemius

Soleus

Peroneus longus

(Achilles tendon)

Flexor digitorum longus

(Calcaneus)

Anterior view

Posterior view

Figure 7-17   Muscles that move the foot. Associated structures are labeled in parentheses.

▶ Effects of Aging on Muscles

Beginning at about 40 years of age, there is a gradual loss of muscle cells with a resulting decrease in the size of each individual muscle. There is also a loss of power, notably in the extensor muscles, such as the large sacrospinalis near the vertebral column. This causes the "bent over" appearance of a hunchback (kyphosis), which in women is often referred to as the *dowager's hump*. Sometimes, there is a tendency to bend (flex) the

---

Box 7-3 · Health Professions

Careers in Physical Therapy

Physical therapy restores mobility and relieves back pain, arthritis, and joint and muscle injuries. Individuals with heart disease and brain injury, or those who are recovering from burns or major surgery, may benefit as well.

Physical therapists work closely with physicians, nurses, occupational therapists, speech pathologists, and audiologists. Some treat a wide range of ailments, whereas others specialize in pediatrics, geriatrics, orthopedics, sports medicine, neurology, or cardiology. Regardless of specialty, physical therapists are responsible for examining their patients and developing individualized treatment programs. The examination includes a medical history and tests measuring strength, mobility, balance, coordination, and endurance. The treatment plan may include stretching and exercise to improve mobility; hot packs, cold compresses, and massage to reduce pain; as well

as the use of crutches, prostheses, and wheelchairs. Physical therapist assistants are responsible for implementing the treatment plan, teaching patients exercises and equipment use, and reporting results back to the physical therapist. To perform these duties, both physical therapists and assistants need a thorough understanding of anatomy and physiology. Most physical therapists in the United States have bachelor's or master's degrees and must pass a national licensing exam. Assistants typically train in a two-year program.

Physical therapists and physical therapist assistants practice in hospitals and clinics and may also visit homes and schools. As the American population continues to age and the need for rehabilitative therapy increases, job prospects are good. For more information about careers in physical therapy, contact the American Physical Therapy Association.

hips and knees. In addition to causing the previously noted changes in the vertebral column (see Chapter 6), these effects on the extensor muscles result in a further decrease in the elderly person's height. Activity and exercise throughout life delay and decrease these undesirable effects of aging. Even among the elderly, resistance exercise, such as weight lifting, increases muscle strength and function. See Box 7-3, Careers in Physical Therapy, for information on how physical therapists participate in treatment of muscular disorders.

Word Anatomy

Medical terms are built from standardized word parts (prefixes, roots, and suffixes). Learning the meanings of these parts can help you remember words and interpret unfamiliar terms.

WORD PART	MEANING	EXAMPLE
The Muscular System		
my/o	muscle	The *endomysium* is the deepest layer of connective tissue around muscle cells.
sarc/o	flesh	A *sarcomere* is a contracting subunit of skeletal muscle.
troph/o	nutrition, nurture	Muscles undergo *hypertrophy*, an increase in size, under the effects of resistance training.
vas/o	vessel	*Vasodilation* (widening) of the blood vessels in muscle tissue during exercise brings more blood into the tissue.
iso-	same, equal	In an *isotonic* contraction, muscle tone remains the same, but the muscle shortens.
ton/o	tone, tension	See preceding example.
metr/o	measure	In an *isometric* contraction, muscle length remains the same, but muscle tension increases.
The Mechanics of Muscle Movement		
brachi/o	arm	The biceps *brachii* and triceps *brachii* are in the arm.
erg/o	work	*Synergists* are muscles that work together.
Skeletal Muscle Groups		
quadr/i	four	The *quadriceps* muscle group consists of four muscles.

Summary

I. Types of muscle
A. Smooth muscle
  1. In walls of hollow organs, vessels, and respiratory passageways
  2. Cells tapered, single nucleus, nonstriated
  3. Involuntary; produces peristalsis; contracts and relaxes slowly
B. Cardiac muscle
  1. Muscle of heart wall
  2. Cells branch; single nucleus; lightly striated
  3. Involuntary; self-excitatory
C. Skeletal muscle
  1. Most attached to bones and move skeleton
  2. Cells long, cylindrical; multiple nuclei; heavily striated
  3. Voluntary; contracts and relaxes rapidly

II. Muscular system
  1. Functions
    a. Movement of skeleton
    b. Maintenance of posture
    c. Generation of heat
A. Structure of a muscle
  1. Held by connective tissue
    a. Endomysium around individual fibers
    b. Perimysium around fascicles (bundles)
    c. Epimysium around whole muscle
B. Muscle cells in action
  1. Neuromuscular junction
    a. Point where nerve fiber stimulates muscle cell
    b. Neurotransmitter is acetylcholine (ACh)
      (1) Generates an action potential
    c. Motor end plate—membrane of muscle cell
  2. Contraction—sliding together of filaments to shorten muscle
    a. Actin—thin and light
    b. Myosin—thick and dark with projecting heads
  3. Role of calcium—uncovers binding sites so crossbridges can form between actin and myosin
D. Energy sources
  1. ATP—supplies energy
    a. Myoglobin—stores oxygen
    b. Glycogen—stores glucose
    c. Creatine phosphate—stores energy
  2. Oxygen consumption
    a. Oxygen debt—develops during strenuous exercise
      (1) Anaerobic metabolism

(2) Yields lactic acid—causes muscle fatigue
   b. Recovery oxygen consumption
     (1) Removes lactic acid
     (2) Replenishes energy-storing compounds
E. Effects of exercise
  1. Changes in structure and function of muscle cells
  2. Vasodilation brings blood to tissues
  3. Heart strengthened
  4. Breathing improved
F. Types of muscle contractions
  1. Tonus—partially contracted state
  2. Isotonic contractions—muscle shortens to produce movement
  3. Isometric contractions—tension increases, but muscle does not shorten

III. Mechanics of muscle movement

  1. Attachments of skeletal muscles
    a. Tendon—cord of connective tissue that attaches muscle to bone
     (1) Origin—attached to more fixed part
     (2) Insertion—attached to moving part
    b. Aponeurosis—broad band of connective tissue that attaches muscle to bone or other muscle
A. Muscles work together
  1. Prime mover—performs movement
  2. Antagonist—produces opposite movement
  3. Synergists—steady body parts and assist prime mover

B. Levers and body mechanics—muscles function with skeleton as lever systems
  1. Components
    a. Lever—bone
    b. Fulcrum—joint
    c. Force—muscle contraction
  2. Most muscles work as third class levers (fulcrum-effort-weight)

IV. Skeletal muscle groups

  1. Naming of muscles—location, size, shape, direction of fibers, number of heads, action
A. Muscles of the head
B. Muscles of the neck
C. Muscles of the upper extremities
  1. Muscles that move the shoulder and arm
  2. Muscles that move the forearm and hand
D. Muscles of the trunk
  1. Muscles of respiration
  2. Muscles of the abdomen and pelvis
  3. Deep muscles of the back
E. Muscles of the lower extremities
  1. Muscles that move the thigh and leg
  2. Muscles that move the foot

V. Effects of aging on muscles

  1. Decrease in size of muscles
  2. Weakening of muscles, especially extensors

Questions for Study and Review

Building Understanding

Fill in the blanks

1. Individual muscle fibers are arranged in bundles called _____.

2. The point at which a nerve fiber contacts a muscle cell is called the _____.

3. A contraction in which there is no change in muscle length but there is a great increase in muscle tension is _____.

4. A contracting subunit of skeletal muscle is called a _____.

5. Widening of the blood vessels, as occurs during exercise, is termed _____.

Matching

Match each numbered item with the most closely related lettered item.

___ 6. Extends vertebral column to produce erect posture

___ 7. Elevates ribs and enlarges thoracic cavity

___ 8. Flattens cheeks

___ 9. Aids in defecation

___ 10. Closes eye

    a. levator ani
    b. buccinator
    c. orbicularis oris
    d. erector spinae
    e. intercostal muscles

Multiple choice

___ 11. From superficial to deep, the correct order of muscle structure is

a. deep fascia, epimysium, perimysium, and endomysium

b. epimysium, perimysium, endomysium, and deep fascia

c. deep fascia, endomysium, perimysium, and epimysium

d. endomysium, perimysium, epimysium, and deep fascia

___ 12. The function of calcium ions in skeletal muscle contraction is to:

a. bind to receptors on the motor end plate to stimulate muscle contraction.

b. cause a pH change in the cytoplasm to trigger muscle contraction.

c. bind to the myosin binding sites on actin so that myosin will have something to attach to.

d. bind to regulatory proteins so that the myosin binding sites on the actin can be exposed.

___ 13. A broad flat extension that attaches muscle to bone is called a(n)

a. tendon

b. fascicle

c. aponeurosis

d. motor end plate

___ 14. Flexion of the forearm is due to a

a. first-class lever

b. second-class lever

c. third-class lever

d. fourth-class lever

___ 15. The most important muscle involved in the act of breathing is the

a. sternocleidomastoid

b. pectoralis major

c. intercostal

d. diaphragm

Understanding Concepts

16. Compare smooth, cardiac, and skeletal muscle with respect to location, structure, and function. Briefly explain how each type of muscle is specialized for its function.

17. Describe three substances stored in skeletal muscle cells that are used to manufacture a constant supply of ATP.

18. Describe the events in a muscular contraction.

19. Name and describe muscle(s) that

a. open and close the eye

b. close the jaw

c. flex and extend the head

d. flex and extend the forearm

e. flex and extend the hand and fingers

f. flex and extend the leg

g. flex and extend the foot and toes

20. During a cesarean section, a transverse incision is made through the abdominal wall. Name the muscles incised and state their functions.

21. What effect does aging have on muscles? What can be done to resist these effects?

Conceptual Thinking

22. Recall that the neurotransmitter acetylcholine initiates skeletal muscle contraction. Normally, acetylcholine is broken down shortly after its release into the synaptic cleft by the enzyme acetylcholinesterase. Many insecticides contain chemicals called organophosphates, which interfere with acetylcholinesterase activity. Based on this information, what could happen to an individual exposed to high concentrations of organophosphates?

23. Margo recently began "working out" and jogs three times a week. After her jog she is breathless and her muscles ache. From your understanding of muscle physiology, describe what has happened inside of Margo's skeletal muscle cells. How do Margo's muscles recover from this? If Margo continues to exercise, what changes would you expect to occur in her muscles?

24. Alfred suffered a mild stroke, leaving him partially paralyzed on his left side. Physical therapy was ordered to prevent left-sided muscle weakness. Prescribe some exercises for Alfred's shoulder and thigh.

unit III

Coordination and Control

*T*wo chapters in this unit describe the nervous system and some of its many parts and complex functions. The organs of special sense and other sensory receptors are described in a separate chapter. The last chapter in this unit discusses hormones and the organs that produce them. Working with the nervous system, these hormones play an important role in coordination and control.

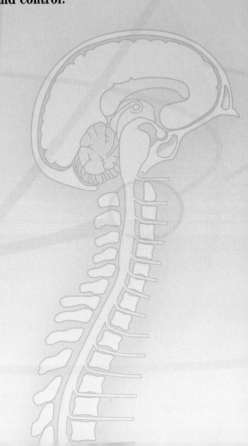

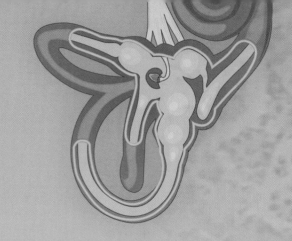

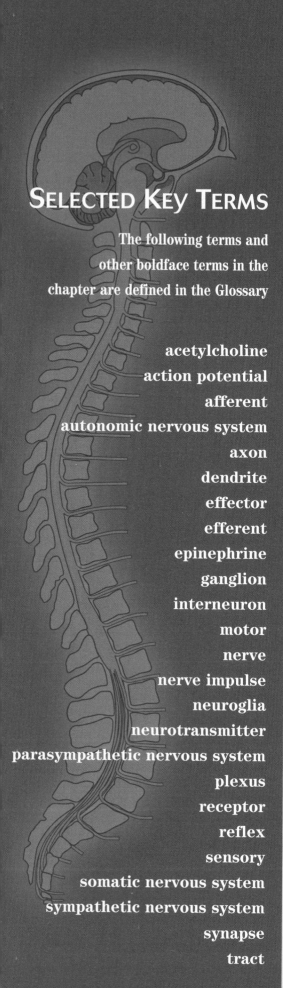

SELECTED KEY TERMS

The following terms and other boldface terms in the chapter are defined in the Glossary

acetylcholine

action potential

afferent

autonomic nervous system

axon

dendrite

effector

efferent

epinephrine

ganglion

interneuron

motor

nerve

nerve impulse

neuroglia

neurotransmitter

parasympathetic nervous system

plexus

receptor

reflex

sensory

somatic nervous system

sympathetic nervous system

synapse

tract

LEARNING OUTCOMES

After careful study of this chapter, you should be able to:

1. Describe the organization of the nervous system according to structure and function

2. Describe the structure of a neuron

3. Describe how neuron fibers are built into a nerve

4. Explain the purpose of neuroglia

5. Diagram and describe the steps in an action potential

6. Briefly describe the transmission of a nerve impulse

7. Explain the role of myelin in nerve conduction

8. Briefly describe transmission at a synapse

9. Define *neurotransmitter* and give several examples of neurotransmitters

10. Describe the distribution of gray and white matter in the spinal cord

11. List the components of a reflex arc

12. Define a simple reflex and give several examples of reflexes

13. Describe and name the spinal nerves and three of their main plexuses

14. Compare the location and functions of the sympathetic and parasympathetic nervous systems

15. Show how word parts are used to build words related to the nervous system (see Word Anatomy at the end of the chapter)

The Nervous System: The Spinal Cord and Spinal Nerves

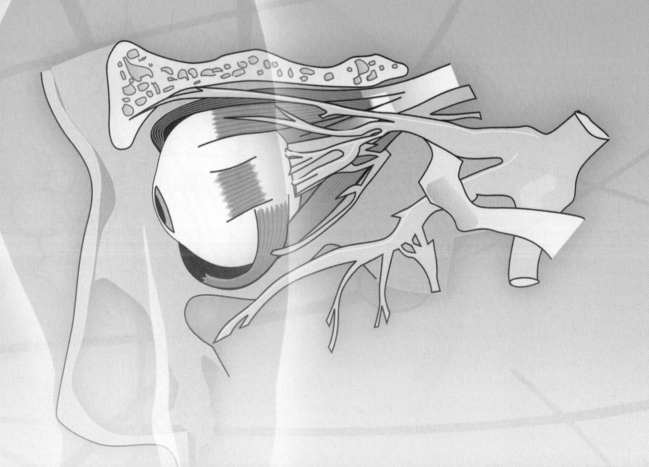

▶ Role of the Nervous System

None of the body systems is capable of functioning alone. All are interdependent and work together as one unit to maintain normal conditions, termed *homeostasis*. The nervous system serves as the chief coordinating agency for all systems. Conditions both within and outside the body are constantly changing. The nervous system must detect and respond to these changes (known as *stimuli*) so that the body can adapt itself to new conditions. The nervous system has been compared with a telephone exchange, in that the brain and the spinal cord act as switching centers and the nerves act as cables for carrying messages to and from these centers.

Although all parts of the nervous system work in coordination, portions may be grouped together on the basis of either structure or function.

Structural Divisions

The anatomic, or structural, divisions of the nervous system are as follows (Fig. 8-1):

▶ The **central nervous system** (CNS) includes the brain and spinal cord.
▶ The **peripheral** (per-IF-er-al) **nervous system** (PNS) is made up of all the nerves outside the CNS. It includes all the **cranial nerves** that carry impulses to and from the brain and all the **spinal nerves** that carry messages to and from the spinal cord.

The CNS and PNS together include all of the nervous tissue in the body.

Functional Divisions

Functionally, the nervous system is divided according to whether control is voluntary or involuntary and according to what type of tissue is stimulated (Table 8-1). Any tissue or organ that carries out a command from the nervous system is called an **effector**, all of which are muscles or glands.

The **somatic nervous system** is controlled voluntarily (by conscious will), and all its effectors are skeletal muscles (described in Chapter 6). The involuntary division of the nervous system is called the **autonomic nervous system** (ANS), making reference to its automatic activity. It is also called the **visceral nervous system** because it controls smooth muscle, cardiac muscle, and glands, much of which make up the soft body organs, the viscera.

The ANS is further subdivided into a **sympathetic nervous system** and a **parasympathetic nervous system** based on organization and how each affects specific organs. The ANS is described later in this chapter.

Although these divisions are helpful for study purposes, the lines that divide the nervous system according to function are not as distinct as those that classify the system structurally. For example, the diaphragm, a skeletal muscle, typically functions in breathing without conscious thought. In addition, we have certain rapid reflex responses involving skeletal muscles—drawing the hand away from a hot stove, for example—that do not involve the brain. In contrast, people can be trained to consciously control involuntary functions, such as blood pressure, heart rate, and breathing rate, by techniques known as *biofeedback*.

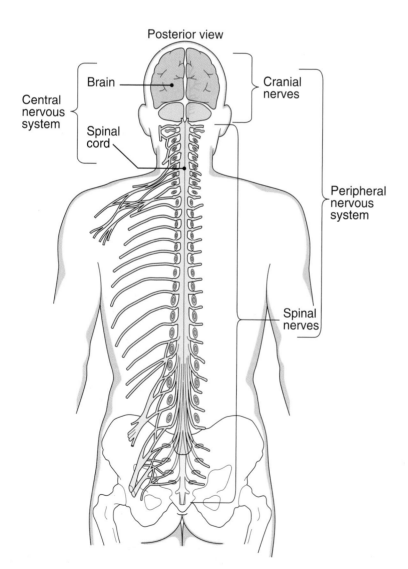

Posterior view

Brain

Cranial nerves

Central nervous system

Spinal cord

Peripheral nervous system

Spinal nerves

Figure 8-1 Anatomic divisions of the nervous system.

Table 8•1	Functional Divisions of the Nervous System			
	CHARACTERISTICS			
DIVISION	**CONTROL**	**EFFECTORS**	**SUBDIVISIONS**	
Somatic nervous system	Voluntary	Skeletal muscle	None	
Autonomic nervous system	Involuntary	Smooth muscle, cardiac muscle, and glands	Sympathetic and parasympathetic systems	

Checkpoint 8-1 What are the two divisions of the nervous system based on structure?

Checkpoint 8-2 The nervous system can be divided functionally into two divisions based on type of control and effectors. What division is voluntary and controls skeletal muscle, and what division is involuntary and controls involuntary muscles and glands?

▶ Neurons and Their Functions

The functional cells of the nervous system are highly specialized cells called **neurons** (Fig. 8-2). These cells have a unique structure related to their function.

Structure of a Neuron

The main portion of each neuron, the cell body, contains the nucleus and other organelles typically found in cells. A distinguishing feature of the neurons, however, are the long, threadlike fibers that extend out from the cell body and carry impulses across the cell (Fig. 8-3). There are two kinds of fibers: dendrites and axons.

▶ **Dendrites** are neuron fibers that conduct impulses *to* the cell body. Most dendrites have a highly branched, treelike appearance (see Fig. 8-2). In fact, the name comes from a Greek word meaning "tree." Dendrites function as **receptors** in the nervous system. That is, they receive the stimulus that begins a neural pathway. In Chapter 10, we describe how the dendrites of the sensory system may be modified to respond to a specific type of stimulus.
▶ **Axons** (AK-sons) are neuron fibers that conduct impulses *away from* the cell body (see Fig. 8-2). These impulses may be delivered to another neuron, to a muscle, or to a gland. An axon is a single fiber, which may be quite long and which branches at its end.

The Myelin Sheath Some axons are covered with a fatty material called **myelin** that insulates and protects the fiber (see Fig. 8-2). In the PNS, this covering is produced by special connective tissue cells called **Schwann** (shvahn) **cells** that wrap around the axon like a jelly roll, depositing layers of myelin (Fig. 8-4). When the sheath is complete, small spaces remain between the individual

cells. These tiny gaps, called **nodes** (originally, nodes of Ranvier), are important in speeding the conduction of nerve impulses.

The outermost membranes of the Schwann cells form a thin coating known as the **neurilemma** (nu-rih-LEM-mah). This covering is a part of the mechanism by which some peripheral nerves repair themselves when injured. Under some circumstances, damaged nerve cell fibers may regenerate by growing into the sleeve formed by the neurilemma. Cells of the brain and the spinal cord are myelinated, not by Schwann cells, but by

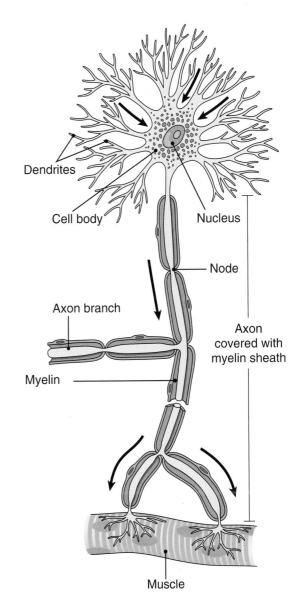

Dendrites
Cell body
Nucleus
Node
Axon branch
Axon covered with myelin sheath
Myelin
Muscle

Figure 8-2 Diagram of a motor neuron. The break in the axon denotes length. The arrows show the direction of the nerve impulse. *ZOOMING IN ✦ Is the neuron shown here a sensory or a motor neuron?*

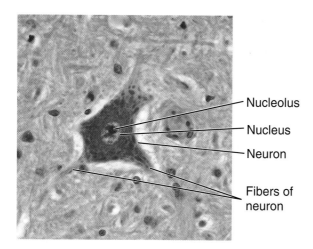

Figure 8-3 A typical neuron as seen under the microscope. The nucleus, nucleolus, and multiple fibers of the neuron are visible. (Reprinted with permission from Cormack DH. Essential Histology. 2nd ed. Philadelphia: Lippincott Williams & Wilkins, 2001.)

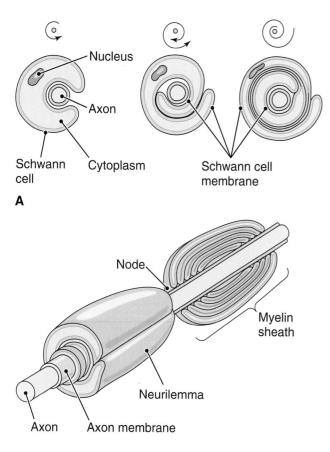

Figure 8-4 Formation of a myelin sheath. (A) Schwann cells wrap around the axon, creating a myelin coating. **(B)** The outermost layer of the Schwann cell forms the neurilemma. Spaces between the cells are the nodes (of Ranvier).

other types of connective tissue cells. As a result, they have no neurilemma. If they are injured, the damage is permanent. Even in the peripheral nerves, however, repair is a slow and uncertain process.

Myelinated axons, because of myelin's color, are called **white fibers** and are found in the **white matter** of the brain and spinal cord as well as in the nerve trunks in all parts of the body. The fibers and cell bodies of the **gray matter** are not covered with myelin.

> **Checkpoint 8-3** The neuron, the functional unit of the nervous system, has long fibers extending from the cell body. What is the name of the fiber that carries impulses toward the cell body, and what is the name of the fiber that carries impulses away from the cell body?

> **Checkpoint 8-4** Myelin is a substance that covers and protects some axons. What color describes myelinated fibers, and what color describes unmyelinated tissue of the nervous system?

Types of Neurons

The job of neurons in the PNS is to relay information constantly either to or from the CNS. Neurons that conduct impulses *to* the spinal cord and brain are described as **sensory neurons**, also called **afferent neurons.** Those cells that carry impulses *from* the CNS out to muscles and glands are **motor neurons**, also called **efferent neurons.** Neurons that relay information within the CNS are **interneurons**, also called *central* or *association neurons.*

Nerves and Tracts

Everywhere in the nervous system, neuron fibers are collected into bundles of varying size (Fig. 8-5). A bundle of fibers located within the PNS is a **nerve.** A similar grouping, but located within the CNS, is a **tract.** Tracts are located both in the brain and in the spinal cord, where they conduct impulses to and from the brain.

A nerve or tract can be compared with an electric cable made up of many wires. The "wires," the nerve cell fibers, in a nerve or tract are bound together with connective tissue, just like muscle fibers in a muscle. As in muscles, the individual fibers are organized into subdivisions called *fascicles.* The names of the connective tissue layers are similar to their names in muscles, but the root *neur/o*, meaning "nerve" is substituted for the muscle root *my/o*, as follows:

▶ Endoneurium is around an individual fiber.
▶ Perineurium is around a fascicle.
▶ Epineurium is around the whole nerve.

A nerve may contain all sensory fibers, all motor fibers, or a combination of both types of fibers. A few of the cranial nerves contain only sensory fibers conducting impulses toward the brain. These are described as **sensory (afferent) nerves.** A few of the cranial nerves contain only motor fibers conducting impulses away from the brain, and

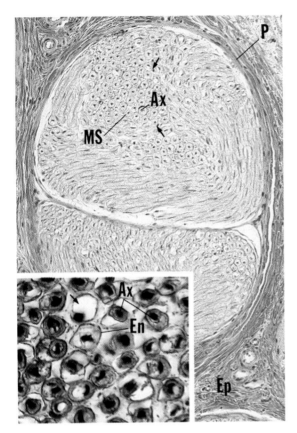

Figure 8-5 Cross section of a nerve as seen under the microscope (×132). Two fascicles (subdivisions) are shown. Perineurium (P) surrounds each fascicle. Epineurium (Ep) is around the entire nerve. Individual axons (Ax) are covered with a myelin sheath (MS), around which is the endoneurium (En) (inset). (Reprinted with permission from Gartner LP, Hiatt JL. Color Atlas of Histology. 3rd ed. Philadelphia: Lippincott Williams & Wilkins, 2000.)

these are classified as **motor (efferent) nerves**. However, most of the cranial nerves and *all* of the spinal nerves contain both sensory *and* motor fibers and are referred to as **mixed nerves**. Note that in a mixed nerve, impulses may be traveling in two directions (toward or away from the CNS), but each individual fiber in the nerve is carrying impulses in one direction only. Think of the nerve as a large highway. Traffic may be going north and south, for example, but each car is going forward in only one direction.

> **Checkpoint 8-5** Nerves are bundles of neuron fibers in the PNS. These nerves may be carrying impulses either toward or away from the CNS. What name is given to nerves that convey impulses toward the CNS, and what name is given to nerves that transport away from the CNS?

▶ Neuroglia

In addition to conducting tissue, the nervous system contains cells that serve for support and protection. Collectively, these cells are called **neuroglia** (nu-ROG-le-ah) or **glial (GLI-al) cells**, from a Greek word meaning "glue." There are different types of neuroglia, each with specialized functions, some of which are the following:

▶ Protect nervous tissue.
▶ Support nervous tissue and bind it to other structures.
▶ Aid in repair of cells.
▶ Act as phagocytes to remove pathogens and impurities.
▶ Regulate the composition of fluids around and between cells.

Neuroglia appear throughout the central and peripheral nervous systems. The Schwann cells that produce the myelin sheath in the peripheral nervous system are one type of neuroglia. Another example is shown in Figure 8-6. These cells are astrocytes, named for their starlike appear-

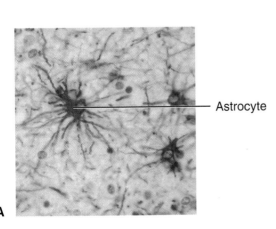

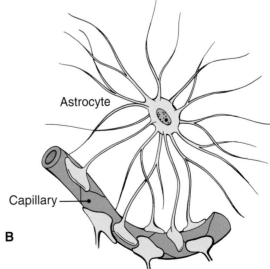

Figure 8-6 Examples of neuroglia. (A) Astrocytes in the white matter of the brain. **(B)** Astrocytes attach to capillaries and help to protect the brain from harmful substances. (Reprinted with permission from Ross MH, Kaye GI, Pawlina W. Histology. 4th ed. Philadelphia: Lippincott Williams & Wilkins, 2003.)

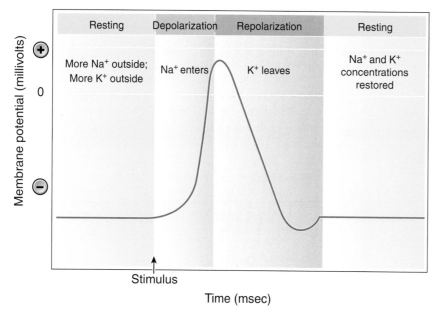

Figure 8-7 The action potential. In depolarization, Na$^+$ membrane channels open and Na$^+$ enters the cell. In repolarization, K$^+$ membrane channels open and K$^+$ leaves the cell. During and after repolarization, the Na$^+$/K$^+$ pump returns ion concentrations to their original concentrations so the membrane can be stimulated again.

ized. As in a battery, the separation of charges on either side of the membrane creates a possibility (potential) for generating energy. If there is a way for the charges to move toward each other, electricity will be generated.

A **nerve impulse** starts with a local reversal in the membrane potential caused by changes in the ion concentrations on either side. This sudden electrical change at the membrane is called an **action potential**, as described in Chapter 7 on the muscles. A simple description of the events in an action potential is as follows (Fig. 8-7):

▶ The resting state. In addition to an electrical difference on the two sides of the plasma membrane at rest, there is also a slight difference in the concentration of ions on either side. At rest, sodium ions (Na$^+$) are a little more concentrated at the outside of the

ance. In the brain they attach to capillaries (small blood vessels) and help protect the brain from harmful substances.

Unlike neurons, neuroglia continue to multiply throughout life. Because of their capacity to reproduce, most tumors of the nervous system are tumors of neuroglial tissue and not of nervous tissue itself.

> **Checkpoint 8-6** The nonconducting cells of the nervous system serve in protection and support. What are these cells called?

▶ The Nervous System at Work

The nervous system works by means of electrical impulses sent along neuron fibers and transmitted from cell to cell at highly specialized junctions.

The Nerve Impulse

The mechanics of nerve impulse conduction are complex but can be compared with the spread of an electric current along a wire. What follows is a brief description of the electrical changes that occur as a resting neuron is stimulated and transmits a nerve impulse.

The plasma membrane of an unstimulated (resting) neuron carries an electrical charge, or **potential**. This resting potential is maintained by ions (charged particles) concentrated on either side of the membrane. At rest, the inside of the membrane is negative as compared with the outside. In this state, the membrane is said to be *polar-*

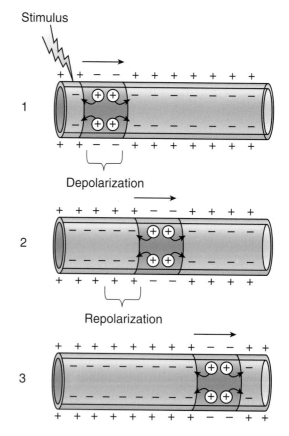

Figure 8-8 A nerve impulse. From a point of stimulation, a wave of depolarization followed by repolarization travels along the membrane of a neuron. This spreading action potential is a nerve impulse.

membrane. At the same time, potassium ions (K^+) are a little more concentrated at the inside of the membrane.

▸ Depolarization. A stimulus of adequate force, such as electrical, chemical, or mechanical energy, causes specific channels in the membrane to open and allow Na^+ ions to flow into the cell. (Remember that substances flow by diffusion from an area where they are in higher concentration to an area where they are in lower concentration.) As these positive ions enter, they raise the charge on the inside of the membrane, a change known as **depolarization** (see Fig. 8-7).

▸ Repolarization. In the next step of the action potential, K^+ channels open to allow K^+ to leave the cell. As the electrical charge returns to its resting value, the membrane is undergoing **repolarization**. At the same time that the membrane is repolarizing, the cell uses active transport to move Na^+ and K^+ back to their original concentrations on either side of the membrane so that the membrane can be stimulated again. This activity is described as the **Na^+/K^+ pump**.

The action potential occurs rapidly—in less than 1/1000 of a second, and is followed by a rapid return to the resting state (Fig. 8-8). However, this local electrical change in the membrane stimulates an action potential at an adjacent point along the membrane. In scientific terms, the channels in the membrane are "voltage dependent," that is, they respond to an electrical stimulus. And so, the action potential spreads along the membrane as a wave of electrical current. The spreading action potential is the nerve impulse, and in fact, the term *action potential* is used to mean the nerve impulse. A stimulus is any force that can start an action potential by opening membrane channels and allowing Na^+ to enter the cell.

The Role of Myelin in Conduction
As previously noted, some axons are coated with the fatty material myelin. If a fiber is not myelinated, the action potential spreads continuously along the membrane of the cell (see Fig. 8-4). When myelin is present on an axon, however, it insulates the fiber against the spread of current. This would appear to slow or stop conduction along these fibers, but in fact, the myelin sheath speeds conduction. The reason is that the action potential must "jump" like a spark from node (space) to node along the sheath (see Fig. 8-3), and this type of conduction is actually faster than continuous conduction.

The Synapse

Neurons do not work alone; impulses must be transferred between neurons to convey information within the nervous system. The point of junction for transmitting the nerve impulse is the **synapse** (SIN-aps), a term that comes from a Greek word meaning "to clasp" (Fig. 8-9).

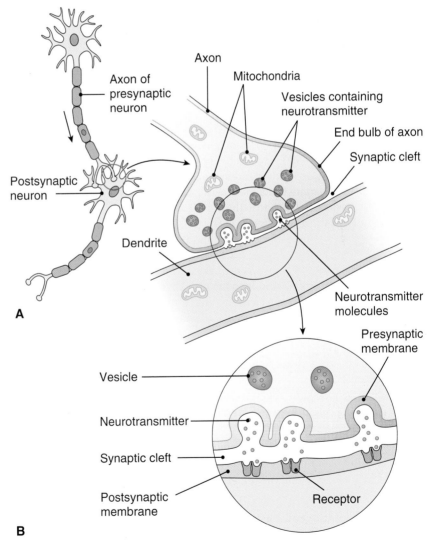

Figure 8-9 A synapse. (A) The end-bulb of the presynaptic (transmitting) axon has vesicles containing neurotransmitter, which is released into the synaptic cleft to the membrane of the postsynaptic (receiving) cell. **(B)** Close-up of a synapse showing receptors for neurotransmitter in the postsynaptic cell membrane.

At a synapse, transmission of an impulse usually occurs from the axon of one cell, the **presynaptic cell**, to the dendrite of another cell, the **postsynaptic cell**.

As described in Chapter 7, information must be passed from one cell to another at the synapse across a tiny gap between the cells, the **synaptic cleft**. Information usually crosses this gap in the form of a chemical known as a **neurotransmitter**. While the cells at a synapse are at rest, the neurotransmitter is stored in many small vesicles (bubbles) within the enlarged endings of the axons, usually called *end-bulbs* or *terminal knobs*, but known by several other names as well.

When a nerve impulse traveling along a neuron membrane reaches the end of the presynaptic axon, some of these vesicles fuse with the membrane and release their neurotransmitter into the synaptic cleft (an example of exocytosis, as described in Chapter 3). The neurotransmitter then acts as a chemical signal to the postsynaptic cell.

On the postsynaptic receiving membrane, usually that of a dendrite, but sometimes another part of the cell, there are special sites, or **receptors**, ready to pick up and respond to specific neurotransmitters. Receptors in the postsynaptic cell membrane influence how or if that cell will respond to a given neurotransmitter.

Neurotransmitters Although there are many known neurotransmitters, the main ones are **epinephrine** (ep-ih-NEF-rin), also called **adrenaline**; a related compound, **norepinephrine** (nor-ep-ih-NEF-rin), or **noradrenaline**; and **acetylcholine** (as-e-til-KO-lene). Acetylcholine (ACh) is the neurotransmitter released at the neuromuscular junction, the synapse between a neuron and a muscle cell. All three of the above neurotransmitters function in the ANS. It is common to think of neurotransmitters as stimulating the cells they reach; in fact, they have been described as such in this discussion. Note, however, that some of these chemicals inhibit the postsynaptic cell and keep it from reacting, as will be demonstrated later in discussions of the autonomic nervous system.

The connections between neurons can be quite complex. One cell can branch to stimulate many receiving cells, or a single cell may be stimulated by a number of different axons (Fig. 8-10). The cell's response is based on the total effects of all the neurotransmitters it receives at any one time.

After its release into the synaptic cleft, the neurotransmitter may be removed by several methods:

▸ It may slowly diffuse away from the synapse.
▸ It may be destroyed rapidly by enzymes in the synaptic cleft.
▸ It may be taken back into the presynaptic cell to be used again, a process known as *Reuptake*.

The method of removal helps determine how long a neurotransmitter will act.

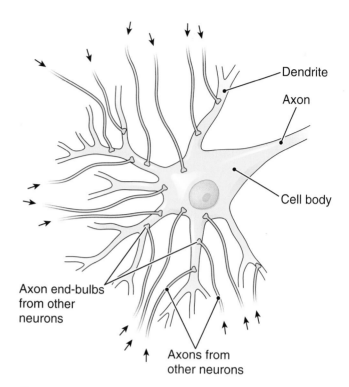

Figure 8-10 **The effects of neurotransmitters on a neuron.** A single neuron is stimulated by axons of many other neurons. The cell responds according to the total of all the excitatory and inhibitory neurotransmitters it receives.

Electrical Synapses Not all synapses are chemically controlled. In smooth muscle, cardiac muscle, and also in the CNS there is a type of synapse in which electrical energy travels directly from one cell to another. The membranes of the presynaptic and postsynaptic cells are close together and an electrical charge can spread directly between them. These electrical synapses allow more rapid and more coordinated communication. In the heart, for example, it is important that large groups of cells contract together for effective pumping action.

▸ The Spinal Cord

The spinal cord is the link between the peripheral nervous system and the brain. It also helps to coordinate impulses within the CNS. The spinal cord is contained in and protected by the vertebrae, which fit together to form a continuous tube extending from the occipital bone to the coccyx (Fig. 8-11). In the embryo, the spinal cord occupies the entire spinal canal, extending down into the tail portion of the vertebral column. The column of bone grows much more rapidly than the nerve tissue of the cord, however, and eventually, the end of the spinal cord no longer reaches the lower part of the spinal canal. This disparity in growth continues to increase, so that in adults, the spinal cord ends in the region just below the area to which the last rib attaches (between the first and second lumbar vertebrae).

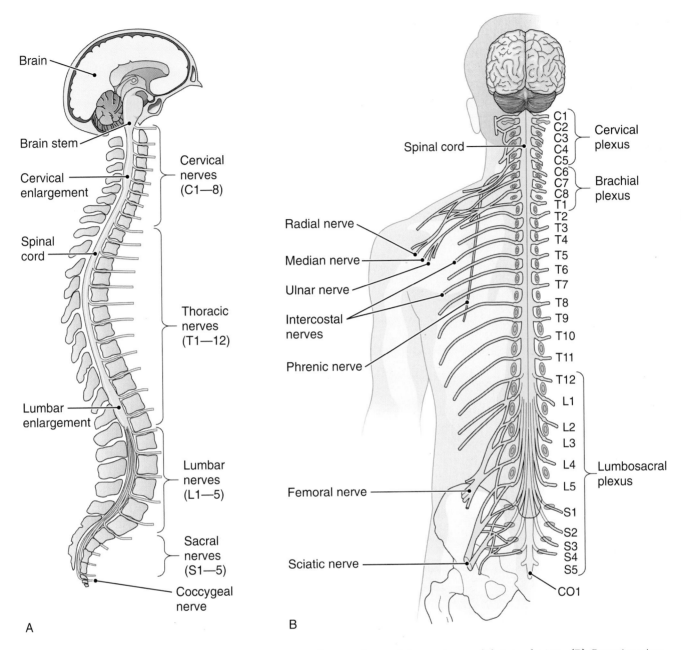

Figure 8-11 Spinal cord and spinal nerves. Nerve plexuses (networks) are shown. **(A)** Lateral view. **(B)** Posterior view. *ZOOMING IN ✦ Is the spinal cord the same length as the spinal column? How does the number of cervical vertebrae compare with the number of cervical spinal nerves?*

Structure of the Spinal Cord

The spinal cord has a small, irregularly shaped internal section of gray matter (unmyelinated tissue) surrounded by a larger area of white matter (myelinated axons) (Fig. 8-12). The internal gray matter is arranged so that a column of gray matter extends up and down dorsally, one on each side; another column is found in the ventral region on each side. These two pairs of columns, called the **dorsal horns** and **ventral horns,** give the gray matter an H-shaped appearance in cross-section. The bridge of gray matter that connects the right and left horns is the **gray commissure** (KOM-ih-shure). In the center of the gray

commissure is a small channel, the **central canal,** that contains cerebrospinal fluid, the liquid that circulates around the brain and spinal cord. A narrow groove, the **posterior median sulcus** (SUL-kus), divides the right and left portions of the posterior white matter. A deeper groove, the **anterior median fissure** (FISH-ure), separates the right and left portions of the anterior white matter.

Ascending and Descending Tracts The spinal cord is the pathway for sensory and motor impulses traveling to and from the brain. These impulses are carried in the thousands of myelinated axons in the white matter of

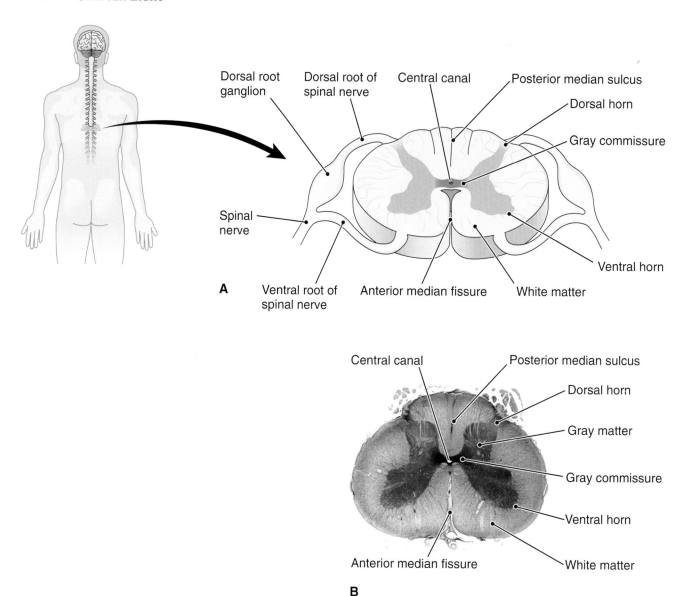

A

Dorsal root ganglion
Dorsal root of spinal nerve
Central canal
Posterior median sulcus
Dorsal horn
Gray commissure
Spinal nerve
Ventral horn
Ventral root of spinal nerve
Anterior median fissure
White matter

B

Central canal
Posterior median sulcus
Dorsal horn
Gray matter
Gray commissure
Ventral horn
Anterior median fissure
White matter

Figure 8-12 **The spinal cord. (A)** Cross-section of the spinal cord showing the organization of the gray and white matter. The roots of the spinal nerves are also shown. **(B)** Microscopic view of the spinal cord in cross-section (×5). (B, Reprinted with permission from Ross MH, Kaye GI, Pawlina W. Histology. 4th ed. Philadelphia: Lippincott Williams & Wilkins, 2003.)

the spinal cord, which are subdivided into tracts (groups of fibers). Sensory (afferent) impulses entering the spinal cord are transmitted toward the brain in **ascending tracts** of the white matter. Motor (efferent) impulses traveling from the brain are carried in **descending tracts** toward the peripheral nervous system. Damage to these tracts prevents transmission of impulses along the spinal cord. Box 8-1, Spinal Cord Injury: Crossing the Divide, contains information on treatment of these injuries.

> **Checkpoint 8-10** The spinal cord contains both gray and white matter. How is this tissue arranged in the spinal cord?

> **Checkpoint 8-11** What is the purpose of the tracts in the white matter of the spinal cord?

The Reflex Arc

As the nervous system functions, it receives, interprets, and acts on both external and internal stimuli. The spinal cord is also a relay center for coordinating neural pathways. A complete pathway through the nervous system from stimulus to response is termed a **reflex arc** (Fig. 8-13). This is the basic functional pathway of the nervous system. The basic parts of a reflex arc are the following (Table 8-2):

1. **Receptor**—the end of a dendrite or some specialized receptor cell, as in a special sense organ, that detects a stimulus.
2. **Sensory neuron,** or afferent neuron—a cell that transmits impulses *toward* the CNS. Sensory impulses enter the dorsal horn of the gray matter in the spinal cord.

Box 8-1	Hot Topics

Spinal Cord Injury: Crossing the Divide

Approximately 11,000 new cases of spinal cord injury occur each year in the United States, the majority involving males ages 16 to 30. Because neurons show little, if any, capacity to repair themselves, spinal cord injuries almost always result in a loss of sensory or motor function (or both), and therapy has focused on injury management rather than cure. However, scientists are investigating four improved treatment approaches:

▶ *Minimizing spinal cord trauma after injury.* Intravenous injection of the steroid methylprednisolone shortly after injury reduces swelling at the site of injury and improves recovery.

▶ *Using **neurotrophins** to induce repair in damaged nerve tissue.* Certain types of neuroglia produce chemicals called neurotrophins (*e.g.*, nerve growth factor) that have promoted nerve regeneration in experiments.
▶ *Regulation of inhibitory factors that keep neurons from dividing.* "Turning off" these factors (produced by neuroglia) in the damaged nervous system may promote tissue repair. The factor called Nogo is an example.
▶ *Nervous tissue transplantation.* Successfully transplanted donor tissue may take over the damaged nervous system's functions.

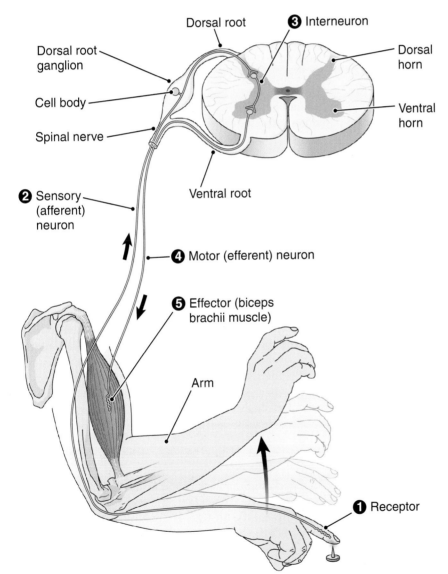

3. **Central nervous system**—where impulses are coordinated and a response is organized. One or more interneurons may carry impulses to and from the brain, may function within the brain, or may distribute impulses to different regions of the spinal cord. Almost every response involves connecting neurons in the CNS.
4. **Motor neuron,** or efferent neuron—a cell that carries impulses *away from* the CNS. Motor impulses leave the cord through the ventral horn of the spinal cord gray matter.
5. **Effector**—a muscle or a gland outside the CNS that carries out a response.

At its simplest, a reflex arc can involve just two neurons, one sensory and one motor, with a synapse in the CNS. Few reflex arcs require only this minimal number of neurons. (The knee-jerk reflex described below is one of the few examples in humans.) Most reflex arcs involve many more, even hundreds, of connecting neurons within the CNS. The many intricate patterns that make the nervous system so responsive and adaptable also make it difficult to study, and investigation of the nervous system is one of the most active areas of research today.

Figure 8-13 **Typical reflex arc.** Numbers show the sequence of impulses through the spinal cord (solid arrows). Contraction of the biceps brachii results in flexion of the arm at the elbow. *ZOOMING IN* ✦ *Is this a somatic or an autonomic reflex arc? What type of neuron is located between the sensory and motor neuron in the CNS?*

Checkpoint 8-12 What name is given to a pathway through the nervous system from a stimulus to an effector?

Table 8·2	Components of a Reflex Arc	
COMPONENT	**FUNCTION**	
Receptor	End of a dendrite or specialized cell that responds to a stimulus	
Sensory neuron	Transmits a nerve impulse toward the CNS	
Central nervous system	Coordinates sensory impulses and organizes a response; usually requires interneurons	
Motor neuron	Carries impulses away from the CNS toward the effector, a muscle, or a gland	
Effector	A muscle or gland outside the CNS that carries out a response	

Such stretch reflexes may be evoked by appropriate tapping of most large muscles (such as the triceps brachii in the arm and the gastrocnemius in the calf of the leg). Because reflexes are simple and predictable, health professionals use them in physical examinations to test the condition of the nervous system. Box 8-2, Careers in Occupational Therapy, describes professions related to care of people with nervous system injuries.

Reflex Activities Although reflex pathways may be quite complex, a **simple reflex** is a rapid, uncomplicated, and automatic response involving very few neurons. Reflexes are specific; a given stimulus always produces the same response. When you fling out an arm or leg to catch your balance, withdraw from a painful stimulus, or blink to avoid an object approaching your eyes, you are experiencing reflex behavior. A simple reflex arc that passes through the spinal cord alone and does not involve the brain is termed a **spinal reflex**.

The **stretch reflex**, in which a muscle is stretched and responds by contracting, is one example of a spinal reflex. If you tap the tendon below the kneecap (the patellar tendon), the muscle of the anterior thigh (quadriceps femoris) contracts, eliciting the knee-jerk reflex (Fig. 8-14).

The Spinal Nerves

There are 31 pairs of spinal nerves, each pair numbered according to the level of the spinal cord from which it arises (see Fig. 8-11). Each nerve is attached to the spinal cord by two roots: the **dorsal root** and the **ventral root** (see Fig. 8-12). On each dorsal root is a marked swelling of gray matter called the **dorsal root ganglion**, which contains the cell bodies of the sensory neurons. A **ganglion** (GANG-le-on) is any collection of nerve cell bodies located outside the CNS. Fibers from sensory receptors throughout the body lead to these dorsal root ganglia.

The ventral roots of the spinal nerves are a combination of motor (efferent) fibers that supply muscles and glands (effectors). The cell bodies of these neurons are located in the ventral gray matter (ventral horns) of the cord. Because the dorsal (sensory) and ventral (motor) roots are combined to form the spinal nerve, all spinal nerves are mixed nerves.

Branches of the Spinal Nerves

Each spinal nerve continues only a short distance away from the spinal cord and then branches into small posterior divisions and larger anterior divisions. The larger anterior branches interlace to form networks called **plexuses** (PLEK-sus-eze), which then distribute branches to all parts of the body (see Fig. 8-11). The three main plexuses are described as follows:

- The **cervical plexus** supplies motor impulses to the muscles of the neck and receives sensory impulses from the neck and the back of the head. The phrenic nerve, which activates the diaphragm, arises from this plexus.
- The **brachial** (BRA-ke-al) **plexus** sends numerous branches to the shoulder, arm, forearm, wrist, and hand. The radial nerve emerges from the brachial plexus.
- The **lumbosacral** (lum-bo-SA-kral) **plexus** supplies nerves to the pelvis and legs. The largest branch in this plexus is the **sciatic** (si-AT-ik) **nerve**, which leaves the dorsal part of the pelvis, passes beneath the gluteus

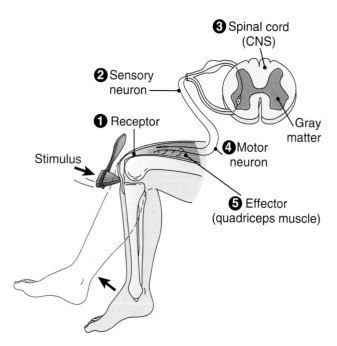

Figure 8-14 **The patellar (knee-jerk) reflex.** Numbers indicate the sequence of a reflex arc. *ZOOMING IN ✦ How many total neurons are involved in this spinal reflex? What neurotransmitter is released at the synapse shown by number 5?*

maximus muscle, and extends down the back of the thigh. At its beginning, it is nearly 1 inch thick, but it soon branches to the thigh muscles; near the knee, it forms two subdivisions that supply the leg and the foot.

Dermatomes Sensory neuron from all over the skin, except for the skin of the face and scalp, feed information into the spinal cord through the spinal nerves. The skin surface can be mapped into distinct regions that are supplied by a single spinal nerve. Each of these regions is called a **dermatome** (DER-mah-tome) (Fig. 8-15).

Sensation from a given dermatome is carried over its corresponding spinal nerve. This information can be used to identify the spinal nerve or spinal segment that is involved in an injury. In some areas, the dermatomes are not absolutely distinct. Some dermatomes may share a nerve supply with neighboring regions. For this reason, it is necessary to numb several adjacent dermatomes to achieve successful anesthesia.

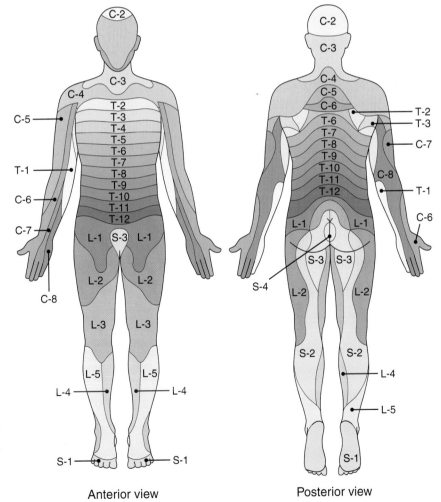

Anterior view   Posterior view

Figure 8-15 **Dermatomes.** A dermatome is a region of the skin supplied by a single spinal nerve. *ZOOMING IN ✦ Which spinal nerves carry impulses from the skin of the toes? From the anterior hand and fingers?*

Checkpoint 8-13 How many pairs of spinal nerves are there?

The Autonomic Nervous System (ANS)

The autonomic (visceral) nervous system regulates the action of the glands, the smooth muscles of hollow organs and vessels, and the heart muscle. These actions are carried on automatically; whenever a change occurs that calls for a regulatory adjustment, it is made without conscious awareness.

Most studies of the ANS concentrate on the motor (efferent) portion of the system. All autonomic pathways contain two motor neurons connecting the spinal cord with the effector organ. The two neurons synapse in ganglia that serve as relay stations along the way. The first neuron, the preganglionic neuron, extends from the spinal cord to the ganglion. The second neuron, the postganglionic neuron, travels from the ganglion to the effector. This differs from the voluntary (somatic) nervous system, in which each motor nerve fiber extends all the way from the spinal cord to the skeletal muscle with no intervening synapse. Some of the autonomic fibers are within the spinal nerves; some are within the cranial nerves (see Chapter 9).

Checkpoint 8-14 How many neurons are there in each motor pathway of the ANS?

Divisions of the Autonomic Nervous System

The motor neurons of the ANS are arranged in a distinct pattern, which has led to their separation for study purposes into **sympathetic** and **parasympathetic** divisions (Fig. 8-16), as described below and summarized in Table 8-3.

Sympathetic Nervous System The sympathetic motor neurons originate in the spinal cord with cell bodies in the thoracic and lumbar regions, the **thoracolumbar** (tho-rah-ko-LUM-bar) area. These preganglionic fibers arise from the spinal cord at the level of the first thoracic spinal nerve down to the level of the second lumbar spinal nerve. From this part of the cord, nerve fibers extend to ganglia where they synapse with postganglionic neurons, the fibers of which extend to the glands and involuntary muscle tissues.

Many of the sympathetic ganglia form the **sympathetic chains**, two cordlike strands of ganglia that extend along either side of the spinal column from the lower neck to the upper abdominal region. (Note that Figure 8-16 shows only one side for each division of the ANS.)

In addition, the nerves that supply the organs of the abdominal and pelvic cavities synapse in three single **collateral ganglia** farther from the spinal cord. These are the:

▸ Celiac ganglion, which sends fibers mainly to the digestive organs.
▸ Superior mesenteric ganglion, which sends fibers to the large and small intestines.
▸ Inferior mesenteric ganglion, which sends fibers to the distal large intestine and organs of the urinary and reproductive systems.

The postganglionic neurons of the sympathetic system, with few exceptions, act on their effectors by releasing the neurotransmitter epinephrine (adrenaline) and the related compound norepinephrine (noradrenaline). This system is therefore described as **adrenergic**, which means "activated by adrenaline."

Parasympathetic Nervous System The parasympathetic motor pathways begin in the **craniosacral** (kra-ne-o-SAK-ral) areas, with fibers arising from cell bodies in the brainstem (midbrain and medulla) and the lower (sacral) part of the spinal cord. From these centers, the first fibers extend to autonomic ganglia that are usually located near or within the walls of the effector organs and are called **terminal ganglia**. The pathways then continue along postganglionic neurons that stimulate the involuntary tissues.

Table 8·3	Divisions of the Autonomic Nervous System	
CHARACTERISTICS		**DIVISIONS**
	Sympathetic Nervous System	**Parasympathetic Nervous System**
Origin of fibers	Thoracic and lumbar regions of the spinal cord; thoracolumbar	Brain stem and sacral regions of the spinal cord; craniosacral
Location of ganglia	Sympathetic chains and three single collateral ganglia (celiac, superior mesenteric, inferior mesenteric)	Terminal ganglia in or near the effector organ
Neurotransmitter	Adrenaline and noradrenaline; adrenergic	Acetylcholine; cholinergic
Effects (see Table 8-4)	Response to stress; fight-or-flight response	Reverses fight-or-flight (stress) response; stimulates some activities

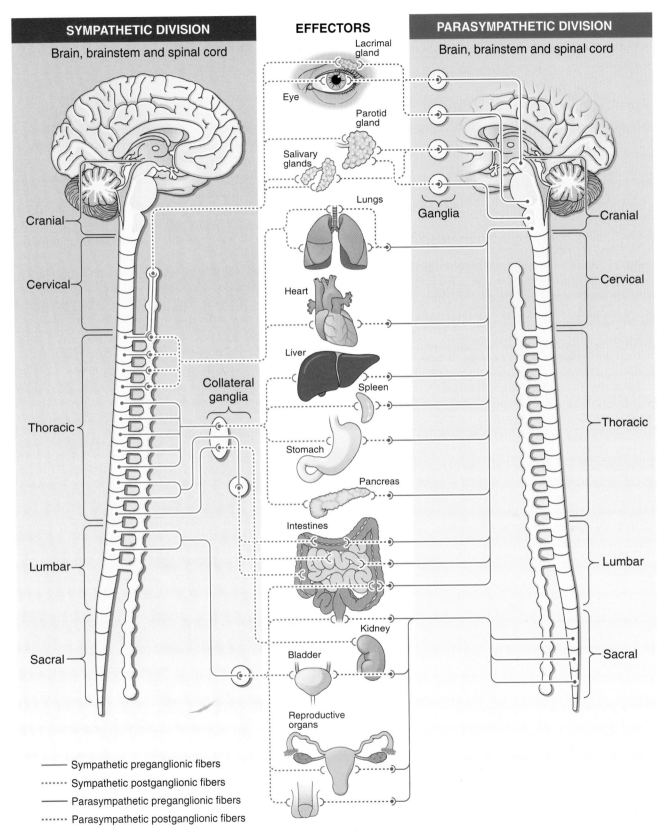

Figure 8-16 Autonomic nervous system. The diagram shows only one side of the body for each division. *ZOOMING IN* ✦ *Which division of the autonomic system has a ganglia closer to the effector organ?*

The neurons of the parasympathetic system release the neurotransmitter acetylcholine, leading to the description of this system as **cholinergic** (activated by acetylcholine).

Functions of the Autonomic Nervous System

Most organs are supplied by both sympathetic and parasympathetic fibers, and the two systems generally have opposite effects. The sympathetic part of the ANS tends to act as an accelerator for those organs needed to meet a stressful situation. It promotes what is called the **fight-or-flight response** because in the most primitive terms, the person must decide to stay and "fight it out" with the enemy or to run away from danger. If you think of what happens to a person who is frightened or angry, you can easily remember the effects of impulses from the sympathetic nervous system:

- Increase in the rate and force of heart contractions.
- Increase in blood pressure due partly to the more effective heartbeat and partly to constriction of small arteries in the skin and the internal organs.
- Dilation of blood vessels to skeletal muscles, bringing more blood to these tissues.
- Dilation of the bronchial tubes to allow more oxygen to enter.
- Stimulation of the central portion of the adrenal gland. This produces hormones, including epinephrine, that prepare the body to meet emergency situations in many ways (see Chap. 11). The sympathetic nerves and hormones from the adrenal gland reinforce each other.

- Increase in basal metabolic rate.
- Dilation of the pupil and decrease in focusing ability (for near objects).

The sympathetic system also acts as a brake on those systems not directly involved in the response to stress, such as the urinary and digestive systems. If you try to eat while you are angry, you may note that your saliva is thick and so small in amount that you can swallow only with difficulty. Under these circumstances, when food does reach the stomach, it seems to stay there longer than usual.

The parasympathetic part of the ANS normally acts as a balance for the sympathetic system once a crisis has passed. The parasympathetic system brings about constriction of the pupils, slowing of the heart rate, and constriction of the bronchial tubes. It also stimulates the formation and release of urine and activity of the digestive tract. Saliva, for example, flows more easily and profusely, and its quantity and fluidity increase.

Most organs of the body receive both sympathetic and parasympathetic stimulation, the effects of the two systems on a given organ generally being opposite. Table 8-4 shows some of the actions of these two systems. Box 8-3, Cell Receptors: Getting the Message, stresses the role of receptors in regulating the activities of the sympathetic and parasympathetic systems.

Checkpoint 8-15 Which division of the ANS stimulates a stress response, and which division reverses the stress response?

Table 8·4 Effects of the Sympathetic and Parasympathetic Systems on Selected Organs

Effector	Sympathetic System	Parasympathetic System
Pupils of eye	Dilation	Constriction
Sweat glands	Stimulation	None
Digestive glands	Inhibition	Stimulation
Heart	Increased rate and strength of beat	Decreased rate of beat
Bronchi of lungs	Dilation	Constriction
Muscles of digestive system	Decreased contraction (peristalsis)	Increased contraction
Kidneys	Decreased activity	None
Urinary bladder	Relaxation	Contraction and emptying
Liver	Increased release of glucose	None
Penis	Ejaculation	Erection
Adrenal medulla	Stimulation	None
Blood vessels to:		
Skeletal muscles	Dilation	Constriction
Skin	Constriction	None
Respiratory system	Dilation	Constriction
Digestive organs	Constriction	Dilation

Box 8-3	A Closer Look

Cell Receptors: Getting the Message

Neurons use neurotransmitters to communicate with other cells at synapses. Just as important, however, are the "docking sites," the receptors on the receiving (postsynaptic) cell membranes. A neurotransmitter fits into its receptor like a key in a lock. Once the neurotransmitter binds, the receptor initiates events that change the postsynaptic cell's activity. Different receptors' responses to the same neurotransmitter may vary, and a cell's response depends on the receptors it contains.

Among the many different classes of identified receptors, two are especially important and well-studied. The first is the cholinergic receptors, which bind acetylcholine (ACh). Cholinergic receptors are further subdivided into two types, each named for drugs that bind to them and mimic ACh's effects:

▶ Nicotinic receptors (which bind nicotine) are found on skeletal muscle cells and stimulate muscle contraction when ACh is present.
▶ Muscarinic receptors (which bind muscarine, a poison) are

found on effector cells of the parasympathetic nervous system. ACh can either stimulate or inhibit muscarinic receptors depending on the effector organ. For example, ACh stimulates digestive organs but inhibits the heart.

The second class of receptors is the adrenergic receptors, which bind norepinephrine and epinephrine. They are found on effector cells of the sympathetic nervous system. They are further subdivided into alpha (α) and beta (β), each with several subtypes (*e.g*, α_1, α_2, β_1, and β_2). When norepinephrine (or epinephrine) binds to adrenergic receptors, it can either stimulate or inhibit, depending on the organ. For example, norepinephrine stimulates the heart and inhibits the digestive organs. With some exceptions, α_1 and β_1 receptors usually stimulate, whereas α_2 and β_2 receptors inhibit.

Some drugs block specific receptors. For example, "beta-blockers" regulate the heart in cardiac disease by preventing β_1 receptors from binding epinephrine, the neurotransmitter that increases the rate and strength of heart contractions.

Word Anatomy

Medical terms are built from standardized word parts (prefixes, roots, and suffixes). Learning the meanings of these parts can help you remember words and interpret unfamiliar terms.

WORD PART	MEANING	EXAMPLE
The Nervous System as a Whole		
soma-	body	The *somatic* nervous system controls skeletal muscles that move the body.
aut/o	self	The *autonomic* nervous system is automatically controlled and is involuntary.
neur/i	nerve, nervous tissue	The *neurilemma* is the outer membrane of the myelin sheath around an axon.
-lemma	sheath	See preceding example.

WORD PART	MEANING	EXAMPLE
The Nervous System at Work		
de-	remove	*Depolarization* removes the charge on the plasma membrane of a cell.
re-	again, back	*Repolarization* restores the charge on the plasma membrane of a cell.
post-	after	The *postsynaptic* cell is located after the synapse and receives neurotransmitter from the presynaptic cell.

Summary

I. Role of the nervous system
A. Structural divisions—anatomic
  1. Central nervous system (CNS)—brain and spinal cord
  2. Peripheral nervous system (PNS)—spinal and cranial nerves
B. Functional divisions—physiologic
  1. Somatic nervous system—voluntary; supplies skeletal muscles
  2. Autonomic (visceral) nervous system—involuntary; supplies smooth muscle, cardiac muscle, glands

II. Neurons and their functions
A. Structure of a neuron
  1. Cell body
  2. Cell fibers
    a. Dendrite—carries impulses to cell body
    b. Axon—carries impulses away from cell body
  3. Myelin sheath
    a. Covers and protects some axons
    b. Speeds conduction
    c. Made by Schwann cells in PNS; other cells in CNS
      (1) Neurilemma—outermost layer of Schwann cell; aids axon repair
    d. White matter—myelinated tissue; gray matter—unmyelinated tissue
B. Types of neurons
  1. Sensory (afferent)—carry impulses toward CNS
  2. Motor (efferent)—carry impulses away from CNS
  3. Interneurons—in CNS
C. Nerves and tracts—bundles of neuron fibers
  1. Nerve—in peripheral nervous system
    a. Held together by connective tissue
      (1) Endoneurium—around a single fiber
      (2) Perineurium—around each fascicle
      (3) Epineurium—around whole nerve
    b. Types of nerves
      (1) Sensory (afferent) nerve—contains only fibers that carry impulses toward the CNS (from a receptor)
      (2) Motor (efferent) nerve—contains only fibers that carry impulses away from the CNS (to an effector)
      (3) Mixed nerve—contains both sensory and motor fibers
  2. Tract—in central nervous system

III. Neuroglia
  1. Nonconducting cells
  2. Protect and support nervous tissue

IV. The nervous system at work
A. Nerve impulse
  1. Potential—electrical charge on the plasma membrane of neuron
  2. Action potential
    a. Depolarization—reversal of charge
    b. Repolarization—return to normal
    c. Involves changes in concentrations of Na^+ and K^+
  3. Nerve impulse—spread of action potential along membrane
  4. Myelin sheath speeds conduction
B. Synapse—junction between neurons
  1. Nerve impulse transmitted from presynaptic neuron to postsynaptic neuron
  2. Neurotransmitter—carries impulse across synapse
  3. Receptors—in postsynaptic membrane; pick up neurotransmitters
  4. Neurotransmitter removed by diffusion, destruction by enzyme, return to presynaptic cell (reuptake)
  5. Electrical synapses—in smooth muscle, cardiac muscle, CNS

V. Spinal cord
  1. In vertebral column
  2. Ends between first and second lumbar vertebrae
A. Structure of the spinal cord
  1. H-shaped area of gray matter
  2. White matter around gray matter
    a. Ascending tracts—carry impulses toward brain
    b. Descending tracts—carry impulses away from brain
B. Reflex arc—pathway through the nervous system
  1. Components
    a. Receptor—detects stimulus
    b. Sensory neuron—receptor to CNS
    c. Central neuron—in CNS
    d. Motor neuron—CNS to effector
    e. Effector—muscle or gland that responds
  2. Reflex activities—simple reflex is rapid, automatic response using few neurons
    a. Examples—stretch reflex, eye blink, withdrawal reflex
    b. Spinal reflex—coordinated in spinal cord

VI. Spinal nerves—31 pairs
  1. Roots
    a. Dorsal (sensory)
    b. Ventral (motor)
  2. Spinal nerve—combines sensory and motor fibers (mixed nerve)
A. Branches of the spinal nerves
  1. Plexuses: networks formed by anterior branches
    a. Cervical plexus
    b. Brachial plexus
    c. Lumbosacral plexus
  2. Dermatome—region of the skin supplied by a single spinal nerve

VII. Autonomic nervous system (visceral nervous system)
  1. Involuntary
  2. Controls glands, smooth muscle, heart (cardiac) muscle
  3. Two motor neurons (preganglionic and postganglionic)
A. Divisions of the autonomic nervous system
  1. Sympathetic nervous system
    a. Thoracolumbar
    b. Adrenergic—uses adrenaline
    c. Synapses in sympathetic chains and three collateral ganglia (celiac, superior mesenteric, inferior mesenteric)

2. Parasympathetic system
   a. Craniosacral
   b. Cholinergic—uses acetylcholine
   c. Synapses in terminal ganglia in or near effector organs

B. Functions of the autonomic nervous system
   1. Sympathetic—stimulates fight-or-flight (stress) response
   2. Parasympathetic—returns body to normal
   3. Usually have opposite effects on an organ

Questions for Study and Review

Building Understanding

Fill in the blanks
1. The brain and spinal cord make up the _____ nervous system.
2. Action potentials are conducted away from the neuron cell body by the _____.
3. During an action potential the flow of Na^+ into the cell causes _____.
4. In the spinal cord, sensory information travels in _____ tracts.
5. With few exceptions, the sympathetic nervous system uses the neurotransmitter _____ to act on effector organs.

Matching
Match each numbered item with the most closely related lettered item.
___ 6. Cells that carry impulses from the CNS
___ 7. Cells that carry impulses to the CNS
___ 8. Cells that carry impulses within the CNS
___ 9. Cells that detect a stimulus
___ 10. Cells that carry out a response to a stimulus

    a. receptors
    b. effectors
    c. sensory neurons
    d. motor neurons
    e. interneurons

Multiple choice
___ 11. Skeletal muscles are voluntarily controlled by the
    a. central nervous system
    b. somatic nervous system
    c. parasympathetic nervous system
    d. sympathetic nervous system
___ 12. The cells involved in most nervous system tumors are called
    a. motor neurons
    b. sensory neurons
    c. interneurons
    d. neuroglia
___ 13. The correct order of synaptic transmission is
    a. postsynaptic neuron, synapse, and presynaptic neuron
    b. presynaptic neuron, synapse, and postsynaptic neuron
    c. presynaptic neuron, postsynaptic neuron, and synapse
    d. postsynaptic neuron, presynaptic neuron, and synapse
___ 14. Afferent nerve fibers enter the part of the spinal cord called the
    a. dorsal horn
    b. ventral horn

    c. gray commisure
    d. central canal
___ 15. The "fight-or-flight" response is promoted by the
    a. sympathetic nervous system
    b. parasympathetic nervous system
    c. somatic nervous system
    d. reflex arc

Understanding Concepts

16. Differentiate between the terms in each of the following pairs:
    a. neurons and neuroglia
    b. vesicle and receptor
    c. gray matter and white matter
    d. nerve and tract
17. Describe an action potential. How does conduction along a myelinated fiber differ from conduction along an unmyelinated fiber?
18. Discuss the structure and function of the spinal cord.
19. Explain the reflex arc using stepping on a tack as an example.
20. Describe the anatomy of a spinal nerve. How many pairs of spinal nerves are there?
21. Define a *plexus*. Name the three main spinal nerve plexuses.

22. Differentiate between the functions of the sympathetic and parasympathetic divisions of the autonomic nervous system.

Conceptual Thinking

23. Clinical depression is associated with abnormal serotonin levels. Medications that block the removal of this neurotransmitter from the synapse can control the disorder. Based on this information, is clinical depression associated with increased or decreased levels of serotonin? Explain your answer.

24. Mr. Hayward visits his dentist for a root canal and is given Novocain, a local anesthetic, at the beginning of the procedure. Novocain reduces membrane permeability to Na^+. What effect does this have on action potential?

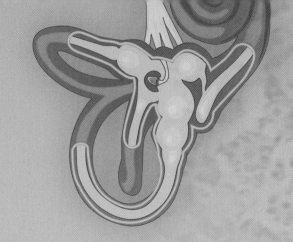

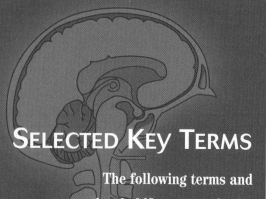

SELECTED KEY TERMS

The following terms and other boldface terms in the chapter are defined in the Glossary

brain stem
cerebellum
cerebral cortex
cerebrospinal fluid (CSF)
cerebrum
diencephalon
electroencephalograph (EEG)
gyrus (pl., gyri)
hypothalamus
medulla oblongata
meninges
midbrain
pons
sulcus (pl., sulci)
thalamus
ventricle

LEARNING OUTCOMES

After careful study of this chapter, you should be able to:

1. Give the location and functions of the four main divisions of the brain
2. Name and describe the three meninges
3. Cite the function of cerebrospinal fluid and describe where and how this fluid is formed
4. Name and locate the lobes of the cerebral hemispheres
5. Cite one function of the cerebral cortex in each lobe of the cerebrum
6. Name two divisions of the diencephalon and cite the functions of each
7. Locate the three subdivisions of the brain stem and give the functions of each
8. Describe the cerebellum and cite its functions
9. Name some techniques used to study the brain
10. Cite the names and functions of the 12 cranial nerves
11. Show how word parts are used to build words related to the nervous system (see Word Anatomy at the end of the chapter)

The Nervous System: The Brain and Cranial Nerves

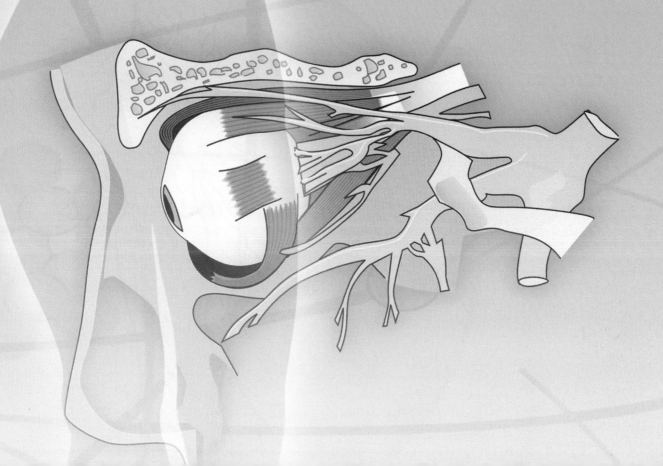

The Brain

The brain occupies the cranial cavity and is covered by membranes, fluid, and the bones of the skull. Although the brain's various regions communicate and function together, the brain may be divided into distinct areas for ease of study (Fig. 9-1, Table 9-1):

- The **cerebrum** (SER-e-brum) is the largest part of the brain. It is divided into right and left **cerebral** (SER-e-bral) **hemispheres** by a deep groove called the **longitudinal fissure** (Fig. 9-2). Each hemisphere is further subdivided into lobes.
- The **diencephalon** (di-en-SEF-ah-lon) is the area between the cerebral hemispheres and the brain stem. It includes the thalamus and the hypothalamus.
- The **brain stem** connects the cerebrum and diencephalon with the spinal cord. The superior portion of the brain stem is the **midbrain**. Inferior to the midbrain is the **pons** (ponz), followed by the **medulla oblongata** (meh-DUL-lah ob-long-GAH-tah). The pons connects the midbrain with the medulla, whereas the medulla connects the brain with the spinal cord through a large opening in the base of the skull (foramen magnum).
- The **cerebellum** (ser-eh-BEL-um) is located immediately below the posterior part of the cerebral hemispheres and is connected with the cerebrum, brain stem, and spinal cord by means of the pons. The word *cerebellum* means "little brain."

Each of these divisions is described in greater detail later in this chapter. Damage to any of these brain structures can have severe consequences on brain function (see Box 9-1, Brain Injury: A Heads-Up).

> **Checkpoint 9-1** What are the main divisions of the brain?

Protective Structures of the Brain and Spinal Cord

The **meninges** (men-IN-jez) are three layers of connective tissue that surround both the brain and spinal cord to form a complete enclosure (Fig. 9-3). The outermost of these membranes, the **dura mater** (DU-rah MA-ter), is the thickest and toughest of the meninges. (*Mater* is from the Latin meaning "mother," referring to the protective function of the meninges; *dura* means "hard.") Around the brain, the dura mater is in two layers, and the outer layer is fused to the bones of the cranium. In certain places, these two layers separate to provide venous channels, called **dural sinuses**, for the drainage of blood coming from the brain tissue.

The middle layer of the meninges is the **arachnoid** (ah-RAK-noyd). This membrane is loosely attached to the deepest of the meninges by weblike fibers, allowing a space for

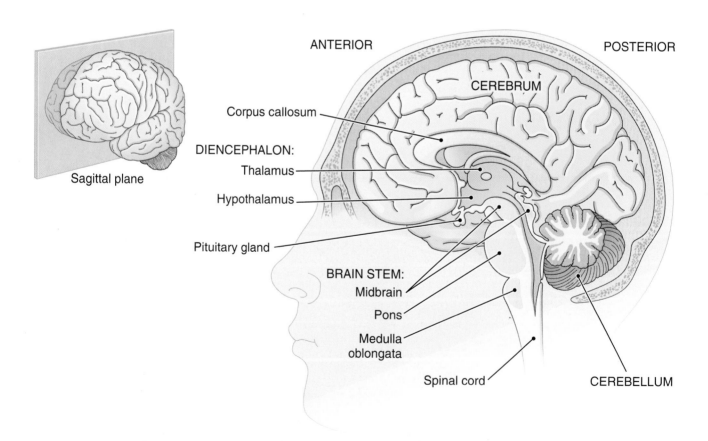

Figure 9-1 Brain, sagittal section. Main divisions are shown.

Table 9·1	Organization of the Brain	
DIVISION	**DESCRIPTION**	**FUNCTIONS**
Cerebrum	Largest and uppermost portion of the brain Divided into two hemispheres, each subdivided into lobes	Cortex (outer layer) is site for conscious thought, memory, reasoning, and abstract mental functions, all localized within specific lobes
Diencephalon	Between the cerebrum and the brain stem Contains the thalamus and hypothalamus	Thalamus sorts and redirects sensory input; hypothalamus maintains homeostasis, controls autonomic nervous system and pituitary gland
Brain stem	Anterior region below the cerebrum	Connects cerebrum and diencephalon with spinal cord
Midbrain	Below the center of the cerebrum	Has reflex centers concerned with vision and hearing; connects cerebrum with lower portions of the brain
Pons	Anterior to the cerebellum	Connects cerebellum with other portions of the brain; helps to regulate respiration
Medulla oblongata	Between the pons and the spinal cord	Links the brain with the spinal cord; has centers for control of vital functions, such as respiration and the heartbeat
Cerebellum	Below the posterior portion of the cerebellum Divided into two hemispheres	Coordinates voluntary muscles; maintains balance and muscle tone

the movement of cerebrospinal fluid (CSF) between the two membranes. (The arachnoid is named from the Latin word for spider because of its weblike appearance).

The innermost layer around the brain, the **pia mater** (PI-ah MA-ter), is attached to the nervous tissue of the brain and spinal cord and follows all the contours of these structures (see Fig. 9-3). It is made of a delicate connec-

tive tissue (*pia* meaning "tender" or "soft"). The pia mater holds blood vessels that supply nutrients and oxygen to the brain and spinal cord.

Checkpoint 9-2 The meninges are protective membranes around the brain and spinal cord. What are the names of the three layers of the meninges from the outermost to the innermost?

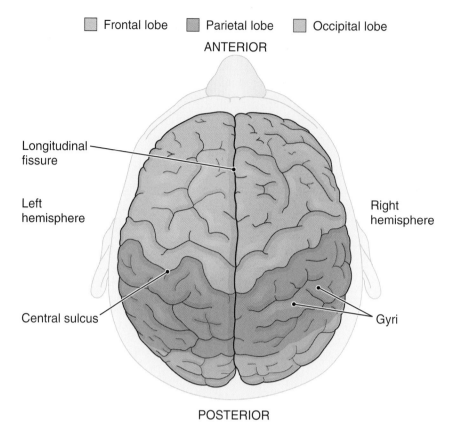

Frontal lobe Parietal lobe Occipital lobe

ANTERIOR

Longitudinal fissure

Left hemisphere

Right hemisphere

Central sulcus

Gyri

POSTERIOR

Figure 9-2 External surface of the brain, superior view. The division into two hemispheres and into lobes is visible.

Box 9-1   Clinical Perspectives

Brain Injury: A Heads-Up

Traumatic brain injury is a leading cause of death and disability in the United States. Each year, approximately 1.5 million Americans sustain a brain injury, of whom about 50,000 will die and 80,000 will suffer long-term or permanent disability. The leading causes of traumatic brain injury are motor vehicle accidents, gunshot wounds, and falls. Other causes include shaken baby syndrome (caused by violent shaking of an infant or toddler) and second impact syndrome (when a second head injury occurs before the first has fully healed).

Brain damage occurs either from penetrating head trauma or acceleration-deceleration events where a head in motion suddenly comes to a stop. Nervous tissue, blood vessels, and possibly the meninges may be bruised, torn, lacerated, or ruptured, which may lead to swelling, hemorrhage, and hematoma. The best protection from brain injury is to prevent it. The following is a list of safety tips:

▶ Always wear a seat belt and secure children in approved car seats.
▶ Never drive after using alcohol or drugs or ride with an impaired driver.

▶ Always wear a helmet during activities such as biking, motorcycling, in-line skating, horseback riding, football, ice hockey, and batting and running bases in baseball and softball.
▶ Inspect playground equipment and supervise children using it. Never swing children around to play "airplane," nor vigorously bounce or shake them.
▶ Allow adequate time for healing after a head injury before resuming potentially dangerous activities.
▶ Prevent falls by using a nonslip bathtub or shower mat and using a step stool to reach objects on high shelves. Use a safety gate at the bottom and top of stairs to protect young children (and adults with dementia or other disorienting conditions).
▶ Keep unloaded firearms in a locked cabinet or safe and store bullets in a separate location.

For more information, contact the Brain Injury Association of America.

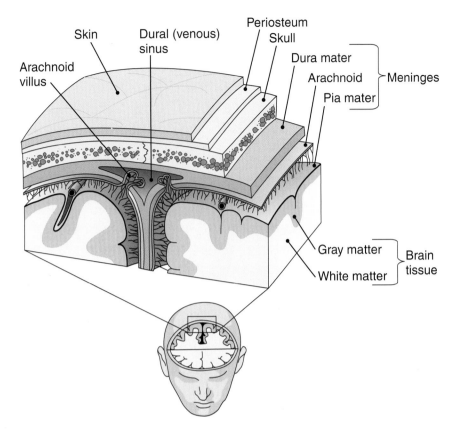

Figure 9-3 Frontal (coronal) section of the top of the head. The meninges and related parts are shown. *ZOOMING IN ✦ What is located in the spaces where the dura mater divides into two layers?*

Cerebrospinal Fluid

Cerebrospinal (ser-e-bro-SPI-nal) **fluid** is a clear liquid that circulates in and around the brain and spinal cord (Fig. 9-4). The function of the CSF is to support nervous tissue and to cushion shocks that would otherwise injure these delicate structures. This fluid also carries nutrients to the cells and transports waste products from the cells.

CSF flows freely through passageways in and around the brain and spinal cord and finally flows out into the subarachnoid space of the meninges. Much of the fluid then returns to the blood through projections called *arachnoid villi* in the dural sinuses (see Figs. 9-3 and 9-4).

Ventricles CSF forms in four spaces within the brain called **ventricles** (VEN-trih-klz) (Fig. 9-5). A vascular network in each ventricle, the **choroid** (KOR-oyd) **plexus**, forms CSF by filtration of the blood and by cellular secretion.

The four ventricles that produce CSF extend somewhat irregularly into the various parts of the brain. The largest are the lateral ventricles in the two cerebral hemispheres. Their extensions into the lobes of the cerebrum are called **horns**. These paired ventricles communicate with a midline space, the third ventricle, by means of openings called **foramina** (fo-RAM-in-ah). The third ventricle is surrounded by the diencephalon. Continuing down from the third ventricle, a small canal, called the **cerebral aqueduct**, extends through the midbrain into the fourth ventricle,

which is located between the brain stem and the cerebellum. This ventricle is continuous with the central canal of the spinal cord. In the roof of the fourth ventricle are three openings that allow the escape of CSF to the area that surrounds the brain and spinal cord.

Box 9-2, The Blood-Brain Barrier: Access Denied, presents information on protecting the brain.

Checkpoint 9-3 In addition to the meninges, CSF helps to support and protect the brain and spinal cord. Where is CSF produced?

❱ The Cerebral Hemispheres

Each cerebral hemisphere is divided into four visible **lobes** named for the overlying cranial bones. These are the frontal, parietal, temporal, and occipital lobes (Fig. 9-6). In addition, there is a small fifth lobe deep within each hemisphere that cannot be seen from the surface. Not much is known about this lobe, which is called the **insula** (IN-su-lah).

The outer nervous tissue of the cerebral hemispheres is gray matter that makes up the **cerebral cortex** (see Fig. 9-3). This thin layer of gray matter (2–4 mm thick) is the most highly evolved portion of the brain and is responsible for conscious thought, reasoning, and abstract mental functions. Specific functions are localized in the cortex of the different lobes, as described in greater detail later.

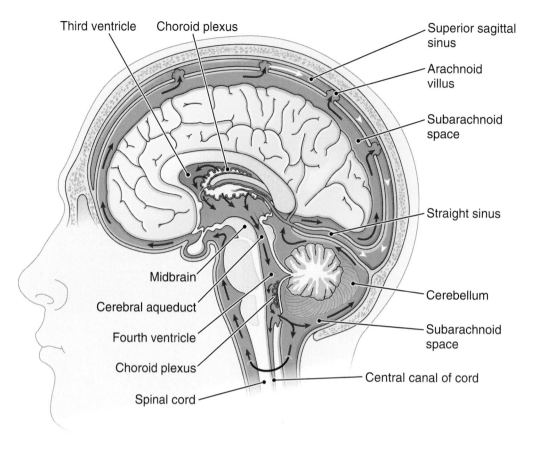

Figure 9-4 Flow of cerebrospinal fluid (CSF). Black arrows show the flow of CSF from the choroid plexuses and back to the blood in dural sinuses; white arrows show the flow of blood. (The actual passageways through which the CSF flows are narrower than those shown here, which have been enlarged for visibility.) *ZOOMING IN ✦ Which ventricle is continuous with the central canal of the spinal cord?*

Box 9-2	A Closer Look

The Blood-Brain Barrier: Access Denied

Neurons in the central nervous system (CNS) function properly only if the composition of the extracellular fluid bathing them is carefully regulated. The semipermeable blood-brain barrier helps maintain this stable environment by allowing some substances to cross it while blocking others. Whereas it allows glucose, amino acids, and some electrolytes to cross, it prevents passage of hormones, drugs, neurotransmitters, and other substances that might adversely affect the brain.

Structural features of CNS capillaries create this barrier. In most parts of the body, capillaries are lined with simple squamous epithelial cells that are loosely attached to each other. The small spaces between cells let materials move between the bloodstream and the tissues. In CNS capillaries, the simple squamous epithelial cells are joined by tight junctions that limit passage of materials between them. Astrocytes—specialized neuroglial cells that wrap around capillaries and limit their permeability—also contribute to this barrier.

The blood-brain barrier excludes pathogens, although some viruses, including poliovirus and herpesvirus, can bypass it by traveling along peripheral nerves into the CNS. Some streptococci also can breach the tight junctions. Disease processes, such as hypertension, ischemia (lack of blood supply), and inflammation, can increase the blood-brain barrier's permeability.

The blood-brain barrier is an obstacle to delivering drugs to the brain. Some antibiotics can cross it, whereas others cannot. Neurotransmitters also pose problems. In Parkinson disease, the neurotransmitter dopamine is deficient in the brain. Dopamine itself will not cross the barrier, but a related compound, L-dopa, will. L-dopa crosses the blood-brain barrier and is then converted to dopamine. Mixing a drug with a concentrated sugar solution and injecting it into the bloodstream is another effective delivery method. The solution's high osmotic pressure causes water to osmose out of capillary cells, shrinking them and opening tight junctions through which the drug can pass.

The cortex is arranged in folds forming elevated portions known as **gyri** (JI-ri), singular *gyrus*. These raised areas are separated by shallow grooves called **sulci** (SUL-si), *singular sulcus* (Fig. 9-7). Although there are many sulci, the following two are especially important landmarks:

▸ The **central sulcus,** which lies between the frontal and parietal lobes of each hemisphere at right angles to the longitudinal fissure (see Figs. 9-2 and 9-6).
▸ The **lateral sulcus,** which curves along the side of each hemisphere and separates the temporal lobe from the frontal and parietal lobes (see Fig. 9-6).

Internally, the cerebral hemispheres are made largely of white matter and a few islands of gray matter. The white matter consists of myelinated fibers that connect the cortical areas with each other and with other parts of the nervous system.

Basal nuclei, also called **basal ganglia,** are masses of gray matter located deep within each cerebral hemisphere. These groups of neurons work with the cerebral cortex to regulate body movement and the muscles of facial expression. The neurons of the basal nuclei secrete the neurotransmitter **dopamine** (DO-pah-mene).

The **corpus callosum** (kah-LO-sum) is an important band of white matter located at the bottom of the longitudinal fissure (see Fig. 9-1). This band is a bridge between the right and left hemispheres, permitting impulses to cross from one side of the brain to the other.

The **internal capsule** is a compact band of myelinated fibers that carries impulses between the cerebral hemispheres and the brain stem. The vertical fibers that make up the internal capsule travel between the thalamus and some of the basal nuclei on each side and then radiate toward the cerebral cortex.

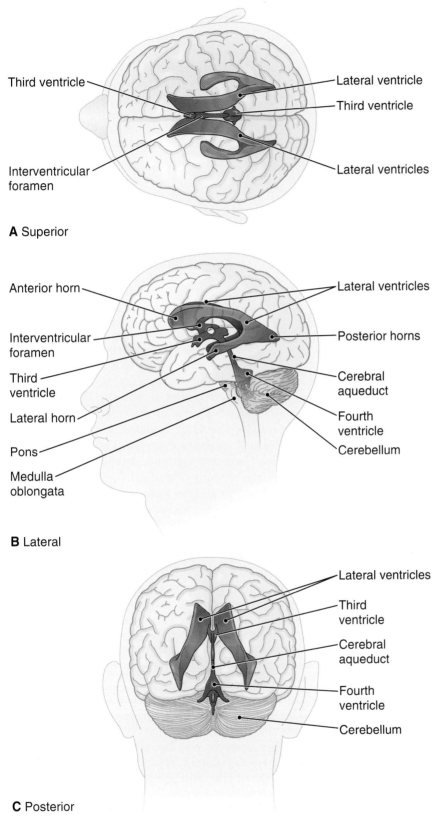

A Superior

B Lateral

C Posterior

Figure 9-5 **Ventricles of the brain.** Three views are shown. *ZOOMING IN ✦ Which are the largest ventricles?*

Checkpoint 9-4 What are the four surface lobes of each cerebral hemisphere?

☐ Frontal lobe   ▨ Parietal lobe   ☐ Temporal lobe   ☐ Occipital lobe

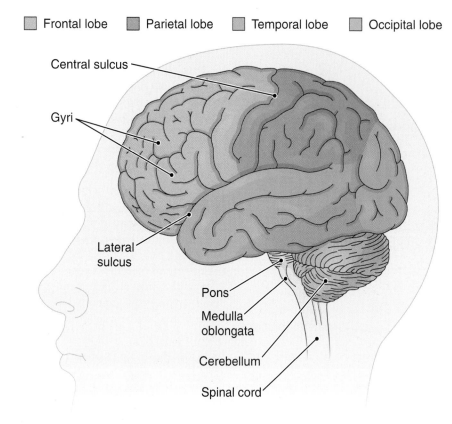

Figure 9-6   External surface of the brain, lateral view. The lobes and surface features of the cerebrum are visible.   *ZOOMING IN* ✦ *What structure separates the frontal from the parietal lobe?*

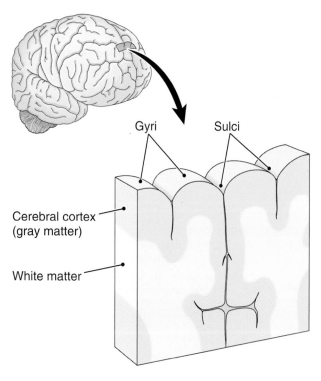

Figure 9-7   Section of the cerebrum. Labels point out surface features, the cerebral cortex, and the white matter. *ZOOMING IN* ✦ *How is the cortex provided with increased surface area?*

Functions of the Cerebral Cortex

It is within the cerebral cortex, the layer of gray matter that forms the surface of each cerebral hemisphere, that impulses are received and analyzed. These activities form the basis of knowledge. The brain "stores" information, much of which can be recalled on demand by means of the phenomenon called *memory*. It is in the cerebral cortex that thought processes such as association, judgment, and discrimination take place. Conscious deliberation and voluntary actions also arise from the cerebral cortex.

Although the various brain areas act in coordination to produce behavior, particular functions are localized in the cortex of each lobe (Fig. 9-8). Some of these are described below:

▶ The **frontal lobe,** which is relatively larger in humans than in any other organism, lies anterior to the central sulcus. The gyrus just anterior to the central sulcus in this lobe contains a **primary motor area**, which provides conscious control of skeletal muscles. Note that the more detailed the action, the greater the amount of cortical tissue involved (Fig. 9-9). The frontal lobe also contains two areas important in speech (the speech centers are discussed later).

▶ The **parietal lobe** occupies the superior part of each hemisphere and lies posterior to the central sulcus. The gyrus just behind the central sulcus in this lobe contains the **primary sensory area,** where impulses from the skin, such as touch, pain, and temperature, are interpreted. The estimation of distances, sizes, and shapes also takes place here. As with the motor cortex, the greater the intensity of sensation from a particular area, the tongue or fingers, for example, the more area of the cortex is involved.

▶ The **temporal lobe** lies inferior to the lateral sulcus and folds under the hemisphere on each side. This lobe contains the **auditory area** for receiving and interpreting impulses from the ear. The **olfactory area,** concerned with the sense of smell, is located in the medial part of the temporal lobe; it is stimulated by impulses arising from receptors in the nose.

▶ The **occipital lobe** lies posterior to the parietal lobe and extends over the cerebellum. The visual area of this lobe contains the **visual receiving area** and the **visual association area** for interpreting impulses arising from the retina of the eye.

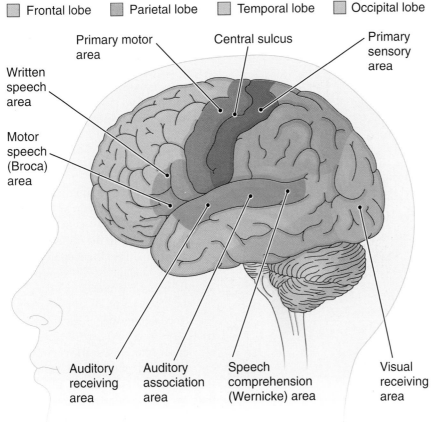

☐ Frontal lobe ☐ Parietal lobe ☐ Temporal lobe ☐ Occipital lobe

Primary motor area

Central sulcus

Primary sensory area

Written speech area

Motor speech (Broca) area

Auditory receiving area

Auditory association area

Speech comprehension (Wernicke) area

Visual receiving area

Figure 9-8 **Functional areas of the cerebral cortex.** *ZOOMING IN ✦ What cortical area is posterior to the central sulcus? What area is anterior to the central sulcus?*

Checkpoint 9-5 Higher functions of the brain occur in a thin layer of gray matter on the surface of the cerebral hemispheres. What is the name of this outer layer of gray matter?

Communication Areas

The ability to communicate by written and verbal means is an interesting example of the way in which areas of the cerebral cortex are interrelated (see Fig. 9-8). The development and use of these areas are closely connected with the process of learning.

▶ The **auditory areas** lie in the temporal lobe. One of these areas, the **auditory receiving area**, detects sound impulses transmitted from the environment, whereas the surrounding area, the **auditory association area**, interprets the sounds. Another region of the auditory cortex, the **speech comprehension area**, or **Wernicke** (VER-nih-ke) **area**, functions in speech recognition and the meaning of words. Someone who suffers damage in this region of the brain, as by a stroke, will have difficulty in understanding the meaning of speech. The beginnings of language are learned by hearing; thus, the auditory areas for understanding sounds are near the auditory receiving area of the cortex. Babies often appear to understand what is being said long before they do any talking

themselves. It is usually several years before children learn to read or write words.

▶ The **motor areas** for spoken and written communication lie anterior to the most inferior part of the frontal lobe's motor cortex. The speech muscles in the tongue, the soft palate, and the larynx are controlled here, in a region named the **motor speech area**, or **Broca** (bro-KAH) **area** (see Fig. 9-8). A person who suffers damage to this area may have difficulty in producing speech (motor aphasia). Similarly, the written speech center lies anterior to the cortical area that controls the arm and hand muscles. The ability to write words is usually one of the last phases in the development of learning words and their meanings.

▶ The **visual areas** of the occipital lobe's cortex are also involved in communication. Here, visual images of language are received. The visual area that lies anterior to the receiving cortex then interprets these visual impulses as words. The ability to read with understanding also develops in this area. You might *see* writing in the Japanese language, for example, but this would involve only the visual receiving area in the occipital lobe unless you could also *understand* the words.

There is a functional relation among areas of the brain. Many neurons must work together to enable a person to receive, interpret, and respond to verbal and written messages as well as to touch (tactile stimulus) and other sensory stimuli.

Memory and the Learning Process

Memory is the mental faculty for recalling ideas. In the initial stage of the memory process, sensory signals (*e.g.,* visual, auditory) are retained for a very short time, perhaps only fractions of a second. Nevertheless, they can be used for further processing. **Short-term memory** refers to the retention of bits of information for a few seconds or perhaps a few minutes, after which the information is lost unless reinforced. **Long-term memory** refers to the storage of information that can be recalled at a later time. There is a tendency for a memory to become more fixed the more often a person repeats the remembered experience; thus, short-term memory signals can lead to long-term memories. Furthermore, the more often a memory is recalled, the more indelible it becomes; such a memory can be so deeply fixed in the brain that it can be recalled immediately.

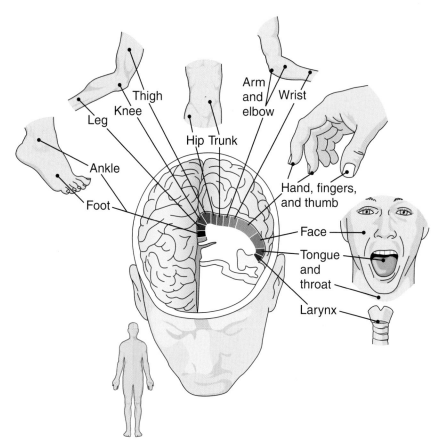

Figure 9-9 Motor areas of the cerebral cortex (frontal lobe). The amount of cortex involved in control of a body part is proportional to the degree of coordination needed in movement. The small figure indicates that control is contralateral. The right hemisphere controls the left side of the body and the left hemisphere controls the right side of the body.

Careful anatomic studies have shown that tiny extensions called *fibrils* form at the synapses in the cerebral cortex, enabling impulses to travel more easily from one neuron to another. The number of these fibrils increases with age. Physiologic studies show that rehearsal (repetition) of the same information again and again accelerates and potentiates the degree of transfer of short-term

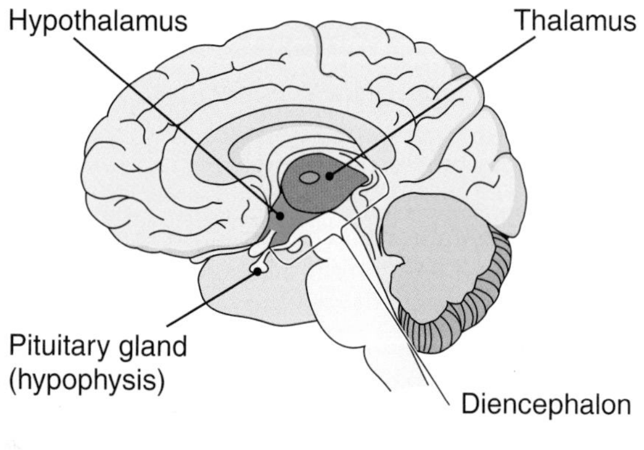

Figure 9-10 Regions of the diencephalon. The figure shows the relationship among the thalamus, hypothalamus, and pituitary gland (hypophysis). *ZOOMING IN ✦ To what part of the brain is the pituitary gland attached?*

memory into long-term memory. A person who is wide awake memorizes far better than does a person who is in a state of mental fatigue. It has also been noted that the brain is able to organize information so that new ideas are stored in the same areas in which similar ones had been stored before.

▶ The Diencephalon

The **diencephalon**, or interbrain, is located between the cerebral hemispheres and the brain stem. One can see it by cutting into the central section of the brain. The diencephalon includes the **thalamus** (THAL-ah-mus) and the **hypothalamus** (Fig. 9-10).

The two parts of the thalamus form the lateral walls of the third ventricle (see Figs. 9-1 and 9-5). Nearly all sensory impulses travel through the masses of gray matter that form the thalamus. The role of the thalamus is to sort out the impulses and direct them to particular areas of the cerebral cortex.

The hypothalamus is located in the midline area inferior to the thalamus and forms the floor of the third ventricle. It helps to maintain homeostasis by controlling body temperature, water balance, sleep, appetite, and some emotions, such as fear and pleasure. Both the sympathetic and parasympathetic divisions of the autonomic nervous system are under the control of the hypothalamus, as is the pituitary gland. The hypothalamus thus influences the heartbeat, the contraction and relaxation of blood vessels, hormone secretion, and other vital body functions.

> **Checkpoint 9-6** What are the two main portions of the diencephalon and what do they do?

The Limbic System

Along the border between the cerebrum and the diencephalon is a region known as the **limbic system**. This system is involved in emotional states and behavior. It includes the **hippocampus** (shaped like a sea horse), located under the lateral ventricles, which functions in learning and the formation of long-term memory. It also includes regions that stimulate the **reticular formation**, a network that extends along the brain stem and governs wakefulness and sleep. The limbic system thus links the conscious functions of the cerebral cortex and the automatic functions of the brain stem.

▶ The Brain Stem

The brain stem is composed of the midbrain, the pons, and the medulla oblongata (see Fig. 9-1). These structures connect the cerebrum and diencephalon with the spinal cord.

The Midbrain

The **midbrain,** inferior to the center of the cerebrum, forms the superior part of the brain stem. Four rounded masses of gray matter that are hidden by the cerebral hemispheres form the superior part of the midbrain. These four bodies act as centers for certain reflexes involving the eye and the ear, for example, moving the eyes in order to track an image or to read. The white matter at the anterior of the midbrain conducts impulses between the higher centers of the cerebrum and the lower centers of the pons, medulla, cerebellum, and spinal cord. Cranial nerves III and IV originate from the midbrain.

The Pons

The **pons** lies between the midbrain and the medulla, anterior to the cerebellum (see Fig. 9-1). It is composed largely of myelinated nerve fibers, which connect the two halves of the cerebellum with the brain stem as well as with the cerebrum above and the spinal cord below. (Its name means "bridge.")

The pons is an important connecting link between the cerebellum and the rest of the nervous system, and it contains nerve fibers that carry impulses to and from the centers located above and below it. Certain reflex (involuntary) actions, such as some of those regulating respiration, are integrated in the pons. Cranial nerves V through VIII originate from the pons.

The Medulla Oblongata

The **medulla oblongata** of the brain stem is located between the pons and the spinal cord (see Fig. 9-1). It appears white externally because, like the pons, it contains many myelinated nerve fibers. Internally, it contains collections of cell bodies (gray matter) called **nuclei,** or *centers.* Among these are vital centers, such as the following:

- The **respiratory center** controls the muscles of respiration in response to chemical and other stimuli.
- The **cardiac center** helps regulate the rate and force of the heartbeat.
- The **vasomotor** (vas-o-MO-tor) **center** regulates the contraction of smooth muscle in the blood vessel walls and thus controls blood flow and blood pressure.

The ascending sensory fibers that carry messages through the spinal cord up to the brain travel through the medulla, as do descending motor fibers. These groups of fibers form tracts (bundles) and are grouped together according to function.

The motor fibers from the motor cortex of the cerebral hemispheres extend down through the medulla, and most of them cross from one side to the other (decussate) while going through this part of the brain. The crossing of motor fibers in the medulla results in contralateral control—the right cerebral hemisphere controls muscles in the left side of the body and the left cerebral hemisphere controls muscles in the right side of the body, a characteristic termed *contralateral* (opposite side) *control.*

The medulla is an important reflex center; here, certain neurons end, and impulses are relayed to other neurons. The last four pairs of cranial nerves (IX through XII) are connected with the medulla.

Checkpoint 9-7 What are the three subdivisions of the brain stem?

▶ The Cerebellum

The **cerebellum** is made up of three parts: the middle portion (vermis) and two lateral hemispheres, the left and right (Fig. 9-11). Like the cerebral hemispheres, the cerebellum has an outer area of gray matter and an inner portion that is largely white matter. However, the white matter is distributed in a treelike pattern. The functions of the cerebellum are as follows:

- Help coordinate voluntary muscles to ensure smooth, orderly function. Disease of the cerebellum causes muscular jerkiness and tremors.
- Help maintain balance in standing, walking, and sitting as well as during more strenuous activities. Messages from the internal ear and from sensory receptors in tendons and muscles aid the cerebellum.
- Help maintain muscle tone so that all muscle fibers are slightly tensed and ready to produce changes in position as quickly as necessary.

Checkpoint 9-8 What are some functions of the cerebellum?

▶ Brain Studies

Some of the imaging techniques used to study the brain are described in Box 1-2, Medical Imaging: Seeing Without Making a Cut, in Chapter 1. These techniques include:

- CT (computed tomography) scan, which provides photographs of the bone, soft tissue, and cavities of the brain (Fig. 9-12 A). Anatomic lesions, such as tumors or scar tissue accumulations, are readily seen.
- MRI (magnetic resonance imaging), which gives more views of the brain than CT and may reveal tumors, scar tissue, and hemorrhaging not shown by CT (see Fig. 9-12 B).
- PET (positron emission tomography), which visualizes the brain in action (see Fig. 9-12 C).

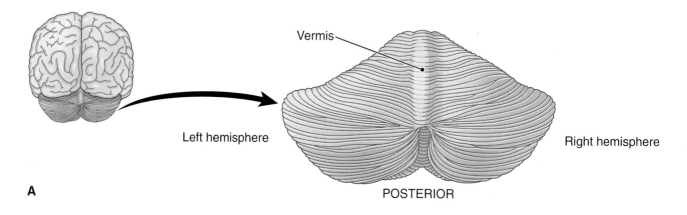

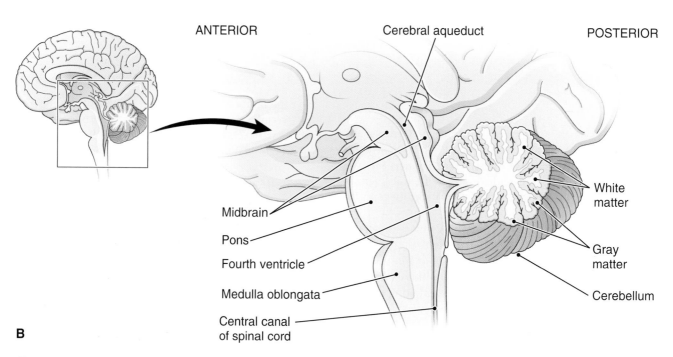

Figure 9-11   **The cerebellum.** (A) Posterior view showing the two hemispheres. (B) Midsagittal section showing the distribution of gray and white matter. The three parts of the brain stem (midbrain, pons, and medulla oblongata) are also labeled.

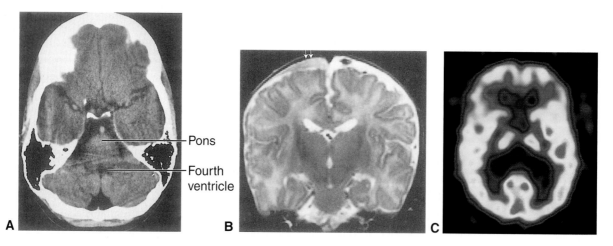

Figure 9-12   **Imaging the brain.** (A) CT scan of a normal adult brain at the level of the fourth ventricle. (B) MRI of the brain showing a point of injury (arrows). (C) PET scan. (A and B, reprinted with permission from Erkonen WE. Radiology 101. Philadelphia: Lippincott Williams & Wilkins, 1998. C, Courtesy of Newport Diagnostic Center, Newport Beach, CA.)

The Electroencephalograph

The interactions of the brain's billions of nerve cells give rise to measurable electric currents. These may be recorded using an instrument called the **electroencephalograph** (e-lek-tro-en-SEF-ah-lo-graf). Electrodes placed on the head pick up the electrical signals produced as the brain functions. These signals are then amplified and recorded to produce the tracings, or brain waves, of an electroencephalogram (EEG).

The electroencephalograph is used to study sleep patterns, to diagnose disease, such as epilepsy, to locate tumors, to study the effects of drugs, and to determine brain death. Figure 9-13 shows some typical normal tracings.

❱ Cranial Nerves

There are 12 pairs of cranial nerves (in this discussion, when a cranial nerve is identified, a pair is meant). They are numbered, usually in Roman numerals, according to their connection with the brain, beginning anteriorly and proceeding posteriorly (Fig. 9-14). Except for the first two pairs, all the cranial nerves arise from the brain stem. The first 9 pairs and the 12th pair supply structures in the head.

From a functional point of view, we may think of messages the cranial nerves handle as belonging to one of four categories:

❱ **Special sensory impulses**, such as those for smell, taste, vision, and hearing located in special sense organs in the head.

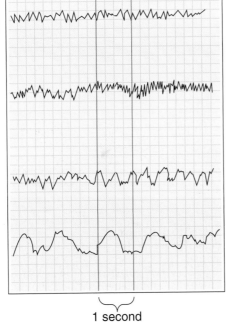

Figure 9-13 Electroencephalography. Normal brain waves.

Alpha waves-Normal, relaxed adult

Beta waves-State of excitement, intense concentration

Theta waves-Children

Delta waves-Deep sleep

1 second

❱ **General sensory impulses**, such as those for pain, touch, temperature, deep muscle sense, pressure, and vibrations. These impulses come from receptors that are widely distributed throughout the body.
❱ **Somatic motor impulses** resulting in voluntary control of skeletal muscles.
❱ **Visceral motor impulses** producing involuntary control of glands and involuntary muscles (cardiac and smooth muscle). These motor pathways are part of the autonomic nervous system, parasympathetic division.

Names and Functions of the Cranial Nerves

A few of the cranial nerves (I, II, and VIII) contain only sensory fibers; some (III, IV, VI, XI, and XII) contain all or mostly motor fibers. The remainder (V, VII, IX, and X) contain both sensory and motor fibers; they are known as *mixed nerves*. All 12 nerves are listed below and summarized in Table 9-2:

I. The **olfactory nerve** carries smell impulses from receptors in the nasal mucosa to the brain.
II. The **optic nerve** carries visual impulses from the eye to the brain.
III. The **oculomotor nerve** is concerned with the contraction of most of the eye muscles.
IV. The **trochlear** (TROK-le-ar) **nerve** supplies one eyeball muscle.
V. The **trigeminal** (tri-JEM-in-al) **nerve** is the great sensory nerve of the face and head. It has three branches that transport general sense impulses (*e.g.,* pain, touch, temperature) from the eye, the upper jaw, and the lower jaw. Motor fibers to the muscles of mastication (chewing) join the third branch. It is branches of the trigeminal nerve that a dentist anesthetizes to work on the teeth without causing pain.
VI. The **abducens** (ab-DU-senz) **nerve** is another nerve sending controlling impulses to an eyeball muscle.
VII. The **facial nerve** is largely motor. The muscles of facial expression are all supplied by branches from the facial nerve. This nerve also includes special sensory fibers for taste (anterior two-thirds of the tongue), and it contains secretory fibers to the smaller salivary glands (the submandibular and sublingual) and to the lacrimal (tear) gland.
VIII. The **vestibulocochlear** (ves-tib-u-lo-KOK-le-ar) **nerve** carries sensory impulses for hearing and equilibrium from the inner ear. This nerve was formerly called the auditory or acoustic nerve.
IX. The **glossopharyngeal** (glos-o-fah-RIN-je-al) **nerve** contains general sensory fibers from the back of the tongue and the pharynx (throat). This nerve also contains sensory fibers for taste from the posterior third of the tongue, secretory fibers that supply the largest salivary gland (parotid), and motor nerve fibers to control the swallowing muscles in the pharynx.

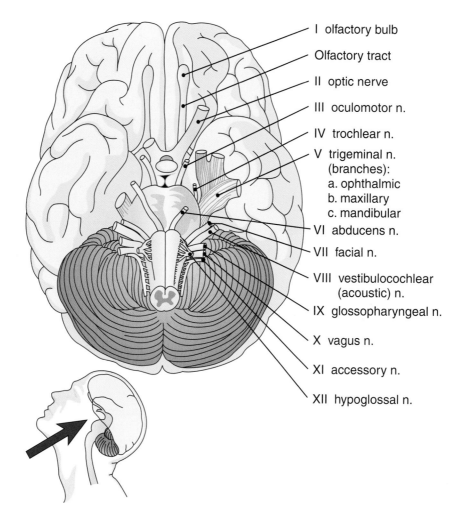

Figure 9-14 **Cranial nerves** on the base of the brain, inferior view.

Table 9•2	The Cranial Nerves and Their Functions	

NERVE (ROMAN NUMERAL DESIGNATION)	NAME	FUNCTION
I	Olfactory	Carries impulses for the sense of smell toward the brain
II	Optic	Carries visual impulses from the eye to the brain
III	Oculomotor	Controls contraction of eye muscles
IV	Trochlear	Supplies one eyeball muscle
V	Trigeminal	Carries sensory impulses from eye, upper jaw and lower jaw toward the brain
VI	Abducens	Controls an eyeball muscles
VII	Facial	Controls muscles of facial expression; carries sensation of taste; stimulates small salivary glands and lacrimal (tear) gland
VIII	Vestibulocochlear	Carries sensory impulses for hearing and equilibrium from the inner ear toward the brain
IX	Glossopharyngeal	Carries sensory impulses from tongue and pharynx (throat); controls swallowing muscles and stimulates the parotid salivary gland
X	Vagus	Supplies most of the organs in the thoracic and abdominal cavities; carries motor impulses to the larynx (voice box) and pharynx
XI	Accessory	Controls muscles in the neck and larynx
XII	Hypoglossal	Controls muscles of the tongue

X. The **vagus** (VA-gus) **nerve** is the longest cranial nerve. (Its name means "wanderer.") It supplies most of the organs in the thoracic and abdominal cavities. This nerve also contains motor fibers to the larynx (voice box) and pharynx and to glands that produce digestive juices and other secretions.

XI. The **accessory nerve** (formerly called the *spinal accessory nerve*) is a motor nerve with two branches. One branch controls two muscles of the neck, the trapezius and sternocleidomastoid; the other supplies muscles of the larynx.

XII. The **hypoglossal nerve**, the last of the 12 cranial nerves, carries impulses controlling the muscles of the tongue.

It has been traditional in medical schools for students to use mnemonics (ne-MON-iks), or memory devices, to remember anatomical lists. As an aside, part of the tradition was that these devices be bawdy. The original mnemonic for the names of the cranial nerves no longer applies, as a few of the names have been changed. Can you and your classmates make up a mnemonic phrase using the first letter of each cranial nerve? You can also check the Internet for sites where medical mnemonics are shared.

Checkpoint 9-9 How many pairs of cranial nerves are there?

Checkpoint 9-10 The cranial nerves are classified as being sensory, motor, or mixed. What is a mixed nerve?

Aging of the Nervous System

The nervous system is one of the first systems to develop in the embryo. By the beginning of the third week of development, the rudiments of the central nervous system have appeared. Beginning with maturity, the nervous system begins to undergo changes. The brain begins to decrease in size and weight due to a loss of cells, especially in the cerebral cortex, accompanied by decreases in synapses and neurotransmitters. The speed of processing information decreases, and movements are slowed. Memory diminishes, especially for recent events. Changes in the vascular system throughout the body with a narrowing of the arteries (atherosclerosis) reduce blood flow to the brain. Degeneration of vessels increases the likelihood of stroke.

Much individual variation is possible, however, with regard to location and severity of changes. Although age might make it harder to acquire new skills, tests have shown that practice enhances skill retention. As with other body systems, the nervous system has vast reserves, and most elderly people are able to cope with life's demands.

Word Anatomy

Medical terms are built from standardized word parts (prefixes, roots, and suffixes). Learning the meanings of these parts can help you remember words and interpret unfamiliar terms.

WORD PART	MEANING	EXAMPLE
The Brain and its Protective Structures		
cerebr/o	brain	*Cerebrospinal* fluid circulates around the brain and spinal cord.
chori/o	membrane	The *choroid* plexus is the vascular membrane in the ventricle that produces CSF.
gyr/o	circle	A *gyrus* is a circular raised area on the surface of the brain.
encephal/o	brain	The *diencephalon* is the part of the brain located between the cerebral hemispheres and the brain stem.
contra-	opposed, against	The cerebral cortex has *contralateral* control of motor function.
later/o	lateral, side	See preceding example.
Imaging the Brain		
tom/o	cut	*Tomography* is a method for viewing sections as if cut through the body.
Cranial Nerves		
gloss/o	tongue	The *hypoglossal* nerve controls muscles of the tongue.

Summary

I. The brain
1. Main parts—cerebrum, diencephalon, brain stem, cerebellum

II. Protective structures of the brain and spinal cord
1. Meninges
   a. Dura mater—tough outermost layer
   b. Arachnoid—weblike middle layer
   c. Pia mater—vascular innermost layer
A. Cerebrospinal fluid (CSF)
1. Circulates around and within brain and spinal cord
2. Cushions and protects
3. Ventricles—four spaces within brain where CSF is produced
   a. Choroid plexus—vascular network in ventricle that produces CSF

III. Cerebral hemispheres
1. Lobes—frontal, parietal, temporal, occipital, insula
2. Cortex—outer layer of gray matter
   a. In gyri (folds) and sulci (grooves)
   b. Specialized functions—interpretation, memory, conscious thought, judgment, voluntary actions
3. Basal nuclei (ganglia)—regulate movement and facial expression
4. Corpus callosum—band of white matter connecting cerebral hemispheres
5. Internal capsule—connects each cerebral hemisphere to lower parts of brain
A. Functions of cerebral cortex
B. Communication areas
C. Memory and the learning process

IV. Diencephalon—area between cerebral hemispheres and brain stem
1. Thalamus—directs sensory impulses to cortex
2. Hypothalamus—maintains homeostasis, controls pituitary
A. Limbic system
1. Contains parts of cerebrum and diencephalon
2. Controls emotion and behavior

V. Brain stem
A. Midbrain—involved in eye and ear reflexes
B. Pons—connecting link for other divisions
C. Medulla oblongata
1. Connects with spinal cord
2. Contains vital centers for respiration, heart rate, vasomotor activity

VI. The cerebellum—regulates coordination, balance, muscle tone

VII. Brain studies
1. Imaging—computed tomography (CT), magnetic resonance imaging (MRI), positron emission tomography (PET)
A. Electroencephalograph (EEG)—measures electrical waves produced as brain functions

VIII. Cranial nerves
1. 12 pairs attached to brain
A. Names and functions of the cranial nerves
1. Functions
   a. Carry special and general sensory impulses
   b. Carry somatic and visceral motor impulses
   c. Sensory (I, II, VIII)
   d. Motor (III, IV, VI, XI, XII)
   e. Mixed (V, VII, IX, X)

IX. Aging of the nervous system

Questions for Study and Review

Building Understanding

Fill in the blanks

1. The thickest and toughest layer of the meninges is the _____.

2. The third and fourth ventricles are connected by a small canal called the _____.

3. The muscles of speech are controlled by a region named _____.

4. The band of white matter that permits impulses to cross from one hemisphere to the other is called the _____.

5. The thalamus and hypothalamus are parts of the division of the brain termed the _____.

Matching
Match each numbered item with the most closely related lettered item.
____ 6. The sensory nerve of the face
____ 7. The motor nerve of the muscles of facial expression
____ 8. The sensory nerve for hearing and equilibrium
____ 9. The motor nerve for swallowing
____ 10. The motor nerve for digestion

a. trigeminal nerve
b. facial nerve
c. vestibulocochlear nerve
d. glossopharyngeal nerve
e. vagus nerve

Multiple choice

___ 11. The cerebrum is divided into left and right
hemispheres by the
a. central sulcus
b. lateral sulcus
c. longitudinal fissure
d. insula

___ 12. The primary sensory area interprets all of the
following sensations except
a. vision
b. pain
c. touch
d. temperature

___ 13. The brain structure involved in learning and
memory is the
a. hypothalamus
b. hippocampus
c. internal capsule
d. basal ganglia

___ 14. An imaging technique capable of visualizing the
brain in action is called
a. computed tomography
b. electroencephalography
c. positron emission tomography
d. radiography

___ 15. Pain messages are classified as
a. special sensory impulses
b. general sensory impulses
c. somatic motor impulses
d. visceral motor impulses

Understanding Concepts

16. Briefly describe the effects of injury to the following
brain areas:
a. cerebrum

b. diencephalon
c. brain stem
d. cerebellum

17. A neurosurgeon has drilled a hole through her patient's skull and is preparing to remove a cerebral glioma.
List, in order, the membranes she must cut through to
reach the cerebral cortex.

18. Compare and contrast the functions of the following
structures:
a. frontal lobe and parietal lobe
b. temporal lobe and occipital lobe
c. thalamus and hypothalamus

19. What is the function of the limbic system? Describe
the effect of damage to the hippocampus.

20. Compare and contrast short-term memory and long-
term memory.

21. The term cerebellum means "little cerebrum." Why is
this an appropriate term?

22. Describe the four different kinds of messages carried
by the cranial nerves.

23. Make a table of the 12 cranial nerves and their functions. According to your table, which ones are sensory,
motor, or mixed?

Conceptual Thinking

24. The parents of Molly R (2-month-old Caucasian female) are informed that their daughter requires a shunt to
drain excess CSF from her brain. What would happen to
Molly's brain if the shunt was not put in place?

25. Mr. Wong has suffered a brain stem injury and his
healthcare team does not expect him to survive. Why is
damage to the brain stem life-threatening?

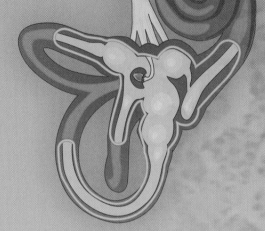

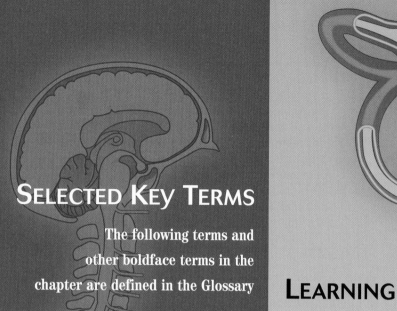

LEARNING OUTCOMES

After careful study of this chapter, you should be able to:

1. Describe the function of the sensory system

2. Differentiate between the special and general senses and give examples of each

3. Describe the structure of the eye

4. List and describe the structures that protect the eye

5. Define *refraction* and list the refractive parts of the eye

6. Differentiate between the rods and the cones of the eye

7. Compare the functions of the extrinsic and intrinsic muscles of the eye

8. Describe the nerve supply to the eye

9. Describe the three divisions of the ear

10. Describe the receptor for hearing and explain how it functions

11. Compare static and dynamic equilibrium and describe the location and function of these receptors

12. Explain the function of proprioceptors

13. List several methods for treatment of pain

14. Describe sensory adaptation and explain its value

15. Show how word parts are used to build words related to the sensory system (see Word Anatomy at the end of the chapter)

The Sensory System

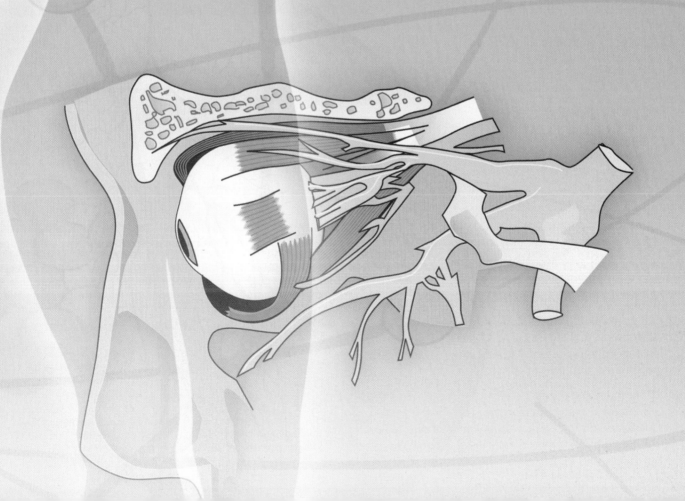

The Senses

The sensory system protects a person by detecting changes in the environment. An environmental change becomes a *stimulus* when it initiates a nerve impulse, which then travels to the central nervous system (CNS) by way of a sensory (afferent) neuron. A stimulus becomes a sensation—something we experience—only when a specialized area of the cerebral cortex interprets the nerve impulse it generates. Many stimuli arrive from the external environment and are detected at or near the body surface. Others, such as stimuli from the viscera, originate internally and help to maintain homeostasis.

Sensory Receptors

The part of the nervous system that detects a stimulus is the **sensory receptor.** In structure, a sensory receptor may be one of the following:

- The free dendrite of a sensory neuron, such as the receptors for pain.
- A modified ending, or **end-organ,** on the dendrite of an afferent neuron, such as those for touch and temperature.
- A specialized cell associated with an afferent neuron, such as the rods and cones of the retina of the eye and the receptors in the other special sense organs.

Receptors can be classified according to the type of stimulus to which they respond:

- Chemoreceptors, such as receptors for taste and smell, detect chemicals in solution.
- Photoreceptors, located in the retina of the eye, respond to light.
- Thermoreceptors detect change in temperature. Many of these receptors are located in the skin.
- Mechanoreceptors respond to movement, such as stretch, pressure, or vibration. These include pressure receptors in the skin, receptors that monitor body position, and the receptors of hearing and equilibrium in the ear, which are activated by the movement of cilia on specialized receptor cells.

Any receptor must receive a stimulus of adequate intensity, that is, at least a **threshold stimulus,** in order to respond and generate a nerve impulse.

Special and General Senses

Another way of classifying the senses is according to the distribution of their receptors. A **special sense** is localized in a special sense organ; a **general sense** is widely distributed throughout the body.

- **Special senses:**
  - **Vision** from receptors in the eye.
  - **Hearing** from receptors in the internal ear.
  - **Equilibrium** from receptors in the internal ear.
  - **Taste** from the tongue receptors.
  - **Smell** from receptors in the upper nasal cavities.
- **General senses:**
  - **Pressure, temperature, pain,** and **touch** from receptors in the skin and internal organs.
  - Sense of **position** from receptors in the muscles, tendons, and joints.

The Eye and Vision

In the embryo, the eye develops as an outpocketing of the brain. It is a delicate organ, protected by a number of structures:

- The skull bones form the walls of the eye orbit (cavity) and protect more than half of the posterior part of the eyeball.
- The upper and lower eyelids aid in protecting the eye's anterior portion (Fig. 10-1). The eyelids can be closed to keep harmful materials out of the eye, and blinking helps to lubricate the eye. A muscle, the levator palpebrae, is attached to the upper eyelid. When this muscle contracts, it keeps the eye open. If the muscle becomes weaker with age, the eyelids may droop and interfere with vision, a condition called *ptosis.*
- The eyelashes and eyebrow help to keep foreign matter out of the eye.
- A thin membrane, the **conjunctiva** (kon-junk-TI-vah), lines the inner surface of the eyelids and covers the visible portion of the white of the eye (sclera). Cells within the conjunctiva produce mucus that aids in lubricating the eye. Where the conjunctiva folds back from the eyelid to the anterior of the eye, a sac is formed. The lower portion of the conjunctival sac can be used to instill drops of medication. With age, the conjunctiva often thins and dries, resulting in inflammation and enlarged blood vessels.

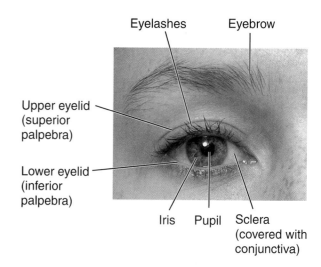

Figure 10-1 **Protective structures of the eye.** (Reprinted with permission from Bickley LS. Bates' Guide to Physical Examination and History Taking. 8th ed. Philadelphia: Lippincott Williams & Wilkins, 2003.)

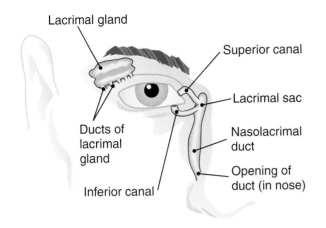

Figure 10-2 The lacrimal apparatus. The lacrimal (tear) gland and its associated ducts are shown.

▶ Tears, produced by the **lacrimal** (LAK-rih-mal) **glands** (Fig. 10-2), lubricate the eye and contain an enzyme that protects against infection. As tears flow across the eye from the lacrimal gland, located in the upper lateral part of the orbit, they carry away small particles that may have entered the eye. The tears then flow into ducts near the nasal corner of the eye where they drain into the nose by way of the **nasolacrimal** (na-zo-LAK-rih-mal) **duct** (see Fig. 10-2). An excess of tears causes a "runny nose"; a greater overproduction of them results in the spilling of tears onto the cheeks. With age, the lacrimal glands produce less secretion, but tears still may overflow onto the cheek if the nasolacrimal ducts become plugged.

Checkpoint 10-1 What are some structures that protect the eye?

Coats of the Eyeball

The eyeball has three separate coats, or tunics (Fig. 10-3). The outermost tunic, called the **sclera** (SKLE-rah), is made of tough connective tissue. It is commonly referred to as the *white of the eye*. It appears white because of the collagen it contains and because it has no blood vessels to add color. (Reddened or "bloodshot" eyes result from inflammation and swelling of blood vessels in the conjunctiva).

The second tunic of the eyeball is the **choroid** (KO-royd). This coat is composed of a delicate network of connective tissue interlaced with many blood vessels. It also contains much dark brown pigment. The choroid may be compared to the dull black lining of a camera in that it prevents incoming light rays from scattering and reflecting off the inner surface of the eye. The blood vessels at the posterior, or fundus, of the eye can reveal signs of disease, and visualization of these vessels with an **ophthalmoscope** (of-THAL-mo-skope) is an important part of a medical examination.

The innermost tunic, the **retina** (RET-ih-nah), is the actual receptor layer of the eye. It contains light-sensitive cells known as **rods** and **cones**, which generate the nerve impulses associated with vision.

Checkpoint 10-2 What are the names of the tunics of the eyeball?

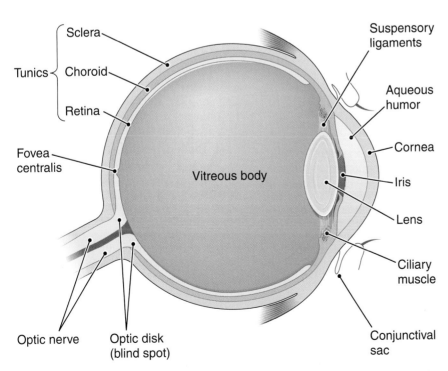

Figure 10-3 The eye. Note the three tunics, the refractive parts of the eye (cornea, aqueous humor, lens, vitreous body), and other structures involved in vision.

Pathway of Light Rays and Refraction

As light rays pass through the eye toward the retina, they travel through a series of transparent, colorless parts described below and seen in Figure 10-3. On the way, they undergo a process known as **refraction**, which is the bending of light rays as they pass from one substance to another substance of different density. (For a simple demonstration of refraction, place a spoon into a glass of water and observe how the handle appears to bend at the surface of the water.) Because of refraction, light from a very large area can be focused on a very small area of the retina. The eye's transparent refracting parts are listed here, in order from exterior to interior:

▶ The **cornea** (KOR-ne-ah) is an anterior continuation of the sclera, but it is transparent and colorless, whereas the rest of the sclera is opaque and white. The cornea is referred to frequently as the *window* of the eye. It bulges forward slightly and is the main refracting structure of the eye. The cornea has no blood vessels; it is nourished by the fluids that constantly wash over it.

▶ The **aqueous** (A-kwe-us) **humor,** a watery fluid that fills much of the eyeball anterior to the lens, helps maintain the slight forward curve of the cornea. The aqueous humor is constantly produced and drained from the eye.

▶ The **lens,** technically called the *crystalline lens,* is a clear, circular structure made of a firm, elastic material. The lens has two bulging surfaces and is thus described as biconvex. The lens is important in light refraction because it is elastic and its thickness can be adjusted to focus light for near or far vision.

▶ The **vitreous** (VIT-re-us) **body** is a soft jellylike substance that fills the entire space posterior to the lens (the adjective *vitreous* means "glasslike"). Like the aqueous humor, it is important in maintaining the shape of the eyeball as well as in aiding in refraction.

Checkpoint 10-3 What are the structures that refract light as it passes through the eye?

Function of the Retina

The retina has a complex structure with multiple layers of cells (Fig. 10-4). The deepest layer is a pigmented layer

just anterior to the choroid. Next are the rods and cones, the receptor cells of the eye, named for their shape. Details on how these two types of cells differ are presented in Table 10-1. Anterior to the rods and cones are connecting neurons that carry impulses toward the optic nerve.

The rods are highly sensitive to light and thus function in dim light, but they do not provide a sharp image. They are more numerous than the cones and are distributed more toward the periphery (anterior portion) of the retina. (If you visualize the retina as the inside of a bowl, the rods would be located toward the lip of the bowl). When you enter into dim light, such as a darkened movie theater, you cannot see for a short period. It is during this time that the rods are beginning to function, a change that is described as **dark adaptation.** When you are able to see again, images are blurred and appear only in shades of gray, because the rods are unable to differentiate colors.

The cones function in bright light, are sensitive to color, and give sharp images. The cones are localized at the center of the retina, especially in a tiny depressed area near the optic nerve that is called the **fovea centralis** (FO-ve-ah sen-TRA-lis) (Fig. 10-5; see also Fig. 10-3). (Note that *fovea* is a general term for a pit or depression.) Because this area contains the highest concentration of cones, it is the point of sharpest vision. The fovea is contained within a yellowish spot, the **macula lutea** (MAK-u-lah LU-te-ah), an area that may show degenerative changes with age.

There are three types of cones, each sensitive to either red, green, or blue light. Color blindness results from a lack of retinal cones. People who completely lack cones are totally colorblind; those who lack one type of cone are partially color blind. This disorder, because of its pattern of inheritance, occurs almost exclusively in males.

The rods and cones function by means of pigments that are sensitive to light. The rod pigment is **rhodopsin** (ro-DOP-sin), or visual purple. Vitamin A is needed for manufacture of these pigments. If a person is lacking in vitamin A, he or she may have difficulty seeing in dim light because there is too little light to activate the rods, a condition termed **night blindness.** Nerve impulses from the rods and cones flow into sensory neurons that eventually merge to form the optic nerve (cranial nerve II) at the eye's posterior (see Figs. 10-3 and 10-5). The impulses travel to the visual center in the occipital cortex of the brain.

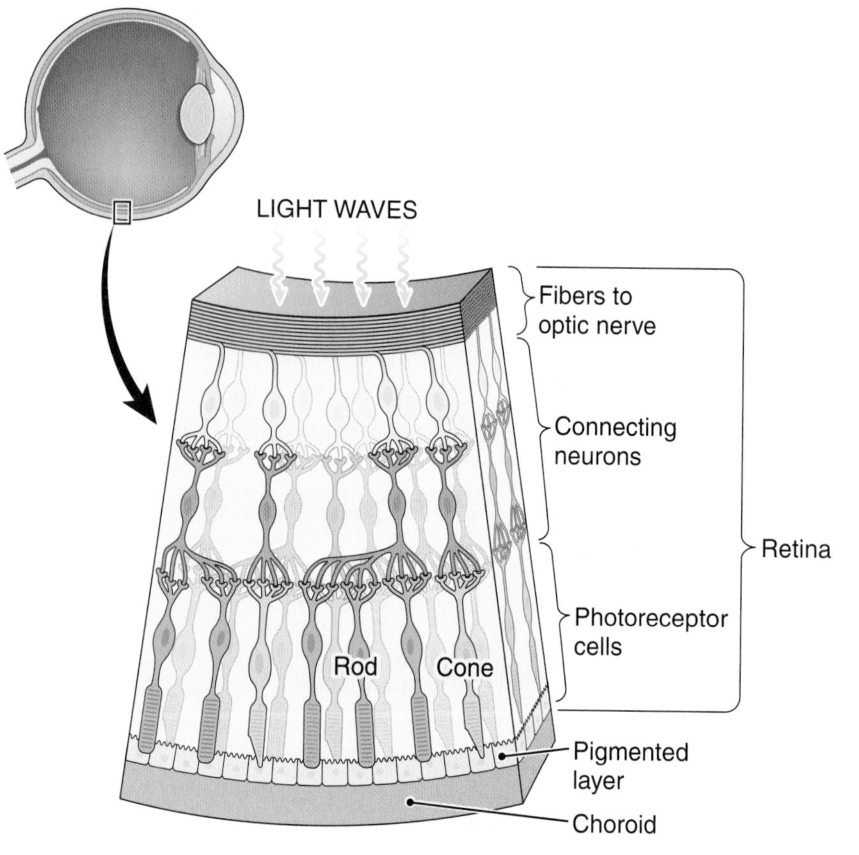

Figure 10-4 Structure of the retina. Rods and cones form a deep layer of the retina, near the choroid. Connecting neurons carry visual impulses toward the optic nerve.

LIGHT WAVES

Fibers to optic nerve

Connecting neurons

Retina

Photoreceptor cells

Rod   Cone

Pigmented layer

Choroid

Table 10·1	Comparison of the Rods and Cones of the Retina	
CHARACTERISTIC	**RODS**	**CONES**
Shape	Cylindrical	Flask shaped
Number	About 120 million in each retina	About 6 million in each retina
Distribution	Toward the periphery (anterior) of the retina	Concentrated at the center of the retina
Stimulus	Dim light	Bright light
Visual acuity (sharpness)	Low	High
Pigments	Rhodopsin (visual purple)	Pigments sensitive to red, green, or blue
Color perception	None; shades of gray	Respond to color

muscles connected with each eye originate on the bones of the orbit and insert on the surface of the sclera (Fig. 10-6). They are named for their location and the direction of the muscle fibers. These muscles pull on the eyeball in a coordinated fashion so that both eyes center on one visual field. This process of **convergence** is necessary to the formation of a clear image on the retina. Having the image come from a slightly different angle from each retina is believed to be important for three-dimensional (stereoscopic) vision, a characteristic of primates.

When an **ophthalmologist** (of-thal-MOL-o-jist), a physician who specializes in treatment of the eye, examines the retina with an ophthalmoscope, he or she can see abnormalities in the retina and in the retinal blood vessels. Some of these changes may signal more widespread diseases that affect the eye, such as diabetes and high blood pressure (hypertension).

Checkpoint 10-4 What are the receptor cells of the retina?

Muscles of the Eye

Two groups of muscles are associated with the eye. Both groups are important in adjusting the eye so that a clear image can form on the retina.

The Extrinsic Muscles The voluntary muscles attached to the eyeball's outer surface are the **extrinsic** (eks-TRIN-sik) **muscles.** The six ribbonlike extrinsic

Checkpoint 10-5 What is the function of the extrinsic muscles of the eye?

The Intrinsic Muscles The involuntary muscles located within the eyeball are the **intrinsic** (in-TRIN-sik) **muscles.** They form two circular structures within the eye, the iris and the ciliary muscle.

The **iris** (I-ris), the colored or pigmented part of the eye, is composed of two sets of muscle fibers that govern the size of the iris's central opening, the **pupil** (PU-pil) (Fig. 10-7). One set of fibers is arranged in a circular fashion, and the other set extends radially like the spokes of a wheel. The iris regulates the amount of light entering the eye. In bright light, the iris's circular muscle fibers contract, reducing the size of the pupil. This narrowing is termed *constriction.* In contrast, in dim light, the radial muscles contract, pulling the opening outward and enlarging it. This enlargement of the pupil is known as *dilation.*

The **ciliary** (SIL-e-ar-e) **muscle** is shaped somewhat like a flattened ring with a central hole the size of the outer edge

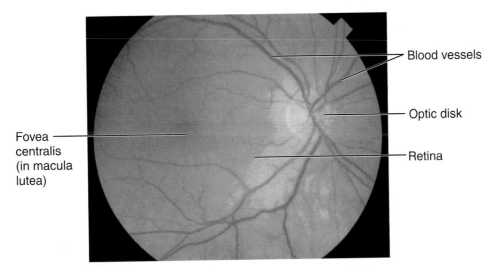

Figure 10-5   The fundus (back) of the eye as seen through an ophthalmoscope. (Reprinted with permission from Moore KL, Dalley AF. Clinically Oriented Anatomy. 4th ed. Baltimore: Lippincott Williams & Wilkins, 1999.)

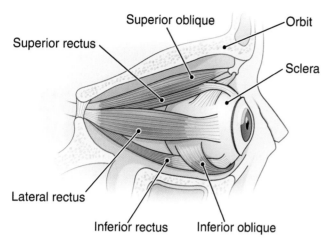

Figure 10-6 **Extrinsic muscles of the eye.** The medial rectus is not shown. *ZOOMING IN ✦ What characteristics are used in naming the extrinsic eye muscles?*

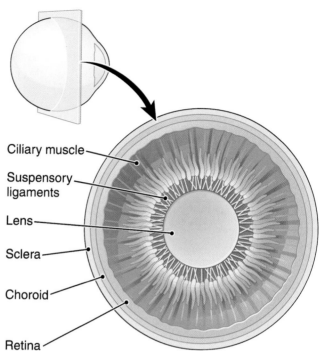

Figure 10-8 **The ciliary muscle and lens (posterior view).** Contraction of the ciliary muscle relaxes tension on the suspensory ligaments, allowing the lens to become more round for near vision. *ZOOMING IN ✦ What structures hold the lens in place?*

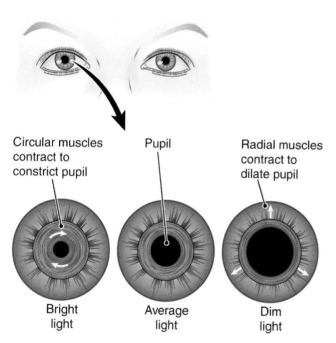

Figure 10-7 **Function of the iris.** In bright light, circular muscles contract and constrict the pupil, limiting the light that enters the eye. In dim light, the radial muscles contract and dilate the pupil, allowing more light to enter the eye. *ZOOMING IN ✦ What muscles of the iris contract to make the pupil smaller? Larger?*

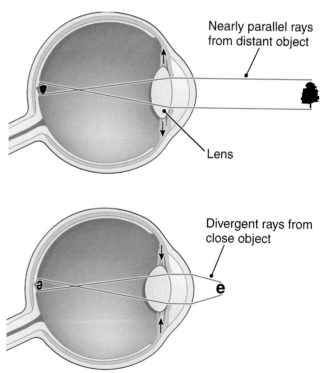

Figure 10-9 **Accommodation for near vision.** When viewing a close object, the lens must become more rounded to focus light rays on the retina.

of the iris. This muscle holds the lens in place by means of filaments, called **suspensory ligaments**, that project from the ciliary muscle to the edge of the lens around its entire circumference (Fig. 10-8). The ciliary muscle controls the shape of the lens to allow for vision at near and far distances. This process of **accommodation** occurs as follows.

The light rays from a close object diverge (separate) more than do the light rays from a distant object (Fig. 10-9). Thus, when viewing something close, the lens must become more rounded to bend the light rays more and focus them on the retina. The ciliary muscle controls the shape of the lens. When this muscle is relaxed, tension on the suspensory ligaments keeps the lens in a more flattened shape. For close vision, the ciliary muscle contracts. This movement draws the ciliary ring forward and relaxes tension on the suspensory ligaments. The elastic lens then recoils and becomes thicker, in much the same way that a rubber band thickens when the pull on it is released. When the ciliary muscle relaxes again, the lens flattens. These actions change the refractive power of the lens to accommodate for near and far vision.

In young people, the lens is elastic, and therefore its thickness can be readily adjusted according to the need for near or distance vision. With aging, the lens loses elasticity and therefore its ability to accommodate for near vision. It becomes difficult to focus clearly on close objects. This condition is called **presbyopia** (pres-be-O-pe-ah), which literally means "old eye." This refractive disorder can be corrected using eye glasses and contacts. Box 10-1 Eye Surgery: A Glimpse of the Cutting Edge, provides information on new methods of treating eye disorders.

Checkpoint 10-6 What is the function of the iris?

Checkpoint 10-7 What is the function of the ciliary muscle?

Nerve Supply to the Eye

Two sensory nerves supply the eye (Fig. 10-10):

▶ The **optic nerve** (cranial nerve II) carries visual impulses from the retinal rods and cones to the brain.
▶ The **ophthalmic** (of-THAL-mik) **branch of the trigeminal nerve** (cranial nerve V) carries impulses of pain, touch, and temperature from the eye and surrounding parts to the brain.

The optic nerve arises from the retina a little toward the medial or nasal side of the eye. There are no retinal rods and cones in the area of the optic nerve. Consequently, no image can form on the retina at this point, which is known as the blind spot or **optic disk** (see Figs. 10-3 and 10-5).

The optic nerve transmits impulses from the retina to the thalamus of the brain, from which they are directed to the occipital cortex. Note that the light rays passing through the eye are actually overrefracted (bent) so that an image falls on the retina upside down and backward (see Figs. 10-9). It is the job of the visual centers of the brain to reverse the images.

Three nerves carry motor impulses to the eyeball muscles:

▶ The **oculomotor nerve** (cranial nerve III) is the largest; it supplies voluntary and involuntary motor impulses to all but two eye muscles.
▶ The **trochlear nerve** (cranial nerve IV) supplies the superior oblique extrinsic eye muscle (see Fig. 10-6).
▶ The **abducens nerve** (cranial nerve VI) supplies the lateral rectus extrinsic eye muscle.

Box 10-1 | **Hot Topics**

Eye Surgery: A Glimpse of the Cutting Edge

Cataracts, glaucoma, and refractive errors are the most common eye disorders affecting Americans. In the past, cataract and glaucoma treatments concentrated on managing the diseases. Refractive errors were corrected using eye glasses and, more recently, contact lenses. Today, laser and microsurgical techniques can remove cataracts, reduce glaucoma, and allow people with refractive errors to put their eyeglasses and contacts away. These cutting-edge procedures include:

▶ *Laser in situ keratomileusis (LASIK)* to correct refractive errors. During this procedure, a laser reshapes the cornea to allow light to refract directly on the retina, rather than in front of or behind it. A microkeratome (surgical knife) is used to cut a flap in the outer layer of the cornea. A computer-controlled laser sculpts the middle layer of the cornea and then the flap is replaced. The procedure takes only a few minutes and patients recover their vision quickly and usually with little postoperative pain.

▶ *Laser trabeculoplasty* to treat glaucoma. This procedure uses a laser to help drain fluid from the eye and lower intraocular pressure. The laser is aimed at drainage canals located between the cornea and iris and makes several burns that are believed to open the canals and allow fluid to drain better. The procedure is typically painless and takes only a few minutes.

▶ *Phacoemulsification* to remove cataracts. During this surgical procedure, a very small incision (approximately 3 mm long) is made through the sclera near the outer edge of the cornea. An ultrasonic probe is inserted through this opening and into the center of the lens. The probe uses sound waves to emulsify the central core of the lens, which is then suctioned out. Then, an artificial lens is permanently implanted in the lens capsule. The procedure is typically painless although the patient may feel some discomfort for 1 to 2 days afterwards.

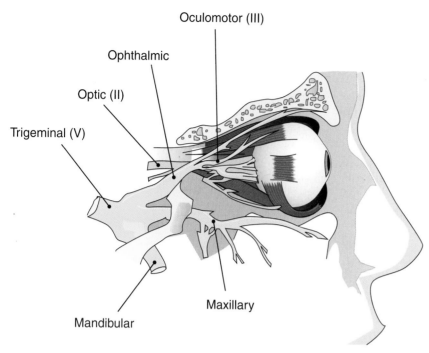

Oculomotor (III)

Ophthalmic

Optic (II)

Trigeminal (V)

Mandibular

Maxillary

Figure 10-10 **Nerves of the eye.** *ZOOMING IN ♦ Which of the nerves shown moves the eye?*

The steps in vision are:

1. Light refracts.
2. The muscles of the iris adjust the pupil.
3. The ciliary muscle adjusts the lens (accommodation).
4. The extrinsic eye muscles produce convergence.
5. Light stimulates retinal receptor cells (rods and cones).
6. The optic nerve transmits impulses to the brain.
7. The occipital lobe cortex interprets the impulses.

Checkpoint 10-8 What is cranial nerve II and what does it do?

▶ The Ear

The ear is the sense organ for both hearing and equilibrium (Fig. 10-11). It is divided into three main sections:

▶ The **outer ear** includes an outer projection and a canal ending at a membrane.
▶ The **middle ear** is an air space containing three small bones.
▶ The **inner ear** is the most complex and contains the sensory receptors for hearing and equilibrium.

The Outer Ear

The external portion of the ear consists of a visible projecting portion, the **pinna** (PIN-nah), also called the **auricle** (AW-rih-kl), and the **external auditory canal,** or **meatus** (me-A-tus), that leads into the deeper parts of the

ear. The pinna directs sound waves into the ear, but it is probably of little importance in humans. The external auditory canal extends medially from the pinna for about 2.5 cm or more, depending on which wall of the canal is measured. The skin lining this tube is thin and, in the first part of the canal, contains many wax-producing **ceruminous** (seh-RU-mih-nus) **glands.** The wax, or **cerumen** (seh-RU-men), may become dried and impacted in the canal and must then be removed. The same kinds of disorders that involve the skin elsewhere—atopic dermatitis, boils, and other infections—may also affect the skin of the external auditory canal.

The **tympanic** (tim-PAN-ik) **membrane,** or eardrum, is at the end of the external auditory canal. It is a boundary between this canal and the middle ear cavity, and it vibrates freely as sound waves enter the ear.

The Middle Ear and Ossicles

The middle ear cavity is a small, flattened space that contains three small bones, or **ossicles** (OS-ih-klz) (see Fig. 10-11). The three ossicles are joined in such a way that they amplify the sound waves received by the tympanic membrane as they transmit the sounds to the inner ear. The first bone is shaped like a hammer and is called the **malleus** (MAL-e-us) (Fig. 10-12). The handlelike part of the malleus is attached to the tympanic membrane, whereas the headlike part is connected to the second bone, the **incus** (ING-kus). The incus is shaped like an anvil, an iron block used in shaping metal, as is used by a blacksmith. The innermost ossicle is shaped somewhat like the stirrup of a saddle and is called the **stapes** (STA-peze). The base of the stapes is in contact with the inner ear.

Checkpoint 10-9 What are the ossicles of the ear and what do they do?

The Eustachian Tube The **eustachian** (u-STA-shun) **tube** (auditory tube) connects the middle ear cavity with the throat, or **pharynx** (FAR-inks) (see Fig. 10-11). This tube opens to allow pressure to equalize on the two sides of the tympanic membrane. A valve that closes the tube can be forced open by swallowing hard, yawning, or blowing with the nose and mouth sealed, as one often does when experiencing pain from pressure changes in an airplane.

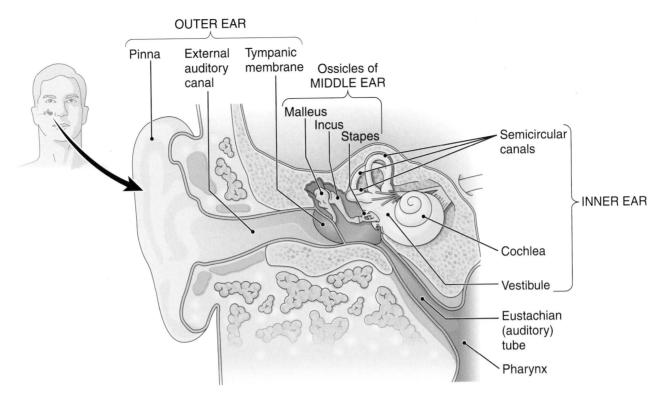

OUTER EAR

Pinna
External auditory canal
Tympanic membrane
Ossicles of MIDDLE EAR
Malleus
Incus
Stapes
Semicircular canals
INNER EAR
Cochlea
Vestibule
Eustachian (auditory) tube
Pharynx

Figure 10-11 **The ear.** Structures in the outer, middle, and inner divisions are shown.

The mucous membrane of the pharynx is continuous through the eustachian tube into the middle ear cavity. At the posterior of the middle ear cavity is an opening into the mastoid air cells, which are spaces inside the mastoid process of the temporal bone (see Fig. 6-5 B).

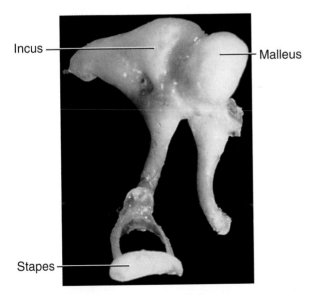

Incus
Malleus
Stapes

Figure 10-12 **The ossicles of the middle ear.** The handle of the malleus is in contact with the tympanic membrane, and the headlike part with the incus. The base of the stapes is in contact with the inner ear (×30). (Reprinted with permission from Ross MH, Kaye GI, Pawlina W. Histology. 4th ed. Philadelphia: Lippincott Williams & Wilkins, 2003.)

The Inner Ear

The most complicated and important part of the ear is the internal portion, which is described as a *labyrinth* (LAB-ih-rinth) because it has a complex mazelike construction. It consists of three separate areas containing sensory receptors. The skeleton of the inner ear is called the **bony labyrinth** (Fig. 10-13). It has three divisions:

▶ The **vestibule** consists of two bony chambers that contain some of the receptors for equilibrium.
▶ The **semicircular canals** are three projecting bony tubes located toward the posterior. Areas at the bases of the semicircular canals also contain receptors for equilibrium.
▶ The **cochlea** (KOK-le-ah) is coiled like a snail shell and is located toward the anterior. It contains the receptors for hearing.

All three divisions of the bony labyrinth contain a fluid called **perilymph** (PER-e-limf).

Within the bony labyrinth is an exact replica of this bony shell made of membrane, much like an inner tube within a tire. The tubes and chambers of this **membranous labyrinth** are filled with a fluid called **endolymph** (EN-do-limf) (see Fig. 10-13). The endolymph is within the membranous labyrinth, and the perilymph surrounds it. These fluids are important to the sensory functions of the inner ear.

Hearing The organ of hearing, called the **organ of Corti** (KOR-te), consists of ciliated receptor cells located inside the membranous cochlea, or **cochlear duct** (Fig. 10-14). Sound waves enter the external auditory canal and cause vibrations in the tympanic membrane. The ossicles amplify

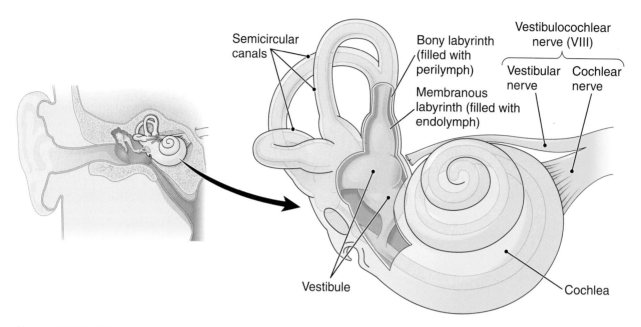

Figure 10-13   The inner ear. The vestibule, semicircular canals, and cochlea are made of a bony shell (labyrinth) with an interior membranous labyrinth. Endolymph fills the membranous labyrinth and perilymph is around it in the bony labyrinth.

these vibrations and finally transmit them from the stapes to a membrane covering the **oval window** of the inner ear.

As the sound waves move through the fluids in these chambers, they set up vibrations in the cochlear duct. As a result, the tiny, hairlike cilia on the receptor cells begin to move back and forth against the **tectorial membrane** above them. (The membrane is named from a Latin word that means "roof.") This motion sets up nerve impulses that travel to the brain in the **cochlear nerve,** a branch of the eighth cranial nerve (formerly called the *auditory* or *acoustic nerve*). Sound waves ultimately leave the ear through another membrane-covered space in the bony labyrinth, the **round window.**

Hearing receptors respond to both the pitch (tone) of sound and its intensity (loudness). The various pitches stim-ulate different regions of the organ of Corti. Receptors detect higher pitched sounds near the base of the cochlea and lower pitched sounds near the top. Loud sounds stimulate more cells and produce more vibrations, sending more nerve impulses to the brain. Exposure to loud noises, such as very loud music, jet plane noise, or industrial noises, can damage the receptors for particular pitches of sound and lead to hearing loss for those tones. Box 10-2 offers information on how audiologists help to treat hearing disorders.

The steps in hearing are:

1. Sound waves enter the external auditory canal.
2. The tympanic membrane vibrates.
3. The ossicles transmit vibrations across the middle ear cavity.

Box 10-2 · Health Professions

Audiologists

Audiologists specialize in preventing, diagnosing, and treating hearing disorders caused by injury, infection, birth defects, noise, or aging. They diagnose hearing disorders by taking a complete history and using specialized equipment to measure hearing acuity. Audiologists design and implement individualized treatment plans, which may include fitting clients with assistive listening devices, such as a hearing aids or cochlear implants and educating them about their use, or teaching alternate communication skills, such as lip reading. Audiologists also measure workplace and community noise levels and teach the public how to prevent hearing loss. To perform these duties, audiologists need a thorough understanding of anatomy and physiology. Most audiologists in the U.S. have master's degrees or the equivalent from an accredited college or university and must pass a national licensing exam.

Audiologists work in a variety of settings, such as hospitals, nursing care facilities, schools, and clinics. Job prospects are good, as the need for audiologists' specialized skills will increase as the American population ages. For more information, contact the American Academy of Audiology.

7. Impulses travel to the brain in the VIIIth cranial nerve.
8. The temporal lobe cortex interprets the impulses.

Checkpoint 10-10 What is the name of the organ of hearing and where is it located?

Equilibrium The other sensory receptors in the inner ear are those related to equilibrium (balance). They are located in the vestibule and the semicircular canals. Receptors for the sense of equilibrium are also ciliated cells. As the head moves, a shift in the position of the cilia within the thick fluid around them generates a nerve impulse.

Receptors located in the two small chambers of the vestibule sense the position of the head or the position of the body when moving in a straight line, as in a moving vehicle or when tilting the head. This form of equilibrium is termed **static equilibrium**. Each receptor is called a **macula**. (There is also a macula in the eye, but this is a general term that means "spot.") The fluid above the ciliated cells contains small crystals of calcium carbonate, called **otoliths** (O-to-liths), which add drag to the fluid around the receptor cells and increase the effect of gravity's pull (Fig. 10-15). Similar devices are found in lower animals, such as fish and crustaceans, that help them in balance.

The receptors for **dynamic equilibrium** function when the body is spinning or moving in different directions. The receptors, called **cristae** (KRIS-te), are located at the bases of the semicircular canals (Fig. 10-16). It's easy to remember what these receptors do, because the semicircular canals go off in different directions.

Nerve fibers from the vestibule and from the semicircular canals form the **vestibular** (ves-TIB-u-lar) **nerve**, which joins the cochlear nerve to form the vestibulocochlear nerve, the eighth cranial nerve.

Checkpoint 10-11 Where are the receptors for equilibrium located?

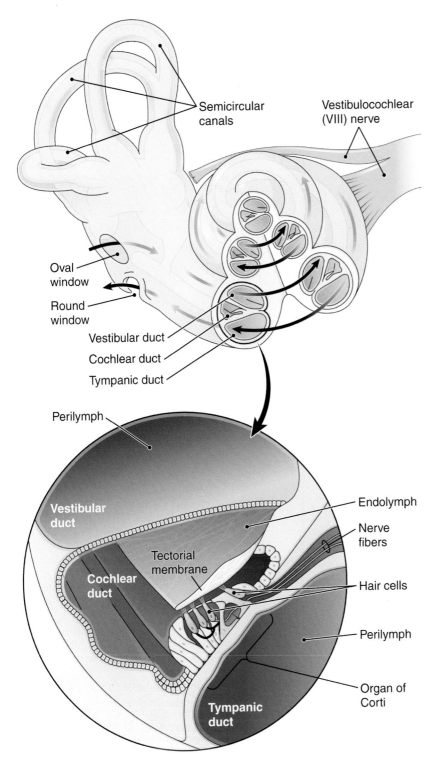

Figure 10-14 Cochlea and the organ of Corti. The arrows show the direction of sound waves in the cochlea.

4. The stapes transmits the vibrations to the inner ear fluid.
5. Vibrations move cilia on hair cells of the organ of Corti in the cochlear duct.
6. Movement against the tectorial membrane generates nerve impulses.

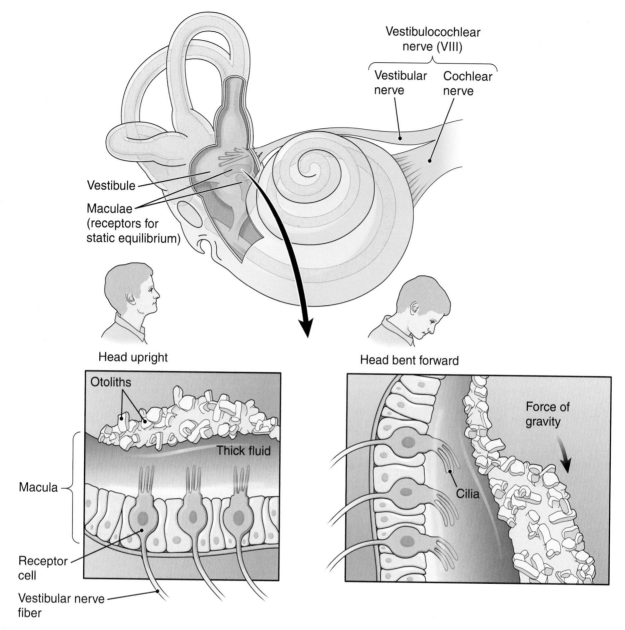

Figure 10-15 **Action of the receptors (maculae) for static equilibrium.** As the head moves, the thick fluid above the receptor cells, weighted with otoliths, pulls on the cilia of the cells, generating a nerve impulse. *ZOOMING IN ✦ What happens to the cilia on the receptor cells when the fluid around them moves?*

Checkpoint 10-12 What are the two types of equilibrium?

Other Special Sense Organs

The sense organs of taste and smell are designed to respond to chemical stimuli.

Sense of Taste

The sense of taste, or **gustation** (gus-TA-shun), involves receptors in the tongue and two different nerves that carry taste impulses to the brain (Fig. 10-17). The taste receptors, known as **taste buds,** are located along the edges of small, depressed areas called **fissures.** Taste buds are stimulated only if the substance to be tasted is in solution or dissolves in the fluids of the mouth. Receptors for four basic tastes are localized in different regions, forming a "taste map" of the tongue (see Fig. 10-17 B):

- **Sweet** tastes are most acutely experienced at the tip of the tongue (hence the popularity of lollipops and ice cream cones).
- **Salty** tastes are most acute at the anterior sides of the tongue.
- **Sour** tastes are most effectively detected by the taste buds located laterally on the tongue.
- **Bitter** tastes are detected at the posterior part of the tongue.

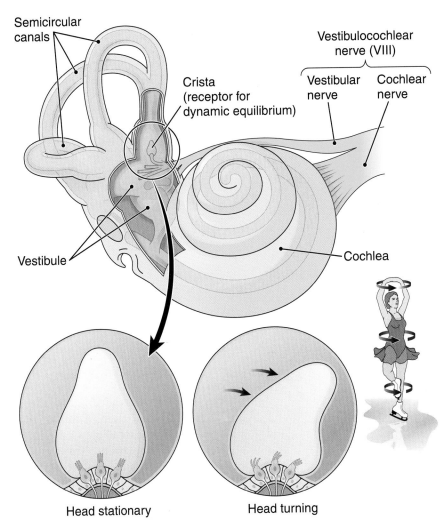

Figure 10-16 Action of the receptors (cristae) for dynamic equilibrium. As the body spins or moves in different directions, the cilia bend as the head changes position, generating nerve impulses.

Taste maps vary among people, but in each person certain regions of the tongue are more sensitive to a specific basic taste. Other tastes are a combination of these four with additional smell sensations. More recently, researchers have identified some other tastes besides these basic four: water, alkaline (basic), and metallic. Another is umami (u-MOM-e), a pungent or savory taste based on a response to the amino acid glutamate. Glutamate is found in MSG (monosodium glutamate), a flavor enhancer used in Asian food. Water taste receptors are mainly in the throat and may help to regulate water balance.

The nerves of taste include the facial and the glossopharyngeal cranial nerves (VII and IX). The interpretation of taste impulses is probably accomplished by the lower frontal cortex of the brain, although there may be no sharply separate gustatory center.

Sense of Smell

The importance of the sense of smell, or **olfaction** (ol-FAK-shun), is often underestimated. This sense helps to detect gases and other harmful substances in the environment and helps to warn of spoiled food. Smells can trigger memories and other psychological responses. Smell is also important in sexual behavior.

The receptors for smell are located in the epithelium of the superior region of the nasal cavity (see Fig. 10-17). Again, the chemicals detected must be in solution in the fluids that line the nose. Because these receptors are high in the nasal cavity, one must "sniff" to bring odors upward in the nose.

The impulses from the receptors for smell are carried by the olfactory nerve (I), which leads directly to the olfactory center in the brain's temporal cortex. The interpretation of smell is closely related to the sense of taste, but a greater variety of dissolved chemicals can be detected by smell than by taste. The smell of foods is just as important in stimulating appetite and the flow of digestive juices as is the sense of taste. When one has a cold, food often seems tasteless and unappetizing because nasal congestion reduces ability to smell the food.

The olfactory receptors deteriorate with age and food may become less appealing. It is important when presenting food to elderly people that the food look inviting so as to stimulate their appetites.

Checkpoint 10-13 What are the special senses that respond to chemical stimuli?

The General Senses

Unlike the special sensory receptors, which are localized within specific sense organs, limited to a relatively small area, the general sensory receptors are scattered throughout the body. These include receptors for touch, pressure, heat, cold, position, and pain (Fig. 10-18).

Sense of Touch

The touch receptors, **tactile** (TAK-til) **corpuscles,** are found mostly in the dermis of the skin and around hair follicles. Sensitivity to touch varies with the number of touch receptors in different areas. They are especially numerous and close together in the tips of the fingers and the toes. The lips and the tip of the tongue also contain many of these receptors and are very sensitive to touch.

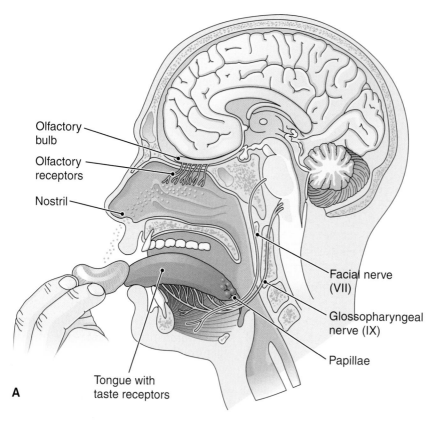

Olfactory
bulb

Olfactory
receptors

Nostril

Facial nerve
(VII)

Glossopharyngeal
nerve (IX)

Papillae

Tongue with
taste receptors

A

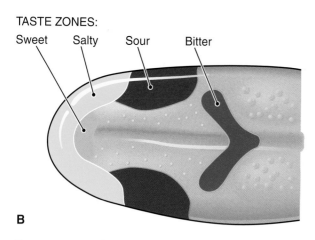

TASTE ZONES:

Sweet   Salty   Sour   Bitter

B

Figure 10-17 **Special senses that respond to chemicals. (A)** Organs of taste (gustation) and smell (olfaction). **(B)** A taste map of the tongue.

Other areas, such as the back of the hand and the back of the neck, have fewer receptors and are less sensitive to touch.

Sense of Pressure

Even when the skin is anesthetized, it can still respond to pressure stimuli. These sensory end-organs for deep pressure are located in the subcutaneous tissues beneath the skin and also near joints, muscles, and other deep tis-

sues. They are sometimes referred to as *receptors for deep touch*.

Sense of Temperature

The temperature receptors are **free nerve endings**, receptors that are not enclosed in capsules, but are merely branchings of nerve fibers. Temperature receptors are widely distributed in the skin, and there are separate receptors for heat and cold. A warm object stimulates only the heat receptors, and a cool object affects only the cold receptors. Internally, there are temperature receptors in the hypothalamus of the brain, which help to adjust body temperature according to the temperature of the circulating blood.

Sense of Position

Receptors located in muscles, tendons, and joints relay impulses that aid in judging one's position and changes in the locations of body parts in relation to each other. They also inform the brain of the amount of muscle contraction and tendon tension. These rather widespread receptors, known as **proprioceptors** (pro-pre-o-SEP-tors), are aided in this function by the equilibrium receptors of the internal ear.

Information received by these receptors is needed for the coordination of muscles and is important in such activities as walking, running, and many more complicated skills, such as playing a musical instrument. They help to provide a sense of body movement, known as **kinesthesia** (kin-es-THE-ze-ah). Proprioceptors play an important part in maintaining muscle tone and good posture. They also help to assess the weight of an object to be lifted so that the right amount of muscle force is used.

The nerve fibers that carry impulses from these receptors enter the spinal cord and ascend to the brain in the posterior part of the cord. The cerebellum is a main coordinating center for these impulses.

Checkpoint 10-14 What are examples of general senses?

Checkpoint 10-15 What are proprioceptors and where are they located?

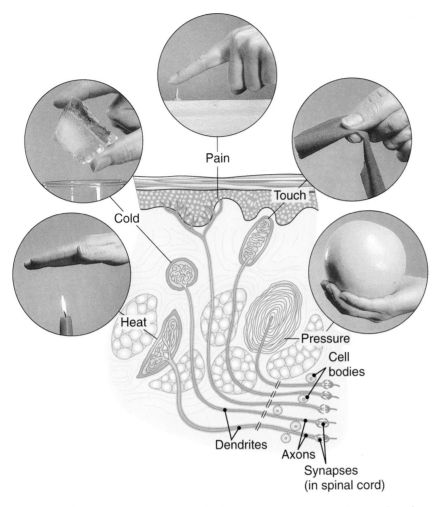

Figure 10-18   **Sensory receptors in the skin.** Synapses are in the spinal cord.

Most of these drugs are commonly known as non-steroidal antiinflammatory drugs (NSAIDs). Examples are ibuprofen (i-bu-PRO-fen) and naproxen (na-PROK-sen).

▸ **Narcotics** act on the CNS to alter the perception and response to pain. Effective for severe pain, narcotics are administered by varied methods, including orally and by intramuscular injection. They are also effectively administered into the space surrounding the spinal cord. An example of a narcotic drug is morphine.

▸ **Anesthetics**. Although most commonly used to prevent pain during surgery, anesthetic injections are also used to relieve certain types of chronic pain.

▸ **Endorphins** (en-DOR-fins) are released naturally from certain regions of the brain and are associated with the control of pain. Massage, acupressure, and electric stimulation are among the techniques that are thought to activate this system of natural pain relief.

▸ **Applications of heat or cold** can be a simple but effective means of pain relief, either alone or in combination with medications. Care must be taken to avoid injury caused by excessive heat or cold.

▸ **Relaxation or distraction techniques** include several methods that reduce perception of pain in the CNS. Relaxation techniques counteract the fight-or-flight response to pain and complement other pain-control methods.

Sense of Pain

Pain is the most important protective sense. The receptors for pain are widely distributed free nerve endings. They are found in the skin, muscles, and joints and to a lesser extent in most internal organs (including the blood vessels and viscera). Two pathways transmit pain to the CNS. One is for acute, sharp pain, and the other is for slow, chronic pain. Thus, a single strong stimulus produces the immediate sharp pain, followed in a second or so by the slow, diffuse, burning pain that increases in severity with the passage of time. Box 10-3 provides information on referred pain.

Sometimes, the cause of pain cannot be remedied quickly, and occasionally it cannot be remedied at all. In the latter case, it is desirable to lessen the pain as much as possible. Some pain relief methods that have been found to be effective include:

▸ **Analgesic drugs.** An analgesic (an-al-JE-zik) is a drug that relieves pain. There are two main categories of such agents:

   ▸ **Nonnarcotic analgesics** act locally to reduce inflammation and are effective for mild to moderate pain.

▸ Sensory Adaptation

When sensory receptors are exposed to a continuous stimulus, receptors often adjust themselves so that the sensation becomes less acute. The term for this phenomenon is **sensory adaptation.** For example, if you immerse your hand in very warm water, it may be uncomfortable; however, if you leave your hand there, soon the water will feel less hot (even if it has not cooled appreciably).

Receptors adapt at different rates. Those for warmth, cold, and light pressure adapt rapidly. In contrast, those for pain do not adapt. In fact, the sensations from the slow pain fibers tend to increase over time. This variation in receptors allows us to save energy by not responding to unimportant stimuli while always heeding the warnings of pain.

| Box 10-3 | Clinical Perspectives |

Referred Pain: More Than Skin Deep

Referred pain is pain that is felt in an outer part of the body, particularly the skin, but actually originates in an internal organ located nearby. Liver and gallbladder disease often cause referred pain in the skin over the right shoulder. Spasm of the coronary arteries that supply the heart may cause pain in the left shoulder and arm. Infection of the appendix is felt as pain of the skin covering the lower right abdominal quadrant.

Apparently, some neurons in the spinal cord have the twofold duty of conducting impulses from visceral pain receptors in the chest and abdomen and from somatic pain receptors in neighboring areas of the skin, resulting in referred pain. The brain cannot differentiate between these two possible sources, but because most pain sensations originate in the skin, the brain automatically assigns the pain to this more likely place of origin. Knowing where visceral pain is referred to in the body is of great value in diagnosing chest and abdominal disorders.

Word Anatomy

Medical terms are built from standardized word parts (prefixes, roots, and suffixes). Learning the meanings of these parts can help you remember words and interpret unfamiliar terms.

WORD PART	MEANING	EXAMPLE
The Eye and Vision		
ophthalm/o	eye	An *ophthalmologist* is a physician who specializes in treatment of the eye.
-scope	instrument for examination	An *ophthalmoscope* is an instrument used to examine the posterior of the eye.
lute/o	yellow	The macula *lutea* is a yellowish spot in the retina that contains the fovea centralis.
presby-	old	*Presbyopia* is farsightedness that occurs with age.
The Ear		
tympan/o	drum	The *tympanic* membrane is the eardrum.
equi-	equal	*Equilibrium* is balance (*equi-* combined with the Latin word *libra* meaning "balance").
ot/o	ear	*Otology* is the study of the ear.
lith	stone	*Otoliths* are small crystals in the inner ear that aid in static equilibrium.
-cusis	hearing	*Presbycusis* is hearing loss associated with age.
The General Senses		
propri/o-	own	*Proprioception* is perception of one's own body position.
kine	movement	*Kinesthesia* is a sense of body movement.
-esthesia	sensation	*Anesthesia* is loss of sensation, as of pain.
-alges/i	pain	An *analgesic* is a drug that relieves pain.
narc/o	stupor	A *narcotic* is a drug that alters the perception of pain.

Summary

I. The senses—protect by detecting changes (stimuli) in the environment

A. Sensory receptors—detect stimuli

   1. Structural types

     a. Free dendrite

     b. End-organ—modified dendrite

     c. Specialized cell—in special sense organs

   2. Types based on stimulus

     a. Chemoreceptors—respond to chemicals

     b. Thermoreceptors—respond to temperature

     c. Photoreceptors—respond to light

     d. Mechanoreceptors—respond to movement

B. Special and general senses

   1. Special senses—vision, hearing, equilibrium, taste, smell

2. General senses—touch, pressure, temperature, position, pain

II. The eye and vision

1. Protection of the eyeball—bony orbit, eyelid, eyelashes, conjunctiva, lacrimal glands (produce tears)
A. Coats of the eyeball
   1. Sclera—white of the eye
      a. Cornea—anterior
   2. Choroid—pigmented; contains blood vessels
   3. Retina—receptor layer
B. Pathway of light rays and refraction
   1. Refraction—bending of light rays as they pass through substances of different density
   2. Refracting parts—cornea, aqueous humor, lens, vitreous body
C. Function of the retina
   1. Cells
      a. Rods—cannot detect color; function in dim light
      b. Cones—detect color; function in bright light
   2. Pigments—sensitive to light; rod pigment is rhodopsin
D. Muscles of the eye
   1. Extrinsic muscles—six move each eyeball
   2. Intrinsic muscles
      a. Iris—colored ring around pupil; regulates the amount of light entering the eye
      b. Ciliary muscle—regulates the thickness of the lens to accommodate for near vision
E. Nerve supply to the eye
   1. Sensory nerves
      a. Optic nerve (II)—carries impulses from retina to brain
      b. Ophthalmic branch of trigeminal (V)
   2. Motor nerves—move eyeball
      a. Oculomotor (III), trochlear (IV), abducens (VI)

III. The ear

A. Outer ear—pinna, auditory canal (meatus), tympanic membrane (eardrum)
B. Middle ear and ossicles
   1. Ossicles—malleus, incus, stapes

2. Eustachian tube—connects middle ear with pharynx to equalize pressure
C. Inner ear
   1. Bony labyrinth—contains perilymph
   2. Membranous labyrinth—contains endolymph
   3. Divisions
      a. Cochlea—contains receptors for hearing (organ of Corti)
      b. Vestibule—contains receptors for static equilibrium (maculae)
      c. Semicircular canals—contain receptors for dynamic equilibrium (cristae)
   4. Receptor cells function by movement of cilia
   5. Nerve—vestibulocochlear (auditory) nerve (VIII)

IV. Other special sense organs

A. Sense of taste (gustation)
   1. Receptors—taste buds on tongue
   2. Basic tastes—sweet, salty, sour, bitter
   3. Nerves—facial (VII) and glossopharyngeal (IX)
B. Sense of smell (olfaction)
   1. Receptors—in upper part of nasal cavity
   2. Nerve—olfactory nerve (I)

V. General senses

A. Sense of touch—tactile corpuscles
B. Sense of pressure
C. Sense of temperature—receptors are free nerve endings
D. Sense of position (proprioception)—receptors are proprioceptors in muscles, tendons, joints
   1. Kinesthesia—sense of movement
E. Sense of pain—receptors are free nerve endings
   1. Relief of pain—analgesic drugs, anesthetics, endorphins, heat, cold, relaxation and distraction techniques

VI. Sensory adaptation—adjustment of receptors so that sensation becomes less acute

---

Questions for Study and Review

Building Understanding

Fill in the blanks

1. The part of the nervous system that detects a stimulus is the _____.
2. The bending of light rays as they pass from air to fluid is called _____.
3. Nerve impulses are carried from the ear to the brain by the _____ nerve.

4. Information about the position of the knee joint is provided by _____.
5. A receptor's ability to decrease its sensitivity to a continuous stimulus is called _____.

Matching

Match each numbered item with the most closely related lettered item.

_____ 6. Consists of ciliated receptor cells sensitive to vibration

_____ 7. The actual receptor layer of the eye

_____ 8. The receptor that senses static equilibrium

_____ 9. The receptor that senses touch

_____ 10. The receptor sensitive to temperature and pain

a. retina
b. free nerve endings
c. macula
d. organ of corti
e. tactile corpuscle

Multiple choice

_____ 11. All of the following are special senses except
    a. smell
    b. taste
    c. equilibrium
    d. pain

_____ 12. From superficial to deep, the order of the eyeball's tunics is
    a. retina, choroid, and sclera
    b. sclera, retina, and choroid
    c. choroid, retina, and sclera
    d. sclera, choroid, and retina

_____ 13. The part of the eye most responsible for light refraction is the
    a. cornea

    b. lens
    c. vitreous body
    d. retina

_____ 14. Information from the retina is carried to the brain by the
    a. ophthalmic nerve
    b. optic nerve
    c. oculomotor nerve
    d. abducens nerve

_____ 15. Receptors in the vestibule sense
    a. muscle tension
    b. sound
    c. light
    d. equilibrium

Understanding Concepts

16. Differentiate between the terms in each of the following pairs:
    a. special sense and general sense
    b. aqueous humor and vitreous body
    c. rods and cones
    d. endolymph and perilymph
    e. static and dynamic equilibrium

17. Trace the path of a light ray from the outside of the eye to the retina.

18. Define convergence and accommodation.

19. List in order the structures that sound waves pass through in traveling through the ear to the receptors for hearing.

20. Compare and contrast static equilibrium and dynamic equilibrium.

21. Name the four basic tastes. Where are the taste receptors? Name the nerves of taste.

22. Trace the pathway of a nerve impulse from the olfactory receptors to the olfactory center in the brain.

23. Name several types of pain-relieving drugs. Describe several methods for relieving pain that do not involve drugs.

Conceptual Thinking

24. Why do you taste eyedrops after applying them to your eyeball?

25. You and a friend have just finished riding the roller coaster at the amusement park. As you walk away from the ride, your friend stumbles and comments that the ride has affected her balance. How do you explain this?

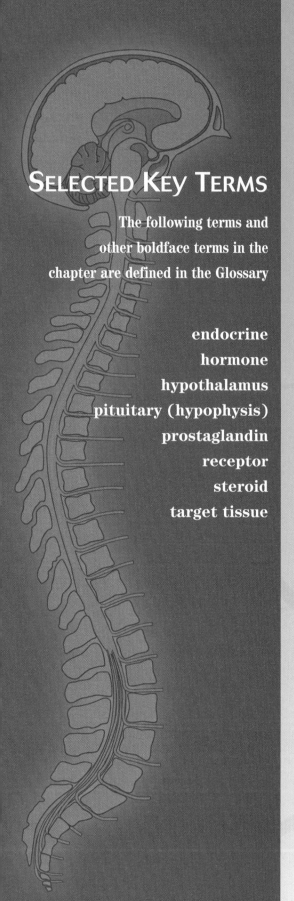
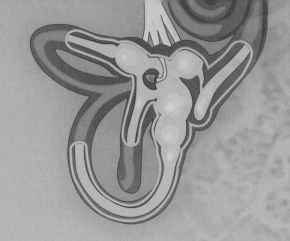

SELECTED KEY TERMS

The following terms and other boldface terms in the chapter are defined in the Glossary

endocrine
hormone
hypothalamus
pituitary (hypophysis)
prostaglandin
receptor
steroid
target tissue

LEARNING OUTCOMES

After careful study of this chapter, you should be able to:

1. Compare the effects of the nervous system and the endocrine system in controlling the body

2. Describe the functions of hormones

3. Explain how hormones are regulated

4. Identify the glands of the endocrine system on a diagram

5. List the hormones produced by each endocrine gland and describe the effects of each on the body

6. Describe how the hypothalamus controls the anterior and posterior pituitary

7. List tissues other than the endocrine glands that produce hormones

8. List some medical uses of hormones

9. Explain how the endocrine system responds to stress

10. Show how word parts are used to build words related to the endocrine system (see Word Anatomy at the end of the chapter)

The Endocrine System: Glands and Hormones

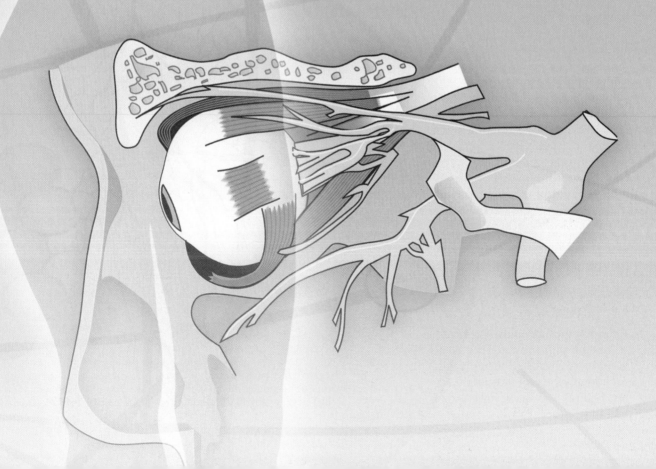

The endocrine system consists of a group of glands that produces regulatory chemicals called **hormones**. The endocrine system and the nervous system work together to control and coordinate all other systems of the body. The nervous system controls such rapid actions as muscle movement and intestinal activity by means of electrical and chemical stimuli. The effects of the endocrine system occur more slowly and over a longer period. They involve chemical stimuli only, and these chemical messengers have widespread effects on the body.

Although the nervous and endocrine systems differ in some respects, the two systems are closely related. For example, the activity of the pituitary gland, which in turn regulates other glands, is controlled by the brain's hypothalamus. The connections between the nervous system and the endocrine system enable endocrine function to adjust to the demands of a changing environment.

▶ Hormones

Hormones are chemical messengers that have specific regulatory effects on certain cells or organs. Hormones from the endocrine glands are released directly into the bloodstream, which carries them to all parts of the body. They regulate growth, metabolism, reproduction, and behavior. Some hormones affect many tissues, for example, growth hormone, thyroid hormone, and insulin. Others affect only specific tissues. For example, one pituitary hormone, thyroid-stimulating hormone (TSH), acts only on the thyroid gland; another, adrenocorticotropic hormone (ACTH), stimulates only the outer portion of the adrenal gland.

The specific tissue acted on by each hormone is the **target tissue**. The cells that make up these tissues have **receptors** in the plasma membrane or within the cytoplasm to which the hormone attaches. Once a hormone binds to a receptor on or in a target cell, it affects cell activities, regulating the manufacture of proteins, changing the permeability of the membrane, or affecting metabolic reactions.

Hormone Chemistry

Chemically, hormones fall into two main categories:

▶ **Amino acid compounds.** These hormones are proteins or related compounds also made of amino acids. All hormones except those of the adrenal cortex and the sex glands fall into this category.

▶ **Steroids.** These hormones are types of lipids derived from the steroid cholesterol. Steroid hormones are produced by the adrenal cortex and the sex glands. Steroid hormones can be recognized by the ending *–one*, as in progesterone, testosterone.

> **Checkpoint 11-1** What are hormones and what are some effects of hormones?

Hormone Regulation

The amount of each hormone that is secreted is normally kept within a specific range. Negative feedback, described in Chapter 1, is the method most commonly used to regulate these levels. In negative feedback, the hormone itself (or the result of its action) controls further hormone secretion. Each endocrine gland tends to oversecrete its hormone, exerting more effect on the target tissue. When the target tissue becomes too active, there is a negative effect on the endocrine gland, which then decreases its secretory action.

We can use as an example the secretion of thyroid hormones (Fig. 11-1). As described in more detail later in the chapter, a pituitary hormone, called *thyroid-stimulating hormone* (TSH), triggers secretion of hormones from the thyroid gland located in the neck. As blood levels of these hormones rise under the effects of TSH, they act as negative feedback messengers to inhibit TSH release from the pituitary. With less TSH, the thyroid releases less hor-

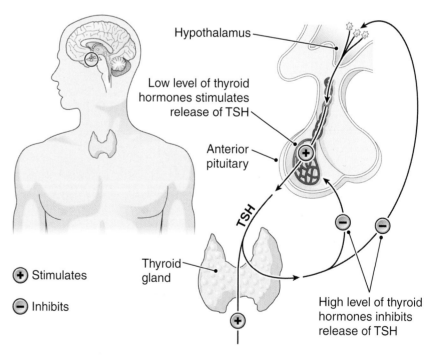

Hypothalamus

Low level of thyroid hormones stimulates release of TSH

Anterior pituitary

TSH

Thyroid gland

⊕ Stimulates

⊖ Inhibits

High level of thyroid hormones inhibits release of TSH

Figure 11-1 Negative feedback control of thyroid hormones. The anterior pituitary releases thyroid stimulating hormone (TSH) when the blood level of thyroid hormones is low. A high level of thyroid hormones inhibits release of TSH and thyroid hormone levels fall.

mone and blood levels drop. When hormone levels fall below the normal range, the pituitary can again begin to release TSH. This is a typical example of the kind of self-regulating system that keeps hormone levels within a set normal range.

Less commonly, some hormones are produced in response to positive feedback. In this case, response to a hormone promotes further hormone release. Examples are the action of oxytocin during labor, as described in Chapter 1, and the release of some hormones in the menstrual cycle, as described in Chapter 20.

The release of hormones may fall into a rhythmic pattern. Hormones of the adrenal cortex follow a 24-hour cycle related to a person's sleeping pattern, with the level of secretion greatest just before arising and least at bedtime. Hormones of the female menstrual cycle follow a monthly pattern.

> Checkpoint 11-2 Hormones levels are normally kept within a specific range. What is the most common method used to regulate secretion of hormones?

▶ The Endocrine Glands and Their Hormones

The remainder of this chapter deals with hormones and the tissues that produce them. Refer to Figure 11-2 to lo-cate each of the endocrine glands as you study them. Table 11-1 summarizes the information on the endocrine glands and their hormones.

Although most of the discussion centers on the endocrine glands, it is important to note that many tissues—other than the endocrine glands—also secrete hormones. That is, they produce substances that act on other tissues, usually at some distance from where they are produced. These tissues include the brain, digestive organs, and kidney. Some of these other tissues will be discussed later in the chapter.

The Pituitary

The **pituitary** (pih-TU-ih-tar-e), or **hypophysis** (hi-POF-ih-sis), is a small gland about the size of a cherry. It is located in a saddlelike depression of the sphenoid bone just posterior to the point where the optic nerves cross. It is surrounded by bone except where it connects with the hypothalmus of the brain by a stalk called the **infundibulum** (in-fun-DIB-u-lum). The gland is divided into two parts, the **anterior lobe** and the **posterior lobe** (Fig. 11-3).

The pituitary is often called the *master gland* because it releases hormones that affect the working of other glands, such as the thyroid, gonads (ovaries and testes), and adrenal glands. (Hormones that stimulate other glands may be recognized by the ending -*tropin,* as in *thyrotropin,* which means "acting on the thyroid gland.") However, the pituitary itself is controlled by the hypothalamus, which sends secretions and nerve impulses to the pituitary through the infundibulum (see Fig. 11-3).

Control of the Pituitary The hormones produced in the anterior pituitary are not released until chemical messengers called **releasing hormones** arrive from the hypothalamus. These releasing hormones travel to the anterior pituitary by way of a special type of circulatory pathway called a **portal system.** By this circulatory "detour," some of the blood that leaves the hypothalamus travels to capillaries in the anterior pituitary before returning to the heart. As the blood circulates through the capillaries, it delivers the hormones that stimulate the release of anterior pituitary secretions. Hypothalamic releasing hormones are indicated with the abbreviation *RH* added to an abbreviation for the name of the

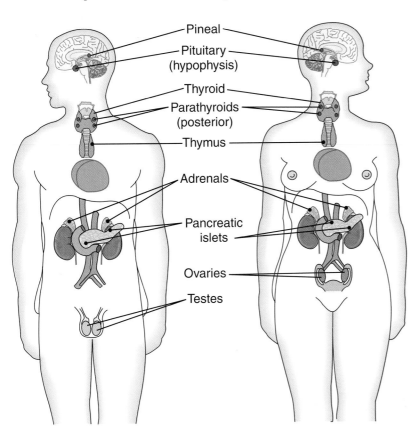

Pineal
Pituitary (hypophysis)
Thyroid
Parathyroids (posterior)
Thymus
Adrenals
Pancreatic islets
Ovaries
Testes

Figure 11-2 The endocrine glands.

Table 11·1 The Endocrine Glands and Their Hormones

GLAND	HORMONE	PRINCIPAL FUNCTIONS
Anterior pituitary	GH (growth hormone)	Promotes growth of all body tissues
	TSH (thyroid-stimulating hormone)	Stimulates thyroid gland to produce thyroid hormones
	ACTH (adrenocorticotropic hormone)	Stimulates adrenal cortex to produce cortical hormones; aids in protecting body in stress situations (injury, pain)
	PRL (prolactin)	Stimulates secretion of milk by mammary glands
	FSH (follicle-stimulating hormone)	Stimulates growth and hormone activity of ovarian follicles; stimulates growth of testes; promotes development of sperm cells
	LH (luteinizing hormone); ICSH (interstitial cell-stimulating hormone) in males	Causes development of corpus luteum at site of ruptured ovarian follicle in female; stimulates secretion of testosterone in male
Posterior pituitary	ADH (antidiuretic hormone)	Promotes reabsorption of water in kidney tubules; at high concentration stimulates constriction of blood vessels
	Oxytocin	Causes contraction of uterine muscle; causes ejection of milk from mammary glands
Thyroid	Thyroxine (T_4) and triiodothyronine(T_3)	Increases metabolic rate, influencing both physical and mental activities; required for normal growth
	Calcitonin	Decreases calcium level in blood
Parathyroids	Parathyroid hormone (PTH)	Regulates exchange of calcium between blood and bones; increases calcium level in blood
Adrenal medulla	Epinephrine and norephinephrine	Increases blood pressure and heart rate; activates cells influenced by sympathetic nervous system plus many not affected by sympathetic nerves
Adrenal cortex	Cortisol (95% of glucocorticoids)	Aids in metabolism of carbohydrates, proteins, and fats; active during stress
	Aldosterone (95% of mineralocorticoids)	Aids in regulating electrolytes and water balance
	Sex hormones	May influence secondary sexual characteristics
Pancreatic islets	Insulin	Needed for transport of glucose into cells; required for cellular metabolism of foods, especially glucose; decreases blood sugar levels
	Glucagon	Stimulates liver to release glucose, thereby increasing blood sugar levels
Testes	Testosterone	Stimulates growth and development of sexual organs (testes, penis) plus development of secondary sexual characteristics, such as hair growth on body and face and deepening of voice; stimulates maturation of sperm cells
Ovaries	Estrogens (e.g., estradiol)	Stimulates growth of primary sexual organs (uterus, tubes) and development of secondary sexual organs, such as breasts, plus changes in pelvis to ovoid, broader shape
	Progesterone	Stimulates development of secretory parts of mammary glands; prepares uterine lining for implantation of fertilized ovum; aids in maintaining pregnancy
Thymus	Thymosin	Promotes growth of T cells active in immunity
Pineal	Melatonin	Regulates mood, sexual development, and daily cycles in response to the amount of light in the environment

hormone stimulated. For example, the releasing hormone that controls growth hormone is GH-RH.

Two anterior pituitary hormones are also regulated by inhibiting hormones (IH) from the hypothalamus. Inhibiting hormones suppress both growth hormone, which stimulates growth and metabolism, and prolactin, which stimulates milk production in the mammary glands. These inhibiting hormones are abbreviated GH-IH (growth hormone-inhibiting hormone) and PIH (prolactin-inhibiting hormone)

The two hormones of the posterior pituitary (antidiuretic hormone, or ADH, and oxytocin) are actually produced in the hypothalamus and stored in the posterior pituitary. Their release is controlled by nerve impulses that travel over pathways (tracts) between the hypothalamus and the posterior pituitary.

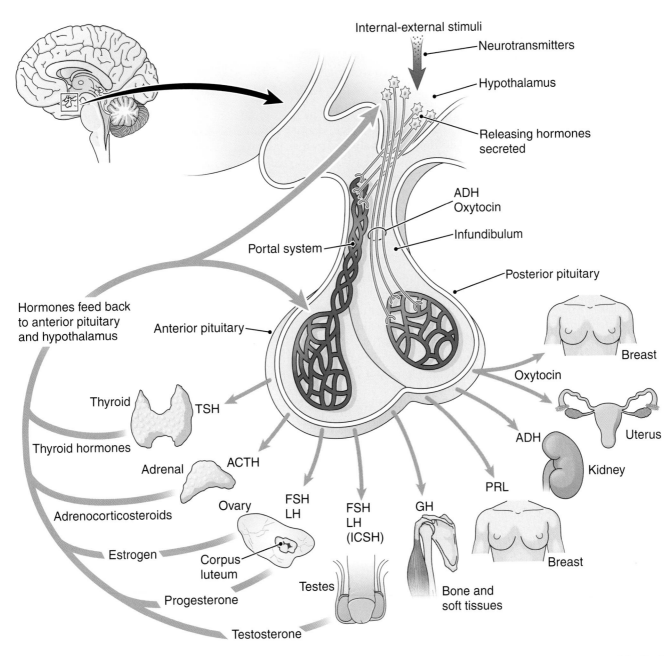

Figure 11-3 **The hypothalamus, pituitary gland, and target tissues.** Arrows indicate the hormones' target issues and feedback pathways. *ZOOMING IN ✦ What two structures does the infundibulum connect?*

Checkpoint 11-3 What part of the brain controls the pituitary?

Hormones of the Anterior Lobe

▶ **Growth hormone (GH),** or **somatotropin** (so-mah-to-TRO-pin), acts directly on most body tissues, promoting protein manufacture that is essential for growth. GH causes increase in size and height to occur in youth, before the closure of the epiphyses of long bones. A young person with a deficiency of GH will re-

main small, though well proportioned, unless treated with adequate hormone. GH is produced throughout life. It stimulates protein synthesis and is needed for maintenance and repair of cells. It also stimulates the liver to release fatty acids for energy in time of stress.

▶ **Thyroid-stimulating hormone (TSH),** or **thyrotropin** (thi-ro-TRO-pin), stimulates the thyroid gland to produce thyroid hormones.

▶ **Adrenocorticotropic** (ad-re-no-kor-te-ko-TRO-pik) **hormone (ACTH)** stimulates the production of hormones in the cortex of the adrenal glands.

▶ **Prolactin** (pro-LAK-tin) **(PRL)** stimulates the production of milk in the breasts.

▶ **Follicle-stimulating hormone (FSH)** stimulates the development of eggs in the ovaries and sperm cells in the testes.

▶ **Luteinizing** (LU-te-in-i-zing) **hormone (LH)** causes ovulation in females and sex hormone secretion in both males and females; in males, the hormone is sometimes called *interstitial cell–stimulating hormone* (ICSH).

FSH and LH are classified as **gonadotropins** (gon-ah-do-TRO-pinz), hormones that act on the gonads to regulate growth, development, and function of the reproductive systems in both males and females.

Hormones of the Posterior Lobe

▶ **Antidiuretic** (an-ti-di-u-RET-ik) **hormone (ADH)** promotes the reabsorption of water from the kidney tubules and thus decreases water excretion. Large amounts of this hormone cause contraction of smooth muscle in blood vessel walls and raise blood pressure. Inadequate amounts of ADH cause excessive water loss and result in a disorder called **diabetes insipidus**. This type of diabetes should not be confused with diabetes mellitus, which is due to inadequate amounts of insulin.

▶ **Oxytocin** (ok-se-TO-sin) causes contractions of the uterus and triggers milk ejection from the breasts. Under certain circumstances, commercial preparations of this hormone are administered during or after childbirth to cause uterine contraction.

Box 11-1 offers information on melanocyte-stimulating hormone, another hormone produced in the pituitary gland.

Checkpoint 11-4 What are the hormones from the anterior pituitary?

Checkpoint 11-5 What hormones are released from the posterior pituitary?

The Thyroid Gland

The **thyroid,** located in the neck, is the largest of the endocrine glands (Fig. 11-4). The thyroid has two roughly oval lateral lobes on either side of the larynx (voice box) connected by a narrow band called an **isthmus** (IS-mus). A connective tissue capsule encloses the entire gland.

Hormones of the Thyroid Gland The thyroid produces two hormones that regulate metabolism. The principal hormone is **thyroxine** (thi-ROK-sin), which is symbolized as T_4, based on the number of iodine atoms in each molecule. The other hormone, which contains three atoms of iodine, is **triiodothyronine** (tri-i-o-do-THI-ro-nene), or T_3. These hormones function to increase the rate of metabolism in body cells. In particular, they increase energy metabolism and protein metabolism. Both thyroid hormones and growth hormone are needed for normal growth.

The thyroid gland needs an adequate supply of iodine to produce its hormones. Iodine deficiency is rare now due to widespread availability of this mineral in iodized salt, vegetables, seafood, dairy products, and processed foods.

Another hormone produced by the thyroid gland is **calcitonin** (kal-sih-TO-nin), which is active in calcium metabolism. Calcitonin lowers the amount of calcium circulating in the blood by promoting the deposit of calcium in bone tissue. Calcitonin works with parathyroid hormone and with vitamin D to regulate calcium metabolism, as described below.

Box 11-1 | **A Closer Look**

Melanocyte-Stimulating Hormone: More Than a Tan?

In amphibians, reptiles, and certain other animals, melanocyte-stimulating hormone (MSH) darkens skin and hair by stimulating melanocytes to manufacture the pigment melanin. In humans, though, MSH levels are usually so low that its role as a primary regulator of skin pigmentation and hair color is questionable. What, then, is its function in the human body?

Recent research suggests that MSH is probably more important as a neurotransmitter in the brain than as a hormone in the rest of the body. When the pituitary gland secretes ACTH, it secretes MSH as well. This is so because pituitary cells do not produce ACTH directly but produce a large pre-cursor molecule, proopiomelanocortin (POMC), which enzymes cut into ACTH and MSH. In Addison disease, the pituitary tries to compensate for decreased glucocorticoid levels by increasing POMC production. The resulting increased levels of ACTH and MSH appear to cause the blotchy skin pigmentation that characterizes the disease.

MSH's roles in the rest of the body include helping the brain to regulate food intake, fertility, and even the immune response. Interestingly, despite MSH's relatively small role in regulating pigmentation, women do produce more MSH during pregnancy and often have darker skin.

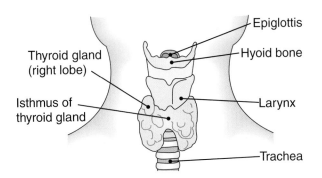

Figure 11-4 **Thyroid gland (anterior view).** The two lobes and isthmus of the thyroid are shown in relation to other structures in the throat. The epiglottis is a cartilage of the larynx. *ZOOMING IN ✦ What structure is superior to the thyroid? Inferior to the thyroid?*

> **Checkpoint 11-6** What is the effect of thyroid hormones on cells?

The Parathyroid Glands

The four tiny **parathyroid glands** are embedded in the posterior capsule of the thyroid (Fig. 11-5). The secretion of these glands, **parathyroid hormone (PTH)**, promotes calcium release from bone tissue, thus increasing the amount of calcium circulating in the bloodstream. PTH also causes the kidney to conserve calcium.

PTH works with calcitonin from the thyroid gland to regulate calcium metabolism. These hormone levels are controlled by negative feedback based on the amount of calcium in the blood. When calcium is high, calcitonin is produced; when calcium is low, PTH is produced.

Calcium Metabolism Calcium balance is required not only for the health of bones and teeth but also for the proper function of the nervous system and muscles. One other hormone is needed for calcium balance in addition

to calcitonin and PTH. This is **calcitriol** (kal-sih-TRI-ol), technically called dihydroxycholecalciferol (di-hi-drok-se-ko-le-kal-SIF-eh-rol), the active form of vitamin D. Calcitriol is produced by modification of vitamin D in the liver and then the kidney. It increases intestinal absorption of calcium to raise blood calcium levels.

Calcitonin, PTH, and calcitriol work together to regulate the amount of calcium in the blood and provide calcium for bone maintenance and other functions.

> **Checkpoint 11-7** What mineral is regulated by calcitonin and parathyroid hormone (PTH)?

The Adrenal Glands

The **adrenals** are two small glands located atop the kidneys. Each adrenal gland has two parts that act as separate glands. The inner area is called the **medulla**, and the outer portion is called the **cortex** (Fig. 11-6).

Hormones From the Adrenal Medulla The hormones of the adrenal medulla are released in response to stimulation by the sympathetic nervous system. The principal hormone produced by the medulla is **epinephrine**, also called **adrenaline**. Another hormone released from the adrenal medulla, **norepinephrine (noradrenalin)**, is closely related chemically and is similar in its actions to epinephrine. These two hormones are referred to as the *fight-or-flight hormones* because of their effects during emergency situations. We have already learned about these hormones in studying the autonomic nervous system. When released from nerve endings instead of being released directly into the bloodstream, they function as neurotransmitters. Some of their effects are as follows:

▶ Stimulation of the involuntary muscle in the walls of the arterioles, causing these muscles to contract and blood pressure to rise accordingly.

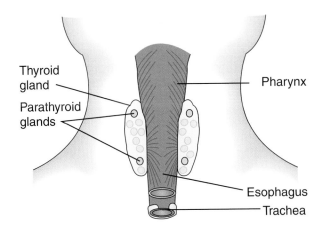

Figure 11-5 **Parathyroid glands (posterior view).** The four small parathyroid glands are embedded in the posterior surface of the thyroid.

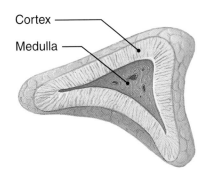

Figure 11-6 **The adrenal gland.** The medulla secretes epinephrine and norepinephrine. The cortex secretes steroid hormones. (Reprinted with permission from Gartner LP, Hiatt JL. *Color Atlas of Histology.* 3rd ed. Philadelphia: Lippincott Williams & Wilkins, 2000.) *ZOOMING IN ✦ What is the outer region of the adrenal gland called? The inner region?*

▶ Conversion of glycogen stored in the liver into glucose. The glucose pours into the blood and travels throughout the body, allowing the voluntary muscles and other tissues to do an extraordinary amount of work.

▶ Increase in the heart rate.

▶ Increase in the metabolic rate of body cells.

▶ Dilation of the bronchioles, through relaxation of the smooth muscle of their walls.

> **Checkpoint 11-8** The main hormone from the adrenal medulla also functions as a neurotransmitter in the sympathetic nervous system. What is the name of this hormone?

Hormones From the Adrenal Cortex There are three main groups of hormones secreted by the adrenal cortex:

▶ **Glucocorticoids** (glu-ko-KOR-tih-koyds) maintain the carbohydrate reserve of the body by stimulating the liver to convert amino acids into glucose (sugar) instead of protein. The production of these hormones increases in times of stress to aid the body in responding to unfavorable conditions. They raise the level of nutrients in the blood, not only glucose, but also amino acids from tissue proteins and fatty acids from fats stored in adipose tissue. Glucocorticoids also have the ability to suppress the inflammatory response and are often administered as medication for this purpose. The major hormone of this group is **cortisol,** which is also called *hydrocortisone.*

▶ **Mineralocorticoids** (min-er-al-o-KOR-tih-koyds) are important in the regulation of electrolyte balance. They control sodium reabsorption and potassium secretion by the kidney tubules. The major hormone of this group is **aldosterone** (al-DOS-ter-one).

▶ **Sex hormones** are secreted in small amounts, having little effect on the body.

> **Checkpoint 11-9** What three categories of hormones are released by the adrenal cortex?

> **Checkpoint 11-10** What effect does cortisol have on glucose levels in the blood?

The Pancreas and Its Hormones

Scattered throughout the **pancreas** are small groups of specialized cells called **islets** (I-lets), also known as **islets of Langerhans** (LAHNG-er-hanz) (Fig. 11-7). These cells make up the endocrine portion of the pancreas. The cells surrounding the islets secrete digestive juices. They make up the exocrine portion of the pancreas, which is independent of the islets and secretes through ducts into the small intestine (see Chapter 17).

The most important hormone secreted by the islets is **insulin** (IN-su-lin). Insulin is active in the transport of glucose across plasma membranes, thus increasing cellular glu-

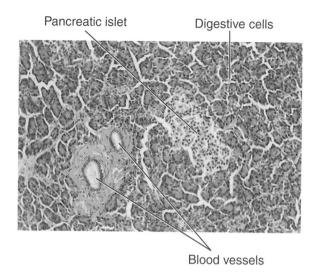

Pancreatic islet   Digestive cells

Blood vessels

Figure 11-7 Microscopic view of pancreatic cells. Light-staining islet cells are visible among the many cells that produce digestive juices. (Courtesy of Dana Morse Bittus and BJ Cohen.)

cose uptake. Once inside a cell, glucose is metabolized for energy. Insulin also increases the rate at which the liver takes up glucose and converts it to glycogen and the rate at which the liver changes excess glucose into fatty acids, which can then be converted to fats and stored in adipose tissue. Through these actions, insulin has the effect of lowering the blood sugar level. Insulin has other metabolic effects as well. It promotes the cellular uptake of amino acids and stimulates the manufacture of these amino acids into proteins. When the islet cells fail to produce enough insulin or body cells do not respond to the insulin, glucose is not transported into the cells and metabolized. Instead the sugar remains in the blood and then must be excreted in the urine. This condition is called **diabetes mellitus** (di-ah-BE-teze mel-LI-tus).

A second hormone produced by the islet cells is **glucagon** (GLU-kah-gon), which works with insulin to regulate blood sugar levels. Glucagon causes the liver to release stored glucose into the bloodstream. Glucagon also increases the rate at which glucose is made from proteins in the liver. In these two ways, glucagon increases blood sugar.

> **Checkpoint 11-11** What two hormones produced by the islets of the pancreas act to regulate glucose levels in the blood?

The Sex Glands

The sex glands, the female ovaries and the male testes, not only produce the sex cells but also are important endocrine organs. The hormones produced by these organs are needed in the development of the sexual characteristics, which usually appear in the early teens, and for the maintenance of the reproductive organs once full development has been attained. Those features that typify a male or female other than the structures directly concerned with reproduction are termed **secondary sex characteristics.** They include a deep voice and facial and

Seasonal Affective Disorder: Seeing the Light

We all sense that long dark days make us blue and sap our motivation. Are these learned responses or is there a physical basis for them? Studies have shown that the amount of light in the environment does have a physical effect on behavior. Evidence that light alters mood comes from people who are intensely affected by the dark days of winter—people who suffer from **seasonal affective disorder**, aptly abbreviated SAD. When days shorten, these people feel sleepy, depressed, and anxious. They tend to overeat, especially carbohydrates. Research suggests that SAD has a genetic basis and may be associated with decreased levels of serotonin.

As light strikes the retina of the eye, it sends impulses that decrease the amount of melatonin produced by the pineal gland in the brain. Because melatonin depresses mood, the final effect of light is to elevate mood. Daily exposure to bright lights has been found to improve the mood of most people with SAD. Exposure for 15 minutes after rising in the morning may be enough, but some people require longer sessions both morning and evening. Other aids include aerobic exercise, stress management techniques, and antidepressant medications.

body hair in males, and wider hips, breast development, and a greater ratio of fat to muscle in females.

Hormones of the Sex Glands The main male sex hormone produced by the testes is **testosterone** (tes-TOS-ter-one). All male sex hormones are classified as **androgens** (AN-dro-jens).

In the female, the hormones that most nearly parallel testosterone in their actions are the **estrogens** (ES-tro-jens), produced by the ovaries. Estrogens contribute to the development of the female secondary sex characteristics and stimulate mammary gland development, the onset of menstruation, and the development and functioning of the reproductive organs.

The other hormone produced by the ovaries, called **progesterone** (pro-JES-ter-one), assists in the normal development of pregnancy (gestation). All the sex hormones are discussed in more detail in Chapter 20.

Checkpoint 11-12 In addition to controlling reproduction, sex hormones confer certain features associated with male and female gender. What are these features called as a group?

The Thymus Gland

The **thymus gland** is a mass of lymphoid tissue that lies in the upper part of the chest superior to the heart. This gland is important in the development of immunity. Its hormone, **thymosin** (THI-mo-sin), assists in the maturation of certain white blood cells known as T cells (T lymphocytes) after they have left the thymus gland and taken up residence in lymph nodes throughout the body.

The Pineal Gland

The **pineal** (PIN-e-al) **gland** is a small, flattened, cone-shaped structure located posterior to the midbrain and connected to the roof of the third ventricle (see Fig. 11-2). The pineal produces the hormone **melatonin** (mel-ah-TO-nin) during dark periods. Little hormone is produced during daylight hours. This pattern of hormone secretion influences the regulation of sleep–wake cycles. (See also Box 11-2, Seasonal Affective Disorder.) Melatonin also appears to delay the onset of puberty.

▶ Other Hormone-Producing Tissues

Originally, the word *hormone* applied to the secretions of the endocrine glands only. The term now includes various body substances that have regulatory actions, either locally or at a distance from where they are produced. Many body tissues produce substances that regulate the local environment. Some of these other hormone-producing organs are the following:

▶ The stomach secretes a hormone that stimulates its own digestive activity.
▶ The small intestine secretes hormones that stimulate the production of digestive juices and help regulate the digestive process.
▶ The kidneys produce a hormone called **erythropoietin** (e-rith-ro-POY-eh-tin), which stimulates red blood cell production in the bone marrow. This hormone is produced when there is a decreased supply of oxygen in the blood.
▶ The brain, as noted, secretes releasing hormones and release-inhibiting hormones that control the anterior pituitary, as well as ADH and oxytocin that are released from the posterior pituitary.
▶ The atria (upper chambers) of the heart produce a substance called **atrial natriuretic** (na-tre-u-RET-ik) **peptide** (ANP) in response to their increased filling with blood. ANP increases loss of sodium by the kidneys and lowers blood pressure.
▶ The **placenta** (plah-SEN-tah) produces several hormones during pregnancy. These cause changes in the

uterine lining and, later in pregnancy, help to prepare the breasts for lactation. Pregnancy tests are based on the presence of placental hormones.

Prostaglandins

Prostaglandins (pros-tah-GLAN-dins) are a group of local hormones made by most body tissues. Their name comes from the fact that they were first discovered in male prostate glands. Prostaglandins are produced, act, and are rapidly inactivated in or close to their sites of origin. A bewildering array of functions has been ascribed to these substances. Some prostaglandins cause constriction of blood vessels, bronchial tubes, and the intestine, whereas others cause dilation of these same structures. Prostaglandins are active in promoting inflammation; certain antiinflammatory drugs, such as aspirin, act by blocking the production of prostaglandins. Some prostaglandins have been used to induce labor or abortion and have been recommended as possible contraceptive agents.

Overproduction of prostaglandins by the uterine lining (endometrium) can cause painful cramps of the uterine muscle. Treatment with prostaglandin inhibitors has been successful in some cases. Much has been written about these substances, and extensive research on them continues.

Checkpoint 11-13 What are some organs other than the endocrine glands that produce hormones?

▶ Hormones and Treatment

Hormones used for medical treatment are obtained from several different sources. Some are extracted from animal tissues. Some hormones and hormonelike substances are available in synthetic form, meaning that they are manufactured in commercial laboratories. A few hormones are produced by the genetic engineering technique of recombinant DNA. In this method, a gene for the cellular manufacture of a given product is introduced in the laboratory into the common bacterium *Escherichia coli*. The organisms are then grown in quantity, and the desired substance is harvested and purified.

A few examples of natural and synthetic hormones used in treatment are:

▶ **Growth hormone** is used for the treatment of children with a deficiency of this hormone. It is also used to strengthen bones and build body mass in the elderly. Adequate supplies are available from recombinant DNA techniques.

▶ **Insulin** is used in the treatment of diabetes mellitus. Types of insulin available include "human" insulin produced by recombinant DNA methods and hormone obtained from animal pancreases.

▶ **Adrenal steroids,** primarily the glucocorticoids, are used for the relief of inflammation in such diseases as rheumatoid arthritis, lupus erythematosus, asthma, and cerebral edema; for immunosuppression after organ transplantation; and for relief of symptoms associated with circulatory shock.

▶ **Epinephrine** (adrenaline) has many uses, including stimulation of the heart muscle when rapid response is required, treatment of asthmatic attacks by relaxation of the small bronchial tubes, and treatment of the acute allergic reaction called **anaphylaxis** (an-ah-fi-LAK-sis).

▶ **Thyroid hormones** are used in the treatment of hypothyroid conditions (cretinism and myxedema) and as replacement therapy after surgical removal of the thyroid gland.

▶ **Oxytocin** is used to cause contractions of the uterus and induce labor.

▶ **Androgens,** including testosterone and androsterone, are used in severe chronic illness to aid tissue building and promote healing.

▶ **Estrogen and progesterone** are used as oral contraceptives (birth control pills; "the pill"). They are highly effective in preventing pregnancy. Occasionally, they give rise to unpleasant side effects, such as nausea. More rarely, they cause serious complications, such as thrombosis (blood clots) or hypertension (high blood pressure). These adverse side effects are more common among women who smoke. Any woman taking birth control pills should have a yearly medical examination.

Preparations of estrogen and progesterone have been used to treat symptoms associated with menopause and protect against adverse changes that occur after menopause. Recent studies on the most popular form of these hormones have raised questions about their benefits and revealed some risks associated with their use. This issue is still under study.

▶ Hormones and Stress

Stress in the form of physical injury, disease, emotional anxiety, and even pleasure calls forth a specific response from the body that involves both the nervous system and the endocrine system. The nervous system response, the "fight-or-flight" response, is mediated by parts of the brain, especially the hypothalamus, and by the sympathetic nervous system, which releases epinephrine. During stress, the hypothalamus also triggers the release of ACTH from the anterior pituitary. The hormones released from the adrenal cortex as a result of ACTH stimulation raise the levels of glucose and other nutrients in the blood and inhibit inflammation. Growth hormone, thyroid hormones, sex hormones, and insulin are also released.

These hormones help the body meet stressful situations. Unchecked, however, they are harmful to the body and may lead to such stress-related disorders as high blood pressure, heart disease, ulcers, back pain, and

Box 11-3 · Health Maintenance

Stress: Mechanisms for Coping

Any event that threatens homeostasis is a form of stress. The body's negative feedback mechanisms can overcome many stressors (such as a drop in body temperature), but some forms of stress require the involvement of the nervous and endocrine systems. Fear, a powerful stressor, activates the nervous system's "fight-or-flight" response, which is often able to counteract the stress.

During long-term stress, such as starvation or prolonged anxiety, the endocrine system releases growth hormone, glucocorticoids, and mineralocorticoids (primarily aldosterone) to restore homeostasis and prevent disease. Research suggests that prolonged secretion of glucocorticoids is responsible for the harmful effects associated with stress. Elevated levels can cause increased blood pressure, muscle atrophy, growth inhi-

bition, and suppression of the immune system, which may lead to disorders such as heart disease, ulcers, cancer, and increased vulnerability to infections. To reduce stress and help prevent these effects:

- Focus on what you can control, let go of what you can't.
- View change as a positive challenge.
- Set realistic goals at home, school, and work.
- Eat well-balanced meals, get enough sleep, and exercise regularly.
- Meditate, practice deep relaxed breathing, and stretch to relieve tension.
- Do activities that help you relax.

headaches. Cortisones decrease the immune response, leaving the body more susceptible to infection. (See Box 11-3, Stress: Mechanisms for Coping.)

Although no one would enjoy a life totally free of stress in the form of stimulation and challenge, unmanaged stress, or "distress," has negative effects on the body. For this reason, techniques such as biofeedback and meditation to control stress are useful. The simple measures of setting priorities, getting adequate periods of relaxation, and getting regular physical exercise are important in maintaining total health.

Checkpoint 11-14 What are some hormones released in time of stress?

▶ Aging and the Endocrine System

Some of the changes associated with aging, such as loss of muscle and bone tissue, can be linked to changes in the endocrine system. The main clinical conditions associated with the endocrine system involve the pancreas and the thyroid.

Many elderly people develop adult-onset diabetes mellitus as a result of decreased secretion of insulin, which is made worse by poor diet, inactivity, and increased body fat. Some elderly people also show the effects of decreased thyroid hormone secretion.

Sex hormones decline during the middle-aged years in both males and females. These changes come from decreased activity of the gonads but also involve the more basic level of the pituitary gland and the secretion of gonadotropic hormones. Decrease in bone mass leading to osteoporosis is one result of these declines. With age, there is also a decrease in growth hormone levels and diminished activity of the adrenal cortex.

Thus far, the only commonly applied treatment for endocrine failure associated with age has been sex hormone replacement therapy for women at menopause. This supplementation has shown some beneficial effects on mucous membranes, the cardiovascular system, bone mass, and mental function.

Word Anatomy

Medical terms are built from standardized word parts (prefixes, roots, and suffixes). Learning the meanings of these parts can help you remember words and interpret unfamiliar terms.

WORD PART	MEANING	EXAMPLE
The Endocrine Glands and Their Hormones		
trop/o	acting on, influencing	*Somatotropin* stimulates growth in most body tissues.
cortic/o	cortex	*Adrenocorticotropic* hormone acts on the adrenal cortex.
lact/o	milk	*Prolactin* stimulates production of milk in the breasts.

ur/o	urine	*Antidiuretic* hormone promotes reabsorption of water in the kidneys and decreases excretion of urine.
oxy	sharp, acute	*Oxytocin* stimulates uterine contractions during labor.
toc/o	labor	
ren/o	kidney	The *adrenal* glands are near (ad-) the kidneys.
nephr/o	kidney	*Epinephrine* is another name for adrenaline.
insul/o	pancreatic islet, island	*Insulin* is a hormone produced by the pancreatic islets.
andr/o	male	An *androgen* is any male sex hormone.

Other Hormone-Producing Tissues

–poiesis	making, forming	*Erythropoietin* is a hormone from the kidneys that stimulates production of red blood cells.
natri	sodium (*L. natrium*)	Atrial *natriuretic* peptide stimulates release of sodium in the urine.

Summary

I. Hormones

1. Functions of hormones
   a. Affect other cells or organs—target tissue
   b. Widespread effects on growth, metabolism, reproduction
   c. Bind to receptors on target cells
A. Hormone chemistry
   1. Amino acid compounds—proteins and related compounds
   2. Steroids
      a. Lipids; derived from cholesterol
      b. Produced by adrenal cortex and sex glands
B. Hormone regulation—mainly negative feedback

II. Endocrine glands and their hormones

A. Pituitary
   1. Regulated by hypothalamus
      a. Anterior pituitary
         (1) Releasing hormones (RH) sent through portal system
         (2) Inhibiting hormones for GH and PRL
      b. Posterior pituitary
         (1) Stores hormones made by hypothalamus
         (2) Released by nervous stimulation
   2. Anterior lobe hormones
      a. Growth hormone (GH)—stimulates growth, tissue repair
      b. Thyroid-stimulating hormone (TSH)
      c. Adrenocorticotropic hormone (ACTH)—acts on cortex of adrenal gland
      d. Prolactin (PRL)—stimulates milk production in mammary glands
      e. Follicle-stimulating hormone (FSH)—acts on gonads
      f. Luteinizing hormone (LH)—acts on gonads
   3. Posterior lobe hormones
      a. Antidiuretic hormone (ADH)—promotes reabsorption of water in the kidneys
      b. Oxytocin—stimulates uterine contractions
B. Thyroid gland
   1. Hormones
      a. Thyroxine (T4) and triiodothyronine (T3) increase metabolic rate
      b. Calcitonin—decreases blood calcium levels
   2. Thyroid function tests—radioactive iodine used
C. Parathyroid glands—secrete parathyroid hormone (PTH), which increases blood calcium levels
D. Adrenal glands
   1. Hormones of adrenal medulla (inner region)
      a. Epinephrine and norepinephrine—act as neurotransmitters
   2. Hormones of adrenal cortex (outer region)
      a. Glucocorticoids—released during stress to raise nutrients in blood; *e.g.*, cortisol
      b. Mineralocorticoids—regulate water and electrolyte balance; *e.g.*, aldosterone
      c. Sex hormones—produced in small amounts
E. Pancreas—islet cells of pancreas secrete hormones
   1. Insulin
      a. Lowers blood glucose
   2. Glucagon
      a. Raises blood glucose
F. Sex glands—needed for reproduction and development of secondary sex characteristics
   1. Testes—secrete testosterone
   2. Ovaries—secrete estrogen and progesterone
G. Thymus gland—secretes thymosin, which aids in development of T lymphocytes
H. Pineal gland—secretes melatonin
   1. Regulates sexual development and sleep–wake cycles
   2. Controlled by environmental light

III. Other hormone-producing tissues

1. Stomach and small intestine—secrete hormones that regulate digestion
2. Kidneys—secrete erythropoietin, which increases production of red blood cells
3. Brain—releasing and inhibiting hormones, ADH, oxytocin
   a. Atria of heart—ANP causes loss of sodium by kidney and lowers blood pressure
   b. Placenta—secretes hormones that maintain pregnancy and prepare breasts for lactation
A. Prostaglandins—other cells throughout body produce prostaglandins, which have varied effects

IV. Hormones and treatment

1. Growth hormone—treatment of deficiency in children, in elderly for bone strength and body mass
2. Insulin—treatment of diabetes mellitus
3. Steroids—reduction of inflammation, suppression of immunity
4. Epinephrine—treatment of asthma, anaphylaxis, shock
5. Thyroid hormone—treatment of hypothyroidism
6. Oxytocin—contraction of uterine muscle
7. Androgens—promote healing
8. Estrogen and progesterone—contraception, symptoms of menopause

V. Hormones and stress

1. Body's response to stress involves nervous and endocrine systems, hormones
2. Fight-or-flight response mediated by brain: hypothalamus, sympathetic nervous system
3. Hormones help body, meet stressful situations
4. Unmanaged stress can be harmful; stress management techniques help maintain overall health

VI. Aging and the endocrine system

1. Aging-associated changes linked with endocrine system changes—loss of muscle and bone tissue
2. Main clinical conditions associated with endocrine system involve pancreas, thyroid
   a. Adult-onset diabetics mellitus
   b. Decline in sex hormones in males and females
      (1) Decreased bone mass—osteoporosis
3. Sex hormone replacement therapy for women at menopause—only common treatment for age-associated endocrine failure

Questions for Study and Review

Building Understanding

Fill in the blanks

1. Chemical messengers carried by the blood are called _____.

2. The part of the brain that regulates endocrine activity is the _____.

3. Red blood cell production in the bone marrow is stimulated by _____.

4. A hormone produced by the heart is _____.

5. Local hormones active in promoting inflammation are _____.

Matching

Match each numbered item with the most closely related lettered item.

___ 6. A hormone produced by the thyroid.
___ 7. A hormone produced by the adrenal gland.
___ 8. A hormone produced by the pancreas.
___ 9. A hormone produced by the testes.
___ 10. A hormone produced by the ovaries.

a. estrogen
b. glucagon
c. aldosterone
d. calcitonin
e. testosterone

Multiple choice

___ 11. A target tissue responds to a hormone only if it has the appropriate
    a. amino acid
    b. transporter
    c. ion channel
    d. receptor

___ 12. Uterine contractions and milk ejection are promoted by
    a. prolactin
    b. oxytocin
    c. estrogen
    d. luteinizing hormone

___ 13. The principal hormone that increases the metabolic rate in body cells is
    a. thyroxine
    b. triiodothyronine
    c. aldosterone
    d. progesterone

___ 14. Epinephrine and norepinephrine are released by the
    a. adrenal cortex
    b. adrenal medulla
    c. kidneys
    d. pancreas

___ 15. Sleep-wake cycles are regulated by the
    a. pituitary
    b. thyroid
    c. thymus
    d. pineal

Understanding Concepts

16. With regard to regulation, what are the main differences between the nervous system and the endocrine system?

17. Explain how the hypothalamus and pituitary gland regulate certain endocrine glands. Use the thyroid as an example.

18. Name the two divisions of the pituitary gland. List the hormones released from each division and describe the effects of each.

19. Compare and contrast the following hormones:
   a. calcitonin and parathyroid hormone
   b. cortisol and aldosterone
   c. insulin and glucagon
   d. testosterone and estrogen

20. Describe the anatomy of the following endocrine glands:
   a. thyroid
   b. pancreas
   c. adrenals

21. Name the hormone released by the thymus gland; by the pineal body. What are the effects of each?

22. List several hormones released during stress. What is the relationship between prolonged stress and disease?

Conceptual Thinking

23. Describe the endocrine activity of the pancreas immediately following a meal and then four hours later.

24. One consequence of decreased blood levels of thyroid hormone is increased blood levels of thyroid stimulating hormone. Why?

unit IV

Circulation and Body Defense

$\mathcal{T}$he chapters in this unit discuss the systems that move materials through the body. The blood is the main transport medium. It circulates through the cardiovascular system, consisting of the heart and the blood vessels. The lymphatic system, in addition to other functions, helps to balance body fluids by bringing substances from the tissues back to the heart. Components of the blood and the lymphatic system are involved in body defenses against infection as part of the immune system.

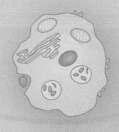

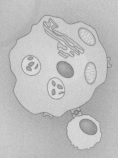

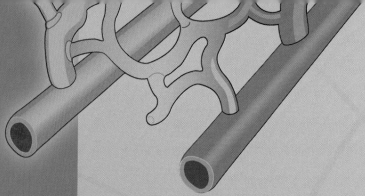

LEARNING OUTCOMES

After careful study of this chapter, you should be able to:

1. List the functions of the blood
2. List the main ingredients in plasma
3. Describe the formation of blood cells
4. Name and describe the three types of formed elements in the blood and give the function of each
5. Characterize the five types of leukocytes
6. Define *hemostasis* and cite three steps in hemostasis
7. Briefly describe the steps in blood clotting
8. Define *blood type* and explain the relation between blood type and transfusions
9. List the possible reasons for transfusions of whole blood and blood components
10. Specify the tests used to study blood
11. Show how word parts are used to build words related to the blood (see Word Anatomy at the end of the chapter)

chapter

12

The Blood

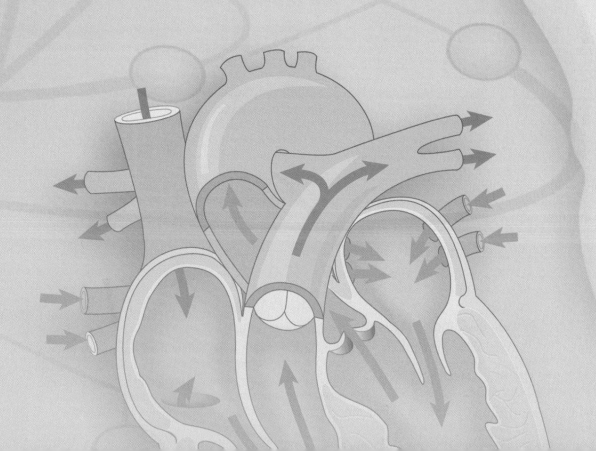

The circulating blood is of fundamental importance in maintaining homeostasis. This life-giving fluid brings nutrients and oxygen to the cells and carries away waste. The heart pumps blood continuously through a closed system of vessels. The heart and blood vessels are described in Chapters 13 and 14.

Blood is classified as a connective tissue because it consists of cells suspended in an intercellular background material, or matrix. Blood cells share many characteristics of origination and development with other connective tissues. However, blood differs from other connective tissues in that its cells are not fixed in position; instead, they move freely in the plasma, the liquid portion of the blood.

Whole blood is a viscous (thick) fluid that varies in color from bright scarlet to dark red, depending on how much oxygen it is carrying. (It is customary in drawings to color blood high in oxygen as red and blood low in oxygen as blue.) The blood volume accounts for approximately 8% of total body weight. The actual quantity of circulating blood differs with a person's size; the average adult male, weighing 70 kg (154 pounds), has about 5 liters (5.2 quarts) of blood.

▶ Functions of the Blood

The circulating blood serves the body in three ways: transportation, regulation, and protection.

Transportation

▶ Oxygen from inhaled air diffuses into the blood through thin membranes in the lungs and is carried by the circulation to all body tissues. Carbon dioxide, a waste product of cell metabolism, is carried from the tissues to the lungs, where it is breathed out.
▶ The blood transports nutrients and other needed substances, such as electrolytes (salts) and vitamins, to the cells. These materials enter the blood from the digestive system or are released into the blood from body reserves.
▶ The blood transports the waste products from the cells to sites where they are removed. For example, the kidney removes excess water, acid, electrolytes, and urea (a nitrogen-containing waste). The liver removes blood pigments, hormones, and drugs, and the lungs eliminate carbon dioxide.
▶ The blood carries hormones from their sites of origin to the organs they affect.

Regulation

▶ Buffers in the blood help keep the pH of body fluids steady at about 7.4. (The actual range of blood pH is 7.35 to 7.45.) Recall that pH is a measure of the acidity or alkalinity of a solution. At an average pH of 7.4, blood is slightly alkaline (basic).

▶ The blood regulates the amount of fluid in the tissues by means of substances (mainly proteins) that maintain the proper osmotic pressure. Recall that osmotic pressure is related to the concentration of dissolved and suspended materials in a solution. Proper osmotic pressure is needed for fluid balance, as described in Chapter 14.
▶ The blood transports heat that is generated in the muscles to other parts of the body, thus aiding in the regulation of body temperature.

Protection

▶ The blood is important in defense against disease. It carries the cells and antibodies of the immune system that protect against pathogens.
▶ The blood contains factors that protect against blood loss from the site of an injury. The process of blood coagulation, needed to prevent blood loss, is described later in this chapter.

Checkpoint 12-1 What are some substances transported in the blood?

Checkpoint 12-2 What is the pH range of the blood?

▶ Blood Constituents

The blood is divided into two main components (Fig. 12-1). The liquid portion is the **plasma**. The **formed elements**, which include cells and cell fragments, fall into three categories, as follows:

▶ **Erythrocytes** (eh-RITH-ro-sites), from *erythro*, meaning "red," are the red blood cells, which transport oxygen.
▶ **Leukocytes** (LU-ko-sites), from *leuko*, meaning "white," are the several types of white blood cells, which protect against infection.
▶ **Platelets**, also called **thrombocytes** (THROM-bo-sites), are cell fragments that participate in blood clotting.

Table 12-1 summarizes information on the different types of formed elements. Figure 12-2 shows all the categories of formed elements in a blood smear, that is, a blood sample spread thinly over the surface of a glass slide, as viewed under a microscope.

Checkpoint 12-3 What are the two main components of blood?

Blood Plasma

About 55% of the total blood volume is plasma. The plasma itself is 91% water. Many different substances, dissolved or suspended in the water, make up the other 9% by weight (see Fig. 12-1). The plasma content may vary somewhat because substances are removed and added as the blood cir-

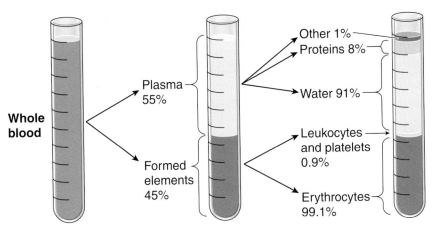

Figure 12-1 **Composition of whole blood.** Percentages show the relative proportions of the different components of plasma and formed elements.

culates to and from the tissues. However, the body tends to maintain a fairly constant level of most substances. For example, the level of glucose, a simple sugar, is maintained at a remarkably constant level of about one tenth of one percent (0.1%) in solution.

After water, the next largest percentage (about 8%) of material in the plasma is **protein**. The plasma proteins include the following:

▸ **Albumin** (al-BU-min), the most abundant protein in plasma, is important for maintaining the osmotic pressure of the blood. This protein is manufactured in the liver.

▸ **Clotting factors**, necessary for blood coagulation, are also manufactured in the liver.

▸ **Antibodies** combat infection. Antibodies are made by certain white blood cells.

▸ **Complement** consists of a group of enzymes that helps antibodies in their fight against pathogens (see Chapter 15).

The remaining 1% of the plasma consists of nutrients, electrolytes, and other materials that must be transported.

With regard to the nutrients, the principal carbohydrate found in the plasma is glucose. This simple sugar is absorbed from digested foods in the intestine. It is also stored as glycogen, mainly in the liver, and released as needed into the blood to supply energy to the cells. Amino acids, the products of protein digestion, also circulate in the plasma. Lipids constitute a small percentage of blood plasma. Lipid components include fats, cholesterol, and lipoproteins, which are proteins bound to cholesterol.

The electrolytes in the plasma appear primarily as chloride, carbonate, or phosphate salts of sodium, potassium, calcium, and magnesium. These salts have a variety of functions, including the formation of bone (calcium and phosphorus), the production of certain hormones (such as iodine for the production of thyroid hormones), and the maintenance of the acid–base balance (such as sodium and potassium carbonates and phosphates present in buffers).

Other materials transported in plasma include vitamins, hormones, waste products, drugs, and dissolved gases, primarily oxygen and carbon dioxide.

Checkpoint 12-4 Next to water, what is the most abundant type of substance in plasma?

The Formed Elements

All of the blood's formed elements are produced in red bone marrow, which is located in the ends of long bones and in the inner mass of all other bones. The ancestors of all the blood cells are called **hematopoietic** (blood-forming) **stem cells**. These cells have the potential to develop

Table 12·1	Formed Elements of Blood		
FORMED ELEMENT	**NUMBER PER μL OF BLOOD**	**DESCRIPTION**	**FUNCTION**
Erythrocyte (red blood cell)	5 million	Tiny (7 μM diameter), biconcave disk without nucleus (anuclear)	Carries oxygen bound to hemoglobin; also carries some carbon dioxide and buffers blood
Leukocyte (white blood cell)	5,000 to 10,000	Larger than red cell with prominent nucleus that may be segmented (granulocyte) or unsegmented (agranulocyte); vary in staining properties	Protects against pathogens; destroys foreign matter and debris; some are active in the immune system; located in blood, tissues, and lymphatic system
Platelet	150,000 to 450,000	Fragment of large cell (megakaryocyte)	Hemostasis; forms a platelet plug and starts blood clotting (coagulation)

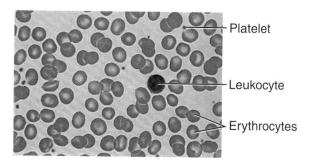

Figure 12-2 Blood cells as viewed under the microscope. All three types of formed elements are visible. *ZOOMING IN ✦ Which cells are the most numerous in the blood?*

into any of the blood cell types produced within the red marrow.

In comparison with other cells, most of those in the blood are short lived. The need for constant blood cell replacement means that normal activity of the red bone marrow is absolutely essential to life.

> **Checkpoint 12-5** Where do blood cells form?

> **Checkpoint 12-6** What type of cell gives rise to all blood cells?

Erythrocytes Erythrocytes, the red blood cells (RBCs, or red cells), measure about 7 μm in diameter. They are disk-shaped bodies with a depression on both sides. This biconcave shape creates a central area that is thinner than the edges (Fig. 12-3). Erythrocytes are different from other cells in that the mature form found in the circulating blood lacks a nucleus (is anuclear) and also lacks most of the other organelles commonly found in cells. As red cells mature, these components are lost, providing more space for the cells to carry oxygen. This vital gas is bound in the red cells to **hemoglobin** (he-mo-GLO-bin), a protein that contains iron (see Box 12-1, Hemoglobin: Door to Door Oxygen Delivery). Hemoglobin, combined with oxygen, gives the blood its characteristic red color. The more oxygen carried by the hemoglobin, the brighter is the red color of the blood. Therefore, the blood that goes from the lungs to the tissues is a bright red because it carries a great supply of oxygen; in contrast, the blood that returns to the lungs is a much darker red because it has given up much of its oxygen to the tissues.

Hemoglobin has two lesser functions in addition to the transport of oxygen. Hemoglobin that has given up its oxygen is able to carry hydrogen ions. In this way, hemoglobin acts as a buffer and plays an important role in acid–base balance (see Chapter 19). Hemoglobin also carries some carbon dioxide from the tissues to the lungs for elimination. The carbon dioxide is bound to a different part of the molecule than the part that holds oxygen, so that it does not interfere with oxygen transport.

Hemoglobin's ability to carry oxygen can be blocked by carbon monoxide. This odorless and colorless but harmful gas combines with hemoglobin to form a stable compound that can severely restrict the erythrocytes' ability to carry oxygen. Carbon monoxide is a byproduct of the incomplete burning of fuels, such as gasoline and other petroleum products and coal, wood, and other carbon-containing materials. It also occurs in cigarette smoke and automobile exhaust.

Erythrocytes are by far the most numerous of the blood cells, averaging from 4.5 to 5 million per microliter (μL) of blood. (A microliter is one millionth of a liter. It is equal to a cubic millimeter or mm^3.) Because mature red cells have no nucleus and cannot divide, they must be replaced constantly. After leaving the bone marrow, they circulate in the bloodstream for about 120 days before their membranes deteriorate and they are destroyed by the liver and spleen. Red cell production is stimulated by the hormone **erythropoietin** (eh-rith-ro-POY-eh-tin) **(EPO)**, which is released from the kidney in response to a decrease in its oxygen supply. The constant production of red cells requires an adequate supply of nutrients, particularly protein, the B vitamins B_{12} and folic acid, required for the production of DNA, and the minerals iron and copper for the production of hemoglobin. Vitamin C is also important for the proper absorption of iron from the small intestine.

> **Checkpoint 12-7** Red cells are modified to carry a maximum amount of hemoglobin. What is the main function of hemoglobin?

Leukocytes The **leukocytes,** or white blood cells (WBCs, or white cells), are different from the erythrocytes in appearance, quantity, and function. The cells themselves are round, but they contain prominent nuclei of varying shapes and sizes. Occurring at a concentration of 5,000 to 10,000 per cubic millimeter of blood, leukocytes are outnumbered by red cells by about 700 to 1. Al-

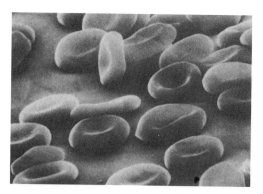

Figure 12-3 Red blood cells as seen under a scanning electron microscope. This type of microscope provides a three-dimensional view of the cells. *ZOOMING IN ✦ Why are these cells described as biconcave?*

Box 12-1   A Closer Look

Hemoglobin: Door to Door Oxygen Delivery

The hemoglobin molecule is a protein made of four chains of amino acids (the globin part of the molecule), each of which holds an iron-containing heme group. Each of the four hemes can bind one molecule of oxygen.

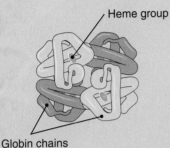

Heme group

Globin chains

Hemoglobin. This protein in red blood cells consists of four amino acid chains (globins), each with an oxygen-binding heme group.

Hemoglobin allows the blood to carry much more oxygen than it could were the oxygen simply dissolved in the plasma. A red blood cell contains about 250 million hemoglobins, each capable of binding four molecules of oxygen. So, a single red blood cell can carry about one billion oxygen molecules! Hemoglobin reversibly binds oxygen, picking it up in the lungs and releasing it in the body tissues. Active cells need more oxygen and also generate heat and acidity. These changing conditions promote the release of oxygen from hemoglobin into metabolically active tissues.

Immature red blood cells (erythroblasts) produce hemoglobin as they mature into erythrocytes in the red bone marrow. When the liver and spleen destroy old erythrocytes they break down the released hemoglobin. Some of its components are recycled, and the remainder leaves the body as a brown fecal pigment called stercobilin. In spite of some conservation, dietary protein and iron are still essential to maintain hemoglobin supplies.

though the red cells have a definite color, the leukocytes tend to be colorless.

The different types of white cells are identified by their size, the shape of the nucleus, and the appearance of granules in the cytoplasm when the cells are stained. The stain commonly used for blood is Wright stain, which is a mixture of dyes that differentiates the various blood cells. The "granules" in the white cells are actually lysosomes and other secretory vesicles. They are present in all white blood cells, but they are more easily stained and more visible in some cells than in others. The relative percentage of the different types of leukocytes is a valuable clue in arriving at a medical diagnosis (Table 12-2).

The granular leukocytes, or **granulocytes** (GRAN-u-lo-sites), are so named because they show visible granules in the cytoplasm when stained (see Fig. 12-4 A-C). Each has a very distinctive, highly segmented nucleus. The different types of granulocytes are named for the type of dyes they take up when stained. They include the following:

▶ **Neutrophils** (NU-tro-fils) stain with either acidic or basic dyes and show lavender granules.
▶ **Eosinophils** (e-o-SIN-o-fils) stain with acidic dyes (eosin is one) and have beadlike, bright pink granules.
▶ **Basophils** (BA-so-fils) stain with basic dyes and have large, dark blue granules that often obscure the nucleus.

The neutrophils are the most numerous of the white cells, constituting approximately 60% of all leukocytes (see Table 12-2). Because the nuclei of the neutrophils have various shapes, these cells are also called **polymorphs** (meaning "many forms") or simply *polys*. Other nicknames are *segs*, referring to the segmented nucleus, and *PMNs*, an abbreviation of **polymorphonuclear neutrophils**. Before reaching full maturity and becoming segmented, the nucleus of the neutrophil looks like a thick, curved band (Fig. 12-5). An increase in the number of these **band cells** (also called *stab* or *staff cells*) is a sign of infection and the active production of neutrophils.

Table 12·2 Leukocytes (White Blood Cells)		
CELL TYPE	RELATIVE PERCENTAGE (ADULT)	FUNCTION
Granulocytes		
Neutrophils	54%–62%	Phagocytosis
Eosinophils	1%–3%	Allergic reactions; defense against parasites
Basophils	< 1%	Allergic reactions; inflammatory reactions
Agranulocytes		
Lymphocytes	25%–38%	Immunity (T cells and B cells)
Monocytes	3%–7%	Phagocytosis

Granulocytes

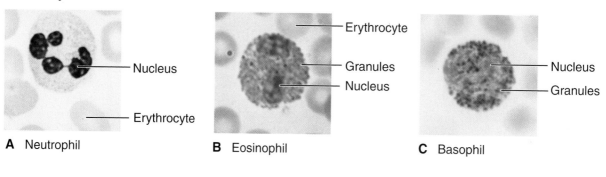

A Neutrophil   B Eosinophil   C Basophil

Agranulocytes

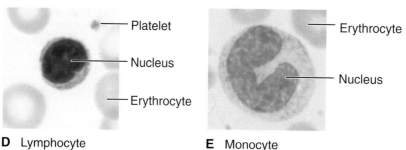

D Lymphocyte   E Monocyte

Figure 12-4 Granulocytes (A-C) and agranulocytes (D, E). (A) The neutrophil has a large, segmented nucleus. **(B)** The eosinophil has many bright pink-staining granules. **(C)** The basophil has large dark blue-staining granules. **(D)** The lymphocyte has a large undivided nucleus. **(E)** The monocyte is the largest of the leukocytes. *ZOOMING IN ✦ Which group of leukocytes has segmented nuclei? Which specific type of leukocyte is largest in size? Smallest in size?*

The eosinophils and basophils make up a small percentage of the white cells but increase in number during allergic reactions.

The agranular leukocytes, or **agranulocytes,** are so named because they lack easily visible granules (see Fig. 12-4 D,E). Their nuclei are round or curved and are not segmented. There are two types of agranular leukocytes:

▶ **Lymphocytes** (LIM-fo-sites) are the second most numerous of the white cells. Although lymphocytes originate in the red bone marrow, they develop to maturity in lymphoid tissue and can multiply in this tissue as

well (see Chapter 15). They circulate in the lymphatic system and are active in immunity.
▶ **Monocytes** (MON-o-sites) are the largest in size. They average about 5% of the leukocytes.

Function of Leukocytes Leukocytes clear the body of foreign material and cellular debris. Most importantly, they destroy pathogens that may invade the body. Neutrophils and monocytes engage in **phagocytosis** (fag-o-si-TO-sis), the engulfing of foreign matter (Fig. 12-6). Whenever pathogens enter the tissues, as through a wound, they are attracted to the area. They squeeze between the cells of the capillary walls and proceed by ameboid (ah-ME-boyd), or amebalike, motion to the area of infection where they engulf the invaders. Lysosomes in the cytoplasm then digest the foreign organisms and the cells eliminate the waste products.

When foreign organisms invade, the bone marrow and lymphoid tissue go into emergency production of white cells, and their number increases enormously as a result. Detection of an abnormally large number of white cells in the blood is an indication of infection. In battling pathogens, leukocytes themselves may be destroyed. A mixture of dead and living

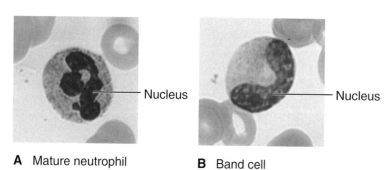

A Mature neutrophil   B Band cell
(immature neutrophil)

Figure 12-5 Stages in neutrophil development. (A) A mature neutrophil has a segmented nucleus. **(B)** An immature neutrophil is called a band cell because the nucleus is shaped like a thick, curved band. (×1325) (Reprinted with permission from Gartner LP, Hiatt JL. Color Atlas of Histology. 3rd ed. Philadelphia: Lippincott Williams & Wilkins, 2000.)

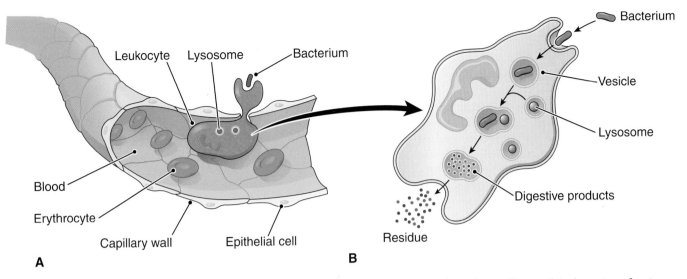

Figure 12-6 **Phagocytosis. (A)** A phagocytic leukocyte (white blood cell) squeezes through a capillary wall in the region of an infection and engulfs a bacterium. **(B)** The bacterium is enclosed in a vesicle and digested by a lysosome. *ZOOMING IN ✦ What type of epithelium makes up the capillary wall?*

bacteria, together with dead and living leukocytes, forms **pus**. A collection of pus localized in one area is known as an **abscess**.

Some monocytes enter the tissues, enlarge, and mature into **macrophages** (MAK-ro-faj-ez), which are highly active in disposing of invaders and foreign material. Although most circulating lymphocytes live only 6 to 8 hours, those that enter the tissues may survive for longer periods—days, months, or even years.

Some lymphocytes become **plasma cells**, active in the production of circulating antibodies needed for immunity. The activities of the various white cells are further discussed in Chapter 15.

Checkpoint 12-8 What are the types of granular leukocytes? Of agranular leukocytes?

Checkpoint 12-9 What is the most important function of leukocytes?

Platelets The blood **platelets** (thrombocytes) are the smallest of all the formed elements (Fig. 12-7 A). These tiny structures are not cells in themselves but rather fragments constantly released from giant bone marrow cells called **megakaryocytes** (meg-ah-KAR-e-o-sites) (Fig. 12-7 B). Platelets do not have nuclei or DNA, but they do contain active enzymes and mitochondria. The number of platelets in the circulating blood has been estimated to range from 150,000 to 450,000 per μL (mm^3). They have a life-span of about 10 days.

Platelets are essential to blood co-agulation (clotting). When blood

comes in contact with any tissue other than the smooth lining of the blood vessels, as in the case of injury, the platelets stick together and form a plug that seals the wound. The platelets then release chemicals that participate in the formation of a clot to stop blood loss. More details on these reactions follow.

Checkpoint 12-10 What is the function of blood platelets?

▶ Hemostasis

Hemostasis (he-mo-STA-sis) is the process that prevents blood loss from the circulation when a blood vessel is ruptured by an injury. Events in hemostasis include the following:

▶ **Contraction** of the smooth muscles in the blood vessel wall. This reduces the flow of blood and loss from the defect in the vessel wall. The term for this reduction in the diameter of a vessel is *vasoconstriction*.
▶ Formation of a **platelet plug**. Activated platelets be-

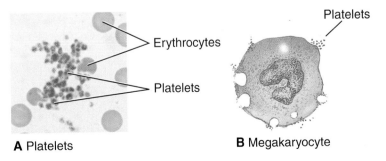

Figure 12-7 **Platelets (thrombocytes). (A)** Platelets in a blood smear. **(B)** A megakaryocyte releases platelets. (B, Reprinted with permission from Gartner LP, Hiatt JL. Color Atlas of Histology. 3rd ed. Philadelphia: Lippincott Williams & Wilkins, 2000.)

come sticky and adhere to the defect to form a temporary plug.

▸ Formation of a **blood clot.**

Blood Clotting

The many substances necessary for blood clotting, or coagulation, are normally inactive in the bloodstream. A balance is maintained between compounds that promote clotting, known as **procoagulants,** and those that prevent clotting, known as **anticoagulants.** In addition, there are chemicals in the circulation that act to dissolve any unnecessary and potentially harmful clots that may form. Under normal conditions, the substances that prevent clotting prevail. When an injury occurs, however, the procoagulants are activated, and a clot is formed.

The clotting process is a well-controlled series of separate events involving 12 different factors, each designated by a Roman numeral. The final step in these reactions is the conversion of a plasma protein called **fibrinogen** (fi-BRIN-o-jen) into solid threads of **fibrin,** which form the clot.

A few of the final steps involved in blood clot formation are described below and diagrammed in Figure 12-8:

▸ Substances released from damaged tissues result in the formation of **prothrombinase** (pro-THROM-bih-nase), a substance that triggers the final clotting mechanism.

▸ Prothrombinase converts prothrombin in the blood to **thrombin.** Calcium is needed for this step.

▸ Thrombin, in turn, converts soluble fibrinogen into insoluble fibrin. **Fibrin** forms a network of threads that entraps plasma and blood cells to form a clot.

Blood clotting occurs in response to injury. Blood also clots when it comes into contact with some surface other than the lining of a blood vessel, for example, a glass or plastic tube used for a blood specimen. In this case, the preliminary steps of clotting are somewhat different and require more time, but the final steps are the same as those described above.

The fluid that remains after clotting has occurred is called **serum** (plural, *sera*). Serum contains all the components of blood plasma *except* the clotting factors, as expressed in the formula:

$$\text{Plasma} = \text{serum} + \text{clotting factors}$$

Several methods used to measure the body's ability to coagulate blood are described later in this chapter.

> **Checkpoint 12-11** What happens when fibrinogen converts to fibrin?

▸ Blood Types

If for some reason the amount of blood in the body is severely reduced, through **hemorrhage** (HEM-eh-rij) (excessive bleeding) or disease, the body cells suffer from lack of oxygen and nutrients. One possible measure to take in such an emergency is to administer blood from another person into the veins of the patient, a procedure called **transfusion.** Care must be taken in transferring blood from one person to another, however, because the patient's plasma may contain substances, called *antibodies* or *agglutinins*, that can cause the red cells of the donor's blood to rupture and release their hemoglobin. Such cells are said to be **hemolyzed** (HE-mo-lized), and the resulting condition can be dangerous.

Certain proteins, called **antigens** (AN-ti-jens) or *agglutinogens*, on the surface of the red cells cause these incompatibility reactions. There are many types of such proteins, but only two groups are particularly likely to cause a transfusion reaction, the so-called A and B antigens and the Rh factor.

The ABO Blood Type Group

There are four blood types involving the A and B antigens: A, B, AB, and O (Table 12-3). These letters indicate the type of antigen present on the red cells. If only the A antigen is present, the person has type A blood; if only the B antigen is present, he or she has type B blood. Type AB red cells have both antigens, and type O have neither. Of course no one has antibodies to his or her own blood type antigens, or their plasma would destroy their own cells. Each person does, however, develop antibodies that react with the AB antigens he or she is lacking. (The reason for the development of these antibodies is not totally understood, because people usually develop antibodies only when they have been exposed to an antigen.) It is these antibodies in the patient's plasma that can react with antigens on the donor's red cells to cause a transfusion reaction.

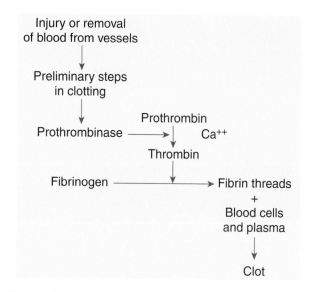

Figure 12-8 Final steps in blood clot formation. *ZOOMING IN ✦ What material in the blood forms a clot?*

Table 12·3 The ABO Blood Group System

BLOOD TYPE	RED BLOOD CELL ANTIGEN	REACTS WITH ANTISERUM	PLASMA ANTIBODIES	CAN TAKE FROM	CAN DONATE TO
A	A	Anti-A	Anti-B	A, O	A, AB
B	B	Anti-B	Anti-A	B, O	B, AB
AB	A, B	Anti-A, Anti-B	None	AB, A, B, O	AB
O	None	None	Anti-A, Anti-B	O	O, A, B, AB

Testing for Blood Type Blood sera containing antibodies to the A or B antigens are used to test for blood type. These antisera are prepared in animals using either the A or the B antigens to induce a response. Blood serum containing antibodies that can agglutinate and destroy red cells with A antigen is called **anti-A serum**; blood serum containing antibodies that can destroy red cells with B antigen is called **anti-B serum**. When combined with a blood sample in the laboratory, each antiserum causes the corresponding red cells to clump together in a process known as **agglutination** (ah-glu-tih-NA-shun). The blood's agglutination pattern when mixed *separately* with these two sera reveals its blood type (Fig. 12-9). Type A reacts with anti-A serum only; type B reacts with anti-B serum only. Type AB agglutinates with both, and type O agglutinates with neither A nor B.

A blood specimen from any person who has had a prior blood transfusion or a pregnancy is tested further for the presence of any less common antibodies. Both the red cells and the serum are tested separately for any possible cross-reactions with donor blood.

> **Checkpoint 12-12** What are the four ABO blood type groups?

Blood Compatibility Heredity determines a person's blood type, and the percentage of people with each of the different blood types varies in different populations. For example, about 45% of the white population of the United States have type O blood, 40% have A, 11% have B and only 4% have AB. The percentages vary within other population groups.

In an emergency, type O blood can be given to any ABO type because the cells lack both A and B antigens and will not react with either A or B antibodies (see Table 12-3). People with type O blood are called *universal donors*. Conversely, type AB blood contains no antibodies to agglutinate red cells, and people with this blood type can therefore receive blood from any ABO type donor. Those with AB blood are described as *universal recipients*. Whenever possible, it is safest to give the same blood type as the recipient's blood.

The Rh Factor

More than 85% of the United States' population has another red cell antigen group called the **Rh factor**, named for *Rhe-*

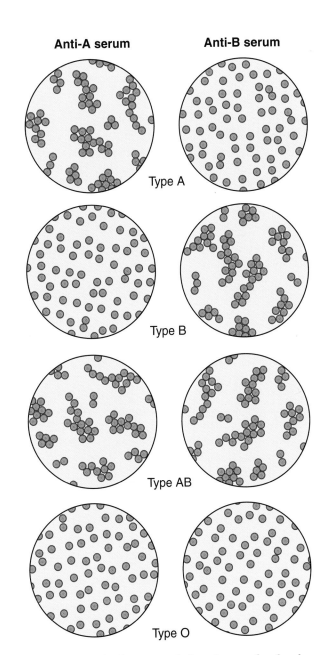

Anti-A serum　　　**Anti-B serum**

Type A

Type B

Type AB

Type O

Figure 12-9 Blood typing. Labels at the top of each column denote the kind of antiserum added to the blood samples. Anti-A serum agglutinates (causes to clump) red cells in type A blood, but anti-B serum does not. Anti-B serum agglutinates red cells in type B blood, but anti-A serum does not. Both sera agglutinate type AB blood cells, and neither serum agglutinates type O blood. *ZOOMING IN ✦ Can you tell from these reactions whether these cells are Rh positive or Rh negative?*

sus monkeys, in which it was first found. Rh is also known as the *D antigen*. People with this antigen are said to be **Rh positive**; those who lack this protein are said to be **Rh negative**. If Rh-positive blood is given to an Rh-negative person, he or she may produce antibodies to the "foreign" Rh antigens. The blood of this "Rh-sensitized" person will then destroy any Rh-positive cells received in a later transfusion.

Rh incompatibility is a potential problem in certain pregnancies. A mother who is Rh negative may develop antibodies to the Rh protein of an Rh-positive fetus (the fetus having inherited this factor from the father). Red cells from the fetus that enter the mother's circulation during pregnancy and childbirth evoke the response. In a subsequent pregnancy with an Rh-positive fetus, some of the anti-Rh antibodies may pass from the mother's blood into the blood of her fetus and destroy the fetus's red cells. This condition is called **hemolytic disease of the newborn** (HDN). An older name is *erythroblastosis fetalis*). HDN is now prevented by administration of immune globulin $Rh_o(D)$, trade name Rho-GAM, to the mother during pregnancy and shortly after delivery. These preformed antibodies clear the mother's circulation of Rh antigens and prevent stimulation of an immune response. In many cases, a baby born with HDN could be saved by a transfusion that replaces much of the baby's blood with Rh-negative blood.

> **Checkpoint 12-13** What are the blood antigens most often involved in incompatibility reactions?

▶ Uses of Blood and Blood Components

Blood can be packaged and kept in blood banks for emergencies. To keep the blood from clotting, a solution such as citrate-phosphate-dextrose-adenine (CPDA-1) is added. The blood may then be stored for up to 35 days. The blood supplies in the bank are dated with an expiration date to prevent the use of blood in which red cells may have disintegrated. Blood banks usually have all types of blood and blood products available. It is important that there be an extra supply of type O, Rh-negative blood because in an emergency this type can be used for any patient. It is normal procedure to test the recipient and give blood of the same type.

A person can donate his or her own blood before undergoing elective (planned) surgery to be used during surgery if needed. This practice eliminates the possibility of incompatibility and of disease transfer as well. Such **autologous** (aw-TOL-o-gus) (self-originating) blood is stored in a blood bank only until the surgery is completed.

Whole Blood Transfusions

The transfer of whole human blood from a healthy person to a patient is often a life-saving process. Whole blood

transfusions may be used for any condition in which there is loss of a large volume of blood, for example:

▶ In the treatment of massive hemorrhage from serious mechanical injuries.
▶ For blood loss during internal bleeding, as from bleeding ulcers.
▶ During or after an operation that causes considerable blood loss.
▶ For blood replacement in the treatment of hemolytic disease of the newborn.

Caution and careful evaluation of the need for a blood transfusion is the rule, however, because of the risk for transfusion reactions and the transmission of viral diseases, particularly hepatitis.

Use of Blood Components

Most often, when some blood ingredient is needed, it is not whole blood but a blood component that is given. Blood can be broken down into its various parts, which may be used for different purposes.

A common method for separating the blood plasma from the formed elements is by use of a **centrifuge** (SEN-trih-fuje), a machine that spins in a circle at high speed to separate components of a mixture according to density. When a container of blood is spun rapidly, all the formed elements of the blood are pulled into a clump at the bottom of the container. They are thus separated from the plasma, which is less dense. The formed elements may be further separated and used for specific purposes, for example, packed red cells alone or platelets alone.

Blood losses to the donor can be minimized by removal of the blood, separation of the desired components, and return of the remainder to the donor. The general term for this procedure is **hemapheresis** (hem-ah-fer-E-sis) (from the Greek word *apheresis* meaning "removal"). If the plasma is removed and the formed elements returned to the donor, the procedure is called **plasmapheresis** (plas-mah-fer-E-sis).

Use of Plasma Blood plasma alone may be given in an emergency to replace blood volume and prevent circulatory failure (shock). Plasma is especially useful when blood typing and the use of whole blood are not possible, such as in natural disasters or in emergency rescues. Because the red cells have been removed from the plasma, there are no incompatibility problems; plasma can be given to anyone. Plasma separated from the cellular elements is usually further separated by chemical means into various components, such as plasma protein fraction, serum albumin, immune serum, and clotting factors.

The packaged plasma that is currently available is actually plasma protein fraction. Further separation yields serum albumin that is available in solutions of 5% or 25% concentration. In addition to its use in treatment of circulatory shock, these solutions are given when plasma proteins are deficient. They increase the osmotic pressure of the blood and thus draw fluids back into circulation. The use of plasma proteins and serum albumin has increased because these blood components can be treated with heat to prevent transmission of viral diseases.

In emergency situations healthcare workers may administer fluids known as *plasma expanders*. These are cell-free isotonic solutions used to maintain blood fluid volume to prevent circulatory shock.

Fresh plasma may be frozen and saved. When frozen plasma is thawed, a white precipitate called **cryoprecipitate** (kri-o-pre-SIP-ih-tate) forms in the bottom of the container. Plasma frozen when it is less than 6 hours old contains all the factors needed for clotting. Cryoprecipitate is especially rich in clotting factor VIII and fibrinogen. These components may be given when there is a special need for these factors.

The gamma globulin fraction of the plasma contains antibodies produced by lymphocytes when they come in contact with foreign agents, such as bacteria and viruses. Antibodies play an important role in the immune system (see Chapter 15). Commercially prepared immune sera are available for administration to patients in immediate need of antibodies, such as infants born to mothers with active hepatitis.

> **Checkpoint 12-14** How is blood commonly separated into its component parts?

◗ Blood Studies

Many kinds of studies can be done on blood, and some of these have become a standard part of a routine physical examination. Machines that are able to perform several tests at the same time have largely replaced manual procedures, particularly in large institutions.

The Hematocrit

The **hematocrit** (he-MAT-o-krit), the volume percentage of red cells in whole blood, is determined by spinning a blood sample in a high-speed centrifuge for 3 to 5 minutes to separate the cellular elements from the plasma (Fig. 12-10).

The hematocrit is expressed as the volume of packed red cells per unit volume of whole blood. For example, "hematocrit, 38%" in a laboratory report means that the patient has 38 mL red cells per 100 mL (dL) of blood; red cells comprise 38% of the total blood volume. For adult men, the normal range is 42% to 54%, whereas for adult women the range is slightly lower, 36% to 46%. These normal ranges, like all normal ranges for humans, may vary depending on the method used and the interpretation of the results by an individual laboratory. Hematocrit values much below or much above these figures point to an abnormality requiring further study.

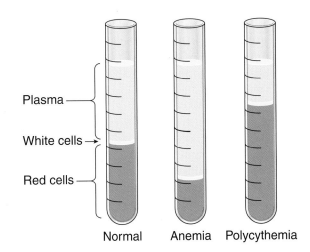

Figure 12-10 **Hematocrit.** The tube on the left shows a normal hematocrit. The middle tube shows that the percentage of red blood cells is low, indicating anemia. The tube on the right shows an excessively high percentage of red cells, as seen in polycythemia. (Reprinted with permission from Cohen BJ. Medical Terminology. 4th ed. Philadelphia: Lippincott Williams & Wilkins, 2004.)

Hemoglobin Tests

A sufficient amount of hemoglobin in red cells is required for adequate oxygen delivery to the tissues. To measure its level, the hemoglobin is released from the red cells, and the color of the blood is compared with a known color scale. Hemoglobin is expressed in grams per 100 mL whole blood. Normal hemoglobin concentrations for adult males range from 14 to 17 g per 100 mL blood. Values for adult women are in a somewhat lower range, at 12 to 15 g per 100 mL blood. A decrease in hemoglobin to below normal levels signifies anemia.

Normal and abnormal types of hemoglobin can be separated and measured by the process of **electrophoresis** (e-lek-tro-fo-RE-sis). In this procedure, an electric current is passed through the liquid that contains the hemoglobin to separate different components based on their electrical charge. This test is useful in the diagnosis of sickle cell anemia and other disorders caused by abnormal types of hemoglobin.

Blood Cell Counts

Most laboratories use automated methods for obtaining the data for blood counts. Visual counts are sometimes done using a **hemocytometer** (he-mo-si-TOM-eh-ter), a ruled slide used to count the cells in a given volume of blood under the microscope.

Red Cell Counts The normal red cell count varies from 4.5 million to 5.5 million cells per µL (mm³) of blood. An increase in the red cell count is called **polycythemia** (pol-e-si-THE-me-ah). A decrease in the red cell count is called **anemia**.

White Cell Counts The leukocyte count varies from 5000 to 10,000 cells per μL of blood. In **leukopenia**, the white count is below 5000 cells per mL. In **leukocytosis** (lu-ko-si-TO-sis), the white cell count exceeds 10,000 cells per mL.

Platelet Counts It is difficult to count platelets visually because they are so small. More accurate counts can be obtained with automated methods. These counts are necessary for the evaluation of platelet loss (thrombocytopenia) such as occurs after radiation therapy or cancer chemotherapy. The normal platelet count ranges from 150,000 to 450,000 per μL of blood, but counts may fall to 100,000 or less without causing serious bleeding problems. If a count is very low, a platelet transfusion may be given.

The Blood Slide (Smear)

In addition to the above tests, the **complete blood count** (CBC) includes the examination of a stained blood slide (see Fig. 12-2). In this procedure, a drop of blood is spread thinly and evenly over a glass slide, and a special stain (Wright) is applied to differentiate the otherwise colorless white cells. The slide is then studied under the microscope. The red cells are examined for abnormalities in size, color, or shape and for variations in the percentage of immature forms, known as reticulocytes (see Box 12-2 to learn about reticulocytes and how their counts are used to diagnose disease). The number of platelets is esti-

mated. Parasites, such as the malarial organism and others, may be found. In addition, a **differential white count** is done. This is an estimation of the percentage of each white cell type in the smear. Because each type has a specific function, changes in their proportions can be a valuable diagnostic aid (see Table 12-2).

> **Checkpoint 12-15** The hematocrit is a common blood test. What is a hematocrit?

Blood Chemistry Tests

Batteries of tests on blood serum are often done by machine. One machine, the Sequential Multiple Analyzer (SMA), can run some 20 tests per minute. Tests for electrolytes, such as sodium, potassium, chloride, and bicarbonate, may be performed at the same time along with tests for blood glucose, and nitrogenous waste products, such as blood urea nitrogen (BUN), and **creatinine** (kre-AT-in-in).

Other tests check for enzymes. Increased levels of **CPK** (creatine phosphokinase), **LDH** (lactic dehydrogenase), and other enzymes indicate tissue damage, such as damage that may occur in heart disease. An excess of **alkaline phosphatase** (FOS-fah-tase) could indicate a liver disorder or metastatic cancer involving bone.

Blood can be tested for amounts of lipids, such as cholesterol, triglycerides (fats), and lipoproteins, or for amounts of plasma proteins. Many of these tests help in

| Box 12-2 | Clinical Perspectives |

Counting Reticulocytes to Diagnose Disease

As erythrocytes mature in the red bone marrow, they go through a series of stages in which they lose their nucleus and most other organelles, maximizing the space available to hold hemoglobin. In one of the last stages of development, small numbers of ribosomes and some rough endoplasmic reticulum remain in the cell and appear as a network, or reticulum, when stained. Cells at this stage are called **reticulocytes**. Reticulocytes leave the red bone marrow and enter the bloodstream where they become fully mature erythrocytes in about 24 to 48 hours. The average number of red cells maturing through the reticulocyte stage at any given time is about 1%-2%. Changes in these numbers can be used in diagnosing certain blood disorders.

When erythrocytes are lost or destroyed, as from chronic bleeding or some form of hemolytic anemia, red blood cell production is "stepped up" to compensate for the loss. Greater numbers of reticulocytes are then released into the blood before reaching full maturity, and counts increase above normal. On the other hand, a decrease in the number of circulating reticulocytes suggests a problem with red blood cell production, as in cases of deficiency anemias or suppression of bone marrow activity.

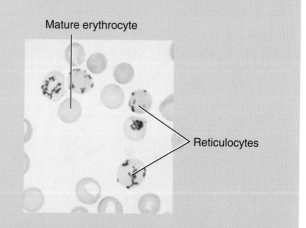

Reticulocytes. Some ribosomes and rough ER appear as a network in a late stage of erythrocyte development. (Reprinted with permission from Cormack DH. Essential Histology. 2nd ed. Philadelphia: Lippincott Williams & Wilkins, 2001.)

Bone Marrow Transplants: Getting the Gift of Life

Large doses of chemotherapy or radiation are sometimes used to destroy abnormal hematopoietic stem cells in the bone marrow of patients with leukemia. Unfortunately, these therapies also destroy normal stem cells in the marrow, hampering the production of new blood cells. A **bone marrow transplant** replaces the hematopoietic cells after aggressive treatment for leukemia. The procedure is also used to treat sickle cell anemia, aplastic anemia, and some immune diseases.

Most patients receive *allogeneic transplants*, stem cells harvested from the bone marrow of a close relative or occasionally from an unrelated donor. It is important that the donor marrow matches the recipient's marrow as closely as possible. For this reason, potential donors undergo blood tests to determine if their marrow antigens are compatible with the recipient's. A poorly matched transplant increases the risk of marrow rejection and graft-versus-host disease (GVHD), a life-threatening complication that occurs when immune cells from the transplanted marrow attack and destroy the patient's

organs. In certain circumstances, the patient's own bone marrow can be harvested, and replaced after treatment. This type of bone marrow transplant is called an *autologous transplant* and is not associated with tissue rejection or GVHD.

When bone marrow is to be harvested, the donor is given general or local anesthesia, a large needle is inserted into the pelvic bone, and the marrow is extracted. Then, it is filtered to remove bone fragments and unwanted blood cells, and either used immediately or stored frozen for later use. The recipient receives the bone marrow transplant intravenously. After entering the bloodstream, the transplanted hematopoietic stem cells travel to the bone marrow, where they begin to produce new blood cells. Complete recovery may take up to several months for an autologous transplant and one to two years for an allogeneic transplant. During this time, the patient is very susceptible to infectious diseases. Despite the risks, bone marrow transplants give patients with life-threatening blood diseases like leukemia a better chance of survival.

---

evaluating disorders that may involve various vital organs. For example, the presence of more than the normal amount of glucose (sugar) dissolved in the blood, a condition called **hyperglycemia** (hi-per-gli-SE-me-ah), is found most frequently in patients with unregulated diabetes. Sometimes, several sugar evaluations are done after the administration of a known amount of glucose. This procedure is called the **glucose tolerance test** and is usually given along with another test that determines the amount of sugar in the urine. This combination of tests can indicate faulty cell metabolism. The list of blood chemistry tests is extensive and is constantly increasing. We may now obtain values for various hormones, vitamins, antibodies, and toxic or therapeutic drug levels.

Coagulation Studies

Before surgery and during treatment of certain diseases, hemophilia for example, it is important to know that coagulation will take place within normal time limits. Because clotting is a complex process involving many reactants, a delay may result from a number of different causes, including lack of certain hormonelike substances, calcium salts, or vitamin K. The amounts of the various clotting factors are evaluated by percentage to aid in the diagnosis and treatment of bleeding disorders.

Additional tests for coagulation include tests for bleeding time, clotting time, capillary strength, and platelet function.

Bone Marrow Biopsy

A special needle is used to obtain a small sample of red marrow from the sternum, sacrum, or iliac crest in a procedure called a **bone marrow biopsy**. If marrow is taken from the sternum, the procedure may be referred to as a **sternal puncture**. Examination of the cells gives valuable information that can aid in the diagnosis of bone marrow disorders, including leukemia and certain kinds of anemia. See Box 12-3, Bone Marrow Transplants: Getting the Gift of Life, for information about the treatment of these disorders.

Word Anatomy

Medical terms are built from standardized word parts (prefixes, roots, and suffixes). Learning the meanings of these parts can help you remember words and interpret unfamiliar terms.

WORD PART	MEANING	EXAMPLE
Blood Constituents		
erythr/o	red, red blood cell	An *erythrocyte* is a red blood cell.
leuk/o	white, colorless	A *leukocyte* is a white blood cell.
thromb/o	blood clot	A *thrombocyte* is a cell fragment that is active in blood clotting.

hemat/o	blood	*Hematopoietic* stem cells form (-poiesis) all of the blood cells.
hemo	blood	*Hemoglobin* is a protein the carries oxygen in the blood.
morph/o	shape	The nuclei of *polymorphs* have many shapes.
lymph/o	lymph, lymphatic system	*Lymphocytes* are white blood cells that circulate in the lymphatic system.
mon/o	single, one	A *monocyte* has a single, unsegmented nucleus.
phag/o	eat, ingest	Certain leukocytes take in foreign matter by the process of *phagocytosis*.
macr/o	large	A *macrophage* takes in large amounts of foreign matter by phago-cytosis.
kary/o	nucleus	A *megakaryocyte* has a very large nucleus.

Hemostasis

-gen	producing, originating	*Fibrinogen* converts to fibrin in the formation of a blood clot.
pro-	before, in front of	Prothrombinase is an enzyme (-ase) that converts *prothrombin* to thrombin.

Blood Types

-lysis	loosening, dissolving, separating	A recipient's antibodies to donated red cells can cause *hemolysis* of the cells.

Uses of Blood and Blood Components

cry/o	cold	*Cryoprecipitate* forms when blood plasma is frozen and then thawed.

Summary

I. Functions of the blood
A. Transportation—of oxygen, carbon dioxide, nutrients, minerals, vitamins, hormones, waste
B. Regulation—of pH, fluid balance, body temperature
C. Protection—against foreign organisms, blood loss

II. Blood constituents
A. Plasma—liquid component
   1. Water—main ingredient
   2. Proteins—albumin, clotting factors, antibodies, complement
   3. Nutrients—carbohydrates, lipids, amino acids
   4. Electrolytes (minerals)
   5. Waste products
   6. Gases—oxygen and carbon dioxide
   7. Hormones and other materials
B. The formed elements—produced in red bone marrow from hematopoietic stem cells
   1. Erythrocytes (red cells)—carry oxygen bound to hemoglobin
   2. Leukocytes (white cells)—destroy invading organisms and remove waste
      a. Granulocytes—neutrophils (polymorphs, segs, PMNs), eosinophils, basophils
      b. Agranulocytes—lymphocytes, monocytes
   3. Platelets (thrombocytes)
      a. Fragments of megakaryocytes
      b. Participate in blood clotting

III. Hemostasis—prevention of blood loss
   1. Contraction of blood vessels
   2. Formation of platelet plug
   3. Formation of blood clot
A. Blood clotting
   1. Regulators
      a. Procoagulants—promote clotting
      b. Anticoagulants—prevent clotting
   2. 12 clotting factors
   3. Final steps in blood clotting
      a. Prothrombinase converts prothrombin to thrombin
      b. Thrombin converts fibrinogen to solid threads of fibrin
      c. Threads form clot
   4. Serum—fluid that remains after blood has clotted

IV. Blood types
A. ABO blood type group—types A, B, AB, and O
   1. Tested by mixing blood sample with antisera to different antigens
   2. Incompatible transfusions cause destruction of donor red cells
B. Rh factor—positive or negative

V. Uses of blood and blood components
   1. Blood banks—store blood
      a. Autologous blood—donated for a person's own use

A. Whole blood transfusions—used only to replace large blood losses
B. Use of blood components—formed elements separated by centrifugation
   1. Use of plasma
      a. Protein fractions
      b. Cryoprecipitate—obtained by freezing; contains clotting factors
      c. Gamma globulin—contains antibodies

B. Hemoglobin tests—color test, electrophoresis
C. Blood cell counts
D. Blood slide (smear)
E. Blood chemistry tests—electrolytes, waste products, enzymes, glucose, hormones
F. Coagulation studies—clotting factor assays, bleeding time, clotting time, capillary strength, platelet function
G. Bone marrow biopsy

VI. Blood studies

A. Hematocrit—measures percentage of packed red cells in whole blood

Questions for Study and Review

Building Understanding

Fill in the blanks

1. The liquid portion of blood is called _____.
2. The ancestors of all blood cells are called _____cells.
3. Platelets are produced by certain giant cells called _____.

4. Some monocytes enter the tissues and mature into phagocytic cells called _____.
5. Erythrocytes have a lifespan of approximately _____ days.

Matching

Match each numbered item with the most closely related lettered item.

____ 6. an increased erythrocyte count
____ 7. a decreased erythrocyte count
____ 8. an increased leukocyte count
____ 9. a decreased leukocyte count
____ 10. a decreased platelet count

a. thrombocytopenia
b. anemia
c. leukopenia
d. leukocytosis
e. polycythemia

Multiple choice

____ 11. Red blood cells transport oxygen that is bound to
   a. erythropoietin
   b. complement
   c. hemoglobin
   d. thrombin
____ 12. All of the following are granulocytes except
   a. lymphocytes
   b. neutrophils
   c. eosinophils
   d. basophils
____ 13. Antibodies are produced by
   a. erythrocytes
   b. macrophages
   c. plasma cells
   d. band cells
____ 14. The correct sequence of hemostatic events is
   a. vessel contraction, plug formation, and blood clot
   b. blood clot, plug formation, vessel contraction

   c. plug formation, blood clot, vessel contraction
   d. vessel contraction, blood clot, plug formation
____ 15. If one wanted to measure the number of eosinophils in a blood sample, he or she would conduct the following test:
   a. hematocrit
   b. electrophoresis
   c. complete blood cell count
   d. differential white blood cell count

Understanding Concepts

16. List the three main functions of blood. What is the average volume of circulating blood in the body?
17. Compare and contrast the following:
   a. formed elements and plasma
   b. erythrocyte and leukocyte
   c. hemorrhage and transfusion
   d. hemapheresis and plasmapheresis

18. List four main types of proteins in blood plasma and state their functions. What are some other substances carried in blood plasma?

19. Describe the structure and function of erythrocytes. State the normal blood cell count for erythrocytes.

20. Construct a chart that compares the structure and function of the five types of leukocytes. State the normal blood cell count for leukocytes

21. Diagram the three final steps in blood clot formation.

22. Name the four blood types in the ABO system. What antigens and antibodies (if any) are found in each type?

Conceptual Thinking

23. J. Regan, a 40-year-old firefighter, has just had his annual physical. He is in excellent health, except for his red blood cell count, which is elevated. How might Mr. Regan's job explain his test results?

24. Nikki has type A blood. Why can she receive a transfusion of type A or type O blood, but not a transfusion of type B or type AB blood?

SELECTED KEY TERMS

The following terms and other boldface terms in the chapter are defined in the Glossary

atrium

coronary

diastole

echocardiograph

electrocardiography

endocardium

epicardium

murmur

myocardium

pacemaker

pericardium

septum

systole

valve

ventricle

LEARNING OUTCOMES

After careful study of this chapter,
you should be able to:

1. Describe the three layers of the heart wall
2. Describe the structure of the pericardium and cite its functions
3. Compare the functions of the right and left sides of the heart
4. Name the four chambers of the heart and compare their functions
5. Name the valves at the entrance and exit of each ventricle and cite the function of the valves
6. Briefly describe blood circulation through the myocardium
7. Briefly describe the cardiac cycle
8. Name and locate the components of the heart's conduction system
9. Explain the effects of the autonomic nervous system on the heart rate
10. List and define several terms that describe variations in heart rates
11. Explain what produces the two main heart sounds
12. Briefly describe four methods for studying the heart
13. Show how word parts are used to build words related to the heart (see Word Anatomy at the end of the chapter)

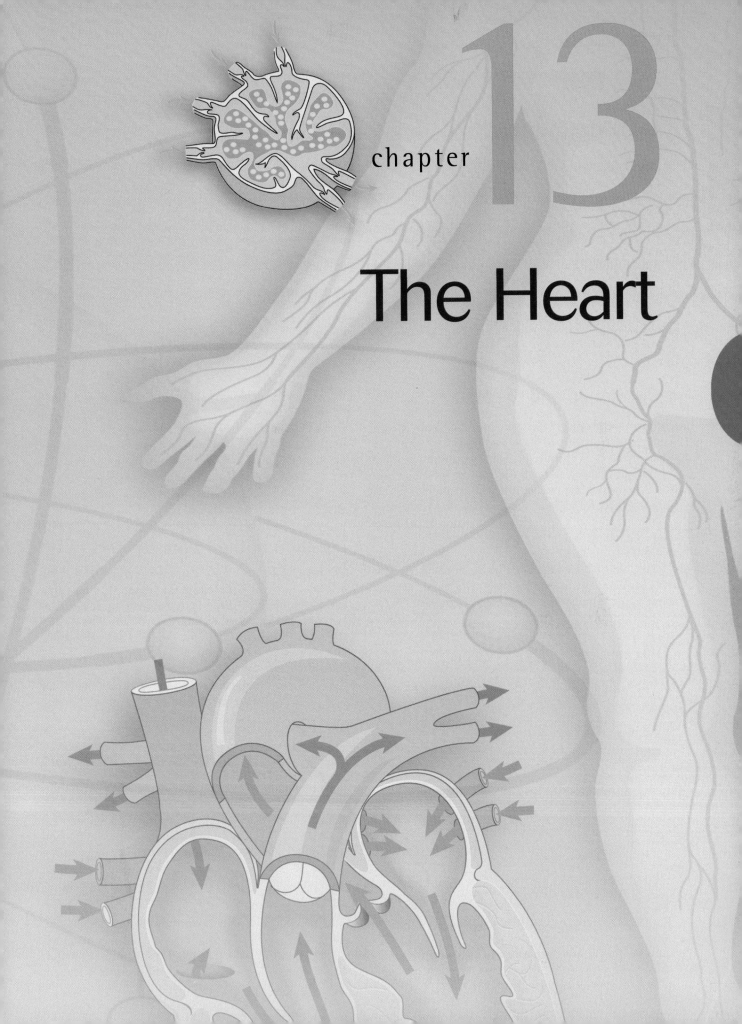

The Heart

| Box 13-1 | Hot Topics |

Artificial Hearts: Saving Lives With Technology

More than 2000 Americans receive a heart transplant each year. Because, unfortunately, the number of individuals waiting to receive a transplant far exceeds the number of donor hearts available, researchers are inventing alternate technologies.

The ventricular assist device (VAD) is a mechanical pump that helps a patient's damaged heart to pump blood. The device is surgically implanted into a patient's chest or abdomen and connected to either the left or right ventricle. Powered by an external battery connected to it by a thin wire, the VAD pulls blood from the ventricle and pumps it to the aorta (in the case of a left VAD) or the pulmonary artery (in the case of a right VAD). These devices were first designed to help a patient survive until a suitable donor heart could be found, but a permanent model has recently been approved for use in the United States.

More than thirty years ago, researchers began experimenting with total artificial hearts, which are designed to completely replace a patient's damaged heart. The best known of these pumps is the Jarvik-7, an air-driven pump that required tubes and wires to remain connected through the skin to a large external unit. Unfortunately, all of the patients who received this device died of complications shortly after surgery and testing was discontinued. Today, researchers are experimenting with a new completely self-contained artificial heart that uses a wireless rechargeable external battery. A computer implanted in the abdomen closely monitors and controls the heart's pumping speed. If the experiments are successful, total artificial hearts may become a real alternative for patients who would otherwise die waiting for a heart transplant.

▶ Circulation and the Heart

The next two chapters investigate how the blood delivers oxygen and nutrients to the cells and carries away the waste products of cell metabolism. The continuous one-way circuit of blood through the body in the blood vessels is known as the **circulation**. The prime mover that propels blood throughout the body is the **heart**. This chapter examines the structure and function of the heart to lay the foundation for the detailed discussion of blood vessels that follows.

The importance of the heart has been recognized for centuries. Strokes (the contractions) of this pump average about 72 per minute and are carried on unceasingly for the whole of a lifetime. The beating of the heart is affected by the emotions, which may explain the frequent references to it in song and poetry. However, the vital functions of the heart are of more practical concern. Failure of the heart to pump sufficient quantities of blood throughout the body may have life-threatening consequences (see Box 13-1, Artificial Hearts: Saving Lives With Technology).

Location of the Heart

The heart is slightly bigger than a person's fist. This organ is located between the lungs in the center and a bit to the left of the midline of the body (Fig. 13-1). It occupies most of the mediastinum, the central region of the thorax. The heart's **apex**, the pointed, inferior portion, is directed toward the left. The broad, superior **base** is the area of attachment for the large vessels carrying blood into and out of the heart.

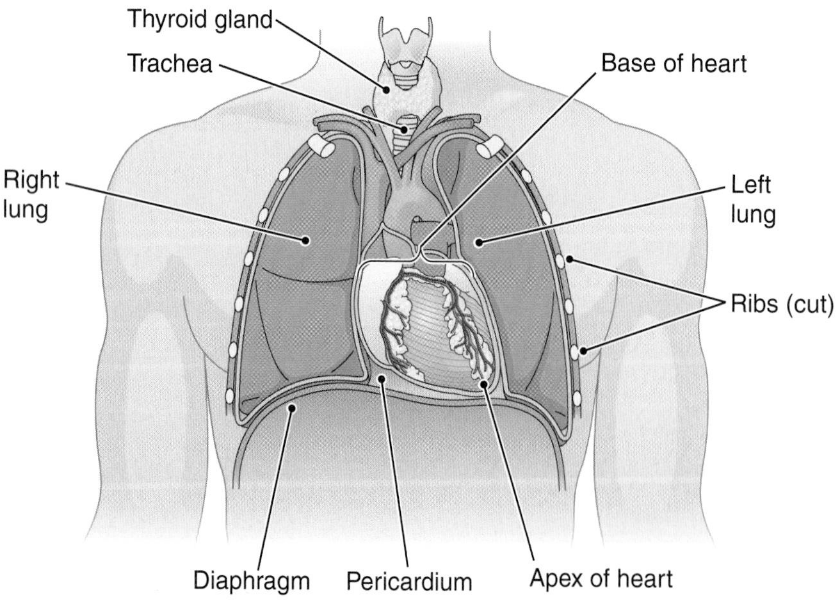

▶ Structure of the Heart

The heart is a hollow organ, with walls formed of three different layers. Just as a warm coat might have a smooth lining, a thick and bulky interlining, and an outer layer of a third fabric, so the heart wall has three tissue layers (Fig. 13-2, Table 13-1). Starting with the innermost layer, these are as follows:

▶ The **endocardium** (en-do-KAR-de-um) is a thin, smooth layer of epithelial cells that lines the heart's interior. The endocardium provides a smooth

Figure 13-1   **The heart in position in the thorax (anterior view).**   *ZOOMING IN*
✦ *Why is the left lung smaller than the right lung?*

Table 13·1 Layers of the Heart Wall

LAYER	LOCATION	DESCRIPTION	FUNCTION
Endocardium	Innermost layer of the heart wall	Thin, smooth layer of epithelial cells	Lines the interior of the chambers and covers the heart valves
Myocardium	Middle layer of the heart wall	Thick layer of cardiac muscle	Contracts to pump blood into the arteries
Epicardium	Outermost layer of the heart wall	Thin serous membrane	Covers the heart and forms the visceral layer of the serous pericardium

surface for easy flow as blood travels through the heart. Extensions of this membrane cover the flaps (cusps) of the heart valves.

▶ The **myocardium** (mi-o-KAR-de-um), the heart muscle, is the thickest layer and pumps blood through the vessels. Cardiac muscle's unique structure is described in more detail next.

▶ The **epicardium** (ep-ih-KAR-de-um) is a serous membrane that forms the thin, outermost layer of the heart wall.

The Pericardium

The **pericardium** (per-ih-KAR-de-um) is the sac that encloses the heart (Fig. 13-2, Table 13-2). The formation of the pericardial sac was described and illustrated in Chapter 4 under a discussion of membranes (see Fig. 4-9). The outermost and heaviest layer of this sac is the fibrous pericardium. Connective tissue anchors this pericardial layer to the diaphragm, located inferiorly; the sternum, located anteriorly; and to other structures surrounding the heart, thus holding the heart in place. A serous membrane lines this fibrous sac and folds back at the base to cover the heart's surface. Anatomically, the outer layer of this serous membrane is called the parietal layer, and the inner layer is the visceral layer, also known as the epicardium, as previously noted. A thin film of fluid between these two layers reduces friction as the heart moves within the pericardium. Normally the visceral and parietal layers are very close together, but fluid may accumulate in the region between them, the pericardial cavity, under certain disease conditions.

Checkpoint 13-1 What are the names of the innermost, middle, and outermost layers of the heart?

Checkpoint 13-2 What is the name of the sac that encloses the heart?

Special Features of the Myocardium

Cardiac muscle cells are lightly striated (striped) based on alternating actin and myosin filaments, as seen in skeletal muscle cells (see Chapter 7). Unlike skeletal muscle cells, however, cardiac muscle cells have a single nucleus instead of multiple nuclei. Also, cardiac muscle tissue is involuntarily controlled. There are specialized partitions between cardiac muscle cells that show faintly under a

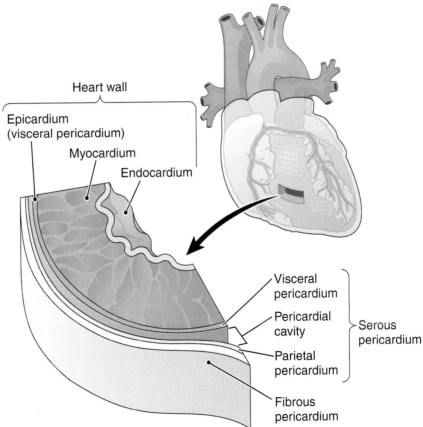

Figure 13-2 **Layers of the heart wall and pericardium.** The serous pericardium covers the heart and lines the fibrous pericardium. *ZOOMING IN ✦ Which layer of the heart wall is the thickest?*

Table 13·2	Layers of the Pericardium		
LAYER	**LOCATION**	**DESCRIPTION**	**FUNCTION**
Fibrous pericardium	Outermost layer	Fibrous sac	Encloses and protects the heart; anchors heart to surrounding structures
Serous pericardium	Between the fibrous pericardium and the myocardium	Doubled membranous sac with fluid between layers	Fluid reduces friction within the pericardium as the heart functions
Parietal layer	Lines the fibrous pericardium	Serous membrane	Forms the outer layer of the serous pericardium
Visceral layer	Surface of the heart	Serous membrane	Forms the inner layer of the serous pericardium; also called the epicardium

microscope (Fig. 13-3). These **intercalated** (in-TER-cah-la-ted) **disks** are actually modified plasma membranes that firmly attach adjacent cells to each other but allow for rapid transfer of electrical impulses between them. The adjective *intercalated* is from Latin and means "inserted between."

Another feature of cardiac muscle tissue is the branching of the muscle fibers (cells). These fibers are interwoven so that the stimulation that causes the contraction of one fiber results in the contraction of a whole group. The intercalated disks and the branching cellular networks allow cardiac muscle cells to contract in a coordinated manner.

Divisions of the Heart

Healthcare professionals often refer to the *right heart* and the *left heart,* because the human heart is really a double pump (Fig. 13-4). The right side pumps blood low in oxygen to the lungs through the **pulmonary circuit.** The left side pumps oxygenated blood to the remainder of the body through the **systemic circuit.** Each side of the heart is divided into two chambers.

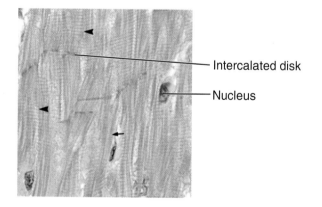
Intercalated disk
Nucleus

Figure 13-3 Cardiac muscle tissue viewed under the microscope (×540). The sample shows light striations (arrowheads), intercalated disks, and branching fibers (arrow). (Reprinted with permission from Gartner LP, Hiatt JL. Color Atlas of Histology. 3ʳᵈ ed. Philadelphia: Lippincott Williams & Wilkins, 2000.)

Four Chambers The upper chambers on the right and left sides, the **atria** (A-tre-ah), are mainly blood-receiving chambers (Fig. 13-5, Table 13-3). The lower chambers on the right and left side, the **ventricles** (VEN-trih-klz) are forceful pumps. The chambers, listed in the order in which blood flows through them, are as follows:

1. The **right atrium** (A-tre-um) is a thin-walled chamber that receives the blood returning from the body tissues. This blood, which is low in oxygen, is carried in veins, the blood vessels leading back to the heart from the body tissues. The superior vena cava brings blood from the head, chest, and arms; the inferior vena cava delivers blood from the trunk and legs. A third vessel that opens into the right atrium brings blood from the heart muscle itself, as described later in this chapter.
2. The **right ventricle** pumps the venous blood received from the right atrium to the lungs. It pumps into a large pulmonary trunk, which then divides into right and left pulmonary arteries, which branch to the lungs. An artery is a vessel that takes blood from the heart to the tissues. Note that the pulmonary arteries in Figure 13-5 are colored blue because they are carrying deoxygenated blood, unlike other arteries, which carry oxygenated blood.
3. The **left atrium** receives blood high in oxygen content as it returns from the lungs in pulmonary veins. Note that the pulmonary veins in Figure 13-5 are colored red because they are carrying oxygenated blood, unlike other veins, which carry deoxygenated blood.
4. The **left ventricle,** which is the chamber with the thickest wall, pumps oxygenated blood to all parts of the body. This blood goes first into the aorta (a-OR-tah), the largest artery, and then into the branching systemic arteries that take blood to the tissues. The heart's apex, the lower pointed region, is formed by the wall of the left ventricle (see Fig. 13-2).

The heart's chambers are completely separated from each other by partitions, each of which is called a **septum.** The **interatrial** (in-ter-A-tre-al) **septum** separates the two atria, and the **interventricular** (in-ter-ven-TRIK-u-lar) **septum** separates the two ventricles. The septa, like the heart wall, consist largely of myocardium.

> **Checkpoint 13-3** The heart is divided into four chambers. What is the upper receiving chamber on each side called? What is the lower pumping chamber called?

Four Valves One-way valves that direct blood flow through the heart are located at the entrance and exit of each ventricle (Fig. 13-6, Table 13-4). The entrance valves are the **atrioventricular** (a-tre-o-ven-TRIK-u-lar) (**AV**) **valves**, so named because they are between the atria and ventricles. The exit valves are the **semilunar** (sem-e-LU-nar) **valves**, so named because each flap of these valves resembles a half-moon. Each valve has a specific name, as follows:

▶ The **right atrioventricular (AV) valve** is also known as the **tricuspid** (tri-KUS-pid) **valve** because it has three cusps, or flaps, that open and close. When this valve is open, blood flows freely from the right atrium into the right ventricle. When the right ventricle begins to contract, however, the valve is closed by blood squeezed backward against the cusps. With the valve closed, blood cannot return to the right atrium but must flow forward into the pulmonary arterial trunk.

▶ The **left atrioventricular** (*AV*) valve is the bicuspid valve, but it is commonly referred to as the **mitral** (MI-tral) **valve** (named for a miter, the pointed, two-sided hat worn by bishops). It has two heavy cusps that permit blood to flow freely from the left atrium into the left ventricle. The cusps close when the left ventricle begins to contract; this closure prevents blood from returning to the left atrium and ensures the forward flow of blood into the aorta. Both the right and left AV valves are attached by means of thin fibrous threads to muscles in the walls of the ventricles. The function of these threads, called the **chordae** tendineae (KOR-de ten-DIN-e-e) (see Fig. 13-6), is to stabilize the valve flaps when the ventricles contract so that the force of the blood will not push them up into the atria. In this man-

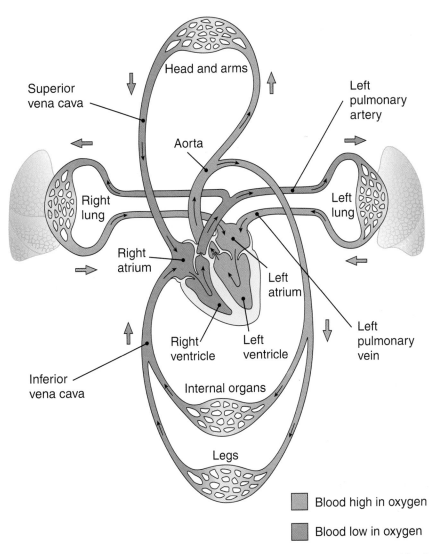

Figure 13-4   The heart as a double pump. The right side of the heart pumps blood through the pulmonary circuit to the lungs to be oxygenated; the left side of the heart pumps blood through the systemic circuit to all other parts of the body. *ZOOMING IN ✦ What vessel carries blood into the systemic circuit?*

ner, they help to prevent a backflow of blood when the heart beats.

▶ The **pulmonary** (PUL-mon-ar-e) **valve**, also called the *pulmonic valve*, is a semilunar valve located between the right ventricle and the pulmonary trunk that leads to the lungs. As soon as the right ventricle begins to relax from a contraction, pressure in that chamber drops. The higher pressure in the pulmonary artery, described as *back pressure*, closes the valve and prevents blood from returning to the ventricle.

▶ The **aortic** (a-OR-tik) **valve** is a semilunar valve located between the left ventricle and the aorta. After contraction of the left ventricle, back pressure closes the aortic valve and prevents the back flow of blood from the aorta into the ventricle.

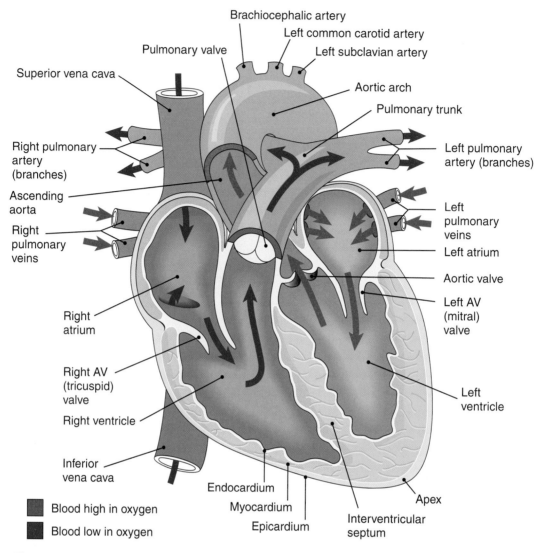

Figure 13-5 **The heart and great vessels.** *ZOOMING IN* ✦ *Which heart chamber has the thickest wall?*

Figure 13-7 traces a drop of blood as it completes a full circuit through the heart's chambers. Note that blood passes through the heart twice in making a trip from the heart's right side through the pulmonary circuit to the lungs and back to the heart's left side to start on its way through the systemic circuit. Although Figure 13-7 follows the path of a single drop of blood in sequence through the heart, the heart's two sides function in unison to pump blood through both circuits at the same time.

Checkpoint 13-4 What is the purpose of valves in the heart?

Table 13·3	Chambers of the Heart	
CHAMBER	**LOCATION**	**FUNCTION**
Right atrium	Upper right chamber	Receives blood from the vena cavae and the coronary sinus; pumps blood into the right ventricle
Right ventricle	Lower right chamber	Receives blood from the right atrium and pumps blood into the pulmonary artery, which carries blood to the lungs to be oxygenated
Left atrium	Upper left chamber	Receives oxygenated blood coming back to the heart from the lungs in the pulmonary veins; pumps blood into the left ventricle
Left ventricle	Lower left chamber	Receives blood from the left atrium and pumps blood into the aorta to be carried to tissues in the systemic circuit

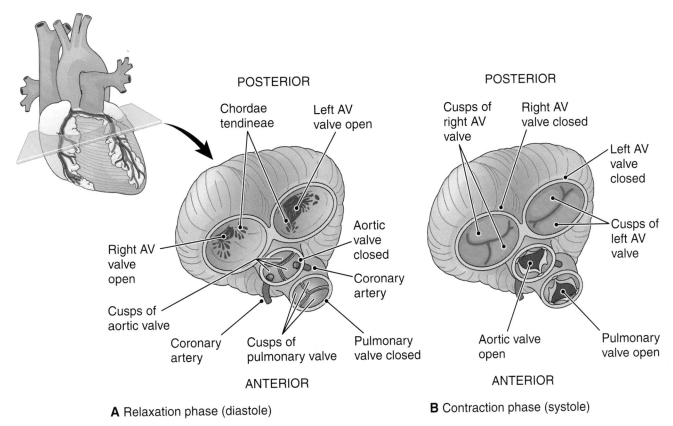

POSTERIOR

Chordae tendineae

Left AV valve open

Aortic valve closed

Right AV valve open

Coronary artery

Cusps of aortic valve

Coronary artery

Cusps of pulmonary valve

Pulmonary valve closed

A Relaxation phase (diastole)

ANTERIOR

POSTERIOR

Cusps of right AV valve

Right AV valve closed

Left AV valve closed

Cusps of left AV valve

Aortic valve open

Pulmonary valve open

B Contraction phase (systole)

ANTERIOR

Figure 13-6   Valves of the heart (superior view from anterior, atria removed). (A) When the heart is relaxed (diastole), the AV valves are open and blood flows freely from the atria to the ventricles. The pulmonary and aortic valves are closed. **(B)** When the ventricles contract, the AV valves close and blood pumped out of the ventricles opens the pulmonary and aortic valves.   *ZOOMING IN* ✦ *How many cusps does the right AV valve have? The left?*

Blood Supply to the Myocardium

Only the endocardium comes into contact with the blood that flows through the heart chambers. Therefore, the myocardium must have its own blood vessels to provide oxygen and nourishment and to remove waste products. Together, these blood vessels provide the **coronary** (KOR-o-na-re) **circulation**. The main arteries that supply blood to the muscle of the heart are the right and left coronary arteries (Fig. 13-8), named because they encircle the heart like a crown. These arteries, which are the first to branch off the aorta, arise just above the cusps of the aortic valve and branch to all regions of the heart muscle. They receive blood when the heart relaxes be-

Table 13·4	Valves of the Heart		
VALVE	**LOCATION**	**DESCRIPTION**	**FUNCTION**
Right AV valve	Between the right atrium and right ventricle	Valve with three cusps; tricuspid valve	Prevents blood from flowing back up into the right atrium when the right ventricle contracts (systole)
Left AV valve	Between the left atrium and left ventricle	Valve with two cusps; bicuspid or mitral valve	Prevents blood from flowing back up into the left atrium when the left ventricle contracts (systole)
Pulmonary semi-lunar valve	At the entrance to the pulmonary artery	Valve with three half-moon shaped cusps	Prevents blood from flowing back into the right ventricle when the right ventricle relaxes (diastole)
Aortic semilunar valve	At the entrance to the aorta	Valve with three half-moon shaped cusps	Prevents blood from flowing back into the left ventricle when the left ventricle relaxes (diastole)

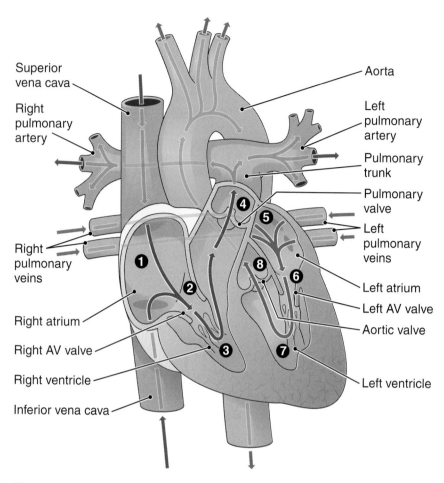

Figure 13-7 Pathway of blood through the heart. Blood from the systemic circuit enters the right atrium (1) through the superior and inferior venae cavae, flows through the right AV (tricuspid) valve (2), and enters the right ventricle (3). The right ventricle pumps the blood through the pulmonary (semilunar) valve (4) into the pulmonary trunk, which divides to carry blood to the lungs in the pulmonary circuit. Blood returns from the lungs in the pulmonary veins, enters the left atrium (5), and flows through the left AV (mitral) valve (6) into the left ventricle (7). The left ventricle pumps the blood through the aortic (semilunar) valve (8) into the aorta, which carries blood into the systemic circuit.

the thin-walled upper chambers, the atria, and is followed by a contraction of the thick muscle of the lower chambers, the ventricles. This active phase is called **systole** (SIS-to-le), and in each case, it is followed by a resting period known as **diastole** (di-AS-to-le). One complete sequence of heart contraction and relaxation is called the **cardiac cycle** (Fig. 13-10). Each cardiac cycle represents a single heart-beat. At rest, one cycle takes an average of 0.8 seconds.

The contraction phase of the cardiac cycle begins with contraction of both atria, which forces blood through the AV valves into the ventricles. The atrial walls are thin, and their contractions are not very powerful. However, they do improve the heart's efficiency by forcing blood into the ventricles before these lower chambers contract. Atrial contraction is completed at the time ventricular contraction begins. Thus, a resting phase (diastole) begins in the atria at the same time that a contraction (systole) begins in the ventricles.

After the ventricles have contracted, all chambers are relaxed for a short period as they fill with blood. Then another cycle begins with an atrial contraction followed by a ventricular contraction. Although both upper and lower chambers have a systolic and diastolic phase in each cardiac cycle, discussions of heart function usually refer to these phases as they occur in the ventricles, because these chambers contract more forcefully and drive blood into the arteries.

cause the aortic valve must be closed to expose the entrance to these vessels (Fig. 13-9). After passing through capillaries in the myocardium, blood drains into a system of cardiac veins that brings blood back toward the right atrium. Blood finally collects in the **coronary sinus**, a dilated vein that opens into the right atrium near the inferior vena cava (see Fig. 13-8).

Checkpoint 13-5 The myocardium must have its own vascular system to supply it with blood. What name is given to this blood supply to the myocardium?

▶ Function of the Heart

Although the heart's right and left sides are separated from each other, they work together. Blood is squeezed through the chambers by a heart muscle contraction that begins in

Cardiac Output

A unique property of heart muscle is its ability to adjust the strength of contraction to the amount of blood received. When the heart chamber is filled and the wall stretched (within limits), the contraction is strong. As less blood enters the heart, contractions become less forceful. Thus, as more blood enters the heart, as occurs during exercise, the muscle contracts with greater strength to push the larger volume of blood out into the blood vessels (see Box 13-2, Cardiac Reserve).

The volume of blood pumped by each ventricle in 1 minute is termed the **cardiac output** (CO). It is the prod-

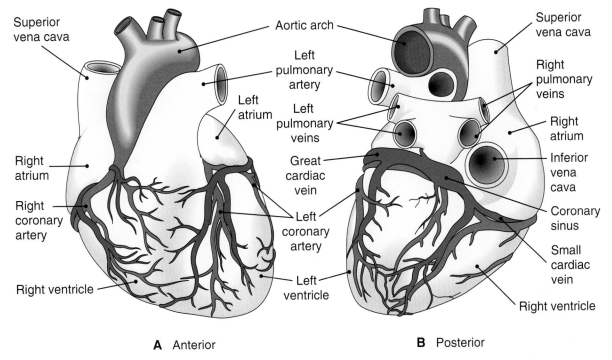

Figure 13-8 **Blood vessels that supply the myocardium.** Coronary arteries and cardiac veins are shown. **(A)** Anterior view. **(B)** Posterior view.

uct of the **stroke volume** (SV)—the volume of blood ejected from the ventricle with each beat—and the **heart rate** (HR)—the number of times the heart beats per minute. To summarize:

$$CO = HR \times SV$$

Checkpoint 13-6 The cardiac cycle consists of an alternating pattern of contraction and relaxation. What name is given to the contraction phase? To the relaxation phase?

Checkpoint 13-7 Cardiac output is the amount of blood pumped by each ventricle in 1 minute. What two factors determine cardiac output?

The Heart's Conduction System

Like other muscles, the heart muscle is stimulated to contract by a wave of electrical energy that passes along the cells. This action potential is generated by specialized tissue within the

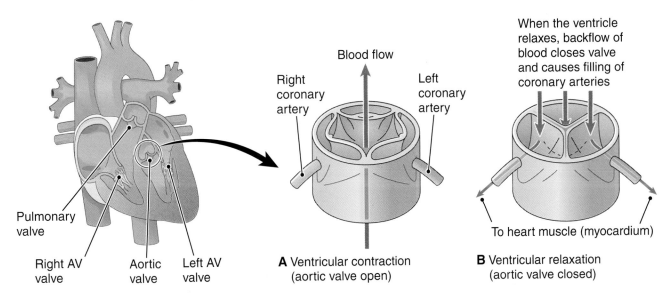

Figure 13-9 **Opening of coronary arteries in the aortic valve (anterior view). (A)** When the left ventricle contracts, the aortic valve opens. The valve cusps prevent filling of the coronary arteries. **(B)** When the left ventricle relaxes, backflow of blood closes the aortic valve and the coronary arteries fill. (Modified with permission from Moore KL, Dalley AF. Clinically Oriented Anatomy. 4th ed. Baltimore: Lippincott Williams & Wilkins, 1999.)

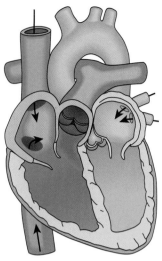

Diastole
Atria fill with blood, which begins to flow into ventricles as soon as their walls relax.

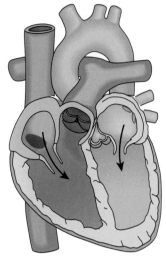

Atrial systole
Contraction of atria pumps blood into the ventricles.

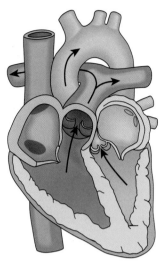

Ventricular systole
Contraction of ventricles pumps blood into aorta and pulmonary arteries.

Figure 13-10 **The cardiac cycle.** *ZOOMING IN ✦ When the ventricles contract, what valves close? What valves open?*

heart and spreads over structures that form the heart's conduction system (Fig. 13-11). Two of these structures are tissue masses called **nodes**, and the remainder consists of specialized fibers that branch through the myocardium.

The **sinoatrial (SA) node** is located in the upper wall of the right atrium in a small depression described as a sinus. This node initiates the heartbeats by generating an action potential at regular intervals. Because the SA node sets the rate of heart contractions, it is commonly called the **pacemaker**. The second node, located in the interatrial septum at the bottom of the right atrium, is called the **atrioventricular (AV) node**.

The **atrioventricular bundle**, also known as the **bundle of His**, is located at the top of the interventricular septum. It has branches that extend to all parts of the ventricular walls. Fibers travel first down both sides of the interventricular septum in groups called the right and left bundle branches. Smaller **Purkinje** (pur-KIN-je) **fibers**, also called *conduction myofibers*, then travel in a branching network throughout the myocardium of the ventricles. Intercalated disks allow the rapid flow of impulses throughout the heart muscle.

The Conduction Pathway The order in which impulses travel through the heart is as follows:

1. The sinoatrial node generates the electrical impulse that begins the heartbeat (see Fig. 13-11).
2. The excitation wave travels throughout the muscle of each atrium, causing the atria to contract. At the same time, impulses also travel directly to the AV node by means of fibers in the wall of the atrium that make up the **internodal pathways**.

Box 13-2 **A Closer Look**

Cardiac Reserve: Extra Output When Needed

Like many other organs, the heart has great reserves of strength. The cardiac reserve is a measure of how many times more than average the heart can produce when needed. Based on a heart rate of 75 beats/minute and a stroke volume of 70 ml/beat, the average cardiac output for an adult at rest is about 5 L/minute. This means that at rest, the heart pumps the equivalent of the total blood volume each minute.

During mild exercise, this volume might double and even double again during strenuous exercise. For most people the cardiac reserve is 4 to 5 times the resting output. This increase in cardiac output is achieved by an increase in either stroke volume, heart rate, or both. In athletes exercising vigorously, the ratio may reach 6 to 7 times the resting output. In contrast, those with heart disease may have little or no cardiac reserve. They may be fine at rest but quickly become short of breath or fatigued when exercising or even when carrying out the simple tasks of daily living.

Cardiac reserve can be measured using an exercise stress test that measures cardiac output while the patient walks on a treadmill or pedals an exercise bicycle. The exercise becomes more and more strenuous until the patient's peak cardiac output (cardiac reserve) is reached.

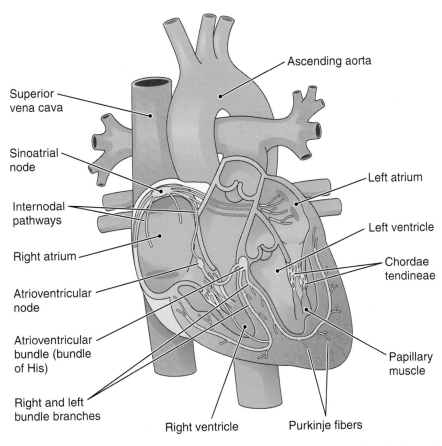

Figure 13-11 **Conduction system of the heart.** The sinoatrial (SA) node, the atrioventricular (AV) node, and specialized fibers conduct the electrical energy that stimulates the heart muscle to contract. *ZOOMING IN ✦ What parts of the conduction system do the internodal pathways connect?*

3. The atrioventricular node is stimulated. A relatively slower rate of conduction through the AV node allows time for the atria to contract and complete the filling of the ventricles before the ventricles contract.

4. The excitation wave travels rapidly through the bundle of His and then throughout the ventricular walls by means of the bundle branches and Purkinje fibers. The entire ventricular musculature contracts almost at the same time.

A normal heart rhythm originating at the SA node is termed a **sinus rhythm**. As a safety measure, a region of the conduction system other than the sinoatrial node can generate a heartbeat if the sinoatrial node fails, but it does so at a slower rate.

Checkpoint 13-8 The heartbeat is started by a small mass of tissue in the upper right atrium. This structure is commonly called the pacemaker, but what is its scientific name?

Control of the Heart Rate

Although the heart's fundamental beat originates within the heart itself, the heart rate can be influenced by the nervous system, hormones and other factors in the internal environment.

The autonomic nervous system (ANS) plays a major role in modifying the heart rate according to need (Fig. 13-12). Sympathetic nervous system stimulation increases the heart rate. During a fight-or-flight response, the sympathetic nerves can boost the cardiac output two to three times the resting value. Sympathetic fibers increase the contraction rate by stimulating the SA and AV nodes. They also increase the contraction force by acting directly on the fibers of the myocardium. These actions translate into increased cardiac output. Parasympathetic stimulation decreases the heart rate to restore homeostasis. The parasympathetic nerve that supplies the heart is the vagus nerve (cranial nerve X). It slows the heart rate by acting on the SA and AV nodes.

These ANS influences allow the heart to meet changing needs rapidly. The heart rate is also affected by substances circulating in the blood, including hormones, ions, and drugs. Regular exercise strengthens the heart and increases the amount of blood ejected with each beat. Consequently, the circulatory needs of the body at rest can be met with a lower heart rate. Trained athletes usually have a low resting heart rate.

Variations in Heart Rates

▶ **Bradycardia** (brad-e-KAR-de-ah) is a relatively slow heart rate of less than 60 beats/ minute. During rest and sleep, the heart may beat less than 60 beats/minute, but the rate usually does not fall below 50 beats/minute.

▶ **Tachycardia** (tak-e-KAR-de-ah) refers to a heart rate of more than 100 beats/minute. Tachycardia is normal during exercise or stress but may also occur under abnormal conditions.

▶ **Sinus arrhythmia** (ah-RITH-me-ah) is a regular variation in heart rate caused by changes in the rate and depth of breathing. It is a normal phenomenon.

▶ **Premature beat,** also called *extrasystole,* is a beat that comes before the expected normal beat. In healthy people, they may be initiated by caffeine, nicotine, or psychological stresses. They are also common in people with heart disease.

Heart Sounds

The normal heart sounds are usually described by the syllables "lubb" and "dupp." The first, "lubb," is a longer,

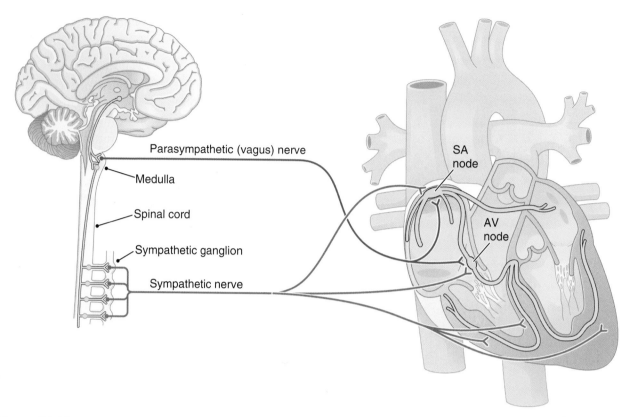

Figure 13-12 **Autonomic nervous system regulation of the heart.** The ANS affects the rate and force of heart contractions. *ZOOMING IN ♦ What parts of the conduction system does the autonomic nervous system affect?*

lower-pitched sound that occurs at the start of ventricular systole. It is probably caused by a combination of events, mainly closure of the atrioventricular valves. This action causes vibrations in the blood passing through the valves and in the tissue surrounding the valves. The second, or "dupp," sound is shorter and sharper. It occurs at the beginning of ventricular relaxation and is caused largely by sudden closure of the semilunar valves.

Murmurs An abnormal sound is called a **murmur** and is usually due to faulty action of a valve. For example, if a valve fails to close tightly and blood leaks back, a murmur is heard. Another condition giving rise to an abnormal sound is the narrowing (stenosis) of a valve opening.

The many conditions that can cause abnormal heart sounds include congenital (birth) defects, disease, and physiologic variations. An abnormal sound caused by any structural change in the heart or the vessels connected with the heart is called an **organic murmur**. Certain normal sounds heard while the heart is working may also be described as murmurs, such as the sound heard during rapid filling of the ventricles. To differentiate these from abnormal sounds, they are more properly called **functional murmurs**.

> **Checkpoint 13-9** What system exerts the main influence on the rate and strength of heart contractions?

> **Checkpoint 13-10** What is a heart murmur?

▶ The Heart in the Elderly

There is much individual variation in the way the heart ages, depending on heredity, environmental factors, diseases, and personal habits. However, some of the changes that may occur with age are as follows. The heart becomes smaller, and there is a decrease in the strength of heart muscle contraction. The valves become less flexible, and incomplete closure may produce an audible murmur. By 70 years of age, the cardiac output may decrease by as much as 35%. Damage within the conduction system can produce abnormal rhythms, including extra beats, rapid atrial beats, and slowing of ventricular rate. Temporary failure of the conduction system (heart block) can cause periodic loss of consciousness. Because of the decrease in the reserve strength of the heart, elderly people are often limited in their ability to respond to physical or emotional stress.

◗ Maintaining Heart Health

Prevention of heart ailments is based on identification of cardiovascular risk factors and modification of those factors that can be changed. Risk factors that cannot be modified include the following:

◗ Age. The risk of heart disease increases with age.
◗ Gender. Until middle age, men have greater risk than women. Women older than 50 years or past menopause have risk equal to that of males.
◗ Heredity. Those with immediate family members with heart disease are at greater risk.
◗ Body type, particularly the hereditary tendency to deposit fat in the abdomen or on the chest surface, increases risk.

Risk factors that can be changed include the following:

◗ Smoking, which leads to spasm and hardening of the arteries. These arterial changes result in decreased blood flow and poor supply of oxygen and nutrients to heart muscle.
◗ Physical inactivity. Lack of exercise weakens the heart muscle and decreases the efficiency of the heart. It also decreases the efficiency of the skeletal muscles, which further taxes the heart.
◗ Weight over the ideal increases risk.
◗ Saturated fat in the diet. Elevated fat levels in the blood lead to blockage of the coronary arteries by plaque (see Box 13-3, Lipoproteins).
◗ High blood pressure (hypertension) damages heart muscle.
◗ Diabetes and gout. Both diseases cause damage to small blood vessels.

Efforts to maintain a healthy heart should include having regular physical examinations and minimizing the controllable risk factors.

◗ Heart Studies

Experienced listeners can gain much information about the heart using a **stethoscope** (STETH-o-skope). This relatively simple instrument is used to convey sounds from within the patient's body to an examiner's ear.

The **electrocardiograph** (**ECG** or **EKG**) is used to record electrical changes produced as the heart muscle contracts. (The abbreviation EKG comes from the German spelling of the word.) The ECG may reveal certain myocardial injuries. Electrodes (leads) placed on the skin surface pick up electrical activity, and the ECG tracing, or electrocardiogram, represents this activity as **waves**. The P wave represents the activity of the atria; the QRS and T waves represent the activity of the ventricles (Fig. 13-13). Changes in the waves and the intervals between them are used to diagnose heart damage and arrhythmias.

Many people with heart disease undergo **catheterization** (kath-eh-ter-i-ZA-shun). In right heart catheterization, an extremely thin tube (catheter) is passed through the veins of the right arm or right groin and then into the right side of heart. A **fluoroscope** (flu-OR-o-scope), an instrument for examining deep structures with x-rays, is used to show the route taken by the catheter. The tube is passed all the way through the pulmonary valve into the large lung arteries. Blood samples are obtained along the way for testing, and pressure readings are taken.

In left heart catheterization, a catheter is passed through an artery in the left groin or arm to the heart. Dye

---

Box 13-3	**Clinical Perspectives**

Lipoproteins: What's the Big DL?

Although cholesterol has received a lot of bad press in recent years, it is a necessary substance in the body. It is found in bile salts needed for digestion of fats, in hormones, and in the plasma membrane of the cell. However, high levels of cholesterol in the blood have been associated with atherosclerosis and heart disease.

It now appears that the total amount of blood cholesterol is not as important as the form in which it occurs. Cholesterol is transported in the blood in combination with other lipids and with protein, forming compounds called lipoproteins. These compounds are distinguished by their relative density. High-density lipoprotein (HDL) is about one-half protein, whereas low-density lipoprotein (LDL) has a higher proportion of cholesterol and less protein. VLDLs, or very-low-density lipoproteins, are substances that are converted to LDLs.

LDLs carry cholesterol from the liver to the tissues, making it available for membrane or hormone synthesis. HDLs remove cholesterol from the tissues, such as the walls of the arteries, and carry it back to the liver for reuse or disposal. Thus, high levels of HDLs indicate efficient removal of arterial plaques, whereas high levels of LDLs suggest that arteries will become clogged.

Diet is an important factor in regulating lipoprotein levels. Saturated fatty acids (found primarily in animal fats) raise LDL levels, while unsaturated fatty acids (found in most vegetable oils) lower LDL levels and stimulate cholesterol excretion. Thus, a diet lower in saturated fat and higher in unsaturated fat may reduce the risk of atherosclerosis and heart disease. Other factors that affect lipoprotein levels include cigarette smoking, coffee drinking, and stress, which raise LDL levels, and exercise, which lowers LDL levels.

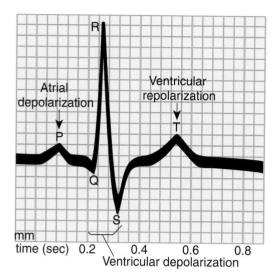

Figure 13-13 Normal ECG tracing. The tracing shows a single cardiac cycle. What is the length of the cardiac cycle shown in this diagram? *ZOOMING IN* ◆ *What is the length of the cardiac cycle shown in this diagram*

can then be injected into the coronary arteries to map damage to the vessels. The tube may also be passed through the aortic valve into the left ventricle for studies of pressure and volume in that chamber.

Ultrasound consists of sound waves generated at a frequency above the range of sensitivity of the human ear. In **echocardiography** (ek-o-kar-de-OG-rah-fe), also known as *ultrasound cardiography*, high-frequency sound waves are sent to the heart from a small instrument on the surface of the chest. The ultrasound waves bounce off the heart and are recorded as they return, showing the heart in action. Movement of the echoes is traced on an electronic instrument called an *oscilloscope* and recorded on film. (The same principle is employed by submarines to detect ships.) The method is safe and painless, and it does not use x-rays. It provides information on the size and shape of heart structures, on cardiac function, and on possible heart defects.

Checkpoint 13-11 What do ECG and EKG stand for?

Word Anatomy

Medical terms are built from standardized word parts (prefixes, roots, and suffixes). Learning the meanings of these parts can help you remember words and interpret unfamiliar terms.

WORD PART	MEANING	EXAMPLE
Structure of the Heart		
cardi/o	heart	The *myocardium* is the heart muscle.
pulmon/o	lung	The *pulmonary* circuit carries blood to the lungs.

WORD PART	MEANING	EXAMPLE
Function of the Heart		
sin/o	sinus	The *sinoatrial* node is in a space (sinus) in the wall of the right atrium.
brady-	slow	*Bradycardia* is a slow heart rate.
tachy-	rapid	*Tachycardia* is a rapid heart rate.
Heart Studies		
steth/o	chest	A *stethoscope* is used to listen to body sounds, such as those heard through the wall of the chest.

Summary

I. Circulation and the heart—heart contractions drive blood through the blood vessels

A. Location of the heart
  1. In mediastinum
  2. Slightly left of the midline; apex pointed toward left

II. Structure of the heart
  1. Layers of the heart wall
    a. Endocardium—thin inner layer of epithelium

  b. Myocardium—thick muscle layer
  c. Epicardium—thin outer layer of serous membrane
    (1) Also called visceral pericardium
A. Pericardium—sac that encloses the heart
  1. Outer layer fibrous
  2. Inner layers—parietal and visceral serous membranes
B. Special features of myocardium
  1. Lightly striated
  2. Intercalated disks
  3. Branching of fibers

C. Divisions of the heart
  1. Two sides divided by septa
  2. Four chambers
      a. Atria—left and right receiving chambers
      b. Ventricles—left and right pumping chambers
  3. Four valves—prevent backflow of blood
      a. Right atrioventricular (AV) valve—tricuspid
      b. Left atrioventricular valve—mitral or bicuspid
      c. Pulmonary (semilunar) valve—at entrance to pulmonary artery
      d. Aortic (semilunar) valve—at entrance to aorta
D. Blood supply to the myocardium
  1. Coronary arteries—first branches of aorta; fill when heart relaxes
  2. Coronary sinus—collects venous blood from heart and empties into right atrium

III. Function of the heart
  1. Cardiac cycle
      a. Diastole—relaxation phase
      b. Systole—contraction phase
A. Cardiac output—volume pumped by each ventricle per minute
  1. Stroke volume—amount pumped with each beat
  2. Heart rate—number of beats per minute
B. Heart's conduction system
  1. Sinoatrial node (pacemaker)—at top of right atrium
  2. Atrioventricular node—between atria and ventricles
  3. Atrioventricular bundle (bundle of His)—at top of interventricular septum
      a. Bundle branches—right and left, on either side of septum
      b. Purkinje fibers—branch through myocardium of ventricles
C. Control of the heart rate
  1. Autonomic nervous system
      a. Sympathetic system—speeds heart rate
      b. Parasympathetic system—slows heart rate through vagus nerve

  2. Others—hormones, ions, drugs
  3. Variations in heart rates
      a. Bradycardia—slower rate than normal; less than 60 beats/minute
      b. Tachycardia—faster rate than normal; more than 100 beats/minute
      c. Sinus arrhythmia—related to breathing changes
      d. Premature beat—extrasystole
D. Heart sounds
  1. Normal
      a. "Lubb"—occurs at closing of atrioventricular valves
      b. "Dupp"—occurs at closing of semilunar valves
  2. Abnormal—murmur

IV. The heart in the elderly
  1. Individual variations in how heart ages
  2. Common variations include:
      a. Decrease in heart size, strength of muscle contraction, flexibility of values, cardiac output
      b. Abnormal rhythms, temporary failure of conduction system

V. Maintaining Heart Health
  1. Risk factors
  2. Preventive measures—physical examination, proper diet, quitting smoking, regular exercise, control of chronic illness

VI. Heart studies
  1. Stethoscope—used to listen to heart sounds
  2. Electrocardiograph (ECG, EKG)—records electrical activity as waves
  3. Catheterization—thin tube inserted into heart for blood samples, pressure readings, and other tests
  4. Fluoroscope—examines deep tissue with x-rays; used to guide catheter
  5. Echocardiography—uses ultrasound to record pictures of heart in action

Questions for Study and Review

Building Understanding

Fill in the blanks

1. The central thoracic region that contains the heart is the _____.
2. The layer of the heart responsible for pumping blood is called the_____.
3. The heart beat is initiated by electrical impulses from the_____.

4. Adjacent cardiac muscle cells are firmly attached to each other by modified plasma membranes called _____.

5. The partition that separates the left ventricle from the right ventricle is called the _____.

Matching

Match each numbered item with the most closely related lettered item.
___ 6. receives deoxygenated blood from the body
___ 7. receives oxygenated blood from the lungs
___ 8. sends deoxygenated blood to the lungs
___ 9. sends oxygenated blood to the body

a. right atrium
b. left atrium
c. right ventricle
d. left ventricle

Multiple choice

___ 10. Rapid transfer of electrical signals between cardiac muscle cells is promoted by
   a. the striated nature of the cells
   b. branching of the cells
   c. the abundance of mitochondria within the cells
   d. intercalated disks between the cells

___ 11. The upper chambers of the heart are separated by the
   a. intercalated disk
   b. interatrial septum
   c. interventricular septum
   d. ductus arteriosus

___ 12. One complete sequence of heart contraction and relaxation is called the
   a. systole
   b. diastole
   c. cardiac cycle
   d. cardiac output

___ 13. The myocardium receives its blood supply from the
   a. superior vena cava
   b. pulmonary artery
   c. aorta
   d. coronary artery

___ 14. The heartbeat is initiated by the
   a. Purkinje fibers
   b. bundle of His
   c. atrioventricular node
   d. sinoatrial node

___ 15. A regular variation in heart rate due to changes in the rate and depth of breathing is called a
   a. murmur
   b. cyanosis
   c. sinus arrhythmia
   d. stent

Understanding Concepts

16. Differentiate between the terms in each of the following pairs:
   a. pulmonary and systemic circuit
   b. coronary artery and coronary sinus
   c. serous pericardium and fibrous pericardium
   d. systole and diastole

17. Explain the purpose of the four heart valves and describe their structure and location. What prevents the valves from opening backwards?

18. Trace a drop of blood from the superior vena cava to the lungs and then from the lungs to the aorta.

19. Describe the order in which electrical impulses travel through the heart. What is an interruption of these impulses in the conduction system of the heart called?

20. Compare the effects of the sympathetic and parasympathetic nervous systems on the working of the heart.

21. What is the difference between electrocardiography (ECG) and echocardiography?

22. List some age-related changes to the heart.

Conceptual Thinking

23. Jim's father has recently passed away following a massive myocardial infarction. At 45 years old, Jim is frightened that he may suffer the same fate. What can Jim do to lower his risk of heart disease? What risk factors can he not change?

24. Three-month-old Hannah R. is brought to the doctor by her parents. They have noticed that when she cries she becomes breathless and turns blue. The doctor examines Hannah and notices that she is lethargic, small for her age, and has a loud mitral valve murmur during systole. With this information, explain the cause of Hannah's symptoms.

LEARNING OUTCOMES

After careful study of this chapter, you should be able to:

1. Differentiate among the five types of blood vessels with regard to structure and function
2. Compare the pulmonary and systemic circuits relative to location and function
3. Name the four sections of the aorta and list the main branches of each section
4. Define *anastomosis.* Cite the function of anastomoses and give several examples
5. Compare superficial and deep veins and give examples of each type
6. Name the main vessels that drain into the superior and inferior venae cavae
7. Define *venous sinus* and give several examples of venous sinuses
8. Describe the structure and function of the hepatic portal system
9. Explain the forces that affect exchange across the capillary wall
10. Describe the factors that regulate blood flow
11. Define *pulse* and list factors that affect pulse rate
12. List the factors that affect blood pressure
13. Explain how blood pressure is commonly measured
14. Show how word parts are used to build words related to the blood vessels and circulation (see Word Anatomy at the end of the chapter)

chapter 14

Blood Vessels and Blood Circulation

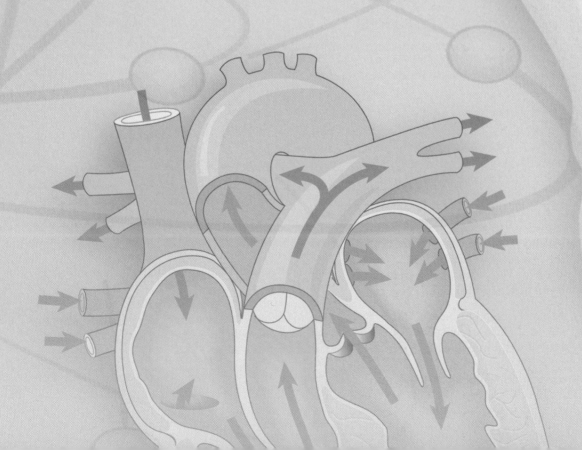

The blood vessels, together with the four chambers of the heart, form a closed system in which blood is carried to and from the tissues. Although whole blood does not leave the vessels, components of the plasma and tissue fluids can be exchanged through the walls of the tiniest vessels, the capillaries.

The vascular system is easier to understand if you refer to the appropriate illustrations in this chapter as the vessels are described. When this information is added to what you already know about the blood and the heart, a picture of the cardiovascular system as a whole will emerge.

▶ Blood Vessels

Blood vessels may be divided into five groups, named below according to the sequence of blood flow from the heart:

▶ **Arteries** carry blood away from the heart and toward the tissues. The heart's ventricles pump blood into the arteries.
▶ **Arterioles** (ar-TE-re-olz) are small subdivisions of the arteries. They carry blood into the capillaries.
▶ **Capillaries** are tiny, thin-walled vessels that allow for exchanges between systems. These exchanges occur between the blood and the body cells and between the blood and the air in the lung tissues. The capillaries connect the arterioles and venules.
▶ **Venules** (VEN-ulz) are small vessels that receive blood from the capillaries and begin its transport back toward the heart.
▶ **Veins** are vessels formed by the merger of venules. They continue the transport of blood until it is returned to the heart

Checkpoint 14-1 What are the five types of blood vessels?

Blood Circuits

The vessels together may be subdivided into two groups, or circuits: pulmonary and systemic. Figure 14-1 shows the vessels in these two circuits; the anatomic relation of the circuits to the heart is shown in Chapter 13's Figure 13-4.

The Pulmonary Circuit
The **pulmonary circuit** delivers blood to the lungs where carbon dioxide is eliminated and oxygen is replenished. The pulmonary vessels that carry blood to and from the lungs include the following:

▶ The pulmonary artery and its branches, which carry blood from the right ventricle to the lungs.
▶ The capillaries in the lungs, through which gases are exchanged.
▶ The pulmonary veins, which carry blood back to the left atrium.

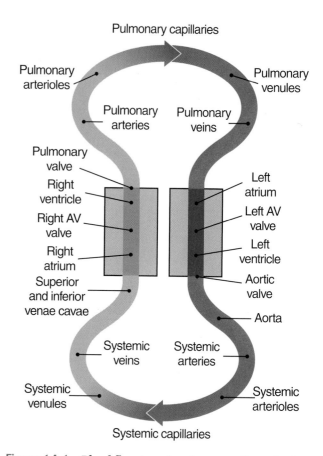

Figure 14-1 Blood flow in a closed system of vessels. Oxygen content changes as blood flows through the capillaries. *ZOOMING IN ✦ Judging from color coding, which vessels pick up oxygen? Which vessels release oxygen?*

The pulmonary vessels differ from those in the systemic circuit in that the pulmonary arteries carry blood that is *low* in oxygen, and the pulmonary veins carry blood that is *high* in oxygen. All the remaining arteries carry highly oxygenated blood, and all remaining veins carry blood that is low in oxygen.

The Systemic Circuit
The **systemic** (sis-TEM-ik) circuit serves the rest of the body. These vessels supply nutrients and oxygen to all the tissues and carry waste materials away from the tissues for disposal. The systemic vessels include the following:

▶ The **aorta** (a-OR-tah), which receives blood from the left ventricle and then branches into the systemic arteries carrying blood to the tissues.
▶ The systemic capillaries, through which materials are exchanged.
▶ The systemic veins, which carry blood back toward the heart. The venous blood flows into the right atrium of the heart through the superior vena cava and inferior vena cava.

Checkpoint 14-2 What are the two blood circuits and what areas does each serve?

Vessel Structure

The arteries have thick walls because they must be strong enough to receive blood pumped under pressure from the heart's ventricles (Fig. 14-2). The three tunics (coats) of the arteries resemble the three tissue layers of the heart:

▶ The innermost membrane of simple, flat epithelial cells makes up the **endothelium** (en-do-THE-le-um), forming a smooth surface over which the blood flows easily.
▶ The middle and thickest layer is made of smooth (involuntary) muscle, which is under the control of the autonomic nervous system.
▶ An outer tunic is made of a supporting connective tissue.

Elastic tissue between the layers of the arterial wall allows these vessels to stretch when receiving blood and then return to their original size. The amount of elastic tissue diminishes as the arteries branch and become smaller.

The small subdivisions of the arteries, the arterioles, have thinner walls in which there is little elastic connective tissue but relatively more smooth muscle. The autonomic nervous system controls this involuntary muscle.

The vessels become narrower (constrict) when the muscle contracts and widen (dilate) when the muscle relaxes. In this manner, the arterioles regulate the amount of blood that enters the various tissues at a given time. Change in the diameter of the arterioles is also a major factor in blood pressure control.

The microscopic capillaries that connect arterioles and venules have the thinnest walls of any vessels: one cell layer. The capillary walls are transparent and are made of smooth, squamous epithelial cells that are a continuation of the lining of the arteries. The thinness of these walls allows for exchanges between the blood and the body cells and between the lung tissue and the outside air. The capillary boundaries are the most important center of activity for the entire circulatory system. Their function is explained later in this chapter (see also Box 14-1).

The smallest veins, the venules, are formed by the union of capillaries, and their walls are only slightly thicker than those of the capillaries. As the venules merge to form veins, the smooth muscle in the vessel walls becomes thicker and the venules begin to acquire the additional layers found in the larger vessels.

The walls of the veins have the same three layers as those of the arteries. However, the middle smooth muscle tunic is relatively thin in the veins. A vein wall is much

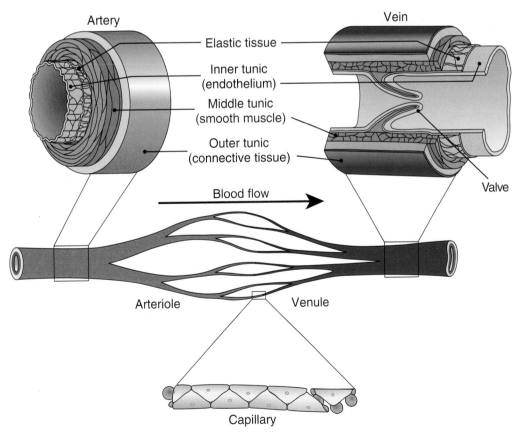

Figure 14-2 **Sections of small blood vessels.** Drawings show the thick wall of an artery, the thin wall of a vein, and the single-layered wall of a capillary. A venous valve also is shown. The arrow indicates the direction of blood flow. *ZOOMING IN* ✦ *Which vessels have valves that control blood flow?*

Capillaries: The Body's Free Trade Zones

The exchange of substances between body cells and the blood occurs along about 50,000 miles (80,000 kilometers) of capillaries. Rates of exchange vary because, based on their structure, different types of capillaries vary in permeability.

Continuous capillaries are the most common type and are found in muscle, connective tissue, the lungs, and the central nervous system (CNS). These capillaries are composed of a continuous layer of endothelial cells. Adjacent cells are loosely attached to each other, with small openings called intercellular clefts between them. Although continuous capillaries are the least permeable, water and small molecules can diffuse easily through their walls. Large molecules, such as plasma proteins and blood cells, cannot. In certain regions of the body, like the CNS, adjacent endothelial cells are joined tightly together, making the capillaries impermeable to many substances (see Box 9-1 in Chapter 9, The Blood Brain Barrier: Access Denied).

Fenestrated (FEN-es-tra-ted) capillaries are much more permeable than continuous capillaries, because they have many holes, or fenestrations, in the endothelium. These sieve-like capillaries are permeable to water and solutes as large as peptides. In the digestive tract, fenestrated capillaries permit rapid absorption of water and nutrients into the bloodstream. In the kidneys, they permit rapid filtration of blood plasma, the first step in urine formation.

Discontinuous capillaries, or sinusoids, are the most permeable. In addition to fenestrations, they have large spaces between endothelial cells that allow the exchange of water, large solutes, such as plasma proteins, and even blood cells. Sinusoids are found in the liver and red bone marrow, for example. Albumin, clotting factors, and other proteins formed in the liver enter the bloodstream through sinusoids. In red bone marrow, newly formed blood cells travel through sinusoids to join the bloodstream.

---

thinner than the wall of a comparably sized artery. These vessels also have less elastic tissue between the layers. As a result, the blood within the veins is carried under much lower pressure. Because of their thinner walls, the veins are easily collapsed. Only slight pressure on a vein by a tumor or other mass may interfere with return blood flow.

Most veins are equipped with one-way valves that permit blood to flow in only one direction: toward the heart (see Fig. 14-2). Such valves are most numerous in the veins of the extremities. Figure 14-3 is a cross-section of an artery and a vein as seen through a microscope.

> Checkpoint 14-3 What type of tissue makes up the middle layer of arteries and veins, and how is this tissue controlled?

> Checkpoint 14-4 How many cell layers make up the wall of a capillary?

▶ Systemic Arteries

The systemic arteries begin with the aorta, the largest artery, which measures about 2.5 cm (1 inch) in diameter. This vessel receives blood from the left ventricle then travels downward through the body, branching to all organs.

The Aorta and Its Parts

The aorta ascends toward the right from the left ventricle. Then it curves posteriorly and to the left. It continues downward posterior to the heart and just anterior to the vertebral column, through the diaphragm, and into the abdomen (Figs. 14-4 and 14-5). The aorta is one continuous artery, but it may be divided into sections:

▶ The **ascending aorta** is near the heart and inside the pericardial sac.
▶ The **aortic arch** curves from the right to the left and also extends posteriorly.
▶ The **thoracic aorta** lies just anterior to the vertebral col-

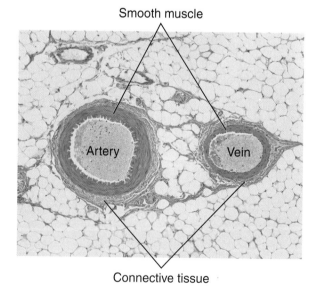

Smooth muscle

Artery   Vein

Connective tissue

Figure 14-3 Cross-section of an artery and vein. The smooth muscle and connective tissue of the vessels are visible in this photomicrograph. (Reprinted with permission from Cormack DH. Essential Histology. 2nd ed. Philadelphia: Lippincott Williams & Wilkins, 2001.) *ZOOMING IN ✦ Which type of vessel shown has a thicker wall?*

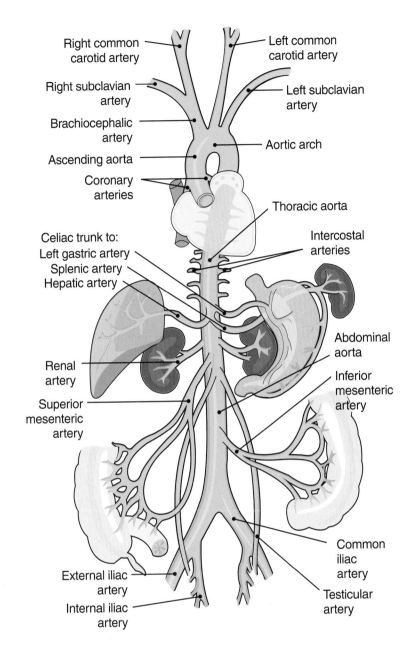

Figure 14-4 The aorta and its branches. *ZOOMING IN ✦ How many brachiocephalic arteries are there?*

umn posterior to the heart and in the space behind the pleura.
▶ The **abdominal aorta** is the longest section of the aorta, spanning the abdominal cavity.

The thoracic and abdominal aorta together make up the descending aorta.

Branches of the Ascending Aorta and Aortic Arch

The first, or ascending, part of the aorta has two branches near the heart, called the **left** and **right coronary arteries,** which supply the heart muscle. These form a crown around the heart's base and give off branches to all parts of the myocardium.

The arch of the aorta, located immediately beyond the ascending aorta, divides into three large branches.

▶ The **brachiocephalic** (brak-e-o-seh-FAL-ik) **artery** is a short vessel that supplies the arm and the head on the right side. After extending upward somewhat less than 5 cm (2 inches), it divides into the **right subclavian** (sub-KLA-ve-an) **artery,** which extends under the right clavicle (collar bone) and supplies the right upper extremity (arm), and the **right common carotid** (kah-ROT-id) **artery,** which supplies the right side of the neck, head and brain. Note that the brachiocephalic artery is unpaired.
▶ The **left common carotid artery** extends upward from the highest part of the aortic arch. It supplies the left side of the neck and the head.
▶ The **left subclavian artery** extends under the left clavicle and supplies the left upper extremity. This is the last branch of the aortic arch.

Branches of the Thoracic Aorta

The thoracic aorta supplies branches to the chest wall, **esophagus** (e-SOF-ah-gus), and bronchi (the subdivisions of the trachea), and their treelike subdivisions in the lungs. There are usually 9 to 10 pairs of **intercostal** (in-ter-KOS-tal) **arteries** that extend between the ribs, sending branches to the muscles and other structures of the chest wall.

Branches of the Abdominal Aorta

As in the case of the thoracic aorta, there are unpaired branches extending anteriorly and paired arteries extending laterally. The unpaired vessels are large arteries that supply the abdominal viscera. The most important of these visceral branches are as follows:

▶ The **celiac** (SE-le-ak) **trunk** is a short artery about 1.25 cm (1/2 inch) long that subdivides into three branches: the **left gastric artery** goes to the stomach, the **splenic** (SPLEN-ik) **artery** goes to the spleen, and the **hepatic** (heh-PAT-ik) **artery** carries oxygenated blood to the liver.
▶ The **superior mesenteric** (mes-en-TER-ik) **artery,** the largest of these branches, carries blood to most of the small intestine and to the first half of the large intestine.
▶ The much smaller **inferior mesenteric artery,** located below the superior mesenteric artery and near the end

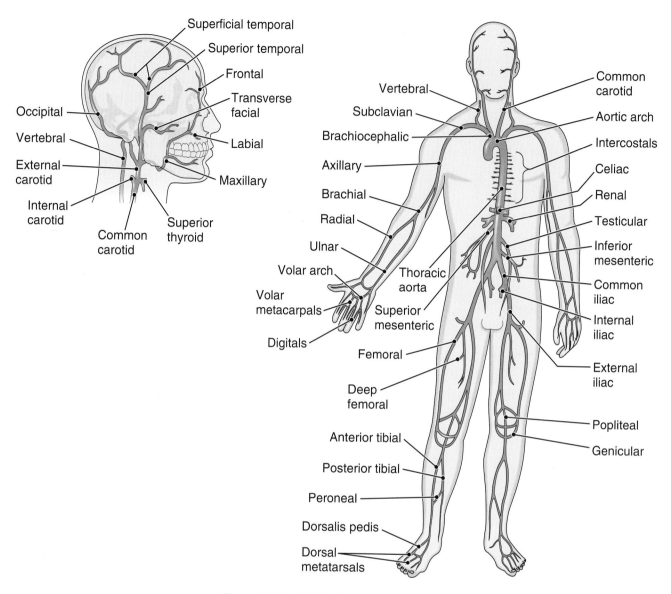

Figure 14-5 **Principal systemic arteries.**

of the abdominal aorta, supplies the second half of the large intestine.

The paired lateral branches of the abdominal aorta include the following right and left vessels:

▶ The **phrenic** (FREN-ik) **arteries** supply the diaphragm.
▶ The **suprarenal** (su-prah-RE-nal) **arteries** supply the adrenal (suprarenal) glands.
▶ The **renal** (RE-nal) **arteries**, the largest in this group, carry blood to the kidneys.
▶ The **ovarian arteries** in women and **testicular** (tes-TIK-u-lar) **arteries** in men (formerly called the spermatic arteries), supply the sex glands.
▶ Four pairs of **lumbar** (LUM-bar) **arteries** extend into the musculature of the abdominal wall.

Checkpoint 14-5 What are the subdivisions of the aorta, the largest artery?

The Iliac Arteries and Their Subdivisions

The abdominal aorta finally divides into two **common iliac** (IL-e-ak) **arteries**. Both of these vessels, which are about 5 cm (2 inches) long, extend into the pelvis, where each one subdivides into an **internal** and an **external iliac artery**.

The internal iliac vessels then send branches to the pelvic organs, including the urinary bladder, the rectum, and some reproductive organs.

Each external iliac artery continues into the thigh as the **femoral** (FEM-or-al) **artery**. This vessel gives rise to branches in the thigh and then becomes the **popliteal** (pop-LIT-e-al) **artery**, which subdivides below the knee. The subdivisions include the posterior and anterior **tibial arteries** and the **dorsalis pedis** (dor-SA-lis PE-dis), which supply the leg and the foot.

Arteries That Branch to the Arm and Head

Each common carotid artery travels along the trachea enclosed in a sheath with the internal jugular vein and the vagus nerve. Just anterior to the angle of the mandible (lower jaw) it branches into the **external** and **internal carotid arteries.** You can feel the pulse of the carotid artery just anterior to the large sternocleidomastoid muscle in the neck and below the jaw. The internal carotid artery travels into the head and branches to supply the eye, the anterior portion of the brain, and other structures in the cranium. The external carotid artery branches to the thyroid gland and to other structures in the head and upper part of the neck.

The **subclavian** (sub-KLA-ve-an) **artery** supplies blood to the arm and hand. Its first branch, however, is the **vertebral** (VER-the-bral) **artery**, which passes though the transverse processes of the first six cervical vertebrae and supplies blood to the posterior portion of the brain. The subclavian artery changes names as it travels through the arm and branches to the arm and hand. It first becomes the **axillary** (AK-sil-ar-e) **artery** in the axilla (armpit). The longest part of this vessel, the **brachial** (BRA-ke-al) **artery**, is in the arm proper. The brachial artery subdivides into two branches near the elbow: the **radial artery**, which continues down the thumb side of the forearm and wrist, and the **ulnar artery**, which extends along the medial or little finger side into the hand.

Just as the larger branches of a tree divide into limbs of varying sizes, so the arterial tree has a multitude of subdivisions. Hundreds of names might be included. We have mentioned only some of them.

Checkpoint 14-6 What arteries are formed by the final division of the abdominal aorta?

Checkpoint 14-7 What areas are supplied by the brachiocephalic artery?

Anastomoses

A communication between two vessels is called an **anastomosis** (ah-nas-to-MO-sis). By means of arterial anastomoses, blood reaches vital organs by more than one route. Some examples of such end-artery unions are as follows:

▶ The **circle of Willis** (Fig. 14-6) receives blood from the two internal carotid arteries and from the **basilar** (BAS-il-ar) **artery,** which is formed by the union of the two vertebral arteries. This arterial circle lies just under the center of the brain and sends branches to the cerebrum and other parts of the brain.

▶ The **superficial palmar arch** is formed by the union of the radial and ulnar arteries in the hand. It sends branches to the hand and the fingers.

▶ The **mesenteric** arches are made of communications between branches of the vessels that supply blood to the intestinal tract.

▶ **Arterial arches** are formed by the union of branches of the tibial arteries in the foot. There are similar anastomoses in other parts of the body.

Arteriovenous anastomoses are blood shunts found in a few areas, including the external ears, the hands, and the feet. In this type of shunt, a small vessel known as a *metarteriole* or *thoroughfare channel,* connects the arterial system directly with the venous system, bypassing the capillaries (Fig. 14-7). This pathway provides a more rapid flow and a greater blood volume to these areas, thus protecting these exposed parts from freezing in cold weather.

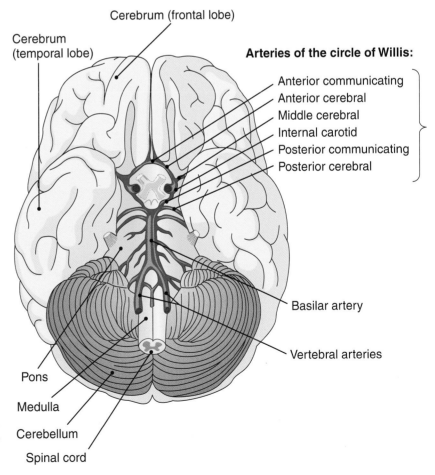

Figure 14-6 Arteries that supply the brain. The bracket at right groups the arteries that make up the circle of Willis.

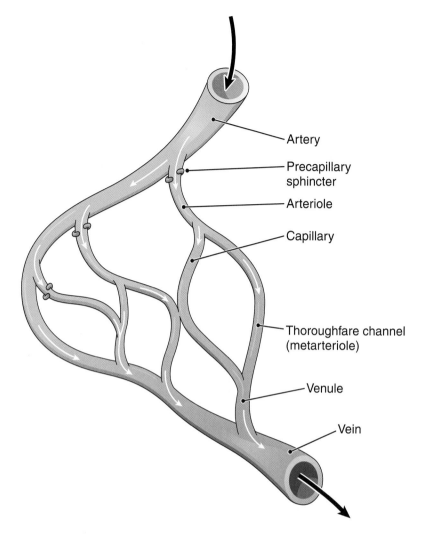

Figure 14-7 **Capillary network showing an arteriovenous shunt (anastomosis).** A connecting vessel, known as a thoroughfare channel or metarteriole, carries blood directly from an arteriole to a venule, bypassing the capillaries.

Artery
Precapillary sphincter
Arteriole
Capillary
Thoroughfare channel (metarteriole)
Venule
Vein

Checkpoint 14-8 What is an anastomosis?

▶ Systemic Veins

Whereas most arteries are located in protected and rather deep areas of the body, many of the principal systemic veins are found near the surface (Fig. 14-8). The most important of the **superficial veins** are in the extremities, and include the following:

▶ The veins on the back of the hand and at the front of the elbow. Those at the elbow are often used for drawing blood for test purposes, as well as for intravenous injections. The largest of this group of veins are the **cephalic** (seh-FAL-ik), the **basilic** (bah-SIL-ik), and the **median cubital** (KU-bih-tal) **veins.**

▶ The **saphenous** (sah-FE-nus) **veins** of the lower extremities, which are the body's longest veins. The great saphenous vein begins in the foot and extends up the medial side of the leg, the knee, and the thigh. It finally empties into the femoral vein near the groin.

The **deep veins** tend to parallel arteries and usually have the same names as the corresponding arteries. Examples of these include the **femoral** and the external and internal **iliac** vessels of the lower part of the body, and the **brachial, axillary,** and **subclavian** vessels of the upper extremities. Exceptions are found in the veins of the head and the neck. The two **jugular** (JUG-u-lar) **veins** on each side of the neck drain the areas supplied by the carotid arteries (*jugular* is from a Latin word meaning "neck"). The larger of the two veins, the internal jugular, receives blood from the large veins (cranial venous sinuses) that drain the head and also from regions of the face and neck. The smaller external jugular drains the areas supplied by the external carotid artery. Both veins empty directly into the subclavian vein on the left and the right. A **brachiocephalic vein** is formed on each side by the union of the subclavian and the jugular veins (see Fig. 14-8). (Remember, there is only *one* brachiocephalic artery.)

The Venae Cavae and Their Tributaries

Two large veins receive blood from the systemic vessels and empty directly into the heart's right atrium. The veins of the head, neck, upper extremities, and chest all drain into the **superior vena cava** (VE-nah KA-vah). This vessel is formed by the union of the right and left brachiocephalic veins, which drain the head, neck, and upper extremities. The unpaired **azygos** (AZ-ih-gos) **vein** drains the veins of the chest wall and empties into the superior vena cava just before the latter empties into the heart (see Fig. 14-8) (*azygous* is from a Greek word meaning "unpaired").

The **inferior vena cava,** which is much longer than the superior vena cava, returns the blood from the parts of the body below the diaphragm. It begins in the lower abdomen with the union of the two common iliac veins. It then ascends along the posterior wall of the abdomen, through a groove in the posterior part of the liver, through the diaphragm, and finally through the lower thorax to empty into the right atrium of the heart.

Drainage into the inferior vena cava is more compli-

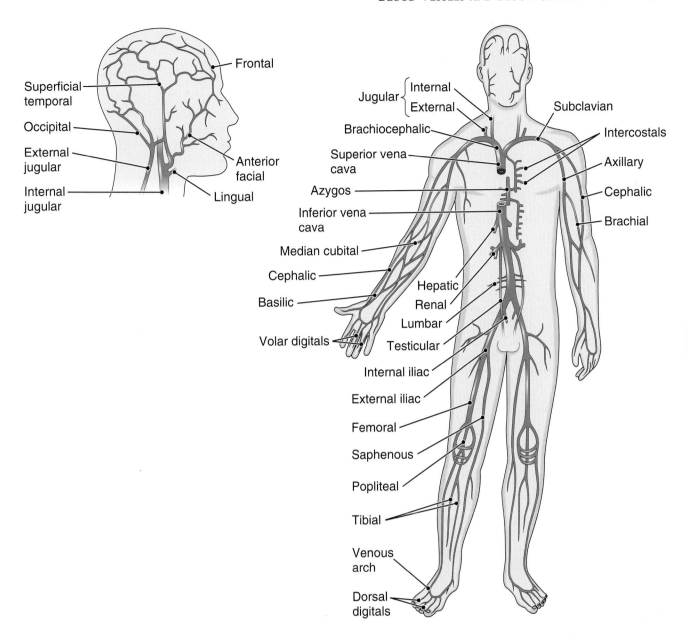

Figure 14-8 Principal systemic veins. *ZOOMING IN ✦ How many brachiocephalic veins are there?*

cated than drainage into the superior vena cava. The large veins below the diaphragm may be divided into two groups:

▶ The right and left veins that drain paired parts and organs. They include the **iliac** veins from near the groin, four pairs of **lumbar veins** from the dorsal part of the trunk and from the spinal cord, the **testicular veins** from the male testes and the **ovarian veins** from the female ovaries, the **renal** and **suprarenal veins** from the kidneys and adrenal glands near the kidneys, and finally the large **hepatic veins** from the liver. For the most part, these vessels empty directly into the inferior vena cava. The left testicular in the male and the left ovarian in the female empty into the left renal vein, which then takes this blood to the inferior vena cava;

these veins thus constitute exceptions to the rule that the paired veins empty directly into the vena cava.

▶ Unpaired veins that come from the spleen and parts of the digestive tract (stomach and intestine) empty into a vein called the **hepatic portal vein.** Unlike other lower veins, which empty into the inferior vena cava, the hepatic portal vein is part of a special system that enables blood to circulate through the liver before returning to the heart. This system, the hepatic portal system, will be described in more detail later.

Checkpoint 14-9 Veins are described as superficial or deep. What does superficial mean?

Checkpoint 14-10 What two large veins drain the systemic blood vessels and empty into the right atrium?

Venous Sinuses

The word *sinus* means "space" or "hollow." A **venous sinus** is a large channel that drains deoxygenated blood, but does not have the usual tubular structure of the veins. One example of a venous sinus is the **coronary sinus,** which receives most of the blood from the heart wall (see Fig. 13-8 in Chapter 13). It lies between the left atrium and left ventricle on the posterior surface of the heart, and empties directly into the right atrium, along with the two venae cavae.

Other important venous sinuses are the **cranial venous sinuses,** which are located inside the skull and drain the veins from all over the brain (Fig. 14-9). The largest of the cranial venous sinuses are the following:

▶ The two **cavernous sinuses,** situated behind the eyeballs, drain the eyes' **ophthalmic** (of-THAL-mik) **veins.** They give rise to the **petrosal** (peh-TRO-sal) **sinuses,** which drain into the jugular veins.

▶ The **superior sagittal** (SAJ-ih-tal) **sinus** is a single long space located in the midline above the brain and in the fissure between the cerebrum's two hemispheres. It ends in an enlargement called the **confluence** (KON-flu-ens) **of sinuses.**

▶ The two **transverse sinuses,** also called the **lateral sinuses,** are large spaces between the layers of the dura mater (the outermost membrane around the brain). They begin posteriorly from the confluence of sinuses and then extend laterally. As each sinus extends around the skull's interior, it receives additional blood, including blood draining through the inferior sagittal sinus and straight sinus. Nearly all of the blood leaving the brain eventually empties into one of the transverse sinuses. Each sinus extends anteriorly to empty into an internal jugular vein, which then passes through a hole in the skull to continue downward in the neck.

> **Checkpoint 14-11** What is a venous sinus?

The Hepatic Portal System

Almost always, when blood leaves a capillary bed, it flows directly back to the heart. In a portal system, however, blood circulates through a second capillary bed, usually in a second organ, before it returns to the heart. A portal system is a kind of detour in the pathway of venous return that transports materials directly from one organ to another. Chapter 11 described the small local portal system that carries secretions from the hypothalamus to the pituitary gland. A much larger portal system is the **hepatic portal system,** which carries blood from the abdominal organs to the liver (Fig. 14-10).

The hepatic portal system includes the veins that drain blood from capillaries in the spleen, stomach, pancreas, and intestine. Instead of emptying their blood directly into the inferior vena cava, they deliver it through the hepatic portal vein to the liver. The portal vein's largest tributary is the **superior mesenteric vein,** which drains blood from the proximal portion of the intestine. It is joined by the **splenic vein** just under the liver. Other tributaries of the portal circulation are the **gastric, pancreatic,** and **inferior mesenteric veins.** As it enters the liver, the portal vein divides and subdivides into ever smaller branches.

Eventually, the portal blood flows into a vast network of sinuslike vessels called **sinusoids** (SI-nus-oyds). These enlarged capillary channels allow liver

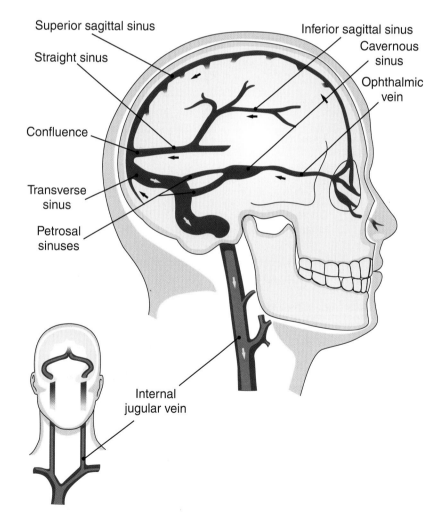

Figure 14-9 Cranial venous sinuses. The inset shows the paired transverse sinuses, which carry blood from the brain to the jugular veins.

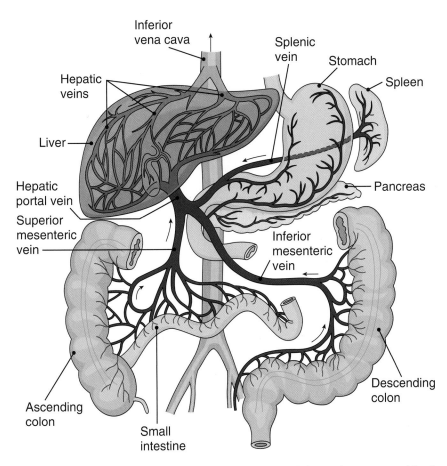

Figure 14-10 Hepatic portal system. Veins from the abdominal organs carry blood to the hepatic portal vein leading to the liver. Arrows show the direction of blood flow. *ZOOMING IN ✦ What vessel do the hepatic veins drain into?*

through capillaries surrounding the air sacs in the lungs, it picks up oxygen and unloads carbon dioxide. Later, when this oxygenated blood is pumped to capillaries in other parts of the body, it unloads the oxygen and picks up carbon dioxide and other substances generated by the cells (Fig. 14-11). The microscopic capillaries are of fundamental importance in these activities. It is only through and between the cells of these thin-walled vessels that the necessary exchanges can occur.

All living cells are immersed in a slightly salty liquid called **tissue fluid**, or **interstitial fluid**. Looking again at Figure 14-11, one can see how this fluid serves as "middleman" between the capillary membrane and the neighboring cells. As water, oxygen, and other necessary cellular materials pass through the capillary walls, they enter the tissue fluid. Then, these substances make their way by diffusion to the cells. At the same time, carbon dioxide and other end products of metabolism leave the cells and move in the opposite direction. These substances enter the capillaries and are carried away in the bloodstream for processing in other organs or elimination from the body.

cells close contact with the blood coming from the abdominal organs. (Similar blood channels are found in the spleen and endocrine glands, including the thyroid and adrenals.) After leaving the sinusoids, blood is finally collected by the hepatic veins, which empty into the inferior vena cava.

The purpose of the hepatic portal system is to transport blood from the digestive organs and the spleen to the liver sinusoids, so that the liver cells can carry out their functions. For example, when food is digested, most of the end products are absorbed from the small intestine into the bloodstream and transported to the liver by the portal system. In the liver, these nutrients are processed, stored, and released as needed into the general circulation.

> **Checkpoint 14-12** The hepatic portal system takes blood from the abdominal organs to what organ?

❱ The Physiology of Circulation

Circulating blood might be compared to a train that travels around the country, picking up and delivering passengers at each stop on its route. For example, as blood flows

Capillary Exchange

Diffusion is the main process by which substances move between the cells and the capillary blood. Recall that diffusion is the movement of a substance from an area where it is in higher concentration to an area where it is in lower concentration. Diffusion does not require transporters or cellular energy.

An additional force that moves materials from the blood into the tissues is the pressure of the blood as it flows through the capillaries. Blood pressure is the force that filters, or "pushes" water and dissolved materials out of the capillary into the tissue fluid. Fluid is drawn back into the capillary by osmotic pressure, the "pulling force" of substances dissolved and suspended in the blood. Osmotic pressure is maintained by plasma proteins (mainly albumin), which are too large to go through the capillary wall. These processes result in the constant exchange of fluids across the capillary wall.

The movement of blood through the capillaries is relatively slow, owing to the much larger cross-sectional area of the capillaries compared with that of the vessels from which they branch. This slow progress through the capillaries allows time for exchanges to occur.

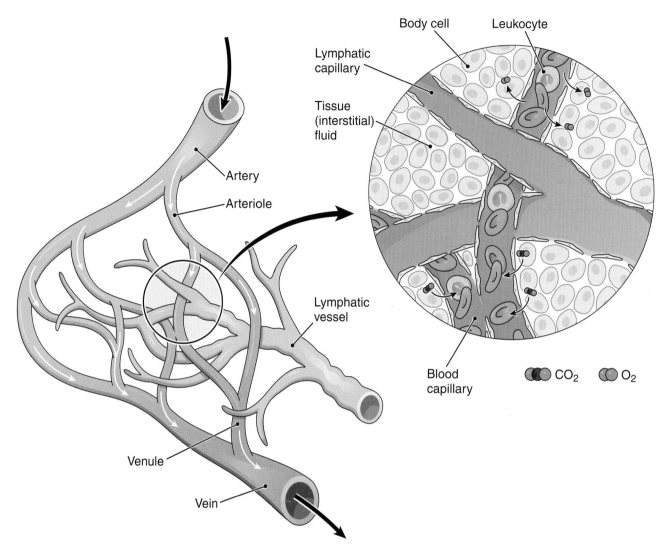

Figure 14-11 **Connection between small blood vessels through capillaries.** The blood delivers oxygen (O_2) to the tissues and picks up carbon dioxide (CO_2) for transport to the lungs. Note the lymphatic capillaries, which aid in tissue drainage.

Note that even when the capillary exchange process is most efficient, some water is left behind in the tissues. Also, some proteins escape from the capillaries into the tissues. The lymphatic system, discussed in Chapter 15, collects this extra fluid and protein and returns them to the circulation (see Fig. 14-11).

Checkpoint 14-13 As materials diffuse back and forth between the blood and tissue fluid across the capillary wall, what force helps to push materials out of the capillary? What force helps to draw materials into the capillary?

The Dynamics of Blood Flow

Blood flow is carefully regulated to supply tissue needs without unnecessary burden on the heart. Some organs, such as the brain, liver, and kidneys, require large quantities of blood even at rest. The requirements of some tissues, such as the skeletal muscles and digestive organs,

increase greatly during periods of activity. For example, the blood flow in muscle can increase 25 times during exercise. The volume of blood flowing to a particular organ can be regulated by changing the size of the blood vessels supplying that organ.

An increase in a blood vessel's diameter is called **vasodilation.** This change allows for the delivery of more blood to an area. **Vasoconstriction** is a decrease in a blood vessel's diameter, causing a decrease in blood flow. These *vasomotor activities* result from the contraction or relaxation of smooth muscle in the walls of the blood vessels, mainly the arterioles. A **vasomotor center** in the medulla of the brain stem regulates vasomotor activities, sending its messages through the autonomic nervous system.

Blood flow into an individual capillary is regulated by a **precapillary sphincter** of smooth muscle that encircles the entrance to the capillary (see Fig. 14-7). This sphincter widens to allow more blood to enter when tissues need more oxygen.

Return of Blood to the Heart Blood leaving the capillary networks returns in the venous system to the heart, and even picks up some speed along the way, despite factors that work against its return. Blood flows in a closed system and must continually move forward as the heart contracts. However, by the time blood arrives in the veins, little force remains from the heart's pumping action. Also, because the veins expand easily under pressure, blood tends to pool in the veins. Considerable amounts of blood are normally stored in these vessels. Finally, the force of gravity works against upward flow from regions below the heart. Several mechanisms help to overcome these forces and promote blood's return to the heart in the venous system. These are:

▸ **Contraction of skeletal muscles.** As skeletal muscles contract, they compress the veins and squeeze blood forward (Fig. 14-12).
▸ **Valves** in the veins prevent back flow and keep blood flowing toward the heart.
▸ **Breathing**. Pressure changes in the abdominal and thoracic cavities during breathing also promote blood return in the venous system. During inhalation, the di-aphragm flattens and puts pressure on the large abdominal veins. At the same time, chest expansion causes pressure to drop in the thorax. Together, these actions serve to both push and pull blood through these cavities and return it to the heart.

As evidence of these effects, if a person stands completely motionless, especially on a hot day when the superficial vessels dilate, enough blood can accumulate in the lower extremities to cause fainting from insufficient oxygen to the brain.

The Pulse

The ventricles regularly pump blood into the arteries about 70 to 80 times a minute. The force of ventricular contraction starts a wave of increased pressure that begins at the heart and travels along the arteries. This wave, called the **pulse,** can be felt in any artery that is relatively close to the surface, particularly if the vessel can be pressed down against a bone. At the wrist, the radial artery passes over the bone on the forearm's thumb side, and the pulse is most commonly obtained here. Other vessels sometimes used for taking the pulse are the carotid artery in the neck and the dorsalis pedis on the top of the foot.

Normally, the pulse rate is the same as the heart rate, but if a heartbeat is abnormally weak, or if the artery is

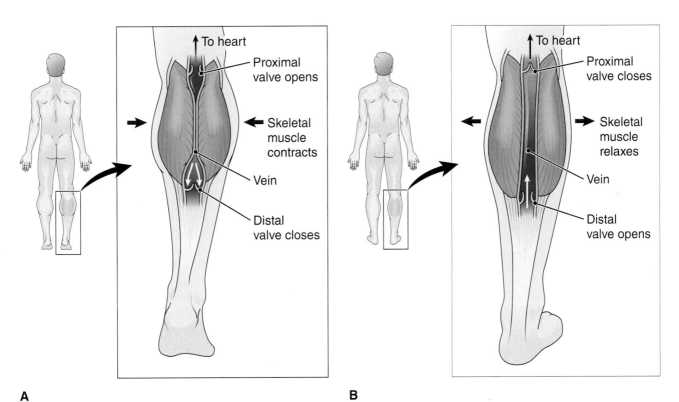

A　　　　　　　　　　　　　　　　　　　　**B**

Figure 14-12　**Role of skeletal muscles and valves in blood return. (A)** Contracting skeletal muscle compresses the vein and drives blood forward, opening the proximal valve, while the distal valve closes to prevent backflow of blood. **(B)** When the muscle relaxes again, the distal valve opens, and the proximal valve closes until blood moving in the vein forces it open again. *ZOOMING IN ✦ Which of the two valves shown is closer to the heart?*

obstructed, the beat may not be detected as a pulse. In checking another person's pulse, it is important to use your second or third finger. If you use your thumb, you may find that you are getting your own pulse. When taking a pulse, it is important to gauge the strength as well as the regularity and rate.

Pulse Rate Various factors may influence the pulse rate. We describe just a few here:

- The pulse is somewhat faster in small people than in large people and usually is slightly faster in women than in men.
- In a newborn infant, the rate may be from 120 to 140 beats/minute. As the child grows, the rate tends to become slower.
- Muscular activity influences the pulse rate. During sleep, the pulse may slow down to 60 beats/minute, whereas during strenuous exercise, the rate may go up to well over 100 beats/minute. For a person in good condition, the pulse does not go up as rapidly as it does in an inactive person, and it returns to a resting rate more quickly after exercise.
- Emotional disturbances may increase the pulse rate.
- In many infections, the pulse rate increases with the increase in temperature.
- An excessive amount of secretion from the thyroid gland may cause a rapid pulse.

Checkpoint 14-16 What is the definition of *pulse?*

Blood Pressure

Blood pressure is the force exerted by the blood against the walls of the vessels. Blood pressure is determined by the heart's output and resistance to blood flow in the vessels. If either of these factors changes and there are no compensating changes, blood pressure will change (Fig. 14-13).

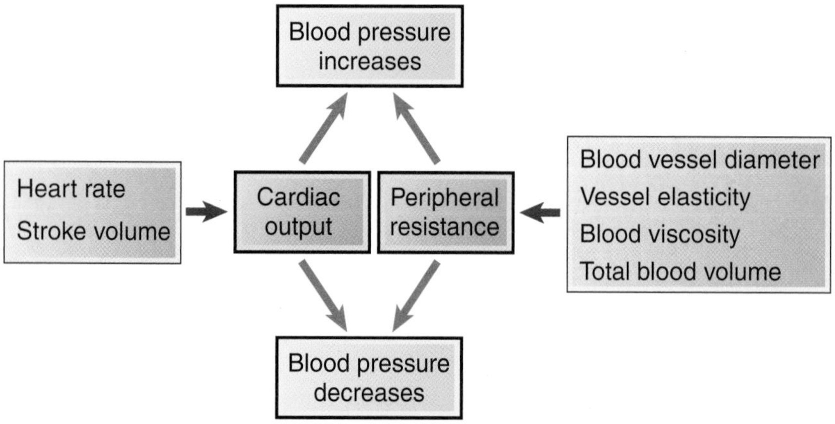

Figure 14-13 **Factors that influence blood pressure.**

Cardiac Output As described in Chapter 13, the output of the heart, or cardiac output (CO), is the volume of blood pumped out of each ventricle in one minute. Cardiac output is the product of two factors:

- **Heart rate**, the number of times the heart beats each minute. The basic heart rate is set internally by the SA node, but can be influenced by the autonomic nervous system, hormones, and other substances circulating in the blood, such as ions.
- **Stroke volume**, the volume of blood ejected from the ventricle with each beat. The sympathetic nervous system can stimulate more forceful heart contractions to increase ejection of blood. Also, if more blood returns to the heart in the venous system, stretching of the heart muscle will promote more forceful contractions.

Resistance to Blood Flow Resistance is opposition to blood flow owing to friction generated as blood slides along the vessel walls. Because the effects of resistance are seen mostly in small arteries and arterioles that are at a distance from the heart and large vessels, this factor is often described as *peripheral resistance*. Resistance in the vessels is affected by the following factors:

- **Vasomotor changes.** A narrow vessel offers more resistance to blood flow than a wider vessel, just as it is harder to draw fluid through a narrow straw than through a wide straw. Thus, vasoconstriction increases resistance to flow and vasodilation lowers resistance.
- **Elasticity of blood vessels.** Arteries normally expand to receive blood and then return to their original size. If vessels lose elasticity, as by atherosclerosis, they offer more resistance to blood flow. You've probably experienced this phenomenon if you've tried to blow up a firm, new balloon. More pressure is generated as you blow, and the balloon is a lot harder to inflate than a soft balloon, which expands easily under pressure. Blood vessels lose elasticity with aging, thus increasing resistance and blood pressure.
- **Viscosity**, or thickness of the blood. Just as a milkshake is harder to suck through a straw than milk is, increased blood viscosity will increase blood pressure. Increased numbers of red blood cells, as in polycythemia, or a loss of plasma volume, as by dehydration, will increase blood viscosity. The hematocrit test described in Chapter 12 is one measure of blood viscosity; it measures the relative percentage of packed cells in whole blood.
- **Total blood volume**, the total amount of blood that is in the vas-

cular system at a given time. A loss of blood volume, as by hemorrhage, will lower blood pressure. An increase in blood volume will generate more pressure within the vessels. It will also increase cardiac output by increasing venous return of blood to the heart.

To summarize, all of these relationships are expressed together by the following equation:

Blood pressure = cardiac output × peripheral resistance

Measurement of Blood Pressure The measurement and careful interpretation of blood pressure may prove a valuable guide in the care and evaluation of a person's health. Because blood pressure decreases as the blood flows from arteries into capillaries and finally into veins, healthcare providers ordinarily measure arterial pressure only, most commonly in the brachial artery of the arm. They use an instrument called a **sphygmomanometer** (sfig-mo-mah-NOM-eh-ter) (Fig. 14-14), or more simply, a blood pressure cuff or blood pressure apparatus. They measure two variables:

▶ **Systolic pressure,** which occurs during heart muscle contraction, averages about 120 and is expressed in millimeters of mercury (mmHg).
▶ **Diastolic pressure,** which occurs during relaxation of the heart muscle, averages about 80 mmHg.

The sphygmomanometer is an inflatable cuff attached to a device for reading pressure. The examiner wraps the cuff around the patient's upper arm and inflates it with air until the brachial artery is compressed and the blood flow is cut off. Then, listening with a stethoscope, he or she slowly lets air out of the cuff until the first pulsations are heard. At this point, the pressure in the cuff is equal to the systolic pressure, and this pressure is read. Then, more air is let out until a characteristic muffled sound indicates the point where the vessel is open and the diastolic pressure is read. Sphygmomanometers originally displayed pressure readings on a graduated column of mercury, but alternate types display the readings on a dial, or measure blood pressure electronically and give a digital reading. Blood pressure is reported as systolic pressure first, then diastolic pressure, separated by a slash, such as 120/80 mmHg.

Considerable experience is required to ensure an accurate blood pressure reading. Often it is necessary to repeat measurements. Note also that blood pressure varies throughout the day and under different conditions, so a single reading does not give a complete picture. Some people typically have a higher reading in a doctor's office because of stress. Those with so-called "white coat hypertension" may need to take their blood pressure at home while relaxed to get a true reading. Box 14-2 explains how cardiac catheterization is used to measure blood pressure with high accuracy.

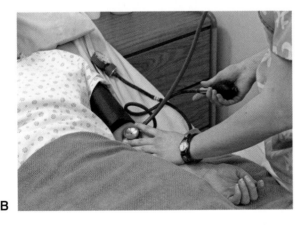

A

B

Figure 14-14 **Measurement of blood pressure. (A)** A sphygmomanometer, or blood pressure cuff. **(B)** Once the cuff is inflated, the examiner releases the pressure and listens for sounds in the vessels with a stethoscope. (A, Reprinted with permission from Bickley LS. Bates' Guide to Physical Examination and History Taking. 8th ed. Philadelphia: Lippincott Williams & Wilkins, 2003; B, reprinted with permission from Taylor C, Lillis C, LeMone P. Fundamentals of Nursing. 5th ed. Philadelphia: Lippincott Williams & Wilkins, 2004.)

Checkpoint 14-17 What is the definition of blood pressure?

Checkpoint 14-18 What two components of blood pressure are measured?

Box 14-2	Clinical Perspectives

Cardiac Catheterization: Measuring Blood Pressure From Within

Because arterial blood pressure decreases as blood flows further away from the heart, measurement of blood pressure with a simple inflatable cuff around the arm is only a reflection of the pressure in the heart and pulmonary arteries. Precise measurement of pressure in these parts of the cardiovascular system is useful in diagnosing certain cardiac and pulmonary disorders.

More accurate readings can be obtained using a catheter (thin tube) inserted directly into the heart and large vessels. One type commonly used is the pulmonary artery catheter (also known as the Swan-Ganz catheter), which has an inflatable balloon at the tip. This device is threaded into the right side of the heart through a large vein. Typically, the right internal jugular vein is used because it is the shortest

and most direct route to the heart, but the subclavian and femoral veins may be used instead. The catheter's position in the heart is confirmed by a chest x-ray and, when appropriately positioned, the atrial and ventricular blood pressures are recorded. As the catheter continues into the pulmonary artery, pressure in this vessel can be read. When the balloon is inflated, the catheter becomes wedged in a branch of the pulmonary artery, blocking blood flow. The reading obtained is called the **pulmonary capillary wedge (PCW) pressure**. It gives information on pressure in the heart's left side and on resistance in the lungs. Combined with other tests, cardiac catheterization can be used to diagnose cardiac and pulmonary disorders such as shock, pericarditis, congenital heart disease, and heart failure.

Word Anatomy

Medical terms are built from standardized word parts (prefixes, roots, and suffixes). Learning the meanings of these parts can help you remember words and interpret unfamiliar terms.

WORD PART	MEANING	EXAMPLE
Systemic Arteries		
brachi/o	arm	The *brachiocephalic* artery supplies blood to the arm and head on the right side.
cephal/o	head	See preceding example.
clav/o	clavicle	The *subclavian* artery extends under the clavicle on each side.
cost/o	rib	The *intercostal* arteries are between the ribs.
celi/o	abdomen	The *celiac* trunk branches to supply blood to the abdominal organs.
gastr/o	stomach	The *gastric* artery goes to the stomach.
splen/o	spleen	The *splenic* artery goes to the spleen.
hepat/o	liver	The *hepatic* artery supplies blood to the liver.
enter/o	intestine	The *mesenteric* arteries supply blood to the intestines.
phren/o	diaphragm	The *phrenic* artery supplies blood to the diaphragm.
ped/o	foot	The dorsalis *pedis* artery supplies blood to the foot.
stoma	mouth	An *anastomosis* is a communication between two vessels.
The Physiology of Circulation		
sphygm/o	pulse	A *sphygmomanometer* is used to measure blood pressure.
man/o	pressure	See preceding example.

Summary

I. Blood vessels

A. Types
1. Arteries—carry blood away from heart
2. Arterioles—small arteries
3. Capillaries—allow for exchanges between blood and tissues, or blood and air in lungs; connect arterioles and venules
4. Venules—small veins
5. Veins—carry blood toward heart

B. Blood circuits
1. Pulmonary circuit—carries blood to and from lungs
2. Systemic circuit—carries blood to and from rest of body

C. Vessel structure
1. Artery walls—layers (tunics)
   a. Innermost—single layer of flat epithelial cells (endothelium)
   b. Middle—thicker layer of smooth muscle and elastic connective tissue
   c. Outer—connective tissue

2. Arterioles—thinner walls, less elastic tissue, more smooth muscle

3. Capillaries—only endothelium; single layer of cells

4. Venules—wall slightly thicker than capillary wall

5. Veins—all three layers; thinner walls than arteries, less elastic tissue

II. Systemic arteries

A. The aorta and its parts
  1. Largest artery
  2. Divisions
    a. Ascending aorta
      (1) Left and right coronary arteries
    b. Aortic arch
      (1) Brachiocephalic artery—branches to arm and head on right
      (2) Left common carotid artery—supplies left side of neck and the head
      (3) Left subclavian artery—supplies left arm
    c. Descending aorta
      (1) Thoracic aorta—branches to chest wall, esophagus, bronchi
      (2) Abdominal aorta—supplies abdominal viscera
B. Iliac arteries and their subdivisions
  1. Final divisions of aorta
  2. Branch to pelvis and legs
C. Arteries that branch to the arm and head—common carotid, subclavian, brachial
D. Anastomoses—communications between vessels

III. Systemic veins

  1. Superficial—near surface
  2. Deep—usually parallel to arteries with same names as corresponding arteries
A. The venae cavae and their tributaries
  1. Superior vena cava—drains upper part of body
    a. Jugular veins drain head and neck
    b. Brachiocephalic veins empty into superior vena cava
  2. Inferior vena cava—drains lower part of body
B. Venous sinuses—enlarged venous channels

C. Hepatic portal system—carries blood from abdominal organs to liver, where it is processed before returning to heart

IV. The physiology of circulation

A. Capillary exchange
  1. Primary method—diffusion
  2. Medium—tissue fluid
  3. Blood pressure—drives fluid into tissues
  4. Osmotic pressure—pulls fluid into capillary
B. Dynamics of blood flow
  1. Vasomotor activities
    a. Vasodilation—increase in diameter of blood vessel
    b. Vasoconstriction—decrease in diameter of blood vessel
    c. Vasomotor center—in medulla; controls contraction and relaxation of smooth muscle in vessel wall
  2. Precapillary sphincter—regulates blood flow into capillary
  3. Return of blood to heart
    a. Pumping action of heart
    b. Pressure of skeletal muscles on veins
    c. Valves in veins
    d. Breathing—changes in pressure move blood toward heart
C. The pulse
  1. Wave of pressure that travels along arteries as ventricles contract
  2. Rate affected by size, age, gender, activity, and other factors
D. Blood pressure
  1. Force exerted by blood against vessel walls
  2. Factors
    a. Cardiac output—stroke volume x heart rate
    b. Resistance to blood flow—vessel diameter, vessel elasticity, blood viscosity, blood volume
  3. Measured in arm with sphygmomanometer
    a. Systolic pressure
      (1) Occurs during heart contraction
      (2) Averages 120 mmHg
    b. Diastolic pressure
      (1) Occurs during heart relaxation
      (2) Averages 80 mmHg

Questions for Study and Review

Building Understanding

Fill in the blanks

1. Blood is delivered to the lungs by the _____ circuit.
2. Capillaries receive blood from vessels called _____.
3. The specific part of the brain that regulates blood pressure is the _____.
4. The flow of blood into an individual capillary is regulated by a(n) _____.
5. The technical name for the instrument that measures blood pressure is _____.

Matching
Match each numbered item with the most closely related lettered item.

___ 6. Supplies blood from the heart to the arm and the head on the right side

___ 7. Supplies blood from the heart to the kidney

___ 8. Returns blood from the brain to the heart

___ 9. Returns blood from the small intestine to the heart

___ 10. Returns blood from the kidney to the heart

a. jugular vein
b. superior mesenteric vein
c. brachiocephalic artery
d. renal artery
e. renal vein

Multiple choice

____ 11. The innermost layer of a blood vessel is composed of
   a. smooth muscle
   b. epithelium
   c. connective tissue
   d. nervous tissue

____ 12. The largest artery in the body is the
   a. aorta
   b. brachiocephalic trunk
   c. splenic artery
   d. superior mesenteric artery

____ 13. The main process by which substances move between the cells and the capillary blood is
   a. endocytosis
   b. exocytosis
   c. osmosis
   d. diffusion

____ 14. The stomach, spleen, and liver receive blood via the
   a. hepatic portal system
   b. superior mesenteric artery
   c. inferior mesenteric artery
   d. celiac trunk

____ 15. Vasomotor activities are regulated by the
   a. medulla
   b. cerebellum
   c. cerebrum
   d. spinal cord

Understanding Concepts

16. Differentiate between the terms in each of the following pairs:
   a. artery and vein
   b. arteriole and venule
   c. anastomosis and venous sinus
   d. vasoconstriction and vasodilation
   e. systolic and diastolic pressure

17. How does the structure of the blood vessels correlate with their function?

18. Trace a drop of blood from the left ventricle to the:
   a. right side of the head and neck
   b. lateral surface of the left hand
   c. right foot
   d. liver
   e. small intestine

19. Trace a drop of blood from capillaries in the wall of the small intestine to the right atrium. What is the purpose of going through the liver on this trip?

20. What physiological factors influence blood pressure?

21. Describe three mechanisms that promote the return of blood to the heart in the venous system.

22. Describe the blood vessels that contribute to the hepatic portal system.

Conceptual Thinking

23. Kidney disease usually results in the loss of protein from the blood into the urine. One common sign of kidney disease is edema. Based on this information and your understanding of capillary exchange, explain why edema is often associated with kidney disease.

24. Cliff C., a 49-year-old self-described "couch potato," has high blood pressure. His doctor suspects that Cliff's lifestyle has resulted in atherosclerosis, a disease of the blood vessels characterized by "narrowing of the arteries." How has this disorder contributed to Cliff's high blood pressure?

SELECTED KEY TERMS

The following terms and other boldface terms in the chapter are defined in the Glossary

adenoids
antibody
antigen
antiserum
B cell
chyle
complement
gamma globulin
immunity
immunization
inflammation
interferon
lymph
lymphatic duct
lymphocyte
lymph node
macrophage
plasma cell
spleen
T cell
thymus
tonsil
vaccine

LEARNING OUTCOMES

After careful study of this chapter, you should be able to:

1. List the functions of the lymphatic system
2. Explain how lymphatic capillaries differ from blood capillaries
3. Name the two main lymphatic ducts and describe the area drained by each
4. List the major structures of the lymphatic system and give the locations and functions of each
5. Describe the composition and function of the reticuloendothelial system
6. Differentiate between nonspecific and specific body defenses and give examples of each
7. Briefly describe the inflammatory reaction
8. List several types of inborn immunity
9. Define *antigen* and *antibody*
10. Compare T cells and B cells with respect to development and type of activity
11. Explain the role of macrophages in immunity
12. Describe some protective effects of an antigen-antibody reaction
13. Differentiate between naturally acquired and artificially acquired immunity
14. Differentiate between active and passive immunity
15. Define the terms *vaccine* and *immune serum*
16. Show how word parts are used to build words related to the lymphatic system (see Word Anatomy at the end of the chapter)

chapter

15

The Lymphatic System and Body Defenses

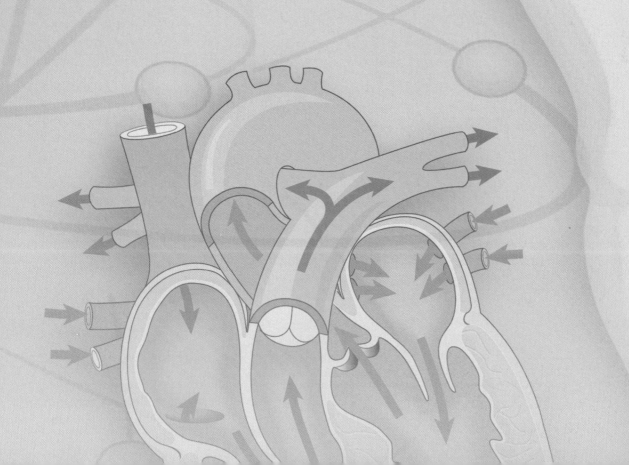

◗ The Lymphatic System

The lymphatic system is a widespread system of tissues and vessels. Its organs are not in continuous order, but are scattered throughout the body, and it services almost all regions. Only bone tissue, cartilage, epithelium and the central nervous system are not in direct communication with this system.

Functions of the Lymphatic System

The functions of the lymphatic system are just as varied as its locations. These functions fall into three categories:

◗ **Fluid balance**. As blood circulates through the capillaries in the tissues, water and dissolved substances are con-

stantly exchanged between the bloodstream and the interstitial (in-ter-STISH-al) fluids that bathe the cells. Ideally, the volume of fluid that leaves the blood should be matched by the amount that returns to the blood. However, there is always a slight excess of fluid left behind in the tissues. In addition, some proteins escape from the blood capillaries and are left behind. This fluid and protein would accumulate in the tissues if not for a second drainage pathway through lymphatic vessels (Fig. 15-1).

In addition to the blood-carrying capillaries, the tissues also contain microscopic lymphatic capillaries. These small vessels pick up excess fluid and protein left behind in the tissues (Fig. 15-2). The capillaries then drain into larger vessels, which eventually return these materials to the venous system near the heart.

The fluid that circulates in the lymphatic system is called **lymph** (limf), a clear fluid similar in composition to interstitial fluid. Although lymph is formed from the components of blood plasma, it differs from the plasma in that it has much less protein.

◗ **Protection from infection**. The lymphatic system is an important component of the immune system, which fights infection. One group of white blood cells, the lymphocytes, can live and multiply in the lymphatic system, where they attack and destroy foreign organisms. Lymphoid tissue scattered throughout the body filters out pathogens, other foreign matter and cellular debris in body fluids.

◗ **Absorption of fats**. Following the chemical and mechanical breakdown of food in the digestive tract, most nutrients are absorbed into the blood through intestinal capillaries. Many digested fats, however, are too large to enter the blood capillaries and are instead absorbed into lymphatic capillaries. These fats are added to the blood when lymph joins the bloodstream. The topic of digestion is covered in Chapter 17.

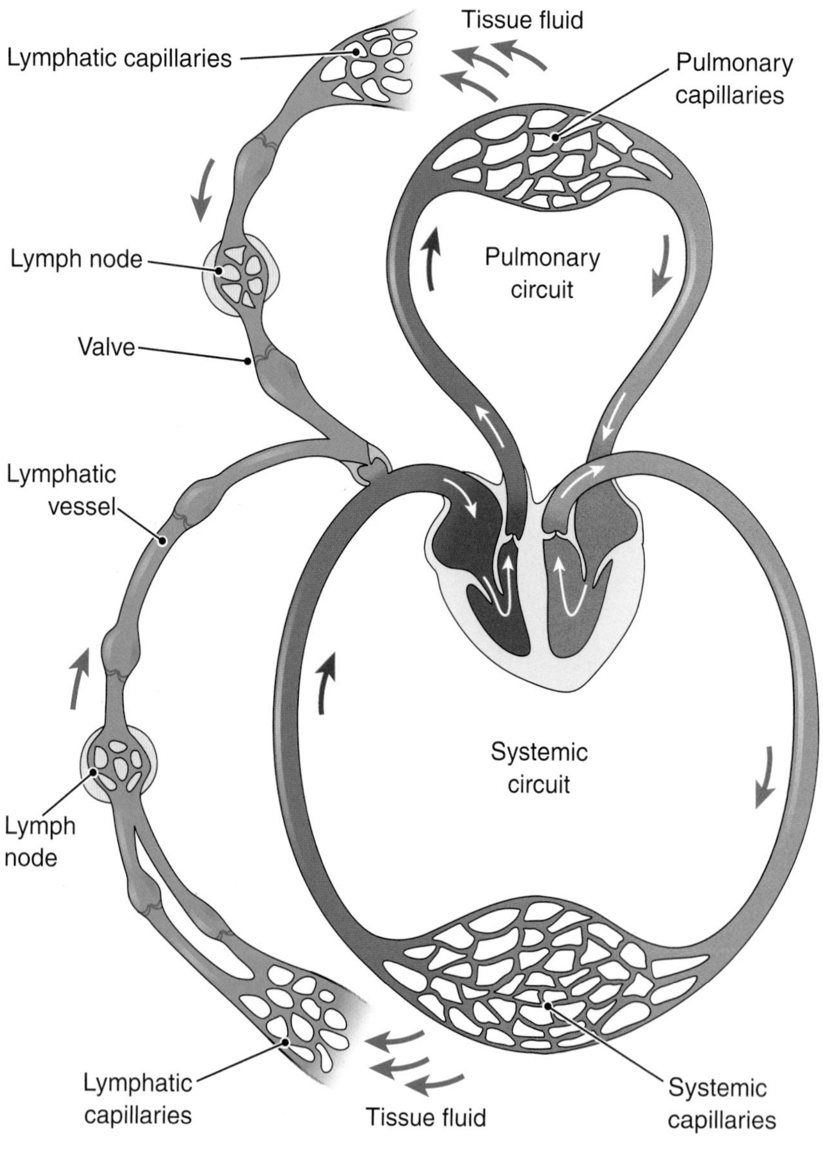

Checkpoint 15-1 What are three functions of the lymphatic system?

Figure 15-1 The lymphatic system in relation to the cardiovascular system. Lymphatic vessels pick up fluid in the tissues and return it to the blood in vessels near the heart. *ZOOMING IN ✦ What type of blood vessel receives lymph collected from the body?*

◗ Lymphatic Circulation

Lymph travels through a network of small and large channels that are in some ways similar to the blood vessels.

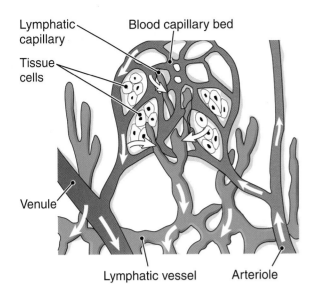

Figure 15-2 **Pathway of lymphatic drainage in the tissues.** Lymphatic capillaries are more permeable than blood capillaries and can pick up fluid and proteins left in the tissues as blood leaves the capillary bed to travel back toward the heart.

However, the system is not a complete circuit. It is a one-way system that begins in the tissues and ends when the lymph joins the blood (see Fig. 15-1).

Lymphatic Capillaries

The walls of the lymphatic capillaries resemble those of the blood capillaries in that they are made of one layer of flattened (squamous) epithelial cells. This thin layer, also called *endothelium*, allows for easy passage of soluble materials and water (Fig. 15-3). The gaps between the endothelial cells in the lymphatic capillaries are larger than

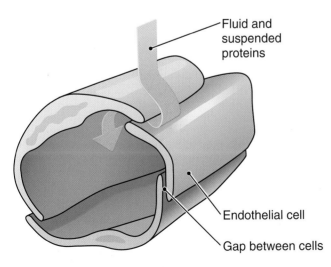

Figure 15-3 **Structure of a lymphatic capillary.** Fluid and proteins can enter the capillary with ease through gaps between the endothelial cells. Overlapping cells act as valves to prevent the material from leaving.

those of the blood capillaries. The lymphatic capillaries are thus more permeable, allowing for easier entrance of relatively large protein particles. The proteins do not move back out of the vessels because the endothelial cells overlap slightly, forming one-way valves to block their return.

Unlike the blood capillaries, the lymphatic capillaries arise blindly; that is, they are closed at one end and do not form a bridge between two larger vessels. Instead, one end simply lies within a lake of tissue fluid, and the other communicates with a larger lymphatic vessel that transports the lymph toward the heart (see Figs. 15-1 and 15-2).

Some specialized lymphatic capillaries located in the lining of the small intestine absorb digested fats. Fats taken into these **lacteals** (LAK-te-als) are transported in the lymphatic vessels until the lymph is added to the blood. More information on the role of the lymphatic system in digestion is found in Chapter 17.

> **Checkpoint 15-2** What are two differences between blood capillaries and lymphatic capillaries?

Lymphatic Vessels

The lymphatic vessels are thin walled and delicate and have a beaded appearance because of indentations where valves are located (see Fig. 15-1). These valves prevent back flow in the same way as do those found in some veins.

Lymphatic vessels (Fig. 15-4) include **superficial** and **deep** sets. The surface lymphatics are immediately below the skin, often lying near the superficial veins. The deep vessels are usually larger and accompany the deep veins.

Lymphatic vessels are named according to location. For example, those in the breast are called **mammary** lymphatic vessels, those in the thigh are called **femoral** lymphatic vessels, and those in the leg are called **tibial** lymphatic vessels. At certain points, the vessels drain through lymph nodes, small masses of lymphatic tissue that filter the lymph. The nodes are in groups that serve a particular region. For example, nearly all the lymph from the upper extremity and the breast passes through the **axillary lymph nodes**, whereas lymph from the lower extremity passes through the **inguinal nodes**. Lymphatic vessels carrying lymph away from the regional nodes eventually drain into one of two terminal vessels, the right lymphatic duct or the thoracic duct, both of which empty into the bloodstream.

The Right Lymphatic Duct The **right lymphatic duct** is a short vessel, about 1.25 cm (1/2 inch) long, that receives only the lymph that comes from the superior right quadrant of the body: the right side of the head, neck, and thorax, as well as the right upper extremity. It empties into the right subclavian vein near the heart (see Fig. 15-4 B). Its opening into this vein is guarded by two

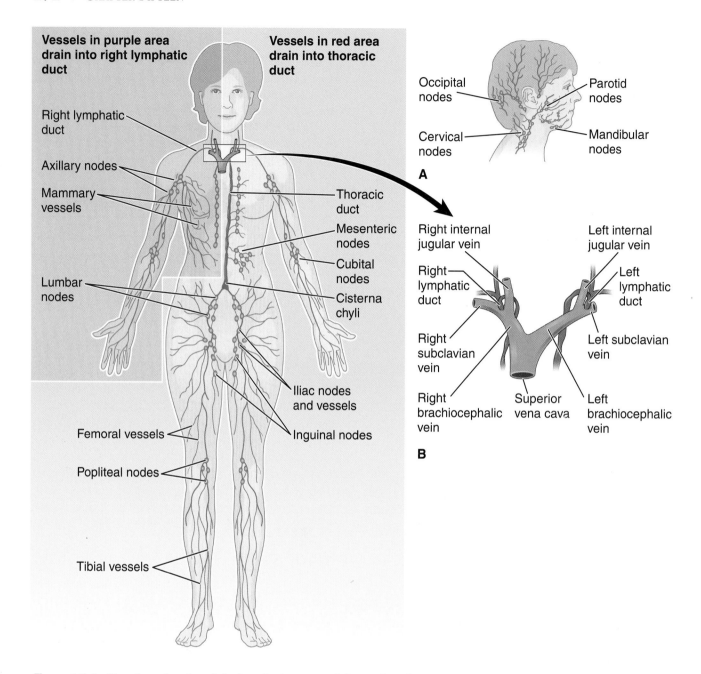

Figure 15-4 **Vessels and nodes of the lymphatic system.** **(A)** Lymph nodes and vessels of the head. **(B)** Drainage of right lymphatic duct and thoracic duct into subclavian veins.

pocket-like semilunar valves to prevent blood from entering the duct. The rest of the body is drained by the thoracic duct.

The Thoracic Duct The **thoracic duct**, or left lymphatic duct, is the larger of the two terminal vessels, measuring about 40 cm (16 inches) in length. As shown in Figure 15-4, the thoracic duct receives lymph from all parts of the body except those above the diaphragm on the right side. This duct begins in the posterior part of the abdominal cavity, below the attachment of the diaphragm. The first part of the duct is enlarged to form a

cistern, or temporary storage pouch, called the **cisterna chyli** (sis-TER-nah KI-li). **Chyle** (kile) is the milky fluid that drains from the intestinal lacteals, and is formed by the combination of fat globules and lymph. Chyle passes through the intestinal lymphatic vessels and the lymph nodes of the mesentery, finally entering the cisterna chyli. In addition to chyle, all the lymph from below the diaphragm empties into the cisterna chyli, passing through the various clusters of lymph nodes. The thoracic duct then carries this lymph into the bloodstream.

The thoracic duct extends upward through the diaphragm and along the posterior wall of the thorax into the base of the neck on the left side. Here, it receives the left jugular lymphatic vessels from the head and neck, the left subclavian vessels from the left upper extremity, and other lymphatic vessels from the thorax and its parts. In addition to the valves along the duct, there are two valves at its opening into the left subclavian vein to prevent the passage of blood into the duct.

> **Checkpoint 15-3** What are the two main lymphatic vessels?

Movement of Lymph

The segments of lymphatic vessels located between the valves contract rhythmically, propelling the lymph along. The contraction rate is related to the volume of fluid in the vessel—the more fluid, the more rapid the contractions.

Lymph is also moved by the same mechanisms that promote venous return of blood to the heart. As skeletal muscles contract during movement, they compress the lymphatic vessels and drive lymph forward. Changes in pressures within the abdominal and thoracic cavities caused by breathing aid the movement of lymph during passage through these body cavities.

▶ Lymphoid Tissue

Lymphoid (LIM-foyd) **tissue** is distributed throughout the body and makes up the specialized organs of the lymphatic system. The lymph nodes have already been described relative to describing lymphatic circulation, but these tissues and other components of the lymphatic system are discussed in greater detail in the next section.

Lymph Nodes

The lymph nodes, as noted, are designed to filter the lymph once it is drained from the tissues (Fig. 15-5). They are also sites where lymphocytes of the immune system multiply and work to combat foreign organisms. The lymph nodes are small, rounded masses varying from pinhead size to as long as 2.5 cm (1 inch). Each has a fibrous connective tissue capsule from which partitions (trabeculae) extend into the substance of the node. At various points in the node's surface, afferent lymphatic vessels pierce the capsule to carry lymph into

the node. An indented area called the **hilum** (HI-lum) is the exit point for efferent lymphatic vessels carrying lymph out of the node. At this region, other structures, including blood vessels and nerves, connect with the node.

Each node is subdivided into lymph-filled spaces (sinuses) and cords of lymphatic tissue. Pulplike nodules in the outer region, or cortex, have germinal centers where certain immune lymphocytes multiply. The inner region,

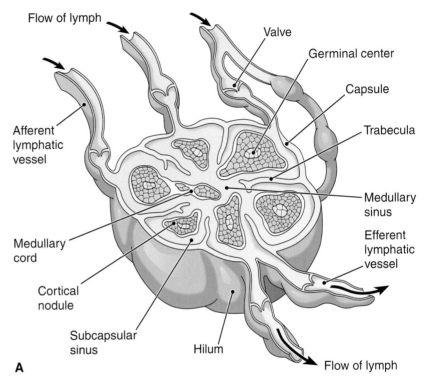

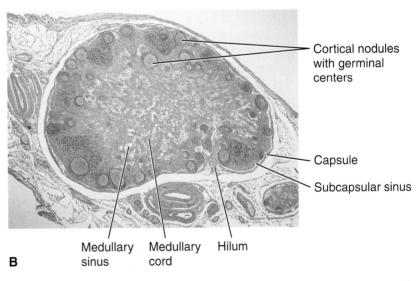

Figure 15-5 Structure of a lymph node. (A) Arrows indicate the flow of lymph through the node. **(B)** Section of a lymph node as seen under the microscope (low power). (B, Reprinted with permission from Cormack DH. Essential Histology. 2nd ed. Philadelphia: Lippincott Williams & Wilkins, 2001.) *ZOOMING IN ✦ What type of lymphatic vessel carries lymph into a node? What type of lymphatic vessel carries lymph out of a node?*

the medulla, has populations of immune cells, including lymphocytes and macrophages (phagocytes) along open channels that lead into the efferent vessels.

Lymph nodes are seldom isolated. As a rule, they are massed together in groups, varying in number from 2 or 3 to well over 100. Some of these groups are placed deeply, whereas others are superficial. The main groups include the following:

▸ **Cervical nodes**, located in the neck in deep and superficial groups, drain various parts of the head and neck. They often become enlarged during upper respiratory infections.
▸ **Axillary nodes**, located in the axillae (armpits), may become enlarged after infections of the upper extremities and the breasts. Cancer cells from the breasts often metastasize (spread) to the axillary nodes.
▸ **Tracheobronchial** (tra-ke-o-BRONG-ke-al) **nodes** are found near the trachea and around the larger bronchial tubes. In people living in highly polluted areas, these nodes become so filled with carbon particles that they are solid black masses resembling pieces of coal.
▸ **Mesenteric** (mes-en-TER-ik) **nodes** are found between the two layers of peritoneum that form the mesentery (membrane around the intestines). There are some 100 to 150 of these nodes.
▸ **Inguinal nodes**, located in the groin region, receive lymph drainage from the lower extremities and from the external genital organs. When they become enlarged, they are often referred to as **buboes** (BU-bose), from which bubonic plague got its name.

Box 15-1 explains lymph node biopsy's role in the treatment of cancer.

Checkpoint 15-4 What is the function of the lymph nodes?

The Spleen

The spleen is an organ that contains lymphoid tissue designed to filter blood. It is located in the superior left hypochondriac region of the abdomen, high up under the dome of the diaphragm, and normally is protected by the lower part of the rib cage (Fig. 15-6). The spleen is a soft, purplish, and somewhat flattened organ, measuring about 12.5 to 16 cm (5 to 6 inches) long and 5 to 7.5 cm (2 to 3 inches) wide. The capsule of the spleen, as well as its framework, is more elastic than that of the lymph nodes. It contains involuntary muscle, which enables the splenic capsule to contract and also to withstand some swelling.

Considering its size, the spleen has an unusually large blood supply. The organ is filled with a soft pulp that filters the blood. It also harbors phagocytes and lymphocytes, which are active in immunity. The spleen is classified as part of the lymphatic system because it contains prominent masses of lymphoid tissue. However, it has wider functions than other lymphatic structures, including the following:

▸ Cleansing the blood of impurities and cellular debris by filtration and phagocytosis.
▸ Destroying old, worn-out red blood cells. The iron and other breakdown products of hemoglobin are carried to the liver by the hepatic portal system to be reused or eliminated from the body.
▸ Producing red blood cells before birth.
▸ Serving as a reservoir for blood, which can be returned to the bloodstream in case of hemorrhage or other emergency.

Box 15-1	Hot Topics

Sentinel Node Biopsy: Finding Cancer Before it Spreads

Ordinarily, the lymphatic system is one of the body's primary defenses against disease. In cancer, though, it can be a vehicle for the spread (metastasis) of disease. When cancer cells enter the lymphatic vessels, they travel to other parts of the body, where they may establish new tumors. Along the way, some cancer cells become lodged in the lymph nodes.

In breast cancer, the degree of invasion of nearby lymph nodes helps determine what treatments are required after surgical removal of the tumor. Until recently, a mastectomy often included the removal of nearby lymphatic vessels and nodes (a procedure called axillary lymph node dissection). Biopsy of the nodes determined whether or not they contained cancerous cells, and if they did, radiation treatment or chemotherapy was required. In many women with early-stage breast cancer, however, the axillary bodies do not contain cancerous cells. In addition, about 20 percent of the women whose lymphatic

vessels and nodes have been removed suffer impaired lymph flow. The results are lymphedema, pain, disability, and an increased risk of infection.

Sentinel node biopsy is a new diagnostic procedure that may minimize the need to perform axillary lymph node dissection, while still detecting metastasis. Surgeons use radioactive tracers to identify the first nodes that receive lymph from the area of a tumor. Biopsy of only these "sentinel nodes" reveals whether tumor cells are present, providing the earliest indication of metastasis. Research shows that sentinel lymph node biopsy is associated with less pain, fewer complications, and faster recovery than axillary lymph node dissection. However, because the procedure is relatively new, more clinical trials are required to determine whether sentinel node biopsy is as successful as axillary dissection in finding cancer before it spreads.

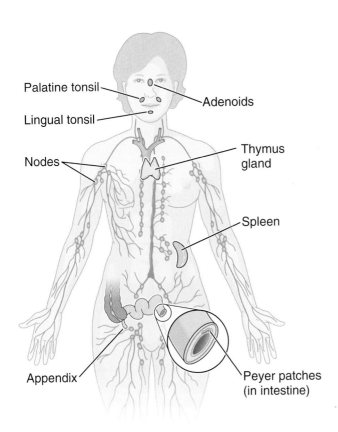

Figure 15-6 Location of lymphoid tissue.

Checkpoint 15-5 What is filtered by the spleen?

The Thymus

Because of its appearance under a microscope, the **thymus** (THI-mus), located in the superior thorax beneath the sternum, traditionally has been considered part of the lymphoid system (see Fig. 15-6). Recent studies, however, suggest that this structure has a much wider function than other lymphoid tissue. It appears that the thymus plays a key role in immune system development before birth and during the first few months of infancy. Certain lymphocytes must mature in the thymus gland before they can perform their functions in the immune system. These T cells (T lymphocytes) develop under the effects of the thymus gland hormone called **thymosin** (THI-mo-sin), which also promotes lymphocyte growth and activity in lymphoid tissue throughout the body. Removal of the thymus causes a decrease in the production of T cells, as well as a decrease in the size of the spleen and of lymph nodes throughout the body.

The thymus is most active during early life. After puberty, the tissue undergoes changes; it shrinks in size and is replaced by connective tissue and fat.

Checkpoint 15-6 What kind of immune system cells develop in the thymus?

The Tonsils

The **tonsils** are masses of lymphoid tissue located in the vicinity of the pharynx (throat) where they remove contaminants from materials that are inhaled or swallowed (Fig. 15-7). The tonsils have deep grooves lined with lymphatic nodules. Lymphocytes attack pathogens trapped in these grooves. The tonsils are located in three areas:

1. The **palatine** (PAL-ah-tine) **tonsils** are oval bodies located at each side of the soft palate. These are generally what is meant when one refers to "the tonsils."
2. The single **pharyngeal** (fah-RIN-je-al) **tonsil** is commonly referred to as the **adenoids** (from a general term that means "gland-like"). It is located behind the nose on the posterior wall of the upper pharynx.
3. The **lingual** (LING-gwal) **tonsils** are little mounds of lymphoid tissue at the back of the tongue.

Any of these tonsils may become so loaded with bacteria that they become reservoirs for repeated infections and their removal is advisable. In children, a slight enlargement of any of them is not an indication for surgery, however, because all lymphoid tissue masses tend to be larger in childhood. A physician must determine whether these masses are abnormally enlarged, taking the patient's age into account, because the tonsils function in immunity during early childhood.

Checkpoint 15-7 Tonsils filter tissue fluid. What is the general location of the tonsils?

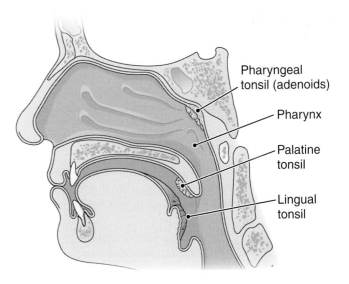

Figure 15-7 Location of the tonsils. All are in the vicinity of the pharynx (throat).

Other Lymphoid Tissue

The **appendix** (ah-PEN-diks) is a fingerlike tube of lymphatic tissue, measuring about about 8 cm (3 in.) long, and is attached, or "appended" to the first portion of the large intestine (see Fig. 15-6). Like the tonsils, it seems to be noticed only when it becomes infected, causing appendicitis. The appendix may, however, figure in the development of immunity, as do the tonsils.

In the mucous membranes lining portions of the digestive, respiratory, and urogenital tracts there are areas of lymphatic tissue that help destroy outside contaminants. By means of phagocytosis and production of antibodies, substances that counteract infectious agents, this **mucosal-associated lymphoid tissue**, or MALT, prevents microorganisms from invading deeper tissues.

Peyer (PI-er) **patches** are part of the MALT system. These clusters of lymphatic nodules are located in the mucous membranes lining the small intestine's distal portion. Peyer patches, along with the tonsils and appendix, are included in the specific network known as GALT, or gut-associated lymphoid tissue. All of these lymphatic tissues associated with mucous membranes are now recognized as an important first barrier against invading microorganisms.

▶ The Reticuloendothelial System

The **reticuloendothelial** (reh-tik-u-lo-en-do-THE-le-al) **system** consists of related cells responsible for the destruction of worn-out blood cells, bacteria, cancer cells, and other foreign substances that are potentially harmful to the body. Included among these cells are monocytes, relatively large white blood cells (see Fig. 12-4 E in Chapter 12) that are formed in the bone marrow and then circulate in the bloodstream to various parts of the body. Upon entering the tissues, monocytes develop into **macrophages** (MAK-ro-faj-ez), a term that means "big eaters."

Macrophages in some organs are given special names; **Kupffer** (KOOP-fer) cells, for example, are located in the lining of the liver sinusoids (blood channels). Other parts of the reticuloendothelial system are found in the spleen, bone marrow, lymph nodes, and brain. Some macrophages are located in the lungs, where they are called *dust cells* because they ingest solid particles that enter the lungs; others are found in soft connective tissues all over the body.

This widely distributed protective system has been called by several other names, including tissue macrophage system, mononuclear phagocyte system, and monocyte-macrophage system. These names describe the type of cells found within this system.

▶ Body Defenses Against Disease

The body is constantly exposed to harmful organisms such as bacteria and viruses. Fortunately, most of us survive contact with these invaders and even become more resistant to disease in the process. The job of protecting us from these harmful agents belongs in part to certain blood cells and to the lymphatic system, which together make up our **immune** system.

The immune system is part of our general body defenses against disease. Some of these defenses are **nonspecific**; that is, they are effective against any harmful agent that enters the body. Other defenses are referred to as **specific**; that is, they act only against a certain agent and no others.

▶ Nonspecific Defenses

The features that protect the body against disease are usually considered as successive "lines of defense," beginning with the relatively simple or outer barriers and proceeding through progressively more complicated responses until the ultimate defense mechanism—immunity—is reached.

Chemical and Mechanical Barriers

Part of the first line of defense against invaders is the skin, which serves as a mechanical barrier as long as it remains intact. A serious danger to burn victims, for example, is the risk of infection as a result of skin destruction.

The mucous membranes that line the passageways leading into the body also act as barriers, trapping foreign material in their sticky secretions. The cilia in membranes in the upper respiratory tract help to sweep impurities out of the body.

Body secretions, such as tears, perspiration, and saliva, wash away microorganisms and may contain acids, enzymes, or other chemicals that destroy invaders. Digestive juices destroy many ingested bacteria and their toxins.

Certain reflexes aid in the removal of pathogens. Sneezing and coughing, for instance, tend to remove foreign matter, including microorganisms, from the upper respiratory tract. Vomiting and diarrhea are ways in which toxins and bacteria may be expelled.

Checkpoint 15-8 What tissues constitute the first line of defense against the invasion of pathogens?

Phagocytosis

Phagocytosis is part of the second line of defense against invaders. In the process of phagocytosis, white blood cells take in and destroy waste and foreign material (see Fig.

12-6 in Chapter 12). Neutrophils and macrophages are the main phagocytic white blood cells. Neutrophils are a type of granular leukocyte. Macrophages are derived from monocytes, a type of agranular leukocyte. Both types of cells travel in the blood to infection sites. Some of the macrophages remain fixed in the tissues, for example, in the skin, liver, lungs, lymphoid tissue, and bone marrow, to fight infection and remove debris.

Natural Killer Cells

The **natural killer (NK) cell** is a type of lymphocyte different from those active in specific immunity, which are described later. NK cells can recognize body cells with abnormal membranes, such as tumor cells and cells infected with virus, and, as their name indicates, can destroy them on contact. NK cells are found in the lymph nodes, spleen, bone marrow, and blood. They destroy abnormal cells by secreting a protein that breaks down the cell membrane, but the way in which they find their targets is not yet completely understood.

Inflammation

Inflammation is the body's effort to get rid of anything that irritates it or, if this is not possible, to limit the harmful effects of the irritant. Inflammation can occur as a result of any irritant, not only microorganisms. Friction, fire, chemicals, x-rays, and cuts or blows all can be classified as irritants. If irritation is caused by pathogenic invasion, the resulting inflammation is termed an **infection.** With the entrance of pathogens and their subsequent multiplication, a whole series of defensive processes begins. This **inflammatory reaction** is accompanied by four classic symptoms: heat, redness, swelling, and pain, as described below.

When tissues are injured, **histamine** (HIS-tah-mene) and other substances are released from the damaged cells, causing the small blood vessels to dilate (widen). More blood then flows into the area, resulting in heat, redness, and swelling.

With the increased blood flow come a vast number of leukocytes. Then a new phenomenon occurs: the walls of the tiny blood vessels become "coarsened" in texture (as does a piece of cloth when it is stretched). Blood flow slows down, and the leukocytes move through these altered walls and into the tissue, where they can reach the irritant directly. Fluid from the blood plasma also leaks out of the vessels into the tissues and begins to clot.

When this response occurs in a local area, it helps prevent the spread of the foreign agent. The mixture of leukocytes and fluid, the **inflammatory exudate,** causes pressure on the nerve endings, which combined with the increased amount of blood in the vessels, causes the pain of inflammation.

As the phagocytes do their work, large numbers of them are destroyed, so that eventually the area becomes filled with dead leukocytes. The mixture of exudate, living and dead white blood cells, pathogens, and destroyed tissue cells is **pus.**

Meanwhile, the lymphatic vessels begin to drain fluid from the inflamed area and carry it toward the lymph nodes for filtration. The regional lymph nodes become enlarged and tender, a sign that they are performing their protective function by working overtime to produce phagocytic cells that "clean" the lymph flowing through them.

Fever

An increase in body temperature above the normal range can be a sign that body defenses are at work. When phagocytes are exposed to infecting organisms, they release substances that raise body temperature. Fever boosts the immune system in several ways. It stimulates phagocytes, increases metabolism, and decreases certain organisms' ability to multiply.

A common misperception is that fever is a dangerous symptom that should always be eliminated. Control of fever in itself does little to alter the course of an illness.

Interferon

Certain cells infected with a virus release a substance that prevents nearby cells from producing more virus. This substance was first found in cells infected with influenza virus, and it was called **interferon** because it "interferes" with multiplication and spread of the virus. Interferon is now known to be a group of substances. Each is abbreviated IFN with a Greek letter, alpha (α), beta (β), or gamma (γ) to indicate the category of interferon and additional letters or numbers to indicate more specific types, such as α2a or β1b.

> **Checkpoint 15-9** What are some nonspecific factors that help to control infection?

▶ Specific Defenses—Immunity

Immunity is the final line of defense against disease. Immunity to disease can be defined as an individual's power to resist or overcome the effects of a *particular* disease agent or its harmful products. In a broader sense, the immune system will recognize *any* foreign material and attempt to rid the body of it, as occurs in tissue transplantation from one individual to another. Immunity is a selective process; that is, immunity to one disease does not necessarily cause immunity to another. This selective characteristic is called **specificity** (spes-ih-FIS-ih-te).

There are two main categories of immunity:

1. **Inborn immunity** is inherited along with other characteristics in a person's genes.
2. **Acquired immunity** develops after birth. Acquired immunity may be obtained by **natural** or **artificial** means; in addition, acquired immunity may be either **active** or **passive**.

Figure 15-8 summarizes the different types of immunity. Refer to this diagram as we investigate each category in turn.

Inborn Immunity

Both humans and animals have what is called a **species immunity** to many of each other's diseases. Although certain diseases found in animals may be transmitted to humans, many infections, such as chicken cholera, hog cholera, distemper, and other animal diseases, do not affect human beings. However, the constitutional differences that make human beings immune to these disorders also make them susceptible to others that do not affect different species. Such infections as measles, scarlet fever and diphtheria do not appear to affect animals who come in contact with infected humans.

Some members of a given group have a more highly developed **individual immunity** to specific diseases. For example, some people are prone to cold sores (fever blisters) caused by herpes virus, whereas others have never shown signs of this type of infection. Newspapers and magazines sometimes feature the advice of an elderly person who is asked to give his or her secret for living to a ripe old age. Some elderly people may say that they lived a carefully regulated life with the right amount of rest, exercise, and work, whereas others may boast of drinking alcohol, smoking, not exercising, and other kinds of unhealthy behavior. However, it is possible that the latter group resisted infection and maintained health despite their habits, rather than because of them, thanks to inherited resistance factors.

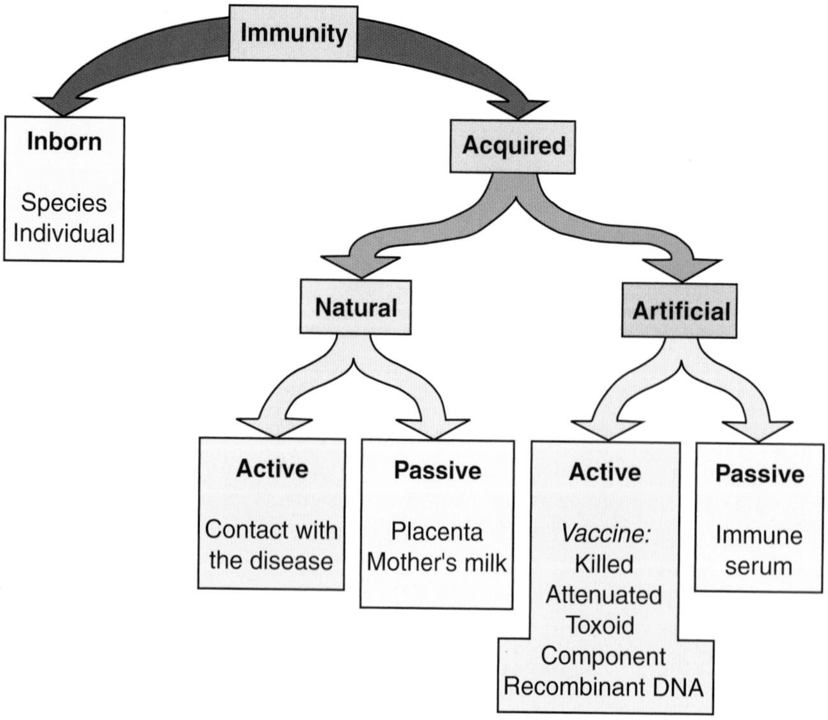

Acquired Immunity

Unlike inborn immunity, which is due to inherited factors, acquired immunity develops during a person's lifetime as that person encounters various specific harmful agents.

If the following description of the immune system seems complex, bear in mind that from infancy on, your immune system is able to protect you from millions of foreign substances, even synthetic substances not found in nature. All the while, the system is kept in check, so that it does not usually overreact to produce allergies or mistakenly attack and damage your own body tissues.

Checkpoint 15-10 What is the difference between inborn and acquired immunity?

Antigens An **antigen** (AN-te-jen) (**Ag**) is any foreign substance that enters the body and induces an immune response. (The word is formed from *anti*body + *gen* because an antigen stimulates production of antibody). Most antigens are large protein molecules, but carbohydrates and some lipids may act as antigens. Antigens may be found on the surface of pathogenic organisms, on the surface of red blood cells and tissue cells, on pollens, in toxins, and in foods. The critical feature of any substance described as an antigen is that it stimulates the activity of certain lymphocytes classified as T or B cells.

T Cells Both T and B cells come from hematopoietic (blood-forming) stem cells in bone marrow, as do all blood cells. The T and B cells differ, however, in their development and their method of action. Some of the immature stem cells migrate to the thymus and become T cells, which constitute about 80% of the lymphocytes in the circulating blood. While in the thymus, these T lymphocytes multiply and become capable of combining with spe-

Figure 15-8 **Types of immunity.**

cific foreign antigens, at which time they are described as **sensitized**. These thymus-derived cells produce an immunity that is said to be **cell-mediated** immunity.

There are several types of T cells, each with different functions. The different types of T cells and some of their functions are as follows:

▶ **Cytotoxic T cells** (T_c) destroy foreign cells directly.
▶ **Helper T cells** (T_h) release substances known as **interleukins** (in-ter-LU-kinz) (IL) that stimulate other lymphocytes and macrophages and thereby assist in the destruction of foreign cells. (These substances are so named because they act between white blood cells). There are several subtypes of these helper T cells, one of which is infected and destroyed by the AIDS virus (HIV). The HIV-targeted T cells have a special surface receptor (CD_4) to which the virus attaches.
▶ **Regulatory T cells** (T_{reg}) suppress the immune response in order to prevent overactivity. These T cells may inhibit or destroy active lymphocytes.
▶ **Memory T cells** remember an antigen and start a rapid response if that antigen is contacted again.

The T cell portion of the immune system is generally responsible for defense against cancer cells, certain viruses, and other pathogens that grow within cells (intracellular parasites), as well as for the rejection of tissue transplanted from another person.

The Role of Macrophages **Macrophages** are phagocytic white blood cells derived from monocytes (their name means "big eater"). They act as processing centers for foreign antigens. They ingest foreign proteins, such as disease organisms, and break them down within phagocytic vesicles (Fig. 15-9). They then insert fragments of the foreign antigen into their plasma membrane. The foreign antigens are displayed on the macrophage's surface

in combination with antigens that a T cell can recognize as belonging to the "self." Self antigens are known as MHC (major histocompatibility complex) antigens because of their importance in cross-matching for tissue transplantation. They are also known as HLAs (human leukocyte antigens), because white blood cells are used in testing tissues for compatibility. Macrophages and other cells that present antigens to T cells are known as APCs (antigen-presenting cells).

For a T cell to react with a foreign antigen, that antigen must be presented to the T cell along with the MHC proteins. A special receptor on the T cell must bind with both the MHC protein and the foreign antigen fragment (see Fig. 15-9). The activated T_h then produces interleukins (ILs), which stimulate other leukocytes, such a s B cells. There are many different types of interleukins, and they participate at different points in the immune response. They are produced by white cells and also by fibroblasts (cells in connective tissue that produce fibers) and by epithelial cells. Because ILs stimulate the cells active in immunity, they are used medically to boost the immune system.

Checkpoint 15-11 What is an antigen?

Checkpoint 15-12 List four types of T cells.

B Cells and Antibodies An **antibody** (**Ab**), also known as an **immunoglobulin** (**Ig**), is a substance produced in response to an antigen. Antibodies are manufactured by **B cells** (B lymphocytes), another type of lymphocyte active in the immune system. These cells must mature in the fetal liver or in lymphoid tissue before becoming active in the blood.

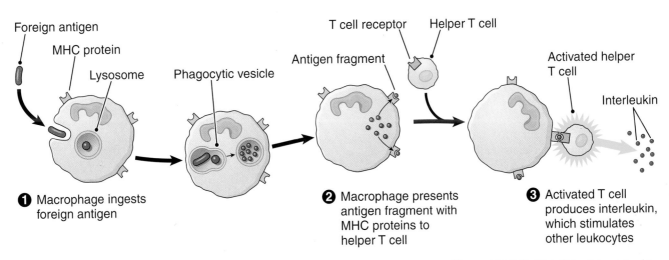

Foreign antigen
MHC protein
Lysosome

Phagocytic vesicle

T cell receptor   Helper T cell
Antigen fragment

Activated helper T cell
Interleukin

❶ Macrophage ingests foreign antigen

❷ Macrophage presents antigen fragment with MHC proteins to helper T cell

❸ Activated T cell produces interleukin, which stimulates other leukocytes

Figure 15-9 **Activation of a helper T cell by a macrophage (antigen-presenting cell).** *ZOOMING IN* ✦ *What is contained in the phagocytic vesicle in step 2?*

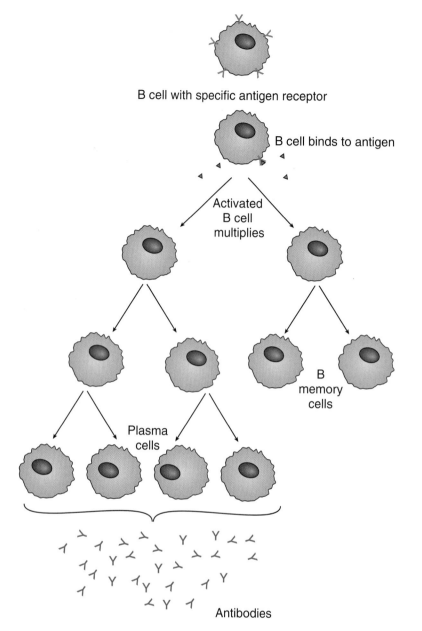

B cell with specific antigen receptor

B cell binds to antigen

Activated
B cell
multiplies

B
memory
cells

Plasma
cells

Antibodies

Figure 15-10 **Activation of B cells.** The B cell combines with a specific antigen. The cell divides to form plasma cells, which produce antibodies. Some of the cells develop into memory cells, which protect against reinfection. *ZOOMING IN ✦ What two types of cells develop from activated B cells?*

B cells have surface receptors that bind with a specific type of antigen (Fig. 15-10). Exposure to the antigen stimulates the cells to multiply rapidly and produce large numbers (clones) of **plasma cells**. Plasma cells produce antibodies against the original antigen and release these antibodies into the blood, providing the form of immunity described as **humoral immunity** (the term humoral refers to body fluids).

Humoral immunity generally protects against circulating antigens and bacteria that grow outside the cells (extracellular pathogens). All antibodies are contained in a portion of the blood plasma called the **gamma globulin** fraction. Box

15-2 provides further information about the different types of antibodies.

Some antibodies produced by B cells remain in the blood to give long-term immunity. In addition, some of the activated B cells do not become plasma cells but, like certain T cells, become memory cells. On repeated contact with an antigen, these cells are ready to produce antibodies immediately. Because of this "immunologic memory," one is usually immune to a childhood disease after having it.

> Checkpoint 15-13 What is an antibody?

> Checkpoint 15-14 What type of cells produce antibodies?

The Antigen–Antibody Reaction

The antibody that is produced in response to a specific antigen, such as a bacterial cell or a toxin, has a shape that matches some part of that antigen, much in the same way that the shape of a key matches the shape of its lock. The antibody can bind specifically to the antigen that caused its production and thereby destroy or inactivate it. Antigen-antibody interactions are illustrated and their protective effects are described in Table 15-1.

Complement The destruction of foreign cells sometimes requires the enzymatic activity of a group of nonspecific proteins in the blood, together called **complement**. Complement proteins are always present in the blood, but they must be activated by antigen-antibody complexes or by foreign cell surfaces. Complement is so named because it assists with immune reactions. Some of the actions of complement are:

▶ It coats foreign cells to help phagocytes recognize and engulf them.
▶ It destroys cells by forming complexes that punch holes in plasma membranes.
▶ It promotes inflammation by increasing capillary permeability.
▶ It attracts phagocytes to an area of inflammation.

> Checkpoint 15-15 What is complement?

Box 15-2	A Closer Look

Antibodies: A Protein Army That Fights Disease

Antibodies are proteins secreted by plasma cells (activated B cells) in response to specific antigens. They are all contained in a fraction of the blood plasma known as gamma globulin. Because the plasma contains other globulins as well, antibodies have become known as immunoglobulins (Ig). Immunologic studies have shown that there are several classes of immunoglobulins that vary in molecular size and in function (see below). Studies of these antibody fractions can be helpful in making a diagnosis. For example, high levels of IgM antibodies, because they are the first to be produced in an immune response, indicate a recent infection.

CLASS	ABUNDANCE	CHARACTERISTICS AND FUNCTION
IgG	75%	Found in the blood, lymph, and intestines
		Enhances phagocytosis, neutralizes toxins, and activates complement
		Crosses the placenta and confers passive immunity from mother to fetus
IgA	15%	Found in glandular secretions such as sweat, tears, saliva, mucus, and digestive juices
		Provides local protection in mucous membranes against bacteria and viruses
		Also found in breast milk, providing passive immunity to newborn
IgM	5%–10%	Found in the blood and lymph
		The first antibody to be secreted after infection
		Stimulates agglutination and activates complement
IgD	<1%	Located on the surface of B cells
IgE	<0.1%	Located on basophils
		Active in allergic reactions and parasitic infections

Naturally Acquired Immunity

Immunity may be acquired naturally through contact with a specific disease organism, in which case, antibodies manufactured by the infected person's cells act against the infecting agent or its toxins. The infection that triggers the immunity may be so mild as to cause no symptoms (subclinical). Nevertheless, it stimulates the host's cells to produce an active immunity.

Each time a person is invaded by disease organisms, his or her cells manufacture antibodies that provide immunity against the infection. Such immunity may last for years, and in some cases for life. Because the host is actively involved in the production of antibodies, this type of immunity is called **active immunity**. See Box 15-3 for information on how stress affects the immune system.

Immunity also may be acquired naturally by the passage of antibodies from a mother to her fetus through the placenta. Because these antibodies come from an outside source, this type of immunity is called **passive immunity**. The antibodies obtained in this way do not last as long as actively produced antibodies, but they do help protect the infant for about 6 months, at which time the child's own immune system begins to function. Nursing an infant can lengthen this protective period because of the presence of specific antibodies in breast milk and colostrum (the first breast secretion). These are the only known examples of naturally acquired passive immunity.

Checkpoint 15-16 What is the difference between the active and passive forms of naturally acquired immunity?

Artificially Acquired Immunity

A person who has not been exposed to repeated small doses of a particular organism has no antibodies against that organism and may be defenseless against. Therefore, medical personnel may use artificial measures to cause a person's immune system to manufacture antibodies. The administration of virulent pathogens obviously would be dangerous. Instead, laboratory workers treat the harmful agent to reduce its virulence before it is administered. In this way, the immune system is made to produce antibodies without causing a serious illness. This protective

Table 15·1	Antigen-Antibody Interactions and Their Effects	
Interaction	**Effects**	
Prevention of attachment	A pathogen coated with antibody is prevented from attaching to a cell.	
Clumping of antigen	Antibodies can link antigens together, forming a cluster that phagocytes can ingest.	
Neutralization of toxins	Antibodies bind to toxin molecules to prevent them from damaging cells.	
Help with phagocytosis	Phagocytes can attach more easily to antigens that are coated with antibody.	
Activation of complement	When complement attaches to antibody on a cell surface, a series of reactions begins that activates complement to destroy cells.	
Activation of NK cells	NK cells respond to antibody adhering to a cell surface and attack the cell.	

process is known as **vaccination** (vak-sin-A-shun), or **immunization**, and the solution used is called a **vaccine** (vak-SENE). Ordinarily, the administration of a vaccine is a preventive measure designed to provide protection in anticipation of invasion by a certain disease organism.

Types of Vaccines Vaccines can be made with live organisms or with organisms killed by heat or chemicals. If live organisms are used, they must be nonvirulent for humans, such as the cowpox virus used for smallpox immunization, or they must be treated in the laboratory to weaken them as human pathogens. An organism weakened for use in vaccines is described as **attenuated**. In some cases, just an antigenic component of the pathogen is used as a vaccine. Another type of vaccine is made from the toxin produced by a disease organism. The toxin is altered with heat or chemicals to reduce its harmfulness, but it can still function as an antigen to induce immunity. Such an altered toxin is called a **toxoid**.

The newest types of vaccines are produced from antigenic components of pathogens or by genetic engineering. By techniques of recombinant DNA, the genes for specific disease antigens are inserted into the genetic material of harmless organisms. The antigens produced by these organisms are extracted

Box 15-3 | **Clinical Perspectives**

Too Much Stress Makes The Immune System Sick

The impact of stress on the immune system is the most wide-ranging and significant of its many effects on the body. Stressors such as trauma, infection, debilitating disease, surgery, pain, extreme environmental conditions, and emotional distress all hamper immune function. The mechanisms responsible for these changes are not yet fully understood. Scientists do know that stress causes the hypothalamus to promote the release of ACTH from the anterior pituitary. This hormone stimulates the adrenal cortex to release the hormone cortisol, which influences a person's immediate ability to overcome any challenge, even stress itself. However, the abnormally high levels of cortisol that appear during periods of intense stress can actually be harmful. Such levels can:

- inhibit histamine release from damaged tissues, thereby blocking inflammation and the arrival of phagocytic leukocytes.
- reduce phagocytosis in damaged tissues, thus preventing antigen presentation to (and activation of) both killer T cells and helper T cells.
- inhibit interleukin secretion from helper T cells, thus preventing the immune system from mounting a coordinated response to infection.

Box 11-3, Stress: Mechanisms for Coping, suggests some strategies for reducing stress.

Table 15·2 Childhood Immunizations[a]

VACCINE	DISEASE(S)	SCHEDULE
DTaP	Diphtheria, tetanus, pertussis (whooping cough)	2, 4, 6, and 15–18 months; booster at 4–6 years; diphtheria and tetanus toxoid (Td) at 11–12 years
Hib	*Haemophilus influenza* type b (spinal meningitis)	2 and 4 months or 2, 4, and 6 months depending on type used
PCV	Pneumococcus (pneumonia, meningitis)	2, 4, 6, and 12–15 months
MMR	Measles, mumps, rubella	15 months and 4–6 years
HBV	Hepatitis B	Birth, 1–2 months, 6–18 months
Polio vaccine (IPV)	Poliomyelitis	2 and 4 months, 6–18 months, and 4–6 years
Varicella	Chicken pox	12–18 months

[a]*Recommended by the Advisory Committee on Immunization Practices (www.cdc.gov/nip/acip), the American Academy of Pediatrics (www.aap.org) and the American Academy of Family Physicians (www.aafp.org). Information available through the National Immunization Program Website (www2a.cdc.gov/nip).*

and purified and used for immunization. The hepatitis B vaccine is produced in this manner.

Boosters In many cases, an active immunity acquired by artificial (or even natural) means does not last a lifetime. Circulating antibodies can decline with time. To help maintain a high titer (level) of antibodies in the blood, repeated inoculations, called *booster shots,* are ad-ministered at intervals. The number of booster injections recommended varies with the disease and with an individual's environment or range of exposure. On occasion, epidemics in high schools or colleges may prompt recommendations for specific boosters. Table 15-2 lists the vaccines currently recommended in the United States for childhood immunizations. The number and timing of doses varies with the different vaccines.

Passive Immunization It takes several weeks to produce a naturally acquired active immunity and even longer to produce an artificial active immunity through the administration of a vaccine. Therefore, a person who receives a large dose of virulent organisms and has no established immunity to them is in great danger. To prevent illness, the person must quickly receive counteracting antibodies from an outside source. This is accomplished through the administration of an **immune serum,** or **antiserum.** The "ready-made" serum gives short-lived but effective protection against the invaders in the form of an artificially acquired passive immunity. Immune sera are used in emergencies, that is, in situations in which there is no time to wait until an active immunity has developed.

Word Anatomy

Medical terms are built from standardized word parts (prefixes, roots and suffixes). Learning the meanings of these parts can help you remember words and interpret unfamiliar terms.

WORD PART	MEANING	EXAMPLE
Lymphoid Tissue		
–oid	like, resembling	*Lymphoid* tissue makes up the specialized organs of the lymphatic system.
aden/o	gland	The *adenoids* are gland-like tonsils.
lingu/o	tongue	The *lingual* tonsils are at the back of the tongue.

Summary

I. Lymphatic system
A. Functions
1. Fluid balance—drains excess fluid and proteins from the tissues and returns them to the blood
2. Protection from infection
   a. Lymphocytes fight foreign organisms
   b. Lymphoid tissue filters body fluids
3. Absorption of fats—lacteals absorb digested fats from small intestine

II. Lymphatic circulation
A. Lymphatic capillaries
1. Made of endothelium (simple squamous epithelium)
2. More permeable than blood capillaries
3. Overlapping cells form one-way valves
B. Lymphatic vessels
1. Superficial and deep sets
2. Right lymphatic duct
   a. Drains upper right part of body
   b. Empties into right subclavian vein
3. Thoracic duct
   a. Drains remainder of body
   b. Empties into left subclavian vein
C. Movement of lymph
1. Valves in vessels
2. Contraction of vessels
3. Skeletal muscle contraction
4. Breathing

III. Lymphoid tissue—distributed throughout body
A. Lymph nodes
1. Along path of lymphatic vessels
2. Filter lymph
B. Spleen
1. Filtration of blood
2. Destruction of old red cells
3. Production of red cells before birth
4. Storage of blood
C. Thymus
1. Processing of T lymphocytes (T cells)
2. Secretion of thymosin—stimulates T lymphocytes in lymphoid tissue
D. Tonsils
1. Filter swallowed and inhaled material
2. Located near pharynx (throat)
   a. Palatine—near soft palate
   b. Pharyngeal (adenoids)—behind nose
   c. Lingual—back of tongue
E. Other
1. Appendix—attached to large intestine
2. Mucosal—associated lymphoid tissue (MALT)
   a. Gut-associated lymphoid tissue (GALT)
      (1) Example—Peyer patches in lining of small intestine

IV. The reticuloendothelial system
1. Cells throughout body that remove impurities
2. Macrophages
   a. From monocytes
   b. Localize and given special names—*e.g.* Kuppfer cells, dust cells

V. Nonspecific defenses
A. Chemical and mechanical barriers
1. Skin
2. Mucous membranes
3. Body secretions
4. Reflexes—coughing, sneezing, vomiting, diarrhea
B. Phagocytosis—mainly by neutrophils and macrophages
C. Natural killer (NK) cells—attack tumor cells and virus-infected cells
D. Inflammation
E. Fever
F. Interferon
1. Substances released from virus-infected cells
2. Prevent virus production in nearby cells
3. Stimulate the immune response non-specifically

VI. Specific defenses—immunity
A. Inborn immunity
1. Inherited
2. Types: species, individual
B. Acquired immunity—develops after birth
1. Antigens—stimulate immune response by lymphocytes
2. T cells (T lymphocytes)
   a. Processed in thymus
   b. Types: cytotoxic, helper, regulatory, memory
   c. Involved in cell-mediated immunity
3. Macrophages
   a. Derived from monocytes
   b. Present antigen to T cells in combination with MHC ("self") proteins
   c. Stimulate the release of interleukins (IL)
4. B cells (B lymphocytes)
   a. Mature in lymphoid tissue
   b. Develop into plasma cells
      (1) Produce circulating antibodies
      (2) Antibodies counteract antigens
   c. Also develop into memory cells
   d. Involved in humoral immunity
C. The antigen–antibody reaction
1. Shape of antibody matches shape of antigen
2. Results
   a. Prevention of attachment
   b. Clumping of antigen
   c. Neutralization of toxins
   d. Help in phagocytosis
   e. Activation of complement
   f. Activation of NK cells
3. Complement
   a. Group of proteins in blood
   b. Actions
      (1) Coats foreign cells
      (2) Damages plasma membranes
      (3) Promotes inflammation
      (4) Attracts phagocytes

D. Naturally acquired immunity
   1. Active—acquired through contact with the disease
   2. Passive—acquired from antibodies obtained through placenta and mother's milk
E. Artificially acquired immunity

   1. Active—immunization with vaccines
     a. Types: live (attenuated), killed, toxoid, recombinant DNA
     b. Boosters—keep antibody titers high
   2. Passive—administration of immune serum (antiserum)

Questions for Study and Review

Building Understanding

Fill in the blanks
1. The fluid that circulates in the lymphatic system is called _____.
2. Digested fats enter the lymphatic circulation through vessels called_____.
3. Fat globules and lymph combine to form a milky fluid called _____.
4. Heat, redness, swelling, and pain are classic signs of _____.
5. All antibodies ae contained in a portion of the blood plasma termed the _____.

Matching
Match each numbered item with the most closely related lettered item.
___ 6. Destroy foreign cells directly
___ 7. Release interleukins, which stimulate other cells to join the immune response
___ 8. Regulate the immune response in order to prevent overactivity.
___ 9. Remember an antigen and start a rapid response if the antigen is contacted again.
___ 10. Manufacture antibodies when activated by antigens.

a. regulatory T cells
b. memory T cells
c. cytotoxic T cells
d. B cells
e. helper T cells

Multiple choice
___ 11. Compared to plasma, lymph contains much less
   a. fat
   b. protein
   c. carbohydrate
   d. water
___ 12. Lymph from the lower extremities returns to the cardiovascular system via the
   a. cisterna chyli
   b. right lymphatic duct
   c. thymus
   d. thoracic duct
___ 13. Macrophages and monocytes found throughout the body make up the
   a. tonsils
   b. Peyer patches
   c. reticuloendothelial system
   d. appendix
___ 14. Damaged cells release a vasodilator substance called
   e. interleukin
   f. interferon
   g. histamine
   h. complement
___ 15. Which of the following cells mature in the thymus?
   a. T cell
   b. B cell
   c. plasma cell
   d. natural killer cell

Understanding Concepts
16. How does the structure of a lymphatic capillary correlate with its function? List some differences between a lymphatic and blood capillary.
17. Trace a globule of fat from a lacteal in the wall of the small intestine to the right atrium.
18. Describe the structure of a typical lymph node.
19. State the location of the spleen and list several of its functions.
20. What causes the symptoms of inflammation?
21. Differentiate between the terms in each of the following pairs:
   a. interferon and interleukin
   b. antibody and complement
   c. inborn immunity and acquired immunity
   d. cell-mediated immunity and humoral immunity
   e. active immunization and passive immunizaton
22. Describe the events that must occur for a T cell to react with a foreign antigen. Once activated, what do the T cells do?
23. What role do antibodies play in immunity? How are they produced? How do they work?
24. Compare and contrast the four types of acquired immunity.

Conceptual Thinking
25. Explain the absence of arteries in the lymphatic circulatory system.
26. Why is HIV's attack on helper T cells so devastating to the entire immune system?

Energy: Supply and Use

The four chapters in this unit show how oxygen and nutrients are processed, taken up by the body fluids, and used by the cells to yield energy. This unit also describes how the stability of body functions (homeostasis) is maintained and how waste products are eliminated.

LEARNING OUTCOMES

After careful study of this chapter, you should be able to:

1. Define *respiration* and describe the three phases of respiration
2. Name and describe all the structures of the respiratory system
3. Explain the mechanism for pulmonary ventilation
4. List the ways in which oxygen and carbon dioxide are transported in the blood
5. Describe nervous and chemical controls of respiration
6. Give several examples of altered breathing patterns
7. Show how word parts are used to build words related to respiration (see Word Anatomy at the end of the chapter)

chapter 16

Respiration

Phases of Respiration

Most people think of respiration simply as the process by which air moves into and out of the lungs, that is, *breathing*. By scientific definition, respiration is the process by which oxygen is obtained from the environment and delivered to the cells. Carbon dioxide is transported to the outside in a reverse pathway (Fig. 16-1).

Respiration includes three phases:

- **Pulmonary ventilation,** which is the exchange of air between the atmosphere and the air sacs (alveoli) of the lungs. This is normally accomplished by the inhalation and exhalation of breathing.
- **External exchange of gases,** which occurs in the lungs as oxygen (O_2) diffuses from the air sacs into the blood and carbon dioxide (CO_2) diffuses out of the blood to be eliminated.
- **Internal exchange of gases,** which occurs in the tissues as oxygen diffuses from the blood to the cells, whereas carbon dioxide passes from the cells into the blood.

Gas exchange requires close association of the respiratory system with the circulatory system, as the circulating blood is needed to transport oxygen to the cells and transport carbon dioxide back to the lungs.

The term *respiration* is also used to describe a related process that occurs at the cellular level. In **cellular respiration,** oxygen is taken into a cell and used in the breakdown of nutrients with the release of energy. Carbon dioxide is the waste product of cellular respiration (see Chapter 18's discussion of metabolism).

> **Checkpoint 16-1** What are the three phases of respiration?

The Respiratory System

The respiratory system is an intricate arrangement of spaces and passageways that conduct air into the lungs

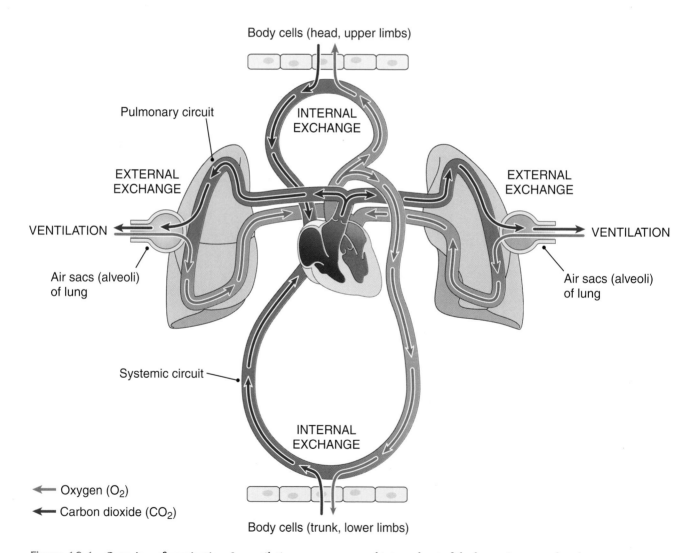

Figure 16-1 **Overview of respiration.** In ventilation, gases are moved into and out of the lungs. In external exchange, gases move between the air sacs (alveoli) of the lungs and the blood. In internal exchange, gases move between the blood and body cells. The circulation transports gases in the blood.

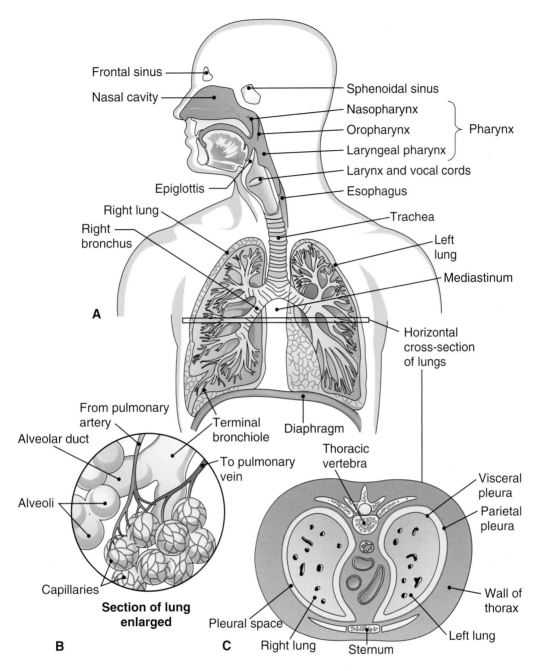

Figure 16-2 The respiratory system. (A) Overview. **(B)** Enlarged section of lung tissue showing the relationship between the alveoli (air sacs) of the lungs and the blood capillaries. **(C)** A transverse section through the lungs. *ZOOMING IN ✦ What organ is located in the medial depression of the left lung?*

(Fig. 16-2). These spaces include the **nasal cavities;** the **pharynx** (FAR-inks), which is common to the digestive and respiratory systems; the voice box, or **larynx** (LAR-inks); the windpipe, or **trachea** (TRA-ke-ah); and the **lungs** themselves, with their conducting tubes and air sacs. The entire system might be thought of as a pathway for air between the atmosphere and the blood.

The Nasal Cavities

Air enters the body through the openings in the nose called the **nostrils,** or **nares** (*NA-reze*) (sing., naris). Im-

mediately inside the nostrils, located between the roof of the mouth and the cranium, are the two spaces known as the **nasal cavities.** These two spaces are separated from each other by a partition, the **nasal septum.** The superior portion of the septum is formed by a thin plate of the ethmoid bone that extends downward, and the inferior portion is formed by the vomer (see Fig. 6-5 A in Chapter 6). An anterior extension of the septum is made of hyaline cartilage. The septum and the walls of the nasal cavity are covered with mucous membrane. On the lateral walls of each nasal cavity are three projections called the **conchae** (KONG-ke) (see Figs. 6-5 A and 6-8 in Chapter 6). The shell-like conchae greatly increase the surface area of the mucous membrane over which air travels on its way through the nasal cavities.

The mucous membrane lining the nasal cavities contains many blood vessels that deliver heat and moisture. The cells of this membrane secrete a large amount of fluid—up to 1 quart each day. The following changes are produced in the air as it comes in contact with the lining of the nose:

▶ Foreign bodies, such as dust particles and pathogens, are filtered out by the hairs of the nostrils or caught in the surface mucus.

▶ Air is warmed by blood in the well-vascularized mucous membrane.

▶ Air is moistened by the liquid secretion.

To allow for these protective changes to occur, it is preferable to breathe through the nose rather than through the mouth.

The **sinuses** are small cavities lined with mucous membrane in the skull bones. They are resonating chambers for the voice and lessen the weight of the skull. The sinuses communicate with the nasal cavities, and they are highly susceptible to infection.

Checkpoint 16-2 What happens to air as it passes over the nasal mucosa?

The Pharynx

The muscular **pharynx,** or throat, carries air into the respiratory tract and carries foods and liquids into the digestive system (see Fig. 16-2). The superior portion, located immediately behind the nasal cavity, is called the **nasopharynx** (na-zo-FAR-inks); the middle section, located posterior to the mouth, is called the **oropharynx** (o-ro-FAR-inks); and the most inferior portion is called the **laryngeal** (lah-RIN-je-al) **pharynx.** This last section opens into the larynx toward the anterior and into the esophagus toward the posterior.

The Larynx

The **larynx,** commonly called the *voice box* (Fig. 16-3), is located between the pharynx and the trachea. It has a framework of cartilage, part of which is the thyroid cartilage that protrudes in the front of the neck. The projection formed by the thyroid cartilage is commonly called the *Adam's apple* because it is considerably larger in the male than in the female.

Folds of mucous membrane used in producing speech are located on both sides at the superior portion of the larynx. These are the vocal folds, or **vocal cords** (Fig. 16-4), which vibrate as air flows over them from the lungs. Variations in the length and tension of the vocal cords and the distance between them regulate the pitch of sound. The amount of air forced over them regulates volume. A difference in the size of the larynx and the vocal cords is what accounts for the difference between adult male and female voices. In general, a man's larynx is larger than a woman's. His vocal cords are thicker and longer, so they vibrate more slowly, resulting in a lower range of pitch. Muscles of the pharynx, tongue, lips, and face also are used to form clear pronunciations. The mouth, nasal cavities, paranasal sinuses, and the pharynx all serve as resonating chambers for speech, just as does the cabinet for an audio speaker.

The space between the vocal cords is called the **glottis** (GLOT-is). This is somewhat open during normal breathing but widely open during forced breathing (see Fig. 16-4). The little leaf-shaped cartilage that covers the larynx during swallowing is called the **epiglottis** (ep-ih-GLOT-is). The glottis and epiglottis help keep food and liquids out of the remainder of the respiratory tract. As the larynx moves upward and forward during swallowing, the epiglottis moves downward, covering the opening into the larynx. You can feel the larynx move upward toward the epiglottis during this process by placing the flat ends of your fingers on your larynx as you swallow. Muscles in the larynx assist in keeping foreign materials out of the respiratory tract by closing the glottis during swallowing. Muscles also close the glottis when one holds his or her breath and strains, as to defecate or lift a heavy weight.

The Trachea

The **trachea,** commonly called the *windpipe,* is a tube that extends from the inferior edge of the larynx to the upper part of the chest superior to the heart. The trachea's purpose is to conduct air between the larynx and the lungs.

A framework of separate cartilages reinforces the trachea and keeps it open. These cartilages, each shaped somewhat like a tiny horseshoe or the letter C, are found along the trachea's entire length. The open sections in the cartilages are lined up at their posterior so that the esophagus can expand into this region during swallowing.

Checkpoint 16-3 What are the scientific names for the throat, voice box, and windpipe?

Checkpoint 16-4 What are the three regions of the pharynx?

The Bronchi

At its inferior end, the trachea divides into two primary, or main-stem, **bronchi** (BRONG-ki), which enter the lungs (see Fig. 16-2). The right bronchus is considerably larger in diameter than the left and extends downward in a more vertical direction. Therefore, if a foreign body is inhaled, it is likely to enter the right lung. Each bronchus enters the lung at a notch or depression called the **hilum** (HI-lum). Blood vessels and nerves also connect with the lung in this region.

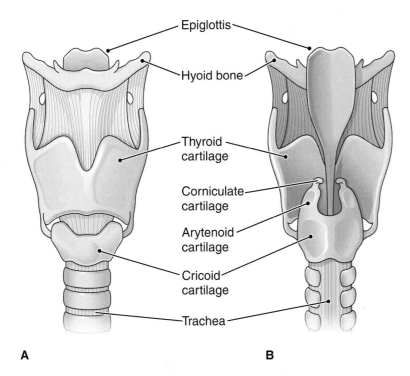

Figure 16-3 **The larynx. (A)** Anterior view. **(B)** Posterior view.

The Lining of the Air Passageways The trachea, bronchi, and other conducting passageways of the respiratory tract are lined with a special type of epithelium (Fig. 16-5). Basically, it is simple columnar epithelium, but the cells are arranged in such a way that they appear stratified. The tissue is thus described as *pseudostratified*, meaning "falsely stratified." These epithelial cells have cilia to filter out impurities and to create fluid movement within the conducting tubes. The cilia beat to drive impurities toward the throat, where they can be swallowed or eliminated by coughing, sneezing, or blowing the nose.

> **Checkpoint 16-5** The cells that line the respiratory passageways help to keep impurities out of the lungs. What feature of these cells enables them to filter impurities and move fluids?

The Lungs

The **lungs** are the organs in which gas diffusion takes place through the extremely thin and delicate lung tissues (see Fig. 16-2). The two lungs are set side by side in the thoracic (chest) cavity. Between them are the heart, the great blood vessels, and other organs of the **mediastinum** (me-de-as-TI-num), the space between the lungs, including the esophagus, trachea, and lymph nodes.

On its medial side, the left lung has an indentation that accommodates the heart. The right lung is subdivided by fissures into three lobes; the left lung is divided into two lobes. Each lobe is then further subdivided into segments and then lobules. These subdivisions correspond to subdivisions of the bronchi as they branch throughout the lungs.

Each primary bronchus enters the lung at the hilum and immediately subdivides. The right bronchus divides into three secondary bronchi, each of which enters one of the three lobes of the right lung. The left bronchus gives rise to two secondary bronchi, which enter the two lobes of the left lung. Because the bronchial subdivisions resemble the branches of a tree, they have been given the common name *bronchial tree*. The bronchi subdivide again and again, becoming progressively smaller as they branch through lung tissue.

The smallest of these conducting tubes are called **bronchioles** (BRONG-ke-oles). The bronchi contain small

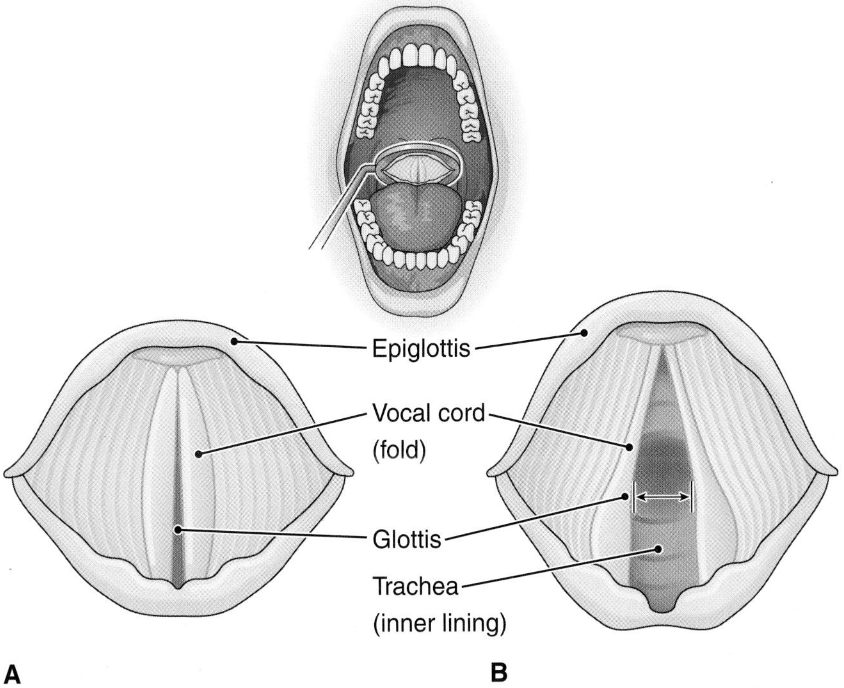

Figure 16-4 **The vocal cords, superior view. (A)** The glottis in closed position. **(B)** The glottis in open position. *ZOOMING IN ✦ What cartilage is named for its position above the glottis?*

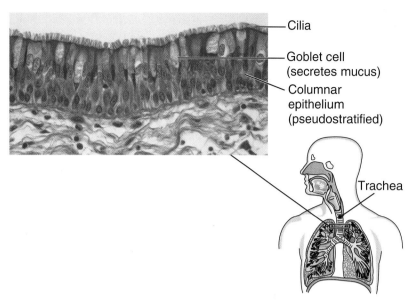

Figure 16-5 **Microscopic view of ciliated epithelium.** Ciliated epithelium lines the respiratory passageways, as shown here in the trachea. (Micrograph reprinted with permission from Cormack DH. Essential Histology. 2ⁿᵈ ed. Philadelphia: Lippincott Williams & Wilkins, 2001.)

bits of cartilage, which give firmness to their walls and hold the passageways open so that air can pass in and out easily. As the bronchi become smaller, however, the cartilage decreases in amount. In the bronchioles, there is no cartilage at all; what remains is mostly smooth muscle, which is under the control of the autonomic (involuntary) nervous system.

The Alveoli At the end of the **terminal bronchioles**, the smallest subdivisions of the bronchial tree, there are clusters of tiny air sacs in which most gas exchange takes place. These sacs are known as **alveoli** (al-VE-o-li) (sing., alveolus) (see Fig. 16-2). The wall of each alveolus is made of a single-cell layer of squamous (flat) epithelium. This thin wall provides easy passage for the gases entering and leaving the blood as the blood circulates through the millions of tiny capillaries covering the alveoli.

Certain cells in the alveolar wall produce **surfactant** (sur-FAK-tant), a substance that reduces the surface tension ("pull") of the fluids that line the alveoli. This surface action prevents collapse of the alveoli and eases expansion of the lungs.

There are about 300 million alveoli in the human lungs. The resulting surface area in contact with gases approximates 60 square meters (some books say even more). This area is equivalent, as an example, to the floor surface of a classroom that measures about 24 by 24 feet. As with many other systems in the body, there is great functional reserve; we have about three times as much lung tissue as is minimally necessary to sustain life. Because of the many air spaces, the lung is light in weight; normally, a piece of lung tissue dropped into a glass of water will float. Figure 16-6 shows a microscopic view of lung tissue.

The pulmonary circuit brings blood to and from the lungs. In the lungs, blood passes through the capillaries around the alveoli, where gas exchange takes place.

The Lung Cavities and Pleura

The lungs occupy a considerable portion of the thoracic cavity, which is separated from the abdominal cavity by the muscular partition known as the **diaphragm**. A continuous doubled sac, the **pleura**, covers each lung. The two layers of the pleura are named according to location. The portion of the pleura that is attached to the chest wall is the **parietal pleura**, and the portion that is attached to the surface of the lung is called the **visceral pleura**. Each closed sac completely surrounds the lung, except in the place where the bronchus and blood vessels enter the lung, a region known as the *root* of the lung.

Between the two layers of the pleura is the **pleural space** containing a thin film of fluid that lubricates the membranes. The effect of this fluid is the same as between two flat pieces of glass joined by a film of water; that is, the surfaces slide easily on each other but strongly resist separation. Thus, the lungs are able to move and enlarge effortlessly in response to changes in the thoracic volume that occur during breathing.

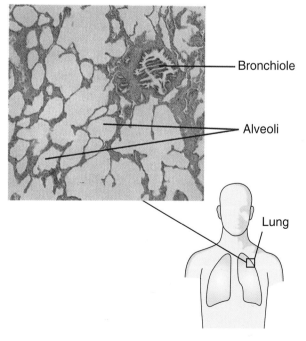

Figure 16-6 **Lung tissue viewed through a microscope.** (Micrograph courtesy of Dana Morse Bittus and BJ Cohen.)

Checkpoint 16-6 In what structures does gas exchange occur in the lung?

Checkpoint 16-7 What is the name of the membrane that encloses the lung?

The Process of Respiration

Respiration involves ventilation of the lungs, exchange of gases, and their transport in the blood. Respiratory needs are met by central and peripheral controls of breathing.

Pulmonary Ventilation

Ventilation is the movement of air into and out of the lungs, normally accomplished by breathing. There are two phases of ventilation (Fig. 16-7):

▶ **Inhalation,** or inspiration, is the drawing of air into the lungs.
▶ **Exhalation,** or expiration, is the expulsion of air from the lungs.

In **inhalation,** the active phase of breathing, respiratory muscles contract to enlarge the thoracic cavity. During quiet breathing, the movement of the diaphragm accounts for most of the increase in thoracic volume. The diaphragm is a strong, dome-shaped muscle attached to the body wall around the base of the rib cage. The contraction and flattening of the diaphragm cause a piston-like downward motion that increases the vertical dimension of the chest. Other muscles that participate in breathing are the external and internal intercostal muscles. These muscles run at different angles in two layers between the ribs. As the external intercostals contract for inhalation, they lift the rib cage upward and outward. Put the palms of your hands on either side of the rib cage to feel this action as you inhale. During forceful inhalation, the rib cage is moved further up and out by contraction of muscles in the neck and chest wall.

As the thoracic cavity increases in size, gas pressure within the cavity decreases. This phenomenon follows a law in physics stating that when the volume of a given amount of gas increases, the pressure of the gas decreases. Conversely, when the volume decreases, the pressure increases. If you blow air into a tight balloon that does not expand very much, the gas particles are in close contact and will hit the wall of the balloon frequently, creating greater pressure (Fig. 16-8). If you tap this balloon, it will spring back to its original shape. When you blow into a soft balloon that expands easily under pressure, the gas particles spread out into a larger area and will not hit the balloon's wall as often. If you tap the balloon, your finger will make an indentation. Thus, pressure in the chest cavity drops as the thorax expands. When the pressure drops to slightly below the air pressure outside the lungs, air is drawn into the lungs, as by suction.

The ease with which one can expand the lungs and thorax is called **compliance**. Normal elasticity of the lung tissue, aided by surfactant, allows the lungs to expand under pressure and fill adequately with air during inhalation. Compliance is decreased when the lungs resist expansion. Conditions that can decrease compliance include diseases that damage or scar lung tissue, fluid accumulation in the lungs, deficiency of surfactant, and interference with the action of breathing muscles.

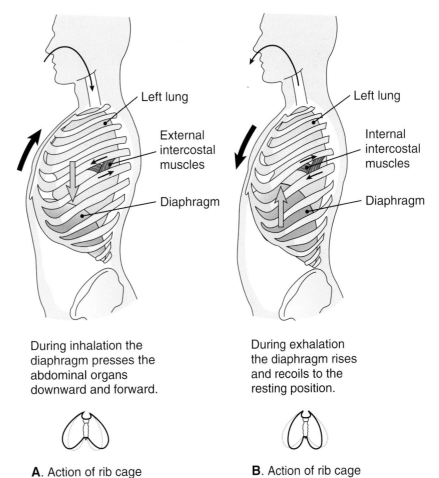

During inhalation the diaphragm presses the abdominal organs downward and forward.

A. Action of rib cage in inhalation

During exhalation the diaphragm rises and recoils to the resting position.

B. Action of rib cage in exhalation

Figure 16-7   Pulmonary ventilation. (A) Inhalation. **(B)** Exhalation. *ZOOMING IN ✦ What muscles are located between the ribs?*

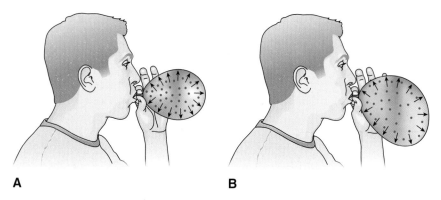

A   **B**

Figure 16-8 The relationship of gas pressure to volume. (A) Inflation of a stiff balloon creates strong air pressure against the wall of the balloon. **(B)** The same amount of air in a soft balloon spreads out into the available space, resulting in lower gas pressure. *ZOOMING IN ◆ What happens to gas pressure as the volume of its container increases?*

Air enters the respiratory passages and flows through the ever-dividing tubes of the bronchial tree. As the air traverses this route, it moves more and more slowly through the great number of bronchial tubes until there is virtually no forward flow as it reaches the alveoli. The incoming air mixes with the residual air remaining in the respiratory passageways, so that the gases soon are evenly distributed. Each breath causes relatively little change in the gas composition of the alveoli, but normal continuous breathing ensures the presence of adequate oxygen and the removal of carbon dioxide.

In **exhalation,** the passive phase of breathing, the respiratory muscles relax, allowing the ribs and diaphragm to return to their original positions. The lung tissues are elastic and recoil to their original size during exhalation.

Surface tension within the alveoli aids in this return to resting size. During forced exhalation, the internal intercostal muscles contract, pulling the bottom of the rib cage in and down. The muscles of the abdominal wall contract, pushing the abdominal viscera upward against the relaxed diaphragm.

Table 16-1 gives the definitions and average values for some of the breathing volumes and capacities that are important in evaluating respiratory function. A lung *capacity* is a sum of volumes. These same values are shown on a graph as they might appear on a tracing made by a **spirometer** (spi-ROM-eh-ter), an instrument for recording lung volumes (Fig. 16-9). The tracing is a **spirogram** (SPI-ro-gram).

Checkpoint 16-8 What are the two phases of breathing? Which is active and which is passive?

Gas Exchange

External exchange is the movement of gases between the alveoli and the capillary blood in the lungs (see Fig. 16-1). The barrier that separates alveolar air from the blood is composed of the alveolar wall and the capillary wall, both of which are extremely thin. This respiratory membrane is not only very thin, it is also moist. The moisture is important because the oxygen and carbon dioxide must go into solution before they can diffuse across the membrane. Recall that **diffusion** refers to the movement of molecules from an area in which they are in higher concentration to an area in which they are in lower concentration. Therefore, the relative concentrations of a gas on the two sides of a membrane determine the direction of diffusion. Normally, inspired air contains about 21% oxygen and 0.04% carbon dioxide; expired air has only 16% oxygen and 3.5% carbon dioxide. These values illustrate that a two-way diffusion takes place through the walls of the alveoli and capillaries (Fig. 16-10).

Internal exchange takes place between the blood and the tissues. In metabolism, the cells constantly consume oxygen and produce carbon dioxide. Based on relative concentrations of these gases, oxygen diffuses out of the blood and carbon dioxide enters.

Table 16·1	Lung Volumes and Capacities	
VOLUME	**DEFINITION**	**AVERAGE VALUE (mL)**
Tidal volume	The amount of air moved into or out of the lungs in quiet, relaxed breathing	500
Residual volume	The volume of air that remains in the lungs after maximum exhalation	1200
Inspiratory reserve volume	The additional amount that can be breathed in by force after a normal inhalation	2600
Expiratory reserve volume	The additional amount that can be breathed out by force after a normal exhalation	900
Vital capacity	The volume of air that can be expelled from the lungs by maximum exhalation after maximum inhalation	4000
Functional residual capacity	The amount of air remaining in the lungs after normal exhalation	2100
Total lung capacity	The total volume of air that can be contained in the lungs after maximum inhalation	5200

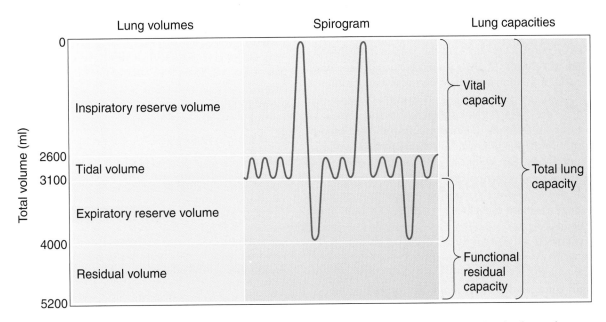

Figure 16-9 **A spirogram.** The tracing of lung volumes is made with a spirometer. *ZOOMING IN ✦ What lung volume cannot be measured with a spirometer?*

At this point, blood returning from the tissues and entering the lung capillaries through the pulmonary circuit is relatively low in oxygen and high in carbon dioxide. Again, the blood will pick up oxygen and give up carbon dioxide. After a return to the left side of the heart, it starts once more on its route through the systemic circuit.

> **Checkpoint 16-9** Gases move between the alveoli and the blood by the process of diffusion. What is the definition of diffusion?

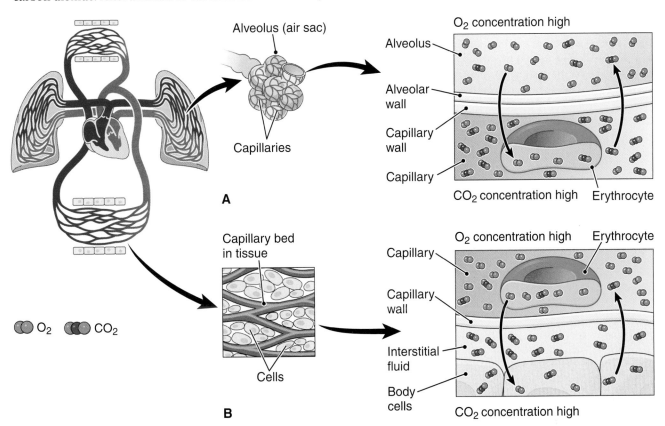

Figure 16-10 **Gas exchange. (A)** External exchange between the alveoli and the blood. Oxygen diffuses into the blood and carbon dioxide diffuses out, based on concentrations of the two gases in the alveoli and in the blood. **(B)** Internal exchange between the blood and the cells. Oxygen diffuses out of the blood and into tissues, while carbon dioxide diffuses from the cells into the blood.

Transport of Oxygen

A very small percentage (1.5%) of the oxygen in the blood is carried in solution in the plasma. (Oxygen does dissolve in water, as shown by the fact that aquatic animals get their oxygen from water.) However, almost all (98.5%) of the oxygen that diffuses into the capillary blood in the lungs binds to **hemoglobin** in the red blood cells. If not for hemoglobin and its ability to hold oxygen in the blood, the heart would have to work much harder to supply enough oxygen to the tissues. The hemoglobin molecule is a large protein with four small iron-containing "heme" regions. Each heme portion can bind one molecule of oxygen.

Oxygenated blood (in systemic arteries and pulmonary veins) is 97% saturated with oxygen. That is, the total hemoglobin in the red cells is holding 97% of the maximum amount that it can hold. Deoxygenated blood (in systemic veins and pulmonary arteries) is usually about 70% saturated with oxygen. This 27% difference represents the oxygen that has been taken up by the cells. Note, however, that even blood that is described as deoxygenated still has a reserve of oxygen. Even under conditions of high oxygen consumption, as in vigorous exercise, for example, the blood is never totally depleted of oxygen.

In clinical practice, gas concentrations are expressed as pressure in millimeters of mercury (mmHg), as is blood pressure. Because air is a mixture of gases, each gas exerts only a portion of the total pressure, or a **partial pressure** (P). The partial pressures of oxygen and carbon dioxide are symbolized as Po_2 and Pco_2 respectively.

To enter the cells, oxygen must separate from hemoglobin. Normally, the bond between oxygen and hemoglobin is easily broken, and oxygen is released as blood travels into areas where the oxygen concentration is relatively low. Cells are constantly using oxygen in metabolism and obtaining fresh supplies by diffusion from the blood.

The poisonous gas, carbon monoxide (CO) at low partial pressure binds with hemoglobin at the same sites as does oxygen. However, it binds more tightly and displaces oxygen. Even a small amount of carbon monoxide causes a serious reduction in the blood's ability to carry oxygen.

For an interesting variation on normal gas transport, see Box 16-1 on liquid ventilation.

> **Checkpoint 16-10** What substance in red blood cells carries almost all of the oxygen in the blood?

Transport of Carbon Dioxide

Carbon dioxide is produced continuously in the tissues as a byproduct of metabolism. It diffuses from the cells into the blood and is transported to the lungs in three ways:

▶ About 10% is dissolved in the plasma and in the fluid within red blood cells. (Carbonated beverages are examples of water in which CO_2 is dissolved.)
▶ About 15% is combined with the protein portion of hemoglobin and plasma proteins.
▶ About 75% is transported as an ion, known as a **bicarbonate ion**, which is formed when carbon dioxide undergoes a chemical change after it dissolves in blood fluids.

The bicarbonate ion is formed slowly in the plasma but much more rapidly inside the red blood cells, where an enzyme called **carbonic anhydrase** (an-HI-drase) increases the speed of the reaction. The bicarbonate formed in the red blood cells moves to the plasma and then is carried to the lungs. In the lungs, the process is reversed as bicarbonate reenters the red blood cells and releases carbon dioxide for diffusion into the alveoli and exhalation. For those with a background in chemistry, the equation for these reactions follows. The arrows going in both directions signify that the reactions are reversible. The

---

Box 16-1   *Clinical Perspectives*

Liquid Ventilation: Breath in a Bottle

Researchers have been attempting for years to develop a fluid that could transport high concentrations of oxygen in the body. Such a fluid could substitute for blood in transfusions or be used to carry oxygen into the lungs. Early work on liquid ventilation climaxed in the mid-1960s when a pioneer in this field submerged a laboratory mouse in a beaker of fluid and the animal survived total immersion for more than 10 minutes. The fluid was a synthetic substance that could hold as much oxygen as does air.

A newer version of this fluid, a fluorine-containing chemical known as PFC, has been tested to ventilate the collapsed lungs of premature babies. In addition to delivering oxygen to the lung alveoli, it also removes carbon dioxide. The fluid is less damaging to delicate lung tissue than is air, which has to be pumped in under higher pressure. Others who might benefit from liquid ventilation include people whose lungs have been damaged by infection, inhaled toxins, asthma, emphysema, and lung cancer, but more clinical research is required. Scientists are also investigating whether liquid ventilation could be used to deliver drugs directly to lung tissue.

upper arrows describe what happens as CO_2 enters the blood; the lower arrows indicate what happens as CO_2 is released from the blood to be exhaled from the lungs.

$$CO_2 + H_2O \longrightarrow H_2CO_3 \longrightarrow H^+ + HCO_3^-$$

| carbon dioxide | water | carbonic acid | hydrogen ion | bicarbonate ion |

Carbon dioxide is important in regulating the blood's pH (acid–base balance). As a bicarbonate ion is formed from carbon dioxide in the plasma, a hydrogen ion (H^+) is also produced. Therefore, the blood becomes more acidic as the amount of carbon dioxide in the blood increases to yield more hydrogen and bicarbonate ions. The exhalation of carbon dioxide shifts the blood's pH more toward the alkaline (basic) range. The bicarbonate ion is also an important buffer in the blood, acting chemically to help keep the pH of body fluids within a steady range of 7.35 to 7.45.

Checkpoint 16-11 What is the main form in which carbon dioxide is carried in the blood?

Regulation of Respiration

Centers in the central nervous system control the fundamental respiratory pattern. This pattern is modified by special receptors that detect changes in the blood's chemical composition.

Nervous Control Regulation of respiration is a complex process that must keep pace with moment-to-moment changes in cellular oxygen requirements and carbon dioxide production. Regulation depends primarily on a respiratory control center located partly in the medulla and partly in the pons of the brain stem. The control center's main part, located in the medulla, sets the basic pattern of respiration. This pattern can be modified by centers in the pons. These areas continuously regulate breathing, so that levels of oxygen, carbon dioxide, and acid are kept within normal limits.

From the respiratory center in the medulla, motor nerve fibers extend into the spinal cord. From the cervical (neck) part of the cord, these nerve fibers continue through the **phrenic** (FREN-ik) **nerve** (a branch of the vagus nerve) to the diaphragm. The diaphragm and the other respiratory muscles are voluntary in the sense that they can be regulated consciously by messages from the higher brain centers, notably the cerebral cortex. It is possible for a person to deliberately breathe more rapidly or more slowly or to hold his or her breath and not breathe at all for a while. In a short time, however, the respiratory center in the brain stem will override the voluntary desire to not breathe, and breathing will resume. Most of the time, we breathe without thinking about it, and the respiratory center is in control.

Checkpoint 16-12 What part of the brain stem sets the basic pattern of respiration?

Checkpoint 16-13 What is the name of the motor nerve that controls the diaphragm?

Chemical Control Of vital importance in the control of respiration are **chemoreceptors** (ke-mo-re-SEP-tors) which, like the receptors for taste and smell, are sensitive to chemicals dissolved in body fluids. The chemoreceptors that regulate respiration are located centrally (near the brain stem) and peripherally (in arteries).

The central chemoreceptors are on either side of the brain stem near the medullary respiratory center. These receptors respond to the CO_2 level in circulating blood, but the gas acts indirectly. CO_2 is capable of diffusing through the capillary blood-brain barrier. It dissolves in CSF (the fluid in and around the brain) and separates into hydrogen ion and bicarbonate ion, as explained previously. It is the presence of hydrogen ion and its effect in lowering pH that actually stimulates the central chemoreceptors. The rise in blood CO_2 level, known as **hypercapnia** (hi-per-KAP-ne-ah), thus triggers ventilation.

The peripheral chemoreceptors that regulate respiration are found in structures called the *carotid* and *aortic bodies*. The carotid bodies are located near the bifurcation (forking) of the common carotid arteries in the neck, whereas the aortic bodies are located in the aortic arch. These bodies contain sensory neurons that respond mainly to a decrease in oxygen supply. They are not usually involved in regulating breathing, because they don't act until oxygen drops to a very low level. Because there is usually an ample reserve of oxygen in the blood, carbon dioxide has the most immediate effect in regulating respiration at the level of the central chemoreceptors. When the carbon dioxide level increases, breathing must be increased to blow off the excess gas. Oxygen only becomes a controlling factor when its level falls considerably below normal.

Checkpoint 16-14 What gas is the main chemical controller of respiration?

Abnormal Ventilation

In **hyperventilation** (hi-per-ven-tih-LA-shun), an increased amount of air enters the alveoli. This condition results from deep and rapid respiration that commonly occurs during anxiety attacks, or when a person is experiencing pain or other forms of stress. Hyperventilation causes an increase in the oxygen level and a decrease in the carbon dioxide level of the blood, a condition called **hypocapnia** (hi-po-KAP-ne-ah). The loss of carbon dioxide increases the blood's pH (alkalosis) by removing acidic products, as shown by the equation cited previously. The change in pH results in dizziness and tingling sensations. Breathing may stop because the respiratory control center is not stimulated. Gradually, the carbon dioxide level returns to normal, and a regular breathing pattern is resumed. In extreme cases, a person may faint, and then breathing will involuntarily return to normal. In assisting a person who is hyperventilating, one should speak calmly, reassure him or her that the situation is not dangerous, and encourage even breathing from the diaphragm.

In **hypoventilation,** an insufficient amount of air enters the alveoli. The many possible causes of this condition include respiratory obstruction, lung disease, injury to the respiratory center, depression of the respiratory center, as by drugs, and chest deformity. Hypoventilation results in an increase in the carbon dioxide concentration in the blood, leading to a decrease in the blood's pH (acidosis), again according to the equation previously mentioned.

Breathing Patterns

Normal rates of breathing vary from 12 to 20 times per minute for adults. In children, rates may vary from 20 to 40 times per minute, depending on age and size. In infants, the respiratory rate may be more than 40 times per minute. Changes in respiratory rates are important in various disorders and should be recorded carefully. To determine the respiratory rate, the healthcare worker counts the client's breathing for at least 30 seconds, usually by watching the chest rise and fall with each inhalation and exhalation. The count is then multiplied to obtain the rate in breaths per minute. It is best if the person does not realize that he or she is being observed because awareness of the measurement may cause a change in the breathing rate.

Some Terms for Altered Breathing The following is a list of terms designating various abnormalities of respiration. These are symptoms, not diseases. Note that the word ending -*pnea* refers to breathing.

▶ **Hyperpnea** (hi-PERP-ne-ah) refers to an abnormal increase in the depth and rate of respiration.
▶ **Hypopnea** (hi-POP-ne-ah) is a decrease in the rate and depth of breathing.
▶ **Tachypnea** (tak-IP-ne-ah) is an excessive rate of breathing that may be normal, as in exercise.
▶ **Apnea** (AP-ne-ah) is a temporary cessation of breathing. Short periods of apnea occur normally during deep sleep. More severe sleep apnea can result from obstruction of the respiratory passageways or, less commonly, by failure in the central respiratory center.
▶ **Dyspnea** (disp-NE-ah) is a subjective feeling of difficult or labored breathing.
▶ **Orthopnea** (or-THOP-ne-ah) refers to a difficulty in breathing that is relieved by sitting in an upright position, either against two pillows in bed or in a chair.

Results of Inadequate Breathing Conditions that may result from decreased respiration include the following:

▶ **Cyanosis** (si-ah-NO-sis) is a bluish color of the skin and mucous membranes caused by an insufficient amount of oxygen in the blood.
▶ **Hypoxia** (hi-POK-se-ah) means a lower than normal oxygen level in the tissues. The term anoxia (ah-NOK-se-ah) is sometimes used instead, but is not as accurate because it means a total lack of oxygen.
▶ **Hypoxemia** (hi-pok-SE-me-ah) refers to a lower than normal oxygen concentration in arterial blood.
▶ **Suffocation** is the cessation of respiration, often the result of a mechanical blockage of the respiratory passages.

Box 16-2 offers information on adjusting to high altitudes and other hypoxic conditions.

▶ Age and the Respiratory Tract

With age, the tissues of the respiratory tract lose elasticity and become more rigid. Similar rigidity in the chest wall, combined with arthritis and loss of strength in the

---

Box 16-2	A Closer Look

Adaptations to High Altitude: Living With Hypoxia

Our bodies work best at low altitudes where oxygen is plentiful. However, people are able to live at high altitudes where oxygen is scarce and can even survive climbing Mount Everest, the tallest peak on our planet, showing that the human body can adapt to hypoxic conditions. This adaptation process compensates for decreased atmospheric oxygen by increasing the efficiency of the respiratory and cardiovascular systems.

The body's immediate response to high altitude is to increase the rate of ventilation (hyperventilation) and raise

heart rate to increase cardiac output. Hyperventilation makes more oxygen available to the cells and increases blood pH (alkalosis), which boosts hemoglobin's capacity to bind oxygen. Over time, the body adapts in additional ways. Hypoxia stimulates the kidneys to secrete erythropoietin, prompting red bone marrow to manufacture more erythrocytes and hemoglobin. Also, capillaries proliferate, increasing blood flow to the tissues. Some people are unable to adapt to high altitudes, and for them, hypoxia and alkalosis lead to potentially fatal **altitude sickness.**

breathing muscles, results in an overall decrease in compliance and in lung capacity. Reduction in protective mechanisms, such as phagocytosis in the lungs, leads to increased susceptibility to infection. The incidence of lung disorders increases with age, hastened by cigarette smoking and by exposure to other environmental irritants. Although there is much individual variation, especially related to one's customary level of activity, these changes gradually lead to reduced capacity for exercise. Respiratory therapists specialize in evaluating and treating breathing disorders. For more information, see Box 16-3, Careers in Respiratory Therapy.

Box 16-3 · Health Professions

Careers in Respiratory Therapy

Respiratory therapists and respiratory therapy technicians specialize in evaluating and treating breathing disorders. Respiratory therapists evaluate the severity of their clients' conditions by taking complete histories and testing respiratory function with specialized equipment. Based on their findings, and in consultation with a physician, therapists design and implement individualized treatment plans, which may include oxygen therapy and chest physiotherapy. They also educate clients on the use of ventilators and other medical devices. Respiratory therapy technicians assist in carrying out evaluations and treatments.

To perform their duties, both types of practitioners need a thorough understanding of anatomy and physiology. Most respiratory therapists in the United States receive their training from an accredited college or university and take a national licensing exam. Respiratory therapists and technicians work in a variety of settings, such as hospitals, nursing care facilities, and private clinics. As the American population continues to age, the prevalence of respiratory ailments is expected to increase. Thus, job prospects are good. For more information about careers in respiratory therapy, contact the American Association for Respiratory Care.

Word Anatomy

Medical terms are built from standardized word parts (prefixes, roots, and suffixes). Learning the meanings of these parts can help you remember words and interpret unfamiliar terms.

WORD PART	MEANING	EXAMPLE
The Respiratory System		
nas/o	nose	The *nasopharynx* is behind the nasal cavity.
or/o	mouth	The *oropharynx* is behind the mouth.
laryng/o	larynx	The *laryngeal* pharynx opens into the pharynx.
pleur/o	side, rib	The *pleura* covers the lung and lines the chest wall (rib cage).
The Process of Respiration		
spir/o	breathing	A *spirometer* is an instrument used to record breathing volumes.
capn/o	carbon dioxide	*Hypercapnia* is a rise in the blood level of carbon dioxide.
-pnea	breathing	*Hypopnea* is a decrease in the rate and depth of breathing.
orth/o-	straight	*Orthopnea* can be relieved by sitting in an upright position.

Summary

I. Phases of Respiration
1. Pulmonary ventilation
2. External gas exchange
3. Internal gas exchange

II. The respiratory system
A. Nasal cavities—filter, warm, and moisten air
B. Pharynx (throat)—carries air into respiratory tract and food into digestive tract
C. Larynx (voice box)—contains vocal cords
  1. Glottis- space between the vocal cords
  2. Epiglottis—covers larynx on swallowing to help prevent food from entering
D. Trachea (windpipe)
E. Bronchi—branches of trachea that enter lungs and then subdivide
  1. Bronchioles—smallest subdivisions
F. Lungs
  1. Organs of gas exchange
  2. Lobes: three on right; two on left
  3. Alveoli
    a. Tiny air sacs where gases are exchanged
    b. Surfactant—reduces surface tension in alveoli; eases expansion of lungs
  4. Pleura—membrane that encloses the lung
    a. Visceral pleura—attached to surface of lung
    b. Parietal pleura—attached to chest wall

c. Pleural space—between layers

5. Mediastinum—space and organs between lungs

III. The process of respiration

A. Pulmonary ventilation
  1. Inhalation—drawing of air into lungs
    a. Compliance—ease with which lungs and thorax can be expanded
  2. Exhalation—expulsion of air from lungs
  3. Lung volumes—used to evaluate respiratory function
B. Gas exchange
  1. Gases diffuse from area of higher concentration to area of lower concentration
  2. In lungs—oxygen enters blood and carbon dioxide leaves (external exchange)
  3. In tissues—oxygen leaves blood and carbon dioxide enters (internal exchange)
C. Oxygen transport
  1. Almost totally bound to heme portion of hemoglobin in red blood cells
  2. Separates from hemoglobin when oxygen concentration is low (in tissues)
    a. Carbon monoxide replaces oxygen on hemoglobin
D. Carbon dioxide transport
  1. Most carried as bicarbonate ion

2. Regulates pH of blood
E. Regulation of respiration
  1. Nervous control—centers in medulla and pons
  2. Chemical control
    a. Central chemoreceptors respond to CO_2, which decreases pH
    b. Peripheral chemoreceptors—respond to low levels of O_2
F. Abnormal ventilation
  1. Hyperventilation—rapid, deep respiration
  2. Hypoventilation—inadequate air in alveoli
G. Breathing patterns
  1. Normal—12 to 20 times per minute in adult
  2. Types of altered breathing
    a. Hyperpnea—increase in depth and rate of breathing
    b. Tachypnea—excessive rate of breathing
    c. Apnea—temporary cessation of breathing
    d. Dyspnea—difficulty in breathing
    e. Orthopnea—difficulty relieved by upright position
  3. Possible results—cyanosis, hypoxia (anoxia) hypoxemia suffocation

IV. Age and the respiratory tract

Questions for Study and Review

Building Understanding

Fill in the blanks

1. The exchange of air between the atmosphere and the lungs is called _____.
2. The space between the vocal cords is the _____.
3. The ease with which the lungs and thorax can be expanded is termed _____.
4. The diaphragm is innervated by the _____ nerve.
5. A lower than normal level of oxygen in the tissues is called _____.

Matching

Match each numbered item with the most closely related item.

___ 6. The amount of air remaining in the lungs after normal exhalation

___ 7. The additional amount of air that can be breathed out by force after a normal inspiration

___ 8. The amount of air moved into or out of the lungs in quiet, relaxed breathing

___ 9. The amount of air remaining in the lungs after maximum exhalation

___10. The amount of air that can be expelled from the lungs by maximum exhalation after maximum inhalation

a. vital capacity
b. functional residual capacity
c. tidal volume
d. residual volume
e. expiratory reserve volume

Multiple choice

___ 11. The bony projections in the nasal cavities that increase surface area are called
   a. nares
   b. septae
   c. conchae
   d. sinuses

___ 12. Which of the following structures produces speech?
   a. pharynx
   b. larynx
   c. trachea
   d. lungs

___ 13. The leaf-shaped cartilage that covers the larynx during swallowing is the
   a. epiglottis
   b. glottis
   c. conchae
   d. sinus

___ 14. Respiration is centrally regulated by the
   a. cerebral cortex
   b. diencephalon
   c. brain stem
   d. cerebellum

___ 15. All of the following are true during forced expiration except
   a. the diaphragm relaxes
   b. the external intercostal muscles contract
   c. the abdominal muscles contract
   d. the volume of the thoracic cavity decreases

Understanding Concepts

16. Differentiate between the terms in each of the following pairs:
   a. internal and external gas exchange
   b. pleura and diaphragm
   c. inhalation and exhalation
   d. spirometer and spirogram

17. Trace the path of air from the nostrils to the lung capillaries.

18. What is the function of the cilia on cells that line the respiratory passageways?

19. What is the relationship of gas pressure to volume? What happens to gas pressure in the lungs when the diaphragm contracts?

20. Compare and contrast the transport of oxygen and carbon dioxide in the blood.

21 Describe the directions in which oxygen and carbon dioxide diffuse during gas exchange. Why do the gases move in these directions?

22. Define hyperventilation and hypoventilation. What is the effect of each on blood CO_2 levels and blood pH?

23. What are chemoreceptors and how do they function to regulate breathing?

Conceptual Thinking

24. Jake, a sometimes exasperating 4-year-old, threatens his mother that he will hold his breath until "he dies." Should his mother be concerned that he might succeed?

25. Why is it important that airplane interiors are pressurized? If the cabin lost pressure, what physiological adaptations to respiration might occur in the passengers?

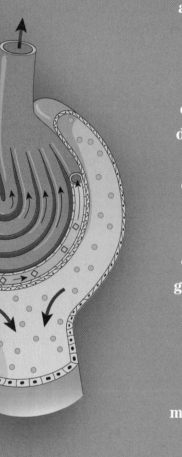

SELECTED KEY TERMS

The following terms and other boldface terms in the chapter are defined in the Glossary

absorption

bile

chyle

chyme

defecation

deglutition

digestion

duodenum

emulsify

enzyme

esophagus

gallbladder

hydrolysis

intestine

lacteal

liver

mastication

pancreas

peristalsis

peritoneum

saliva

stomach

villi

LEARNING OUTCOMES

After careful study of this chapter, you should be able to:

1. Name the three main functions of the digestive system
2. Describe the four layers of the digestive tract wall
3. Differentiate between the two layers of the peritoneum
4. Name and locate the different types of teeth
5. Name and describe the functions of the organs of the digestive tract
6. Name and describe the functions of the accessory organs of digestion
7. Describe how bile functions in digestion
8. Name and locate the ducts that carry bile from the liver into the digestive tract
9. Explain the role of enzymes in digestion and give examples of enzymes
10. Name the digestion products of fats, proteins, and carbohydrates
11. Define *absorption*
12. Define *villi* and state how villi function in absorption
13. Explain the use of feedback in regulating digestion and give several examples
14. List several hormones involved in regulating digestion
15. Show how word parts are used to build words related to digestion (see Word Anatomy at the end of the chapter)

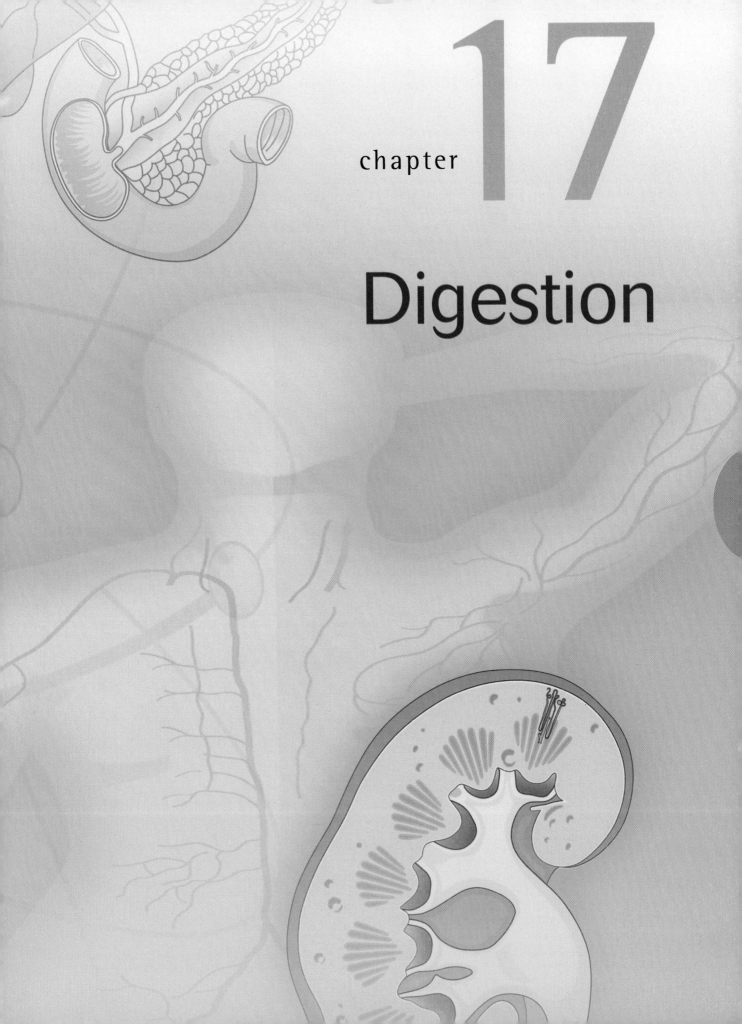

chapter

17

Digestion

❱ Function and Design of the Digestive System

Every body cell needs a constant supply of nutrients. The energy contained in these nutrients is used to do cell work. In addition, the cell rearranges the chemical building blocks of the nutrients to manufacture cellular materials for metabolism, growth, and repair. Food as we take it in, however, is too large to enter the cells. It must first be broken down into particles small enough to pass through the cells' plasma membrane. This breakdown process is known as **digestion**.

After digestion, the circulation must carry nutrients to the cells in every part of the body. The transfer of nutrients into the circulation is called **absorption**. Finally, undigested waste material must be eliminated from the body. Digestion, absorption, and elimination are the three chief functions of the digestive system.

For our purposes, the digestive system may be divided into two groups of organs:

❱ The **digestive tract**, a continuous passageway beginning at the mouth, where food is taken in, and terminating at the anus, where the solid waste products of digestion are expelled from the body.
❱ The **accessory organs**, which are necessary for the digestive process but are not a direct part of the digestive tract. They release substances into the digestive tract through ducts. These organs are the salivary glands, liver, gallbladder, and pancreas.

> **Checkpoint 17-1** Why does food have to be digested before cells can use it?

Before describing the individual organs of the digestive tract, we will pause to discuss the general structure of these organs. We will also describe the large membrane (peritoneum) that lines the abdominopelvic cavity, which contains most of the digestive organs.

The Wall of the Digestive Tract

Although modified for specific tasks in different organs, the wall of the digestive tract, from the esophagus to the anus, is similar in structure throughout. The general pattern consists of four layers:

❱ Mucous membrane
❱ Submucosa
❱ Smooth muscle
❱ Serous membrane

Refer to the diagram of the small intestine in Figure 17-1 as we describe the layers of this wall from the innermost to the outermost surface.

First is the **mucous membrane**, or **mucosa**, so called because its epithelial layer contains many mucus-secreting cells. From the mouth through the esophagus, and also in the anus, the epithelium consists of multiple layers of squamous (flat) cells, which help to protect deeper tissues. Throughout the remainder of the digestive tract, the type of epithelium in the mucosa is simple columnar.

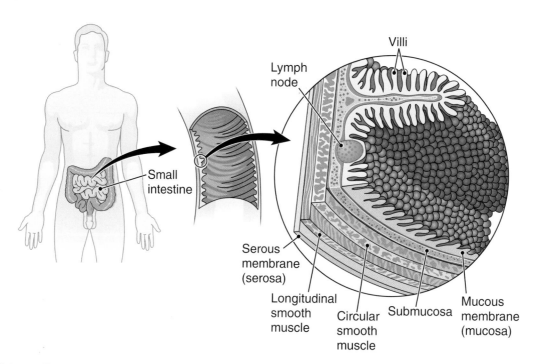

Figure 17-1 Wall of the digestive tract. The mucous membrane of the small intestine shown here has numerous projections called villi. *ZOOMING IN ✦ What type of tissue is between the submucosa and the serous membrane in the digestive tract wall?*

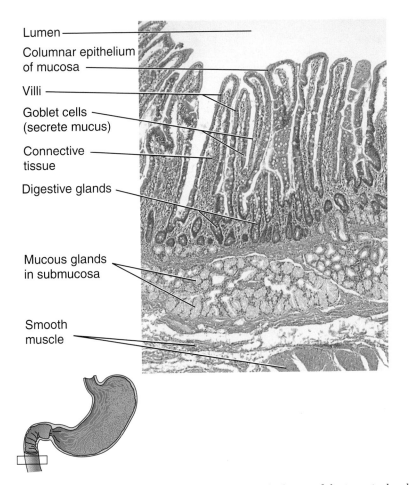

Lumen
Columnar epithelium of mucosa
Villi
Goblet cells (secrete mucus)
Connective tissue
Digestive glands
Mucous glands in submucosa
Smooth muscle

Figure 17-2 Microscopic view of small intestine. The layers of the intestinal wall are visible (except for the serous membrane). (Micrograph reprinted with permission from Cormack DH. Essential Histology. 2nd ed. Philadelphia: Lippincott Williams & Wilkins, 2001.)

peristalsis (per-ih-STAL-sis), that propels food through the digestive tract and mixes it with digestive juices.

The esophagus differs slightly from this pattern in having striated muscle in its upper portion, and the stomach has an additional third layer of smooth muscle in its wall to add strength for churning food.

The digestive organs in the abdominopelvic cavity have an outermost layer of **serous membrane**, or **serosa**, a thin, moist tissue composed of simple squamous epithelium and loose connective tissue. This membrane forms part of the peritoneum (per-ih-to-NE-um). The esophagus above the diaphragm has instead an outer layer composed of fibrous connective tissue.

Checkpoint 17-2 The digestive tract has a wall that is basically similar throughout its length and is composed of four layers. What are the typical four layers of this wall?

The Peritoneum

The abdominopelvic cavity (Fig. 17-3) is lined with a thin, shiny serous membrane that also folds back to cover most of the organs contained within the cavity. The outer portion of this membrane, the layer that lines the cavity, is called the **parietal peritoneum**; that covering the organs is called the **visceral peritoneum**. This slippery membrane allows the organs to slide over each other as they function. The peritoneum also carries blood vessels, lymphatic vessels, and nerves. In some places, it supports the organs and binds them to each other. Subdivisions of the peritoneum around the various organs have special names.

Subdivisions of the Peritoneum The **mesentery** (MES-en-ter-e) is a double-layered portion of the peritoneum shaped somewhat like a fan. The handle portion is attached to the posterior abdominal wall, and the expanded long edge is attached to the small intestine. Between the two membranous layers of the mesentery are the vessels and nerves that supply the intestine. The section of the peritoneum that extends from the colon to the posterior abdominal wall is the **mesocolon** (mes-o-KO-lon).

A large double layer of the peritoneum containing much fat hangs like an apron over the front of the intestine. This **greater omentum** (o-MEN-tum) extends from

Many of the cells that secrete digestive juices are located in the mucosa. Figure 17-2 is a microscopic view of a representative section of the digestive tract taken from the small intestine. Mucus-secreting cells (goblet cells) appear as clear areas between epithelial cells. Note that the small intestine's lining has fingerlike extensions (villi) that aid in the absorption of nutrients, as will be described later.

The layer of connective tissue beneath the mucosa is the **submucosa**, which contains blood vessels and some of the nerves that help regulate digestive activity. In the small intestine, the submucosa has many glands that produce mucus to protect that organ from the highly acidic material it receives from the stomach.

The next layer is composed of **smooth muscle**. Most of the digestive organs have two layers of smooth muscle: an inner layer of circular fibers, and an outer layer of longitudinal fibers. When a section of the circular muscle contracts, the lumen of the organ narrows; when the longitudinal muscle contracts, a section of the wall shortens and the lumen becomes wider. These alternating muscular contractions create the wavelike movement, called

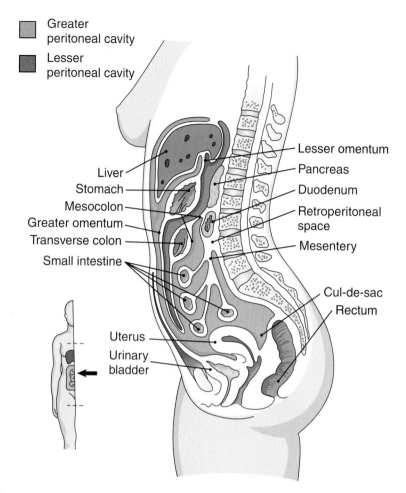

Greater peritoneal cavity

Lesser peritoneal cavity

Liver
Stomach
Mesocolon
Greater omentum
Transverse colon
Small intestine

Lesser omentum
Pancreas
Duodenum
Retroperitoneal space
Mesentery

Cul-de-sac
Rectum

Uterus
Urinary bladder

Figure 17-3 **The abdominopelvic cavity.** Subdivisions of the peritoneum fold over, supporting and separating individual organs. *ZOOMING IN ✦ What part of the peritoneum is around the small intestine?*

the lower border of the stomach into the pelvic part of the abdomen and then loops back up to the transverse colon. A smaller membrane, called the **lesser omentum**, extends between the stomach and the liver.

Checkpoint 17-3 What is the name of the large serous membrane that lines the abdominopelvic cavity and covers the organs it contains?

▶ Organs of the Digestive Tract

As we study the organs of the digestive system, locate each in Figure 17-4.

The digestive tract is a muscular tube extending through the body. It is composed of several parts: the **mouth, pharynx, esophagus, stomach, small intestine,** and **large intestine.** The digestive tract is sometimes called the **alimentary tract,** from the word *aliment,* meaning "food." It is more commonly referred to as the **gastrointestinal (GI) tract** because of the major importance of the stomach and intestine in the process of digestion.

The next section describes the structure and function

of each digestive organ. These descriptions are followed by an overview of how the organs work together in the digestive process.

The Mouth

The **mouth,** also called the **oral cavity,** is where a substance begins its travels through the digestive tract (Fig. 17-5). The mouth has the following digestive functions:

▶ It receives food, a process called **ingestion.**
▶ It breaks food into small portions. This is done mainly by the teeth in the process of chewing or **mastication** (mas-tih-KA-shun), but the tongue, cheeks, and lips are also used.
▶ It mixes the food with **saliva** (sah-LI-vah), which is produced by the salivary glands and secreted into the mouth. Saliva lubricates the food and has a digestive enzyme called *salivary amylase,* which begins starch digestion. The salivary glands will be described with the other accessory organs.
▶ It moves proper amounts of food toward the throat to be swallowed, a process called **deglutition** (deg-lu-TISH-un).

The tongue, a muscular organ that projects into the mouth, is used as an aid in chewing and swallowing, and is one of the principal organs of speech. The tongue has a number of special organs on its surface, called *taste buds,* which can differentiate taste sensations (bitter, sweet, sour, or salty) (see Chapter 10).

The Teeth

The oral cavity also contains the teeth (see Fig. 17-5). A child between 2 and 6 years of age has 20 teeth, known as the baby teeth or **deciduous** (de-SID-u-us) teeth. (The word deciduous means "falling off at a certain time," such as the leaves that fall off the trees in autumn.) A complete set of adult permanent teeth numbers 32. The cutting teeth, or **incisors** (in-SI-sors), occupy the anterior part of the oral cavity. The **cuspids** (KUS-pids), commonly called the *canines* (KA-nines) or *eyeteeth,* are lateral to the incisors. They are pointed teeth with deep roots that are used for more forceful gripping and tearing of food. The **molars** (MO-lars), the larger grinding teeth, are posterior. There are two premolars and three molars. In an adult, each quadrant (quarter) of the mouth, moving from

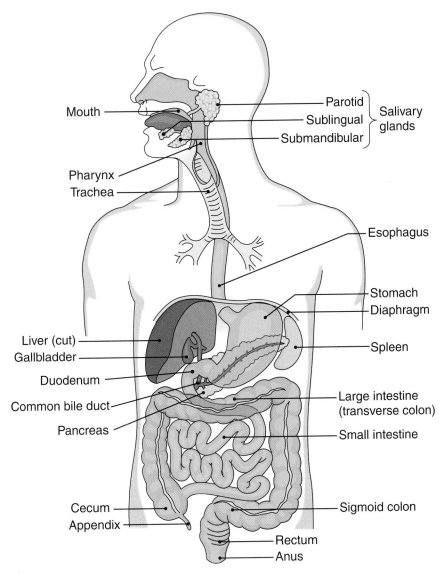

Mouth

Parotid ⎫
Sublingual ⎬ Salivary glands
Submandibular ⎭

Pharynx
Trachea

Esophagus

Stomach
Diaphragm

Liver (cut)
Gallbladder

Spleen

Duodenum
Common bile duct
Pancreas

Large intestine (transverse colon)

Small intestine

Cecum
Appendix

Sigmoid colon

Rectum
Anus

Figure 17-4 **The digestive system.** *ZOOMING IN ✦ What accessory organs of digestion secrete into the mouth?*

anterior to posterior, has two incisors, one cuspid and five molars.

The first eight deciduous (baby) teeth to appear through the gums are the incisors. Later, the cuspids and molars appear. Usually, the 20 baby teeth all have appeared by the time a child has reached the age of 2 to 3 years. During the first 2 years, the permanent teeth develop within the upper jaw (maxilla) and lower jaw (mandible) from buds that are present at birth. The first permanent teeth to appear are the four 6-year molars, which come in before any baby teeth are lost. Because decay and infection of deciduous molars may spread to new, permanent teeth, deciduous teeth need proper care.

As a child grows, the jawbones grow, making space for additional teeth. After the 6-year molars have appeared, the baby incisors loosen and are replaced by permanent incisors. Next, the baby canines (cuspids) are re-

placed by permanent canines, and finally, the baby molars are replaced by the permanent bicuspids (premolars).

At this point, the larger jawbones are ready for the appearance of the 12-year, or second, permanent molar teeth. During or after the late teens, the third molars, or so-called *wisdom teeth,* may appear. In some cases, the jaw is not large enough for these teeth, or there are other abnormalities, so that the third molars may not erupt or may have to be removed. Figure 17-6 shows the parts of a molar.

The main substance of the tooth is **dentin**, a calcified substance harder than bone. Within the tooth is a soft pulp containing blood vessels and nerves. The tooth's crown projects above the gum, the **gingiva** (JIN-jih-vah), and is covered with **enamel**, the hardest substance in the body. The roots of the tooth, below the gum line in a bony socket, are covered with a rigid connective tissue (cementum) that helps to hold the tooth in place. Each root has a canal containing extensions of the pulp.

Checkpoint 17-4 How many baby teeth are there and what is the scientific name for the baby teeth?

The Pharynx

The **pharynx** (FAR-inks) is commonly referred to as the throat (see Fig. 17-5). The oral part of the pharynx, the oropharynx, is visible when you look into an open mouth and depress the tongue. The palatine tonsils may be seen at either side of the oropharynx. The pharynx also extends upward to the nasal cavity, where it is referred to as the nasopharynx and downward to the larynx, where it is called the laryngeal pharynx. The **soft palate** is tissue that forms the posterior roof of the oral cavity. From it hangs a soft, fleshy, V-shaped mass called the **uvula** (U-vu-lah).

In swallowing, the tongue pushes a **bolus** (BO-lus) of food, a small portion of chewed food mixed with saliva, into the pharynx. Once the food reaches the pharynx, swallowing occurs rapidly by an involuntary reflex action. At the same time, the soft palate and uvula are raised to prevent food and liquid from entering the nasal cavity, and the tongue is raised to seal the back of the oral cavity. The entrance of the trachea is guarded during swallowing by a leaf-shaped cartilage, the **epiglottis**, which

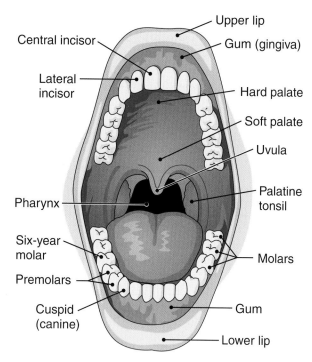

Figure 17-5 **The mouth.** The teeth and tonsils are visible in this view.

covers the opening of the larynx. The swallowed food is then moved into the esophagus.

The Esophagus

The **esophagus** (eh-SOF-ah-gus) is a muscular tube about 25 cm (10 inches) long. In the esophagus, food is lubricated with mucus and moved by peristalsis into the stomach. No additional digestion occurs in the esophagus.

Before joining the stomach, the esophagus must pass through the diaphragm. It travels through a space in the di-

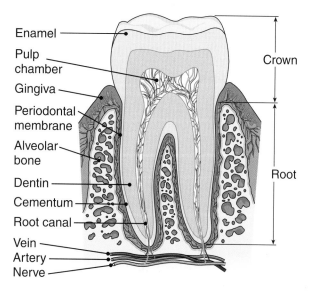

Figure 17-6 **A molar tooth.**

aphragm called the **esophageal hiatus** (eh-sof-ah-JE-al hi-A-tus). If there is a weakness in the diaphragm at this point, a portion of the stomach or other abdominal organ may protrude through the space, a condition called *hiatal hernia.*

The Stomach

The stomach is an expanded J-shaped organ in the upper left region of the abdominal cavity (Fig. 17-7). In addition to the two muscle layers already described, it has a third, inner oblique (angled) layer that aids in grinding food and mixing it with digestive juices. The left-facing arch of the stomach is the **greater curvature**, whereas the right surface forms the **lesser curvature**. The superior rounded portion under the left side of the diaphragm is the stomach's **fundus**.

Sphincters A **sphincter** (SFINK-ter) is a muscular ring that regulates the size of an opening. There are two sphincters that separate the stomach from the organs above and below.

Between the esophagus and the stomach is the **lower esophageal sphincter (LES)**. This muscle has also been called the **cardiac sphincter** because it separates the esophagus from the region of the stomach that is close to the heart. We are sometimes aware of the existence of this sphincter when it does not relax as it should, producing a feeling of being unable to swallow past that point.

Between the distal, or far, end of the stomach and the small intestine is the **pyloric** (pi-LOR-ik) **sphincter**. The region of the stomach leading into this sphincter, the **pylorus** (pi-LOR-us), is important in regulating how rapidly food moves into the small intestine.

Functions of the Stomach The stomach serves as a storage pouch, digestive organ, and churn. When the stomach is empty, the lining forms many folds called **rugae** (RU-je). These folds disappear as the stomach expands. (The stomach can stretch to hold one half of a gallon of food and liquid.) Special cells in the lining of the stomach secrete substances that mix together to form **gastric juice**. Some of the cells secrete a great amount of mucus to protect the stomach lining from digestive secretions. Other cells produce the active components of the gastric juice, which are:

- Hydrochloric acid (HCl), a strong acid that helps break down protein and destroys foreign organisms.
- Pepsin, a protein-digesting enzyme produced in an inactive form and activated only when food enters the stomach and HCl is produced.

Chyme (*kime*), from a Greek word meaning "juice," is the highly acidic, semiliquid mixture of gastric juice and food that leaves the stomach to enter the small intestine.

Checkpoint 17-5 What type of food is digested in the stomach?

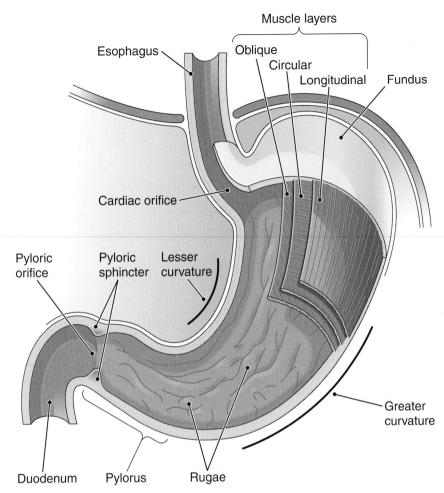

Figure 17-7 Longitudinal section of the stomach. The stomach's interior is visible, along with a portion of the esophagus and the duodenum. *ZOOMING IN ✦ What additional muscle layer is in the wall of the stomach that is not found in the rest of the digestive tract?*

The Small Intestine

The small intestine is the longest part of the digestive tract (Fig. 17-8). It is known as the small intestine because, although it is longer than the large intestine, it is smaller in diameter, with an average width of approximately 2.5 cm (1 inch). After death, when relaxed to its full length, the small intestine is approximately 6 m (20 feet) long. In life, the small intestine averages 3 m (10 feet) in length. The first 25 cm (10 inches) or so of the small intestine make up the **duodenum** (du-o-DE-num) (named for the Latin word for "twelve," based on its length of twelve finger widths). Beyond the duodenum are two more divisions: the **jejunum** (je-JU-num), which forms the next two-fifths of the small intestine, and the **ileum** (IL-e-um), which constitutes the remaining portion.

Functions of the Small Intestine The duodenal mucosa and submucosa contain glands that secrete large amounts of mucus to protect the small intestine from the strongly acidic chyme entering from the stomach. Mucosal cells of the small intestine also secrete enzymes that digest proteins and carbohydrates. In addition, digestive juices from the liver and pancreas enter the small intestine through a small opening in the duodenum. Most of the digestive process takes place in the small intestine under the effects of these juices.

Most absorption of digested food, water, and minerals also occurs through the walls of the small intestine. To increase the organ's surface area for this purpose, the mucosa is formed into millions of tiny, fingerlike projections, called **villi** (VIL-li) (Fig. 17-9), which give the inner surface a velvety appearance (see also Figs. 17-1 and 17-2). The epithelial cells of the villi also have small projecting folds of the plasma membrane known as **microvilli**. These create a remarkable increase in the total surface area available in the small intestine for absorption.

Each villus contains blood vessels through which most digestion products are absorbed into the blood. Each one also contains a specialized lymphatic capillary called a **lacteal** (LAK-tele) through which fats are absorbed into the lymph. Box 17-1 provides more information on the relationship of surface area to absorption.

Checkpoint 17-6 What are the three divisions of the small intestine?

Checkpoint 17-7 How does the small intestine function in the digestive process?

The Large Intestine

The large intestine is approximately 6.5 cm (2.5 inches) in diameter and approximately 1.5 m (5 feet) long (see Fig. 17-8). It is named for its wide diameter, rather than its length. The outer longitudinal muscle fibers in its wall form three separate surface bands (see Fig. 17-8). These bands, known as **teniae** (TEN-e-e) **coli** draw up the organ's wall to give it its distinctive puckered appearance. (Spelling is also *taeniae*; the singular is *tenia* or *taenia*).

Subdivisions of the Large Intestine The large intestine begins in the lower right region of the abdomen. The first part is a small pouch called the **cecum** (SE-kum). Between the ileum of the small intestine and the cecum is a sphincter, the **ileocecal** (il-e-o-SE-kal) **valve**, that prevents food from traveling backward into the small

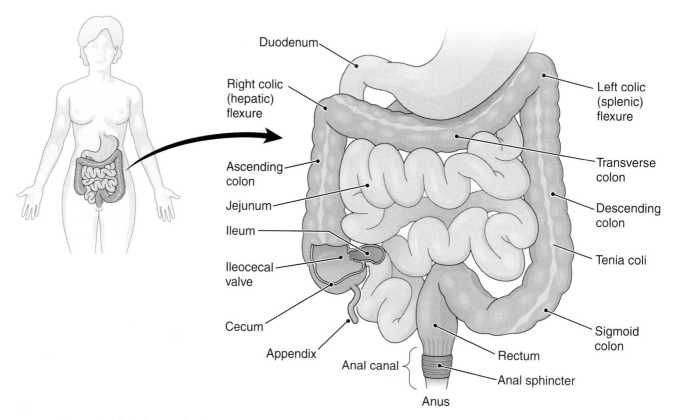

Figure 17-8 **The small and large intestines.** *ZOOMING IN ✦ What part of the small intestine joins the cecum?*

intestine. Attached to the cecum is a small, blind tube containing lymphoid tissue; its full name is **vermiform** (VER-mih-form) **appendix** (*vermiform* means "worm-like"), but usually just "appendix" is used.

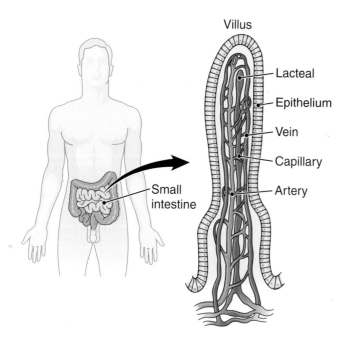

Figure 17-9 **A villus of the small intestine.** Each villus has blood vessels and a lacteal (lymphatic capillary) for absorption of nutrients.

The second portion, the **ascending colon**, extends upward along the right side of the abdomen toward the liver. It bends near the liver at the right colic (hepatic) flexure and extends across the abdomen as the **transverse colon**. It bends again sharply at the left colic (splenic) flexure and extends downward on the left side of the abdomen into the pelvis, forming the **descending colon**. The distal part of the colon bends backward into an S shape forming the **sigmoid colon** (named for the Greek letter *sigma*), which continues downward to empty into the **rectum,** a temporary storage area for indigestible or nonabsorbable food residue (see Fig. 17-8). The narrow portion of the distal large intestine is the **anal canal**, which leads to the outside of the body through an opening called the **anus** (A-nus).

Functions of the Large Intestine

The large intestine secretes a great quantity of mucus, but no enzymes. Food is not digested in this organ, but some water is reabsorbed, and undigested food is stored, formed into solid waste material, called **feces** (FE-seze) or stool, and then eliminated.

At intervals, usually after meals, the involuntary muscles within the walls of the large intestine propel solid waste toward the rectum. Stretching of the rectum stimulates contraction of smooth muscle in the rectal wall. Aided by voluntary contractions of the diaphragm and the abdominal muscles, the feces are eliminated from the body in a process called **defecation** (def-e-KA-shun). An

The Folded Intestine: More Absorption With Less Length

Whenever materials pass from one system to another, they must travel through a cellular membrane. A major factor in how much transport can occur per unit time is the total surface area of the membrane; the greater the surface area, the higher the rate of transport. The problem of packing a large amount of surface into a small space is solved in the body by folding the membranes. We do the same thing in everyday life. Imagine trying to store a bed sheet in the closet without folding it!

In the small intestine, where digested food must absorb into the bloodstream, there is folding of membranes down to the level of single cells.

▶ The 6-meter-long organ is coiled to fit into the abdominal cavity.

▶ The inner wall of the organ is thrown into circular folds called plicae circulares, which not only increase surface area, but aid in mixing.
▶ The mucosal villi project into the lumen, providing more surface area than a flat membrane would.
▶ The individual cells that line the small intestine have microvilli, tiny finger-like folds of the plasma membrane that increase surface area tremendously.

Together, these structural features of the small intestine result in an absorptive surface area estimated to be about 250 square meters! Folding is present in other parts of the digestive system and in other areas of the body as well. Can you name other systems that show this folding pattern?

anal sphincter provides voluntary control over defecation (see Fig. 17-8).

While the food residue is stored in the large intestine, bacteria that normally live in the colon act on it to produce vitamin K and some of the B-complex vitamins. As mentioned, systemic antibiotic therapy may destroy these symbiotic (helpful) bacteria living in the large intestine, causing undesirable side effects.

Checkpoint 17-8 What are the divisions of the large intestine?

Checkpoint 17-9 What are the functions of the large intestine?

▶ The **parotid** (pah-ROT-id) **glands**, the largest of the group, are located inferior and anterior to the ear.
▶ The **submandibular** (sub-man-DIB-u-lar), or **submaxillary** (sub-MAK-sih-ler-e), **glands** are located near the body of the lower jaw.
▶ The **sublingual** (sub-LING-gwal) **glands** are under the tongue.

All these glands empty through ducts into the oral cavity.

Checkpoint 17-10 What are the names of the salivary glands?

▶ The Accessory Organs

The accessory organs (Fig. 17-10) release secretions through ducts into the digestive tract. The salivary glands deliver their secretions into the mouth. All of the others accessory organs release secretions into the duodenum.

The Salivary Glands

While food is in the mouth, it is mixed with **saliva** (sah-LI-vah), which moistens the food and facilitates mastication (chewing) and deglutition (swallowing). Saliva helps to keep the teeth and mouth clean. It also contains some antibodies and an enzyme (lysozyme) that help reduce bacterial growth.

This watery mixture contains mucus and an enzyme called **salivary amylase** (AM-ih-laze), which begins the digestive process by converting starch to sugar. Saliva is manufactured by three pairs of glands (see Fig. 17-4):

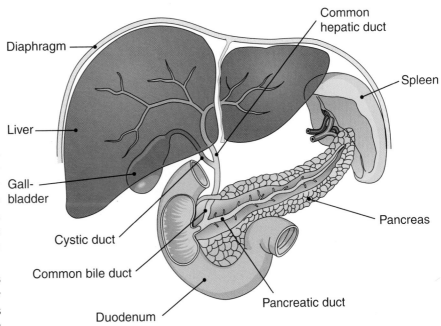

Figure 17-10 Accessory organs of digestion. *ZOOMING IN ✦ Into what part of the intestine do these accessory organs secrete?*

The Liver

The liver, often referred to by the word root *hepat*, is the body's largest glandular organ (see Fig. 17-10). It is located in the upper right portion of the abdominal cavity under the dome of the diaphragm. The lower edge of a normal-sized liver is level with the lower margin of the ribs. The human liver is the same reddish brown color as animal liver seen in the supermarket. It has a large right lobe and a smaller left lobe; the right lobe includes two inferior smaller lobes. The liver is supplied with blood through two vessels: the portal vein and the hepatic artery (the portal system and blood supply to the liver were described in Chapter 14). These vessels deliver about 1.5 quarts (1.6 L) of blood to the liver every minute. The hepatic artery carries oxygenated blood, whereas the venous portal system carries blood that is rich in digestive end products. This most remarkable organ has many functions that affect digestion, metabolism, blood composition, and elimination of waste. Some of its major activities are:

▶ The manufacture of **bile**, a substance needed for the digestion of fats.
▶ The storage of glucose (simple sugar) in the form of **glycogen,** the animal equivalent of the starch found in plants. When the blood sugar level falls below normal, liver cells convert glycogen to glucose, which is released into the blood restoring the normal blood sugar concentration.
▶ The modification of fats so that they can be used more efficiently by cells all over the body.
▶ The storage of some vitamins and iron.
▶ The formation of blood plasma proteins, such as albumin, globulins, and clotting factors.
▶ The destruction of old red blood cells and the recycling or elimination of their breakdown products. One byproduct, a pigment called **bilirubin** (BIL-ih-ru-bin), is eliminated in bile and gives the stool its characteristic dark color.
▶ The synthesis of **urea** (u-RE-ah), a waste product of protein metabolism. Urea is released into the blood and transported to the kidneys for elimination.
▶ The **detoxification** (de-tok-sih-fih-KA-shun) (removal of the poisonous properties) of harmful substances, such as alcohol and certain drugs.

Bile The main digestive function of the liver is the production of bile, a substance needed for the processing of fats. The salts contained in bile act like a detergent to **emulsify** fat, that is, to break up fat into small droplets that can be acted on more effectively by digestive enzymes. Bile also aids in fat absorption from the small intestine.

Bile leaves the lobes of the liver by two ducts that merge to form the **common hepatic** duct. After collecting bile from the gallbladder, this duct, now called the **com-** mon **bile duct,** delivers bile into the duodenum. These and the other accessory ducts are shown in Figure 17-10.

The Gallbladder

The gallbladder is a muscular sac on the inferior surface of the liver that stores bile. Although the liver may manufacture bile continuously, the body needs it only a few times a day. Consequently, bile from the liver flows into the hepatic ducts and then up through the **cystic** (SIS-tik) **duct,** connected with the gallbladder (see Fig. 17-10). When chyme enters the duodenum, the gallbladder contracts, squeezing bile through the cystic duct and into the common bile duct, leading to the duodenum.

The Pancreas

The pancreas is a long gland that extends from the duodenum to the spleen (see Fig. 17-10). The pancreas produces enzymes that digest fats, proteins, carbohydrates, and nucleic acids. The protein-digesting enzymes are produced in inactive forms which must be converted to active forms in the small intestine by other enzymes.

The pancreas also produces large amounts of alkaline (basic) fluid, that neutralizes the acidic chyme in the small intestine, thus protecting the lining of the digestive tract. These juices collect in a main duct that joins the common bile duct or empties into the duodenum near the common bile duct. Most people have an additional smaller duct that opens into the duodenum.

As described in Chapter 11, the pancreas also functions as an endocrine gland, producing the hormones insulin and glucagon that regulate sugar metabolism. These islet cell secretions are released directly into the blood.

Checkpoint 17-11 What is the role of the gallbladder?

Checkpoint 17-12 What is the role of bile in digestion?

▶ Enzymes and the Digestive Process

Although the different organs of the digestive tract are specialized for digesting different types of food, the basic chemical process of digestion is the same for fats, proteins, and carbohydrates. In every case, this process requires enzymes. Enzymes are catalysts, substances that speed the rate of chemical reactions, but are not themselves changed or used up in the reaction.

All enzymes are proteins, and they are highly specific in their actions. In digestion, an enzyme acts only in a certain type of reaction involving a certain type of nutrient molecule. For example, the carbohydrate-digesting enzyme amylase only splits starch into the disaccharide (double sugar) maltose. Another enzyme is required to split maltose into two molecules of the monosaccharide (simple sugar) glucose. Other enzymes split fats into their building blocks, glycerol and fatty acids, and still others split proteins into smaller units called *peptides* and into their building blocks, amino acids.

The Role of Water

Because water is added to nutrient molecules as they are split by enzymes, the process of digestion is referred to chemically as **hydrolysis** (hi-DROL-ih-sis), which means "splitting by means of water." About 7 liters of water are secreted into the digestive tract each day, in addition to the nearly 2 liters taken in with food and drink. You can now understand why so large an amount of water is needed. Water not only is used to produce digestive juices and to dilute food so that it can move more easily through the digestive tract, but also is used in the chemical process of digestion itself.

Digestion, Step by Step

Let us see what happens to a mass of food from the time it is taken into the mouth to the moment that it is ready to be absorbed (see Table 17-1).

In the mouth, the food is chewed and mixed with saliva, softening it so that it can be swallowed easily. Salivary amylase initiates the process of digestion by changing some of the starches into sugar.

Digestion in the Stomach When the food reaches the stomach, it is acted on by gastric juice, with its hydrochloric acid (HCl) and enzymes. The hydrochloric acid has the important function of breaking down proteins and preparing them for digestion. In addition, HCl activates the enzyme pepsin, which is secreted by gastric cells in an inactive form. Once activated by hydrochloric acid, pepsin works to digest protein; this enzyme is the first to digest nearly every type of protein in the diet. The stomach also secretes a fat-digesting enzyme (lipase), but it is of little importance in adults.

The food, gastric juice, and mucus (which is also secreted by cells of the gastric lining) are mixed to form chyme. This semiliquid substance is moved from the stomach to the small intestine for further digestion.

Digestion in the Small Intestine In the duodenum, the first part of the small intestine, chyme is mixed with the greenish yellow bile delivered from the liver and the gallbladder through the common bile duct. Bile does not contain enzymes; instead, it contains salts that emulsify fats to allow the powerful secretions from the pancreas to act on them most efficiently.

Pancreatic juice contains a number of enzymes, including:

▶ **Lipase.** After bile divides fats into tiny particles, the highly active pancreatic enzyme lipase digests almost all of them. In this process, fats are usually broken down into two simpler compounds, glycerol (glycerin) and fatty acids, which are more readily absorbable. If pancreatic lipase is absent, fats are expelled with the feces in undigested form.
▶ **Amylase.** This enzyme changes starch to sugar.
▶ **Trypsin** (TRIP-sin). This enzyme splits proteins into amino acids, which are small enough to be absorbed through the intestine.
▶ **Nucleases** (NU-kle-ases). These enzymes digest the nucleic acids DNA and RNA.

It is important to note that most digestion occurs in the small intestine under the action of pancreatic juice, which has the ability to break down all types of foods. When pancreatic juice is absent, serious digestive disturbances always occur.

The small intestine also produces a number of enzymes, including three that act on complex sugars to transform them into simpler, absorbable forms. These enzymes are **maltase, sucrase,** and **lactase,** which act on the disaccharides maltose, sucrose, and lactose, respectively.

Table 17·1	**Summary of Digestion**		
ORGAN	**ACTIVITY**	**NUTRIENTS DIGESTED**	**ACTIVE SECRETIONS**
Mouth	Chews food and mixes it with saliva; forms into bolus for swallowing	Starch	Salivary amylase
Esophagus	Moves food by peristalsis into stomach	—	—
Stomach	Stores food, churns food, and mixes it with digestive juices	Proteins	Hydrochloric acid, pepsin
Small intestine	Secretes enzymes, neutralizes acidity, receives secretions from pancreas and liver, absorbs nutrients and water into the blood or lymph	Fats, proteins, carbohydrates, nucleic acids	Intestinal enzymes, pancreatic enzymes, bile from liver
Large intestine	Reabsorbs some water; forms, stores, and eliminates stool	—	—

Table 17-2 summarizes the main substances used in digestion. Note that, except for HCl, sodium bicarbonate, and bile salts, all the substances listed are enzymes.

Checkpoint 17-13 What organ produces the most complete digestive secretions?

Table 17·2	Digestive Juices Produced by Digestive Tract Organs and Accessory Organs	
ORGAN	**MAIN DIGESTIVE JUICES SECRETED**	**ACTION**
Salivary glands	Salivary amylase	Begins starch digestion
Stomach	Hydrochloric acid (HCl)^a	Breaks down proteins
	Pepsin	Begins protein digestion
Small intestine	Peptidases	Digests proteins to amino acids
	Lactase, maltase, sucrase	Digests disaccharides to monosaccharides
Pancreas	Sodium bicarbonate^a	Neutralizes HCl
	Amylase	Digests starch
	Trypsin	Digests protein to amino acids
	Lipases	Digests fats to fatty acids and glycerol
	Nucleases	Digests nucleic acids
Liver	Bile salts^a	Emulsifies fats

^{a}Not enzymes

Absorption

The means by which digested nutrients reach the blood is known as **absorption**. Most absorption takes place through the villi in the mucosa of the small intestine (see Fig. 17-9). Within each villus is an arteriole and a venule bridged with capillaries. Simple sugars, small proteins (peptides), amino acids, some simple fatty acids, and most of the water in the digestive tract are absorbed into the blood through these capillaries. From here, they pass by way of the portal system to the liver, to be processed, stored, or released as needed.

Absorption of Fats

Most fats have an alternative method of reaching the blood. Instead of entering the blood capillaries, they are absorbed by the villi's more permeable lymphatic capillaries called **lacteals**. The absorbed fat droplets give the lymph a milky appearance. The mixture of lymph and fat globules that drains from the small intestine after fat has been digested is called **chyle** (kile). Chyle merges with the lymphatic circulation and eventually enters the blood when the lymph drains into veins near the heart. The absorbed fats then circulate to the liver for further processing.

Absorption of Vitamins and Minerals

Minerals and vitamins ingested with food are also absorbed from the small intestine. The minerals and some of the vitamins dissolve in water and are absorbed directly into the blood. Other vitamins are incorporated in fats and are absorbed along with the fats. Vitamin K and some B vitamins are produced by bacterial action in the colon and are absorbed from the large intestine.

Checkpoint 17-14 What is absorption?

Control of Digestion

As food moves through the digestive tract, its rate of movement and the activity of each organ it passes through must be carefully regulated. If food moves too slowly or digestive secretions are inadequate, the body will not get enough nourishment. If food moves too rapidly or excess secretions are produced, digestion may be incomplete or the lining of the digestive tract may be damaged. There are two types of control over digestion: nervous and hormonal. Both illustrate the principles of feedback control.

The nerves that control digestive activity are located in the submucosa and between the muscle layers of the organ walls. Instructions for action come from the autonomic (visceral) nervous system. In general, parasympathetic stimulation increases activity, and sympathetic stimulation decreases activity. Excess sympathetic stimulation, as in stress, can block the movement of food through the digestive tract and inhibit the secretion of mucus, which is crucial in protecting the lining of the digestive tract.

The digestive organs themselves produce the hormones involved in the regulation of digestion. The following is a discussion of some of these controls (Table 17-3).

The sight, smell, thought, taste, or feel of food in the mouth stimulates, through the nervous system, the secretion of saliva and the release of gastric juice. Once in the stomach, food stimulates the release into the blood of the hormone **gastrin,** which promotes stomach secretions and motility (movement).

When chyme enters the duodenum, nerve impulses inhibit movement of the stomach, so that food will not move too rapidly into the small intestine. This action is a good example of negative feedback. At the same time, hormones released from the duodenum not only function in digestion, but also feed back to the stomach to reduce its activity. **Gastric-inhibitory peptide (GIP)** is one such hormone. It acts on the stomach to inhibit the release of gastric juice. Its more important action is to stimulate insulin release from the pancreas when glucose enters the duodenum. Another of these hormones, **secretin** (se-

Table 17·3 Hormones Active in Digestion

HORMONE	SOURCE	ACTION
Gastrin	Stomach	Stimulates release of gastric juice
Gastric-inhibitory peptide (GIP)	Duodenum	Stimulates insulin release from pancreas when glucose enters duodenum; inhibits release of gastric juice
Secretin	Duodenum	Stimulates release of water and bicarbonate from pancreas, stimulates release of bile from liver; inhibits the stomach
Cholecystokinin (CCK)	Duodenum	Stimulates release of digestive enzymes from pancreas, stimulates release of bile from gallbladder; inhibits the stomach

KRE-tin) stimulates the pancreas to release water and bicarbonate to dilute and neutralize chyme. **Cholecystokinin** (ko-le-sis-to-KI-nin) **(CCK)**, stimulates the release of enzymes from the pancreas and causes the gallbladder to release bile.

> **Checkpoint 17-15** What are the two types of control over the digestive process?

Hunger and Appetite

Hunger is the desire for food, which can be satisfied by the ingestion of a filling meal. Hunger is regulated by hypothalamic centers that respond to the levels of nutrients in the blood. When these levels are low, the hypothalamus stimulates a sensation of hunger. Strong, mildly painful contractions of the empty stomach may stimulate a feeling of hunger. Messages received by the hypothalamus reduce hunger as food is chewed and swallowed and begins to fill the stomach. The short-term regulation of food intake works to keep the amount of food eaten within the limits of what the intestine can process. The long-term regulation of food intake maintains appropriate blood levels of certain nutrients.

Appetite differs from hunger in that, although it is basically a desire for food, it often has no relationship to the need for food. Even after an adequate meal that has relieved hunger, a person may still have an appetite for additional food. A variety of factors, such as emotional state, cultural influences, habit, and memories of past food intake, can affect appetite. The regulation of appetite is not well understood (see Box 17-2).

❱ Aging and the Digestive System

With age, receptors for taste and smell deteriorate, leading to a loss of appetite and decreased enjoyment of food. A decrease in saliva and poor gag reflex make swallowing more difficult. Tooth loss or poorly fitting dentures may make chewing food more difficult.

Activity of the digestive organs decreases. These changes can be seen in poor absorption of certain vitamins and poor protein digestion. Slowing of peristalsis in the large intestine and increased consumption of easily chewed, refined foods contribute to the common occurrence of constipation.

The tissues of the digestive system require constant replacement. Slowing of this process contributes to a variety of digestive disorders. As with many body systems, tumors and cancer occur more frequently with age.

Box 17-2   Hot Topics

Leptin: The Weight-Loss Hormone

Despite day-to-day variations in food intake and physical activity, a healthy individual maintains a constant body weight and energy reserves of fat over long periods. Clearly, long-term negative feedback mechanisms are at work, but until recently scientists did not understand them. With the discovery of the hormone **leptin** (from the Greek word *leptos*, meaning thin), researchers have been able to piece together one long-term mechanism for regulating weight. Leptin is produced by adipocytes, the cells in adipose tissue. Fat storage that occurs when food intake exceeds the body's demands stimulates adipocytes to release more leptin into the bloodstream. Centers in the hypothalamus respond to the increased leptin by decreasing food intake and increasing energy expenditure, which result in weight loss. If this feedback mechanism is disrupted, obesity will result. For example, mice with a genetic mutation that prevents them from making leptin are obese. Injecting the mice with leptin causes them to lose weight.

After discovering leptin and demonstrating that it could reverse obesity in genetically obese mice, researchers hoped that leptin could be used to treat obesity in humans. It is now known that unlike genetically obese mice, the vast majority of obese humans are able to make leptin. Human obesity appears to be caused by an inability of the hypothalamus to respond to leptin, rather than our inability to make the hormone.

Summary

Medical terms are built from standardized word parts (prefixes, roots, and suffixes). Learning the meanings of these parts can help you remember words and interpret unfamiliar terms.

WORD PART	MEANING	EXAMPLE
Function and Design of the Digestive System		
ab-	away from	In *absorption*, digested materials are taken from the digestive tract into the circulation.
enter/o	intestine	The *mesentery* is the portion of the peritoneum around the intestine.
mes/o-	middle	The *mesocolon*, like the mesentery, comes from the middle layer of cells in the embryo, the mesoderm.
Organs of the Digestive Tract		
gastr/o	stomach	The *gastrointestinal* tract consists mainly of the stomach and intestine.
The Accessory Organs		
amyl/o	starch	The starch-digesting enzyme in saliva is salivary *amylase*.
lingu/o	tongue	The *sublingual* salivary glands are under the tongue.
hepat/o	liver	The *hepatic* portal system carries blood to the liver.
bil/i	bile	*Bilirubin* is a pigment found in bile.
cyst/o	bladder, sac	The *cystic* duct carries bile into and out of the gallbladder.
Control of Digestion		
chole	bile, gall	*Cholecystokinin* is a hormone that activates the gallbladder (cholecyst/o).

Summary

I. Function and design of the digestive system
1. Functions—digestion, absorption elimination
2. Two groups of organs—digestive tract and accessory organs
A. The wall of the digestive tract—mucous membrane (mucosa), submucosa, smooth muscle, serous membrane (serosa)
B. The peritoneum
  1. Serous membrane that lines the abdominal cavity and folds over organs
  2. Divisions—mesentery, mesocolon, greater omentum, lesser omentum

II. Organs of the digestive tract
A. Mouth
  1. Functions
    a. Ingest food
    b. Begin digestion of starch with salivary amylase
    c. Mastication (chewing)
    d. Deglutition (swallowing)
  2. Tongue—aids mastication and deglutition; has taste buds
B. Teeth
  1. Deciduous (baby) teeth—20 (incisors, canines, molars)
  2. Permanent teeth—32 (incisors, canines, premolars, molars)
C. Pharynx (throat)—moves bolus (portion) of food into esophagus by reflex swallowing
D. Esophagus—long muscular tube that carries food to stomach by peristalsis
E. Stomach
  1. Functions
    a. Storage of food
    b. Breakdown of food by churning to form chyme
    c. Breakdown of protein with hydrochloric acid (HCl)
    d. Digestion of protein with enzyme pepsin
F. Small intestine
  1. Functions
    a. Digestion of food
    b. Absorption of nutrients and water through villi (small projections of intestinal lining)
  2. Divisions—duodenum, jejunum, ileum
G. Large intestine
  1. Divisions—cecum; ascending, transverse, descending, and sigmoid colons; rectum; anus
  2. Functions
    a. Storage and elimination of waste (defecation)
    b. Reabsorption of water

III. Accessory organs
A. Salivary glands—secrete saliva
  1. Functions of saliva
    a. Moistening food—aids chewing and swallowing
    b. Cleaning of mouth and teeth
    c. Digestion of starch with amylase
  2. Three pairs—parotid, submandibular, sublingual

B. Liver
   1. Functions
      a. Manufacture of bile—emulsifies fats
      b. Storage of glucose
      c. Modification of fats
      d. Storage of vitamins and iron
      e. Formation of blood plasma proteins
      f. Destruction of old red blood cells
      g. Synthesis of urea—waste product of proteins
      h. Detoxification of harmful substances
C. Gallbladder
   1. Stores bile until needed for digestion
D. Pancreas
   1. Secretes powerful digestive juice
   2. Secretes alkali (base) to neutralize chyme

IV. Enzymes and the digestive process
   1. Enzymes—catalysts that speed reactions
      a. Products of digestion
         (1) Simple sugars (monosaccharides) from carbohydrates
         (2) Peptides and amino acids from proteins
         (3) Glycerol and fatty acids from fats
A. The role of water
   1. Used to split foods (hydrolysis)

   2. Lubricates and dilutes food
B. Digestion, step-by-step
   1. Mouth—starch
   2. Stomach—protein
   3. Small intestine—remainder of food

V. Absorption—movement of nutrients into the circulation
   1. Nutrients and water from small intestine into blood
A. Absortion of fats
   1. Most fats into lymph through lacteals

VI. Control of digestion
   1. Nervous control
      a. Parasympathetic system—generally increases activity
      b. Sympathetic system—generally decreases activity
   2. Hormonal control
      a. Stimulation of digestive activity
      b. Feedback to inhibit stomach activity
      c. Examples—gastrin, GIP, secretin, CCK
A. Hunger and appetite

VII. Aging and the digestive system

Questions for Study and Review

Building Understanding

Fill in the blanks

1. The wave-like movement of the digestive tract wall is called _____.

2. The small intestine is connected to the posterior abdominal wall by _____.

3. The liver can store glucose in the form of _____.

4. The parotid glands secrete _____.

5. A tooth is composed mainly of a hard calcified substance called _____.

Matching

Match each numbered item with the most closely related lettered item.

____ 6. Digests starch
____ 7. Begins protein digestion
____ 8. Digests fats
____ 9. Digests protein to amino acids
____ 10. Emulsify fats

   a. lipase
   b. amylase
   c. trypsin
   d. pepsin
   e. bile salts

Multiple choice

____ 11. The teeth break up food into small parts by a process called
   a. absorption
   b. deglutition
   c. ingestion
   d. mastication

____ 12. Hydrochloric acid and pepsin are secreted by the
   a. salivary glands
   b. stomach
   c. pancreas
   d. liver

____ 13. The double layer of peritoneum that extends from the lower border of the stomach and hangs over the intestine is the
   a. greater omentum
   b. lesser omentum
   c. mesentery
   d. mesocolon

____ 14. The soft, fleshy V-shaped mass of tissue that hangs from the soft palate is the
   a. epiglottis
   b. esophageal hiatus
   c. uvula
   d. gingiva

___ 15. The entrance of the trachea is guarded during swallowing by the
   a. uvula
   b. epiglottis
   c. gingiva
   d. bolus

Understanding Concepts

16. Differentiate between the terms in each of the following pairs:
   a. digestion and absorption
   b. parietal and visceral peritoneum
   c. gastrin and gastric-inhibitory peptide
   d. secretin and cholecystokinin

17. Name the four layers of the digestive tract. What tissue makes up each layer? What is the function of each layer?

18. Trace the path of a bolus of food through the digestive system.

19. Describe the structure and function of the liver, pancreas, and gallbladder. How are the products of these organs delivered to the digestive tract?

20. Where does absorption occur in the digestive tract, and what structures are needed for absorption? What types of nutrients are absorbed into the blood? Into the lymph?

21. How does the nervous system regulate digestion?

22. Name several hormones that regulate digestion.

Conceptual Thinking

23. Overuse of antacids can inhibit protein digestion. How?

24. Blockage of the common bile duct can cause autodigestion of the pancreas. Why?

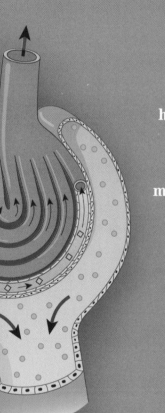

SELECTED KEY TERMS

The following terms and other boldface terms in the chapter are defined in the Glossary

anabolism
catabolism
glucose
glycogen
hypothalamus
kilocalorie
malnutrition
metabolic rate
mineral
oxidation
vitamin

LEARNING OUTCOMES

After careful study of this chapter, you should be able to:

1. Differentiate between catabolism and anabolism
2. Differentiate between the anaerobic and aerobic phases of cellular respiration and give the end products and the relative amount of energy released by each
3. Define *metabolic rate* and name several factors that affect the metabolic rate
4. Explain the roles of glucose and glycogen in metabolism
5. Compare the energy contents of fats, proteins, and carbohydrates
6. Define *essential amino acid*
7. Explain the roles of minerals and vitamins in nutrition and give examples of each
8. List the recommended percentages of carbohydrate, fat and protein in the diet
9. Distinguish between simple and complex carbohydrates, giving examples of each
10. Compare saturated and unsaturated fats
11. List some adverse effects of alcohol consumption
12. Explain how heat is produced and lost in the body
13. Describe the role of the hypothalamus in regulating body temperature
14. Show how word parts are used to build words related to metabolism, nutrition and body temperature (see Word Anatomy at the end of the chapter)

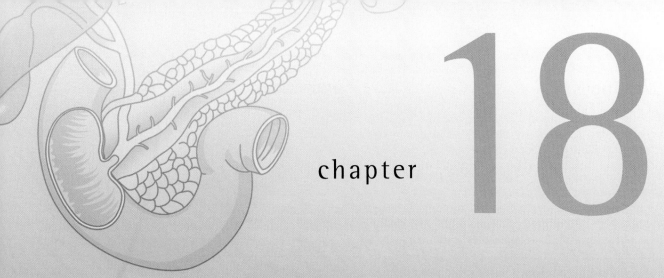

chapter

18

Metabolism, Nutrition, and Body Temperature

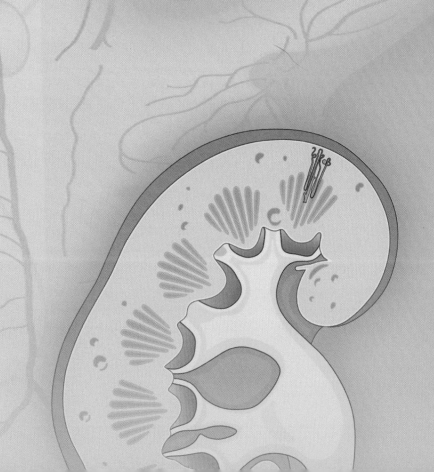

❱ Metabolism

Nutrients absorbed from the digestive tract are used for all the cellular activities of the body, which together make up **metabolism**. These activities fall into two categories:

❱ **Catabolism**, which is the breakdown of complex compounds into simpler compounds. Catabolism includes the digestion of food into small molecules and the release of energy from these molecules within the cell.

❱ **Anabolism**, which is the building of simple compounds into substances needed for cellular activities and for the growth and repair of tissues.

Through the steps of catabolism and anabolism, there is a constant turnover of body materials as energy is consumed, cells function and grow, and waste products are generated.

Checkpoint 18-1 What are the two phases of metabolism?

Cellular Respiration

Energy is released from nutrients in a series of reactions called **cellular respiration** (see Table 18-1 and Fig. 18-1). Early studies on cellular respiration were done with **glucose** as the starting compound. Glucose is a simple sugar that is the main energy source for the body.

The Anaerobic Phase The first steps in the breakdown of glucose do not require oxygen; that is, they are **anaerobic**. This phase of catabolism, known as **glycolysis** (gli-KOL-ih-sis), occurs in the cytoplasm of the cell. It yields a small amount of energy, which is used to make ATP (adenosine triphosphate), the cells' energy compound. Each glucose molecule yields enough energy by this process to produce 2 molecules of ATP.

The anaerobic breakdown of glucose is incomplete and ends with formation of an organic product called **pyruvic** (pi-RU-vik) **acid**. This organic acid is further metabolized in the next phase of cellular respiration, which requires oxygen. In muscle cells operating briefly under anaerobic conditions, pyruvic acid is converted to lactic acid, which accumulates as the cells build up an oxygen debt (described in Chapter 7). Lactic acid induces muscle

ANAEROBIC

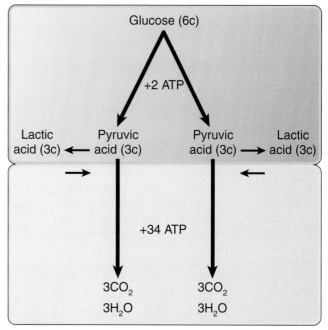

AEROBIC

Figure 18-1   Cellular respiration. This diagram shows the catabolism of glucose without oxygen (anaerobic) and with oxygen (aerobic). (C = carbon atoms in one molecule of a substance.) In cellular respiration, glucose first yields two molecules of pyruvic acid, which will convert to lactic acid under anaerobic conditions, as during intense exercise. (Lactic acid must eventually be converted back to pyruvic acid.) Typically, however, pyruvic acid is broken down aerobically (using oxygen) to CO_2 and H_2O (aerobically).   *ZOOMING IN* ✦ *What does pyruvic acid produce in cellular respiration under anaerobic conditions? Under aerobic conditions?*

fatigue, so the body is forced to rest and recover. During the recovery phase immediately after exercise, breathing restores the oxygen needed to convert lactic acid back to pyruvic acid, which is then metabolized further. During this recovery phase, reserves stored in muscles are also replenished. These compounds are myoglobin, which stores oxygen; glycogen, which can be broken down for glucose; and creatine phosphate, which stores energy.

The Aerobic Phase To generate enough energy for survival, the body's cells must break pyruvic acid down more completely in the second phase of cellular respiration, which requires oxygen. These **aerobic** reactions occur within the mitochondria of the cell. They result in transfer of most of the energy remaining in the nutrients to ATP. On average, about 34 to 36 molecules of ATP can be formed aerobically per glucose molecule—quite an increase over anaerobic metabolism.

During the aerobic steps of cellular respiration, the cells form carbon diox-

	LOCATION IN CELL	END PRODUCT(S)	ENERGY YIELD/GLUCOSE
Table 18·1 **Summary of Cellular Respiration of Glucose**			
PHASE			
Anaerobic (glycolysis)	Cytoplasm	Pyruvic acid	2 ATP
Aerobic	Mitochondria	Carbon dioxide and water	34–36 ATP

ide, which then must be transported to the lungs for elimination. In addition, water is formed by the combination of oxygen with the hydrogen that is removed from nutrient molecules. Because of the type of chemical reactions involved, and because oxygen is used in the final steps, cellular respiration is described as an **oxidation** of nutrients. Note that enzymes are required as catalysts in all the reactions of cellular respiration. Many of the vitamins and minerals described later in this chapter are parts of these enzymes.

Although the oxidation of food is often compared to the burning of fuel, this comparison is inaccurate. Burning fuel results in a sudden and often wasteful release of energy in the form of heat and light. In contrast, metabolic oxidation occurs in small steps, and much of the energy released is stored as ATP for later use by the cells; some of the energy is released as heat, which is used to maintain body temperature, as discussed later in this chapter.

For those who know how to read chemical equations, the net balanced equation for cellular respiration, starting with glucose, is as follows:

$$\underset{\text{glucose}}{C_6 H_{12} O_6} + \underset{\text{oxygen}}{6O_2} \rightarrow \underset{\substack{\text{carbon} \\ \text{dioxide}}}{6CO_2} + \underset{\text{water}}{6H_2O}$$

Checkpoint 18-2 What name is given to the series of cellular reactions that releases energy from nutrients?

Metabolic Rate Metabolic rate refers to the rate at which energy is released from nutrients in the cells. It is affected by a person's size, body fat, sex, age, activity, and hormones, especially thyroid hormone (thyroxine). Metabolic rate is high in children and adolescents and decreases with age. **Basal metabolism** is the amount of energy needed to maintain life functions while the body is at rest.

The unit used to measure energy is the kilocalorie (kcal), which is the amount of heat needed to raise 1 kilogram of water 1°C. To estimate the daily calories needed taking activity level into account, see Box 18-1.

The Use of Nutrients for Energy

As noted, glucose is the main source of energy in the body. Most of the carbohydrates in the diet are converted to glucose in the course of metabolism. Reserves of glucose are stored in liver and muscle cells as **glycogen** (GLI-ko-jen), a compound built from glucose molecules. When glucose is needed for energy, glycogen is broken down to yield glucose. Glycerol and fatty acids (from fat digestion)

Box 18-1 **A Closer Look**

Calorie Counting: Estimating Daily Energy Needs

Basal energy requirements for a day can be estimated with a simple formula. An average woman requires 0.9 kcal/kg/hour, and a man, 1.0 kcal/kg/hour. Multiplying 0.9 by body weight in kilograms* by 24 for a woman, or 1.0 by body weight in kilograms by 24 for a man, yields the daily basal energy requirement. For example, if a woman weighed 132 pounds, the equation would be as follows:

132 pounds ÷ 2.2 pounds/kg = 60 kg

0.9 kcal/kg/hour × 60 kg = 54 kcal/hour

54 kcal/hour × 24 hours/day = 1,296 kcal/day

To estimate total energy needs for a day, a percentage based on activity level ("couch potato" to serious athlete) must also be added to the basal requirement. These percentages are shown in the table below.

The equation to calculate total energy needs for a day is:

Basal energy requirement + (basal energy requirement × activity level)

Using our previous example, and assuming light activity levels, the following equations apply:

At 40% activity:

1,296 kcal/day + (1,296 kcal/day × 40%) = 1,814.4 kcal/day

At 60% activity:

1,296 kcal/day + (1,296 kcal/day × 60%) = 2,073.6 kcal/day

Therefore, the woman in our example would require between 1,814 and 2,073 Kcal/day.

ACTIVITY LEVEL	MALE	FEMALE
Little activity ("couch potato")	25–40%	25–35%
Light activity (*e.g.*, walking to and from class, but little or no intentional exercise)	50–75%	40–60%
Moderate activity (*e.g.*, aerobics several times a week)	65–80%	50–70%
Heavy activity (serious athlete)	90–120%	80–100%

*To convert pounds to kilograms, divide weight in pounds by 2.2.

and amino acids (from protein digestion) can also be used for energy, but they enter the breakdown process at different points.

Fat in the diet yields more than twice as much energy as do protein and carbohydrate (*e.g.*, it is more "fattening"); fat yields 9 kcal of energy per gram, whereas protein and carbohydrate each yield 4 kcal per gram. Calories that are ingested in excess of need are converted to fat and stored in adipose tissue.

Before they are oxidized for energy, amino acids must have their nitrogen (amine) groups removed. This removal, called **deamination** (de-am-ih-NA-shun), occurs in the liver, where the nitrogen groups are then formed into urea by combination with carbon dioxide. The blood transports urea to the kidneys to be eliminated.

There are no specialized storage forms of proteins, as there are for carbohydrates (glycogen) and fats (adipose tissue). Therefore, when one needs more proteins than are supplied in the diet, they must be obtained from body substance, such as muscle tissue or plasma proteins. Drawing on these resources becomes dangerous when needs are extreme. Fats and carbohydrates are described as "protein sparing," because they are used for energy before proteins are and thus spare proteins for the synthesis of necessary body components.

Checkpoint 18-3 What is the main energy source for the cells?

Anabolism

Nutrient molecules are built into body materials by anabolic steps, all of which are catalyzed by enzymes.

Essential Amino Acids Eleven of the 20 amino acids needed to build proteins can be synthesized internally by metabolic reactions. These 11 amino acids are described as *nonessential* because they need not be taken in as food (Table 18-2). The remaining 9 amino acids cannot be made by the body and therefore must be taken in as part of the diet; these are the **essential amino acids**. Note that some nonessential amino acids may become essential under certain conditions, as during extreme physical stress, or in certain hereditary metabolic diseases.

Essential Fatty Acids There are also two essential fatty acids (linoleic acid and linolenic acid) that must be taken in as food. These are easily obtained through a healthful, balanced diet.

Checkpoint 18-4 What is meant when an amino acid or a fatty acid is described as essential?

Minerals and Vitamins

In addition to needing fats, proteins, and carbohydrates, the body requires minerals and vitamins.

Minerals are chemical elements needed for body structure, fluid balance, and such activities as muscle contraction, nerve impulse conduction, and blood clotting. Some minerals are components of vitamins. A list of the main minerals needed in a proper diet is given in Table 18-3. Some additional minerals not listed are also required for good health. Minerals needed in extremely small amounts are referred to as **trace elements**.

Vitamins are complex organic substances needed in very small quantities. Vitamins are parts of enzymes or other substances essential for metabolism, and vitamin deficiencies lead to a variety of nutritional diseases.

The water-soluble vitamins are the B vitamins and vitamin C. These are not stored and must be taken in regularly with food. The fat-soluble vitamins are A, D, E, and K. These vitamins are kept in reserve in fatty tissue. Excess intake of the fat-soluble vitamins can lead to toxicity. A list of vitamins is given in Table 18-4.

Certain substances are valuable in the diet as **antioxidants**. They defend against the harmful effects of **free radicals**, highly reactive and unstable molecules produced from oxygen in the normal course of metabolism (and also from UV radiation, air pollution and tobacco smoke). Free radicals contribute to aging and disease. Antioxidants react with free radicals to stabilize them and minimize their harmful effects on cells. Vitamins C and E and beta carotene, an orange pigment found in plants that is converted to vitamin A, are

Table 18·2 Amino acids			
NONESSENTIAL AMINO ACIDS[a]		**ESSENTIAL AMINO ACIDS**[b]	
Name	Pronunciation	Name[c]	Pronunciation
Alanine	AL-ah-nene	Histidine	HIS-tih-dene
Arginine	AR-jih-nene	Isoleucine	i-so-LU-sene
Asparagine	ah-SPAR-ah-jene	Leucine	LU-sene
Aspartic acid	ah-SPAR-tik AH-sid	Lysine	LI-sene
Cysteine	SIS-teh-ene	Methionine	meh-THI-o-nene
Glutamic acid	glu-TAM-ik AH-sid	Phenylalanine	fen-il-AL-ah-nene
Glutamine	GLU-tah-mene	Threonine	THRE-o-nene
Glycine	GLY-sene	Tryptophan	TRIP-to-fane
Proline	PRO-lene	Valine	VA-lene
Serine	SERE-ene		
Tyrosine	TI-ro-sene		

[a]Nonessential amino acids can be synthesized by the body.
[b]Essential amino acids cannot be synthesized by the body; they must be taken in as part of the diet.
[c]If you are ever called upon to memorize the essential amino acids, the mnemonic (memory device) Pvt. T. M. Hill gives the first letter of each name.

Table 18·3	Minerals		
MINERAL	**FUNCTIONS**	**SOURCES**	**RESULTS OF DEFICIENCY**
Calcium (Ca)	Formation of bones and teeth, blood clotting, nerve conduction, muscle contraction	Dairy products, eggs, green vegetables, legumes (peas and beans)	Rickets, tetany, osteoporosis
Phosphorus (P)	Formation of bones and teeth; found in ATP, nucleic acids	Meat, fish, poultry, egg yolk, dairy products	Osteoporosis, abnormal metabolism
Sodium (Na)	Fluid balance; nerve impulse conduction, muscle contraction	Most foods, especially processed foods, table salt	Weakness, cramps, diarrhea, dehydration
Potassium (K)	Fluid balance, nerve and muscle activity	Fruits, meats, seafood, milk, vegetables, grains	Muscular and neurologic disorders
Chloride (Cl)	Fluid balance, hydrochloric acid in stomach	Meat, milk, eggs, processed foods, table salt	Rarely occurs
Iron (Fe)	Oxygen carrier (hemoglobin, myoglobin)	Meat, eggs, fortified cereals, legumes, dried fruit	Anemia, dry skin, indigestion
Iodine (I)	Thyroid hormones	Seafood, iodized salt	Hypothyroidism, goiter
Magnesium (Mg)	Catalyst for enzyme reactions, carbohydrate metabolism	Green vegetables, grains, nuts, legumes	Spasticity, arrhythmia, vasodilation
Manganese (Mn)	Catalyst in actions of calcium and phosphorus; facilitator of many cell processes	Many foods	Possible reproductive disorders
Copper (Cu)	Necessary for absorption and use of iron in formation of hemoglobin; part of some enzymes	Meat, water	Anemia
Chromium (Cr)	Works with insulin to regulate blood glucose levels	Meat, unrefined food, fats and oils	Inability to use glucose
Cobalt (Co)	Part of vitamin B12	Animal products	Pernicious anemia
Zinc (Zn)	Promotes carbon dioxide transport and energy metabolism; found in enzymes	Meat, fish, poultry, grains, vegetables	Alopecia (baldness); possibly related to diabetes
Fluoride (F)	Prevents tooth decay	Fluoridated water, tea, seafood	Dental caries

antioxidants. There are also many compounds found in plants (*e.g.*, soybeans and tomatoes) that are antioxidants.

Checkpoint 18-5 Both vitamins and minerals are needed in metabolism. What is the difference between vitamins and minerals?

▌ Nutritional Guidelines

The relative amounts of carbohydrates, fats and proteins that should be in the daily diet vary somewhat with the individual. Typical recommendations for the number of calories derived each day from the three types of food are as follows:

▸ Carbohydrate: 55%–60%.
▸ Fat: 30% or less.
▸ Protein: 15%–20%.

It is important to realize that the type as well as the amount of each is a factor in good health. A weight loss diet should follow the same proportions as given above, but with a reduction in portion sizes.

Carbohydrates

Carbohydrates in the diet should be mainly complex, naturally occurring carbohydrates, and simple sugars should be kept to a minimum. Simple sugars are monosaccharides, such as glucose and fructose (fruit sugar), and disaccharides, such as sucrose (table sugar) and lactose (milk sugar). Simple sugars are a source of fast energy because they are metabolized rapidly. However, they boost pancreatic insulin output, and as a result, they cause blood glucose levels to rise and fall rapidly. It is healthier to maintain steady glucose levels, which normally range from approximately 85 to125 mg/dL throughout the day.

The **glycemic effect** is a measure of how rapidly a particular food raises the blood glucose level and stimulates the release of insulin. The effect is generally low for whole grains, fruit and dairy products and high for sweets and refined ("white") grains. Note, however, that the glycemic effect of a food also depends on when it is eaten during the day, and if or how it is combined with other foods.

Complex carbohydrates are polysaccharides. Examples are:

Table 18·4 Vitamins

VITAMINS	FUNCTIONS	SOURCES	RESULTS OF DEFICIENCY
A (retinol)	Required for healthy epithelial tissue and for eye pigments; involved in reproduction and immunity	Orange fruits and vegetables, liver, eggs, dairy products, dark green vegetables	Night blindness; dry, scaly skin; decreased immunity
B1 (thiamin)	Required for enzymes involved in oxidation of nutrients; nerve function	Pork, cereal, grains, meats, legumes, nuts	Beriberi, a disease of nerves
B2 (riboflavin)	In enzymes required for oxidation of nutrients	Milk, eggs, liver, green leafy vegetables, grains	Skin and tongue disorders
B3 (niacin, nicotinic acid)	Involved in oxidation of nutrients	Yeast, meat, liver, grains, legumes, nuts	Pellagra with dermatitis, diarrhea, mental disorders
B6 (pyridoxine)	Amino acid and fatty acid metabolism; formation of niacin; manufacture of red blood cells	Meat, fish, poultry, fruit, grains, legumes, vegetables	Anemia, irritability, convulsions, muscle twitching, skin disorders
Pantothenic acid	Essential for normal growth; energy metabolism	Yeast, liver, eggs, and many other foods	Sleep disturbances, digestive upset
B12 (cyanocobalamin)	Production of cells; maintenance of nerve cells; fatty acid and amino acid metabolism	Animal products	Pernicious anemia
Biotin	Involved in fat and glycogen formation, amino acid metabolism	Peanuts, liver, tomatoes, eggs, and many other foods	Lack of coordination, dermatitis, fatigue
Folate (folic acid)	Required for amino acid metabolism, DNA synthesis, maturation of red blood cells	Vegetables, liver, legumes, seeds	Anemia, digestive disorders, neural tube defects in the embryo
C (ascorbic acid)	Maintains healthy skin and mucous membranes; involved in synthesis of collagen; antioxidant	Citrus fruits, green vegetables, potatoes, orange fruits	Scurvy, poor wound healing, anemia, weak bones
D (calciferol)	Aids in absorption of calcium and phosphorus from intestinal tract	Fatty fish, liver, eggs, fortified milk	Rickets, bone deformities
E (tocopherol)	Protects cell membranes; antioxidant	Seeds, green vegetables, nuts, grains, oils,	Anemia, muscle and liver degeneration, pain
K	Synthesis of blood clotting factors, bone formation	Bacteria in digestive tract, liver, cabbage, and leafy green vegetables	Hemorrhage

▶ Starches, found in grains, legumes, and potatoes.
▶ Fibers, such as cellulose, pectins, and gums, which are the structural materials of plants.

Fiber adds bulk to the stool and promotes elimination of toxins and waste. It also slows the digestion and absorption of carbohydrates, thus regulating the release of glucose. It helps in weight control by providing a sense of fullness and limiting caloric intake. Adequate fiber in the diet lowers cholesterol and helps to prevent diabetes, colon cancer, hemorrhoids, appendicitis, and diverticulitis.

Box 18-2 · Health Maintenance

Dietary Fiber: Bulking Up

Dietary fiber is best known for its ability to improve bowel habits and ease weight loss. But fiber may also help to prevent diabetes, heart disease, and certain digestive disorders such as diverticulitis and gallstones.

Dietary fiber is an indigestible type of carbohydrate found in fruit, vegetables, and whole grains. The amount of fiber recommended for a 2,000-calorie diet is 25 grams per day, but most people in the United States tend to get only half this amount. One should eat fiber-rich foods throughout the day to meet the requirement. It is best to increase fiber in the diet gradually to avoid unpleasant symptoms, such as intestinal bloating and flatulence. If your diet lacks fiber, try adding the following foods over a period of several weeks:

▶ Whole grain breads, cereals, pasta, and brown rice. These add 1 to 3 more grams of fiber per serving than the "white" product.
▶ Legumes, which include beans, peas, and lentils. These add 4 to 12 grams of fiber per serving.
▶ Fruits and vegetables. Whole, raw, unpeeled versions contain the most fiber, and juices, the least. Apple juice has no fiber, whereas a whole apple has 3 grams.
▶ Unprocessed bran. This can be sprinkled over almost any food: cereal, soups, and casseroles. One tablespoon adds 2 grams of fiber. Be sure to take adequate fluids with bran.

Foods high in fiber, such as whole grains, fruits, and vegetables, are also rich in vitamins and minerals (see Box 18-2).

Checkpoint 18-6 What is the normal range of blood glucose?

Fats

Fats are subdivided into saturated and unsaturated forms based on their chemical structure. The fatty acids in **saturated fats** have more hydrogen atoms in their molecules and fewer double bonds between carbons atoms than do those of unsaturated fats (Fig. 18-2). Most saturated fats are from animal sources and are solid at room tempera-

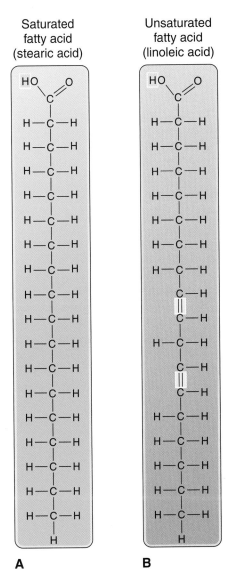

Saturated fatty acid (stearic acid) | Unsaturated fatty acid (linoleic acid)

A   **B**

Figure 18-2 **Saturated and unsaturated fats. (A)** Saturated fatty acids contain the maximum numbers of hydrogen atoms attached to carbons and no double bonds between carbon atoms. **(B)** Unsaturated fatty acids have less than the maximum number of hydrogen atoms attached to carbons and one or more double bonds between carbon atoms (highlighted).

ture, such as butter and lard. Also included in this group are the so-called "tropical oils": coconut oil and palm oil. **Unsaturated fats** are derived from plants. They are liquid at room temperature and are generally referred to as oils, such as corn, peanut, olive and canola oils.

Saturated fats should make up less than one third of the fat in the diet (less than 10% of total calories). Diets high in saturated fats are associated with a higher than normal incidence of cancer, heart disease, and cardiovascular problems, although the relation between these factors is not fully understood.

Many commercial products contain fats that are artificially saturated to prevent rancidity and provide a more solid consistency. These are listed on food labels as partially hydrogenated (HI-dro-jen-a-ted) vegetable oils and are found in baked goods, processed peanut butter, vegetable shortening, and solid margarine. Evidence shows that components of hydrogenated fats, known as *transfatty acids,* may be just as harmful, if not more so, than natural saturated fats and should be avoided.

Proteins

Because proteins, unlike carbohydrates and fats, are not stored in special reserves, protein foods should be taken in on a regular basis, with attention to obtaining the essential amino acids. Most animal proteins supply all of the essential amino acids and are described as complete proteins. Most vegetables are lacking in one or more of the essential amino acids. People on strict vegetarian diets must learn to combine foods, such as legumes (*e.g.,* beans and peas) with grains (*e.g.,* rice, corn, or wheat), to obtain all the essential amino acids each day. Table 18-5 demonstrates the principles of combining two foods, legumes and grains, to supply essential amino acids that might be missing in one food or the other. Legumes are rich in isoleucine and lysine but poor in methonine and tryptophan, while grains are just the opposite. For illustration purposes, the table includes only the 4 missing essential amino acids (there are 9 total). Traditional ethnic diets reflect these healthy combinations, for example, beans with corn or rice in Mexican dishes or chickpeas and lentils with wheat in Middle Eastern fare.

Vitamin and Mineral Supplements

The need for mineral and vitamin supplements to the diet is a subject of controversy. Some researchers maintain that adequate amounts of these substances can be obtained from a varied, healthful diet. Many commercial foods, including milk, cereal and bread, are already fortified with minerals and vitamins. Others hold that pollution, depletion of the soils, and the storage, refining, and processing of foods make additional supplementation beneficial. Most agree, however, that children, elderly people, pregnant and lactating women, and teenagers, who often do not get enough of the proper foods, would profit from additional minerals and vitamins.

Table 18·5	Combining Foods for Essential Amino Acids			
	ESSENTIAL AMINO ACIDS[a]			
	ISOLEUCINE	LYSINE	METHIONINE	TRYPTOPHAN
Legumes	x	x		
Grains			x	x
Legumes and grains combined	x	x	x	x

[a]There are 9 essential amino acids; the table includes 4 for the purposes of illustration.

- Specify portion sizes, which are smaller than most people think.
- Include the need for water.
- Indicate possible need for vitamin supplements.

Governments in the U.S. and other countries will continue to study this topic with input from nutritionists and other scientists. The best nutrition guidelines, however, will be of no benefit unless people are educated and motivated to follow them.

When required, supplements should be selected by a physician or nutritionist to fit an individual's particular needs. Megavitamin dosages may cause unpleasant reactions and in some cases are hazardous. Vitamins A and D have both been found to cause serious toxic effects when taken in excess.

The Food Guide Pyramid

In 1992, the USDA (United States Department of Agriculture) developed a pyramid to represent the quantities of foods in the different food groups recommended each day for good health (Fig. 18-3). This symbol is under revision, and some suggested improvements include:

- Distinguish between unrefined and refined carbohydrates.
- Distinguish between healthful unsaturated fats, which can be eaten in moderation, and less healthful saturated and processed (trans-) fats, which should be restricted.
- Accommodate vegetarians, who may avoid not only meats, but dairy products and eggs as well.

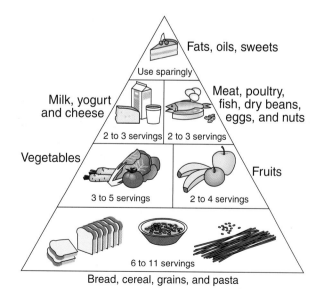

Figure 18-3   **The Food Guide Pyramid.** (From U.S. Department of Agriculture/U.S. Department of Health and Human Services.)

Alcohol

Alcohol yields energy in the amount of 7 kcal per gram, but it is not considered a nutrient because it does not yield useful end products. In fact, alcohol interferes with metabolism and contributes to a variety of disorders.

The body can metabolize about one-half ounce of pure alcohol (ethanol) per hour. This amount translates into one glass of wine, one can of beer, or one shot of hard liquor. Consumed at a more rapid rate, alcohol enters the bloodstream and affects many cells, notably in the brain.

Alcohol is rapidly absorbed through the stomach and small intestine and is detoxified by the liver. When delivered in excess to the liver, alcohol can lead to the accumulation of fat as well as inflammation and scarring of liver tissue. It can eventually cause cirrhosis (sih-RO-sis), which involves irreversible changes in liver structure. Alcohol metabolism ties up enzymes needed for oxidation of nutrients and also results in byproducts that acidify body fluids. Other effects of alcoholism include obesity, malnutrition, cancer, ulcers, and fetal alcohol syndrome. Pregnant women are advised not to drink any alcohol. In addition, alcohol impairs judgment and leads to increased involvement in accidents.

Although alcohol consumption is compatible with good health and may even have a beneficial effect on the cardiovascular system, alcohol should be consumed only in moderation.

Checkpoint 18-7 What are typical recommendations for the relative amounts of carbohydrates, fats, and proteins in the diet?

▶ Nutrition and Aging

With age, a person may find it difficult to maintain a balanced diet. Often, the elderly lose interest in buying and preparing food or are unable to do so. Because metabolism generally slows, and less food is required to meet energy needs, nutritional deficiencies may develop. Medications may interfere with appetite and with the absorption and use of specific nutrients.

It is important for older people to seek out foods that are "nutrient dense," that is, foods that have a high proportion of nutrients in comparison with the number of calories they provide. Exercise helps to boost appetite and maintains muscle tissue, which is more active metabolically. Box 18-3 describes how dietitians and nutritionists can help in planning a healthful diet for people of all ages.

▌ Body Temperature

Heat is an important byproduct of the many chemical activities constantly occurring in body tissues. At the same time, heat is always being lost through a variety of outlets. Under normal conditions, a number of regulatory devices keep body temperature constant within quite narrow limits. Maintenance of a constant temperature despite both internal and external influences is one phase of homeostasis, the tendency of all body processes to maintain a normal state despite forces that tend to alter them.

Heat Production

Heat is a byproduct of the cellular oxidations that generate energy. The amount of heat produced by a given organ varies with the kind of tissue and its activity. While at rest, muscles may produce as little as 25% of total body heat, but when muscles contract, heat production is greatly multiplied, owing to the increase in metabolic rate. Under basal conditions (at rest), the liver and other abdominal organs produce about 50% of total body heat. The brain produces only 15% of body heat at rest, and an increase in nervous tissue activity produces little increase in heat production.

Although it would seem from this description that some parts of the body would tend to become much warmer than others, the circulating blood distributes the heat fairly evenly.

Factors Affecting Heat Production The rate at which heat is produced is affected by a number of factors, including exercise, hormone production, food intake, and age. Hormones, such as thyroxine from the thyroid gland and epinephrine (adrenaline) from the adrenal medulla, increase the rate of heat production.

The intake of food is also accompanied by increased heat production. The nutrients that enter the blood after digestion are available for increased cellular metabolism. In addition, the glands and muscles of the digestive system generate heat as they set to work. These responses do not account for all the increase, however, nor do they account for the much greater increase in metabolism after a meal containing a large amount of protein. Although the reasons are not entirely clear, the intake of food definitely increases metabolism and thus adds to heat production.

Checkpoint 18-8 What are some factors that affect heat production in the body?

Heat Loss

More than 80% of heat loss occurs through the skin. The remaining 15% to 20% is dissipated by the respiratory system and with the urine and feces. Networks of blood vessels in the skin's dermis (deeper part) can bring considerable quantities of blood near the surface, so that heat can be dissipated to the outside. This release can occur in several ways.

- ▌ Heat can be transferred directly to the surrounding air by means **conduction**.
- ▌ Heat also travels from its source as heat waves or rays, a process termed **radiation**.
- ▌ If the air is moving, so that the layer of heated air next to the body is constantly being carried away and replaced with cooler air (as by an electric fan), the process is known as **convection**.

Box 18-3 · Health Professions

Dietitians and Nutritionists

Dietitians and nutritionists specialize in planning and supervising food programs for institutions such as hospitals, schools, and nursing care facilities. They assess their clients' nutritional needs and design individualized meal plans. Dietitians and nutritionists also work in community settings, educating the public about disease prevention through healthy eating. Increased public awareness about food and nutrition has also led to new opportunities in the food manufacturing industry. To perform their duties, dietitians and nutritionists need a thorough understanding of anatomy and physiology. Most dietitians and nutritionists in the United States receive their training from a college or university and take a licensing exam.

Job prospects for dietitians and nutritionists are good. As the American population continues to age, the need for nutritional planning in hospital and nursing care settings is expected to rise. In addition, many people now place an emphasis on healthy eating and may consult nutritionists privately. For more information about this career, contact the American Dietetic Association.

▶ Finally, heat may be lost by **evaporation**, the process by which liquid changes to the vapor state.

To illustrate evaporation, rub some alcohol on your skin; it evaporates rapidly, using so much heat from the skin that your arm feels cold. Perspiration does the same thing, although not as quickly. The rate of heat loss through evaporation depends on the humidity of the surrounding air. When it exceeds 60% or so, perspiration does not evaporate so readily, making one feel generally miserable unless some other means of heat loss is available, such as convection caused by a fan.

Prevention of Heat Loss Factors that play a part in heat loss through the skin include the volume of tissue compared with the amount of skin surface. A child loses heat more rapidly than does an adult. Such parts as fingers and toes are affected most by exposure to cold because they have a great amount of skin compared with total tissue volume.

If the temperature of the surrounding air is lower than that of the body, excessive heat loss is prevented by both natural and artificial means. Clothing checks heat loss by trapping "dead air" in both its material and its layers. This noncirculating air is a good insulator. An effective natural insulation against cold is the layer of fat under the skin. Even when skin temperature is low, this fatty tissue prevents the deeper tissues from losing much heat. On the average, this layer is slightly thicker in females than in males. Naturally, there are individual variations, but as a rule, the degree of insulation depends on the thickness of this subcutaneous fat layer.

Temperature Regulation

Given that body temperature remains almost constant despite wide variations in the rate of heat production or loss, there must be internal mechanisms for regulating temperature.

The Role of the Hypothalamus Many areas of the body take part in heat regulation, but the most important center is the hypothalamus, the area of the brain located just above the pituitary gland. Some of the cells in the hypothalamus control heat production in body tissues, whereas another group of cells controls heat loss. Regulation is based on the temperature of the blood circulating through the brain and also on input from temperature receptors in the skin.

If these two factors indicate that too much heat is being lost, impulses are sent quickly from the hypothalamus to the autonomic (involuntary) nervous system, which in turn causes constriction of the skin blood vessels to reduce heat loss. Other impulses are sent to the muscles to cause shivering, a rhythmic contraction of many muscles, which results in increased heat production. Furthermore, the output of epinephrine may be in-creased if necessary. Epinephrine increases cell metabolism for a short period, and this in turn increases heat production.

If there is danger of overheating, the hypothalamus stimulates the sweat glands to increase their activity. Impulses from the hypothalamus also cause blood vessels in the skin to dilate, so that increased blood flow to the skin will result in greater heat loss. The hypothalamus may also promote muscle relaxation to minimize heat production.

Muscles are especially important in temperature regulation because variations in the activity of these large tissue masses can readily increase or decrease heat generation. Because muscles form roughly one-third of the body, either an involuntary or an intentional increase in their activity can form enough heat to offset a considerable decrease in the temperature of the environment.

Checkpoint 18-9 What part of the brain is responsible for regulating body temperature?

Age Factors Very young and very old people are limited in their ability to regulate body temperature when exposed to environmental extremes. A newborn infant's body temperature decreases if the infant is exposed to a cool environment for a long period. Elderly people also are not able to produce enough heat to maintain body temperature in a cool environment.

With regard to overheating in these age groups, heat loss mechanisms are not fully developed in the newborn. The elderly do not lose as much heat from their skin as do younger people. Both groups should be protected from extreme temperatures.

Normal Body Temperature The normal temperature range obtained by either a mercury or an electronic thermometer may extend from 36.2°C to 37.6°C (97°F to 100°F). Body temperature varies with the time of day. Usually, it is lowest in the early morning because the muscles have been relaxed and no food has been taken in for several hours. Temperature tends to be higher in the late afternoon and evening because of physical activity and consumption of food.

Normal temperature also varies in different parts of the body. Skin temperature obtained in the axilla (armpit) is lower than mouth temperature, and mouth temperature is a degree or so lower than rectal temperature. It is believed that, if it were possible to place a thermometer inside the liver, it would register a degree or more higher than rectal temperature. The temperature within a muscle might be even higher during activity.

Although the Fahrenheit scale is used in the United States, in most parts of the world, temperature is measured with the **Celsius** (SEL-se-us) thermometer. On this scale, the ice point is at 0° and the normal boiling point of water is at 100°, the interval between these two points being divided into 100 equal units. The Celsius scale is also called the **centigrade scale** (think of 100 cents in a dollar). See Appendix 2 for a comparison of the Celsius and Fahrenheit scales and formulas for converting from one to the other.

> Checkpoint 18-10 What is normal body temperature?

Word Anatomy

Medical terms are built from standardized word parts (prefixes, roots, and suffixes). Learning the meanings of these parts can help you remember words and interpret unfamiliar terms.

WORD PART	MEANING	EXAMPLE
Metabolism		
glyc/o	sugar, sweet	*Glycogen* yields glucose molecules when it breaks down.
-lysis	separating, dissolving	*Glycolysis* is the breakdown of glucose for energy.

Summary

I. Metabolism—life-sustaining reactions that occur in the living cell
   1. Catabolism—breakdown of complex compounds into simpler compounds
   2. Anabolism—building of simple compounds into substances needed for cellular activities, growth, and repair
   A. Cellular respiration—a series of reactions in which food is oxidized for energy
      1. Anaerobic phase—does not require oxygen
         a. Location—cytoplasm
         b. Yield—2 ATP per glucose
         c. End product—organic (*i.e.*, pyruvic acid)
      2. Aerobic phase—requires oxygen
         a. Location—mitochondria
         b. Yield—34–36 ATP per glucose
         c. End products—carbon dioxide and water
      3. Metabolic rate—rate at which energy is released from food in the cells
         a. Basal metabolism—amount of energy needed to maintain life functions while at rest
   B. Use of nutrients for energy
      1. Glucose—main energy source
      2. Fats—highest energy yield
      3. Proteins—can be used for energy after removal of nitrogen (deamination)
   C. Anabolism
      1. Essential amino acids and fatty acids must be taken in as part of diet
   D. Minerals and vitamins
      1. Minerals—elements needed for body structure and cell activities
         a. Trace elements—elements needed in extremely small amounts
      2. Vitamins—organic substances needed in small amounts
         a. Antioxidants (*e.g.*, vitamins C and E) protect against free radicals

II. Nutritional guidelines
   A. Carbohydrates
      1. 55%–60% of calories
      2. Should be complex (unrefined) not simple (sugars)
         a. Glycemic effect—how quickly a food raises blood glucose and insulin
         b. Plant fiber important
   B. Fats
      1. 30% or less of calories
      2. Unsaturated healthier than saturated
         a. Hydrogenated fats artificially saturated
   C. Proteins
      1. 15%–20% of calories
      2. Complete—all essential amino acids
         a. Need to combine plant foods
   D. Vitamin and mineral supplements
   E. Food Guide Pyramid (USDA)—under revision
   F. Alcohol—metabolized in liver

III. Nutrition and aging

IV. Body temperature
   A. Heat production
      1. Most heat produced in muscles and glands
      2. Distributed by the circulation
      3. Affected by exercise, hormones, food, age
   B. Heat loss
      1. Avenues—skin, urine, feces, respiratory system
      2. Mechanisms—conduction, radiation, convection, evaporation
      3. Prevention of heat loss—clothing, subcutaneous fat
   C. Temperature regulation
      1. Hypothalamus—main temperature-regulating center
         a. Responds to temperature of blood in brain and temperature receptors in skin

2. Conservation of heat
   a. Constriction of blood vessels in skin
   b. Shivering
   c. Increased release of epinephrine
3. Release of heat
   a. Dilation of skin vessels

    b. Sweating
    c. Relaxation of muscles
4. Age factors
5. Normal body temperature—ranges from 36.2°C to 37.6°C; varies with time of day and location measured

Questions for Study and Review

Building Understanding

Fill in the blanks

1. Building glycogen from glucose is an example of _____.

2. The amount of energy needed to maintain life functions while at rest is _____.

3. Reserves of glucose are stored in liver and muscle as _____.

4. The most important area of the brain for temperature regulation is the _____.

5. Minerals needed in extremely small amounts are referred to as _____.

Matching

Match each numbered item with the most closely related lettered item.

____ 6. Main energy source for the body
____ 7. Chemical element required for normal body function
____ 8. Complex organic substance required for normal body function
____ 9. Energy storage molecule with only single bonds between carbon atoms
____ 10. Energy storage molecule with one or more double bonds between carbon atoms

    a. saturated fat
    b. vitamin
    c. mineral
    d. unsaturated fat
    e. glucose

Multiple choice

____ 11. During amino acid catabolism, nitrogen is removed by
    a. oxidation
    b. the glycemic effect
    c. lysis
    d. deamination

____ 12. Which of the following would have the lowest glycemic effect?
    a. glucose
    b. sucrose
    c. lactose
    d. starch

____ 13. Alcohol is catabolized by the
    a. small intestine
    b. liver
    c. pancreas
    d. spleen

____ 14. Amino acids that cannot be made by metabolism are said to be
    a. essential
    b. nonessential
    c. antioxidants
    d. free radicals

Understanding Concepts

15. In what part of the cell does anaerobic respiration occur and what are its end products? In what part of the cell does aerobic respiration occur? What are its end products?

16. About how many kilocalories are released from a tablespoon of butter (14 grams)? a tablespoon of sugar (12 grams)? a tablespoon of egg white (15 grams)?

17. If you eat 2000 kcal a day, how many kilocalories should come from carbohydrates? from fats? from protein?

18. How is heat produced in the body? What structures produce the most heat during increased activity?

19. Emily's body temperature increased from 36.2°C to 36.5°C and then decreased to 36.2°C Describe the feedback mechanism regulating Emily's body temperature.

20. Differentiate between the terms in the following pairs:
    a. conduction and convection
    b. radiation and evaporation
    c. antioxidants and free radicals
    e. catabolism and anabolism

Conceptual Thinking

21. The oxidation of glucose to form ATP is often compared to the burning of fuel. Why is this analogy inaccurate?

22. It is a hot summer's day and you are trying to keep cool by sitting in front of a fan, but you are still sweating profusely. Describe the two mechanisms of heat loss that you are employing.

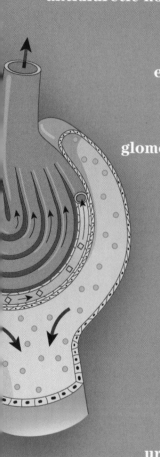

SELECTED KEY TERMS

The following terms and other boldface terms in the chapter are defined in the Glossary

angiotensin
antidiuretic hormone (ADH)
buffer
electrolyte
erythropoietin
excretion
extracellular
glomerular filtrate
glomerulus
interstitial
intracellular
kidney
micturition
nephron
pH
renin
urea
ureter
urethra
urinary bladder
urine

LEARNING OUTCOMES

After careful study of this chapter,
you should be able to:

1. List the systems that eliminate waste and name the substances eliminated by each
2. Describe the parts of the urinary system and give the functions of each
3. Trace the path of a drop of blood as it flows through the kidney
4. Describe a nephron
5. Describe the components and functions of the juxtaglomerular (JG) apparatus
6. Name the four processes involved in urine formation and describe the action of each
7. Identify the role of ADH in urine formation
8. Describe the process of micturition
9. Name three normal constituents of urine
10. Compare intracellular and extrcellular fluids
11. List four types of extracellular fluids
12. Name the systems that are involved in water balance
13. Explain how thirst is regulated
14. Define *electrolytes* and describe some of their functions
15. Describe the role of hormones in electrolyte balance
16. Describe three methods for regulating the pH of body fluids
17. Show how word parts are used to build words related to the urinary system and body fluids (see Word Anatomy at the end of the chapter)

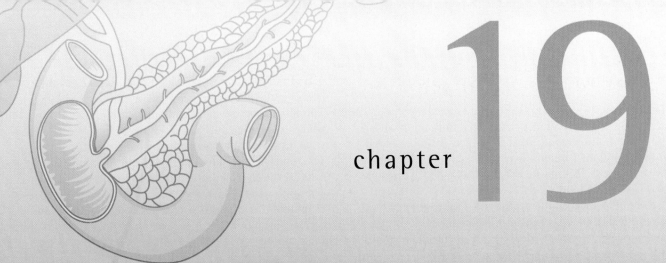

chapter **19**

The Urinary System and Body Fluids

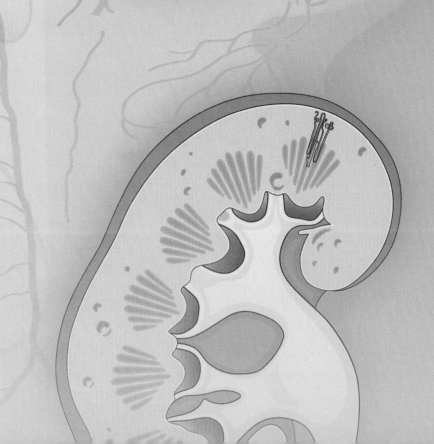

Excretion

The urinary system is also called the *excretory system* because one of its main functions is **excretion**, removal and elimination of metabolic waste products from the blood. It has many other functions as well, including regulation of the volume, acid–base balance (pH), and electrolyte composition of body fluids.

Although the focus of this chapter is the urinary system, certain aspects of other systems are also discussed, because body systems work interdependently to maintain homeostasis (internal balance). The systems active in excretion and some of the substances they eliminate are the following:

▸ The **urinary system** excretes water, nitrogen-containing waste products, and salts. These are all constituents of the urine.
▸ The **digestive system** elimiinates water, some salts, and bile in addition to digestive residue, all of which are contained in the feces. The liver is important in elimi-

nating the products of red blood cell destruction and in breaking down certain drugs and toxins.
▸ The **respiratory system** eliminates carbon dioxide and water. The latter appears as vapor, as can be demonstrated by breathing on a windowpane.
▸ The skin, or **integumentary system**, excretes water, salts, and very small quantities of nitrogenous wastes. These all appear in perspiration, although water also evaporates continuously from the skin without our being conscious of it.

Checkpoint 19-1 The main function of the urinary system is to eliminate waste. What are some other systems that eliminate waste?

Organs of the Urinary System

The main parts of the urinary system, shown in Figure 19-1, are as follows:

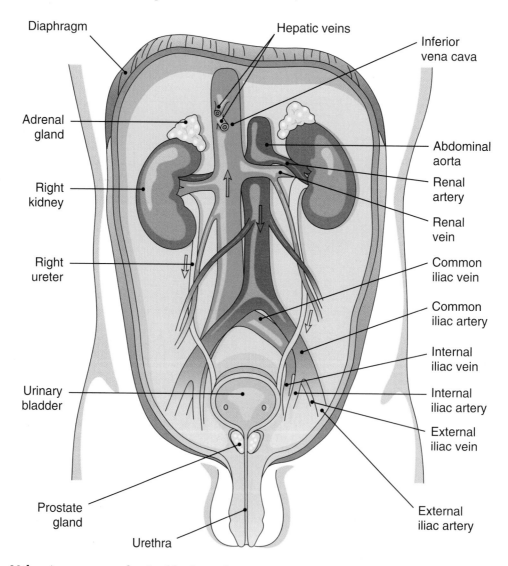

Figure 19-1 Male urinary system, showing blood vessels. *ZOOMING IN ✦ What vessel supplies blood to the kidney? What vessel drains the kidney?*

- Two **kidneys**. These organs extract wastes from the blood, balance body fluids, and form urine.
- Two **ureters** (U-re-ters). These tubes conduct urine from the kidneys to the urinary bladder.
- A single **urinary bladder**. This reservoir receives and stores the urine brought to it by the two ureters.
- A single **urethra** (u-RE-thrah). This tube conducts urine from the bladder to the outside of the body for elimination.

> **Checkpoint 19-2** What are the organs of the urinary system?

▸ The Kidneys

The kidneys lie against the back muscles in the upper abdomen at about the level of the last thoracic and first three lumbar vertebrae. The right kidney is slightly lower than the left to accommodate the liver. Each kidney is firmly enclosed in a membranous **renal capsule** made of fibrous connective tissue. In addition, there is a protective layer of fat called the **adipose capsule** around the organ. An outermost layer of fascia (connective tissue) anchors the kidney to the peritoneum and abdominal wall. The kidneys, as well as the ureters, lie posterior to the peritoneum. Thus, they are not in the peritoneal cavity but rather in an area known as the **retroperitoneal** (ret-ro-per-ih-to-NE-al) **space**.

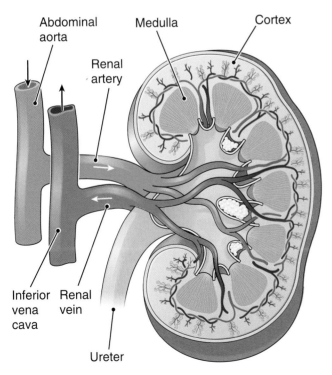

Figure 19-2 **Blood supply and circulation of the kidney.** *ZOOMING IN ✦ What vessel supplies blood to the renal artery? What vessel receives blood from the renal vein?*

Blood Supply to the Kidney

The kidney's blood supply is illustrated in Figure 19-2. Blood is brought to the kidney by a short branch of the abdominal aorta called the **renal artery**.

After entering the kidney, the renal artery subdivides into smaller and smaller branches, which eventually make contact with the functional units of the kidney, the **nephrons** (NEF-ronz). Blood leaves the kidney by vessels that finally merge to form the **renal** vein, which carries blood into the inferior vena cava for return to the heart.

> **Checkpoint 19-3** The kidneys are located in the retroperitoneal space. Where is this space?

> **Checkpoint 19-4** What vessel supplies blood to the kidney and what vessel drains blood from the kidney?

Structure of the Kidney

The kidney is a somewhat flattened organ about 10 cm (4 inches) long, 5 cm (2 inches) wide, and 2.5 cm (1 inch) thick (Fig. 19-3). On the medial border there is a notch called the **hilum**, where the renal artery, the renal vein, and the ureter connect with the kidney. The lateral border is convex (curved outward), giving the entire organ a bean-shaped appearance.

The kidney is divided into two regions: the renal cortex and the renal medulla (Fig. 19-3). The **renal cortex** is the kidney's outer portion. The **renal medulla** contains the tubes in which urine is formed and collected. These tubes form a number of cone-shaped structures called **renal pyramids**. The tips of the pyramids point toward the **renal pelvis**, a funnel-shaped basin that forms the upper end of the ureter. Cuplike extensions of the renal pelvis surround the tips of the pyramids and collect urine; these extensions are called **calyces** (KA-lih-seze; sing., calyx, KA-liks). The urine that collects in the pelvis then passes down the ureters to the bladder.

> **Checkpoint 19-5** What are the outer and inner regions of the kidney called?

The Nephron As is the case with most organs, the most fascinating aspect of the kidney is too small to be seen with the naked eye. This basic unit, which actually does the kidney's work, is the **nephron** (Fig. 19-4). The nephron is essentially a tiny coiled tube with a bulb at one end. This bulb, known as the **glomerular** (Bowman) **capsule**, surrounds a cluster of capillaries called the **glomerulus** (glo-MER-u-lus) (pl., glomeruli [glo-MER-u-li]). Each kidney contains about 1 million nephrons; if all these coiled tubes were separated, straightened out, and laid end to end, they would span some 120 kilometers (75 miles)! Figure 19-5 is a microscopic view of kidney tissue showing several glomeruli, each surrounded by a

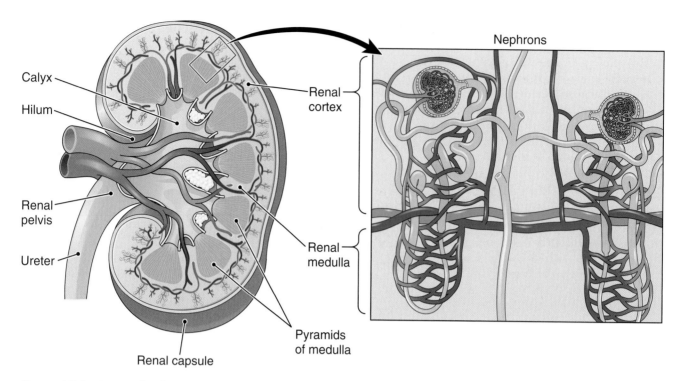

Calyx

Hilum

Renal
pelvis

Ureter

Renal capsule

Pyramids
of medulla

Renal
cortex

Renal
medulla

Nephrons

Figure 19-3 **Longitudinal section through the kidney showing its internal structure (*left*) and an enlarged diagram of nephrons (*right*).** Each kidney contains more than 1 million nephrons. *ZOOMING IN ✦ What is the outer region of the kidney called? What is the inner region of the kidney called?*

glomerular capsule. This figure also shows sections through the tubular portions of the nephrons.

A small blood vessel, the **afferent arteriole**, supplies the glomerulus with blood; another small vessel, called the **efferent arteriole**, carries blood from the glomerulus. When blood leaves the glomerulus, it does not head immediately back toward the heart. Instead, it flows into a capillary network that surrounds the nephron's tubular portion. These **peritubular capillaries**, are named for their location.

The tubular portion of the nephron consists of several parts. The coiled part leading from the glomerular capsule is called the **proximal convoluted** (KON-vo-lu-ted) **tubule** (**PCT**, or just proximal tubule). The tubule then uncoils to form a hairpin-shaped segment called the **loop of Henle**. The first part of the loop, which carries fluid toward the medulla, is the **descending limb** (see Fig. 19-4). The part that continues from the loop's turn and carries fluid away from the medulla, is the **ascending limb**. Continuing from the ascending limb, the tubule coils once again into the **distal convoluted tubule** (**DCT**, or just distal tubule), so called because it is farther along the tubule from the glomerular capsule than is the PCT. The distal end of each tubule empties into a collecting duct, which then continues through the medulla toward the renal pelvis.

The glomerulus, glomerular capsule, and the proximal and distal convoluted tubules of the nephron are within the renal cortex. The loop of Henle and collecting duct extend into the medulla (see Fig. 19-3).

Checkpoint 19-6 What is the functional unit of the kidney called?

Checkpoint 19-7 What name is given to the coil of capillaries in the glomerular (Bowman) capsule?

The Juxtaglomerular (JG) Apparatus The first portion of the DCT curves back toward the glomerulus to pass between the afferent and efferent arterioles (Fig. 19-6). At the point where the DCT makes contact with the afferent arteriole, there are specialized cells in each that together make up the **juxtaglomerular** (juks-tah-glo-MER-u-lar) (**JG**) **apparatus**. The JG apparatus helps to regulate kidney function. When blood pressure falls too low for the kidneys to function effectively, cells in the wall of the afferent arteriole secrete the enzyme **renin** (RE-nin), which raises blood pressure by a mechanism described later.

Functions of the Kidney

The kidneys are involved in the following processes:

▶ Excretion of unwanted substances, such as cellular metabolic waste, excess salts, and toxins. One product of amino acid metabolism is nitrogen-containing waste material, a chief form of which is **urea** (u-RE-ah). After synthesis in the liver, urea is transported in the blood to the kidneys for elimination. The kidneys have a specialized mechanism for the elimination of urea and other nitrogenous (ni-TROJ-en-us) wastes.

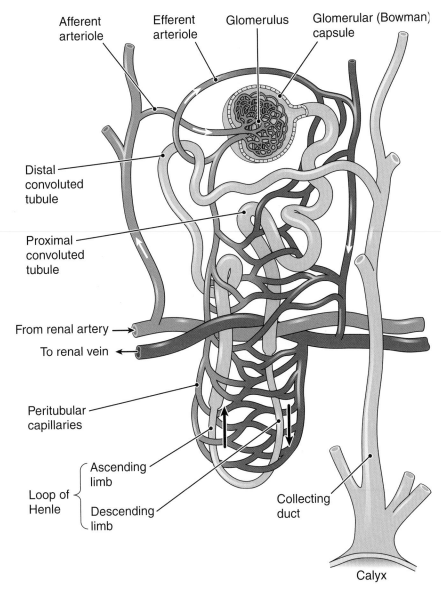

Afferent arteriole
Efferent arteriole
Glomerulus
Glomerular (Bowman) capsule
Distal convoluted tubule
Proximal convoluted tubule
From renal artery
To renal vein
Peritubular capillaries
Ascending limb
Loop of Henle
Descending limb
Collecting duct
Calyx

Figure 19-4 A nephron and its blood supply. The nephron regulates the proportions of water, waste, and other materials according to the body's constantly changing needs. Materials that enter the nephron can be returned to the blood through the surrounding capillaries. *ZOOMING IN ✦ Which of the two convoluted tubules is closer to the glomerular capsule? Which convoluted tubule is farther away?*

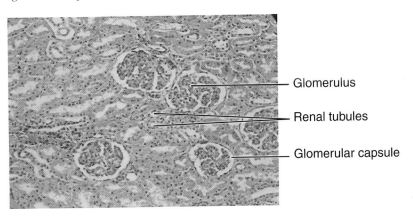

Glomerulus
Renal tubules
Glomerular capsule

Figure 19-5   Microscopic view of the kidney. (Courtesy of Dana Morse Bittus and BJ Cohen.)

- Maintenance of water balance. Although the amount of water gained and lost in a day can vary tremendously, the kidneys can adapt to these variations, so that the volume of body water remains remarkably stable from day to day.
- Regulation of the acid–base balance of body fluids. Acids are constantly being produced by cellular metabolism. Certain foods can yield acids or bases, and people may also ingest antacids, such as bicarbonate. However, if the body is to function normally, the pH of body fluids must remain in the range of 7.35 to 7.45.
- Regulation of blood pressure. The kidneys depend on blood pressure to filter the blood. If blood pressure falls too low for effective filtration, the cells of the JG apparatus release renin. This enzyme activates **angiotensin** (an-je-o-TEN-sin), a blood protein that causes blood vessels to constrict, thus raising blood pressure (Table 19-1). Angiotensin also stimulates the adrenal cortex to produce the hormone aldosterone, which promotes retention of sodium and water, also raising blood pressure. For more information, see Box 19-1, The Renin-Angiotensin Pathway.
- Regulation of red blood cell production. When the kidneys do not get enough oxygen, they produce the hormone **erythropoietin** (eh-rith-ro-POY-eh-tin) **(EPO)**, which stimulates the red cell production in the bone marrow. EPO made by genetic engineering is now available to treat severe anemia, such as occurs in the end stage of kidney failure.

Checkpoint 19-8 What substance is produced by the JG apparatus and under what conditions is it produced?

Formation of Urine

The following explanation of urine formation describes a complex process, involving many back-and-forth exchanges between the bloodstream and the kidney tubules. As fluid filtered from the blood travels slowly through the twists and turns of the nephron, there is ample time for exchanges to take place. These

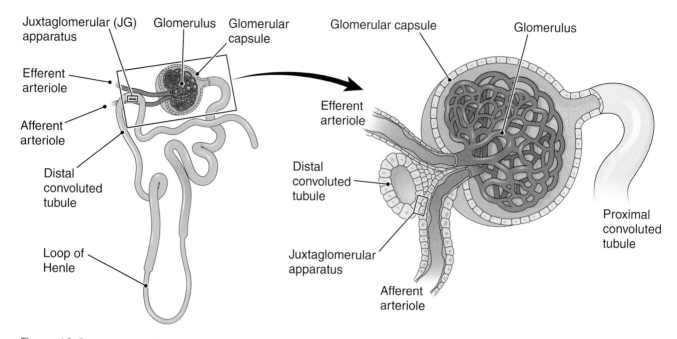

Figure 19-6 **Structure of the juxtaglomerular (JG) apparatus.** Note how the distal convoluted tubule contacts the afferent arteriole (*right*). Cells in these two structures make up the JG apparatus. *ZOOMING IN* ✦ *The JG apparatus is made up of cells from which two structures?*

processes together allow the kidney to "fine tune" body fluids as they adjust the composition of the urine.

Glomerular Filtration The process of urine formation begins with the glomerulus in the glomerular capsule. The walls of the glomerular capillaries are sievelike and permit the free flow of water and soluble materials through them. Like other capillary walls, however, they are impermeable (im-PER-me-abl) to blood cells and large protein molecules, and these components remain in the blood (Fig. 19-7).

Because the diameter of the afferent arteriole is slightly larger than that of the efferent arteriole (see Fig. 19-7), blood can enter the glomerulus more easily than it can leave. Thus, blood pressure in the glomerulus is about three to four times higher than it is in other capillaries. To understand this effect, think of placing your thumb over

the end of a garden hose as water comes through. As you make the diameter of the opening smaller, water is forced out under higher pressure. As a result of increased fluid (hydrostatic) pressure in the glomerulus, materials are constantly being pushed out of the blood and into the nephron's glomerular capsule. As described in Chapter 3, movement of water and dissolved materials through a membrane under pressure is called *filtration*. This movement of materials under pressure from the blood into the capsule is therefore known as **glomerular filtration**.

The fluid that enters the glomerular capsule, called the **glomerular filtrate,** begins its journey along the tubular system of the nephron. In addition to water and the normal soluble substances in the blood, other substances, such as vitamins and drugs, also may be filtered and become part of the glomerular filtrate.

Table 19·1 Substances that Affect Renal Function

SUBSTANCE	SOURCE	ACTION
Renin (RE-nin)	Enzyme produced by renal cells when blood pressure falls too low for effective filtration	Activates angiotensin in the blood
Angiotensin (an-je-o-TEN-sin)	Protein in the blood that is activated by renin	Causes constriction of blood vessels to raise blood pressure; also stimulates release of aldosterone from the adrenal cortex
Aldosterone (al-DOS-ter-one)	Hormone released from the adrenal cortex under effects of angiotensin	Promotes reabsorption of sodium and water in the kidney to conserve water and increase blood pressure
Antidiuretic hormone (an-te-di-u-RET-ik) (ADH)	Made in the hypothalamus and released from the posterior pituitary; released when blood becomes too concentrated	Promotes reabsorption of water from the distal convoluted tubule and collecting duct to concentrate the urine and conserve water

| Box 19-1 | A Closer Look |

The Renin-Angiotensin Pathway: The Kidneys' Route to Blood Pressure Control

In addition to forming urine, the kidneys play an integral role in regulating blood pressure. When blood pressure drops, cells of the juxtaglomerular apparatus secrete the enzyme renin into the blood. Renin acts on another blood protein, **angiotensinogen**, which is manufactured by the liver. Renin converts angiotensinogen into **angiotensin I** by cleaving off some amino acids from the end of the protein. Angiotensin I is then converted into **angiotensin II** by yet another enzyme called angiotensin-converting enzyme (ACE), which is manufactured by capillary endothelium, especially in the lungs. Angiotensin II increases blood pressure in four ways:

▶ It increases cardiac output and stimulates vasoconstriction.
▶ It stimulates the release of aldosterone, a hormone that acts on the kidneys' distal convoluted tubules to increase sodium reabsorption, and secondarily, water reabsorption.

▶ It stimulates the release of antidiuretic hormone, which acts directly on the distal convoluted tubules to increase water reabsorption.
▶ It stimulates thirst centers in the hypothalamus, resulting in increased fluid consumption.

The combined effects of angiotensin II produce a dramatic increase in blood pressure. In fact, angiotensin II is estimated to be four to eight times more powerful than norepinephrine, another potent stimulator of hypertension, and thus is a good target for blood pressure-controlling drugs. One class of drugs used to treat hypertension is the **ACE inhibitors** (angiotensin-converting enzyme inhibitors), which control blood pressure by blocking the production of angiotensin II.

Checkpoint 19-9 The first step in urine formation is glomerular filtration. What is glomerular filtration?

Tubular Reabsorption The kidneys form about 160 to 180 liters of filtrate day. However, only 1 to 1.5 liters of urine are eliminated daily. Clearly, most of the water that enters the nephron is not excreted with the urine, but rather, is returned to the circulation. In addition to water, many other substances the body needs, such as nutrients and ions, pass into the nephron as part of the filtrate, and these also must be returned. Therefore, the process of filtration that occurs in the glomerular capsule is followed by a process of **tubular reabsorption**. As the filtrate travels through the nephron's tubular system, water and other needed substances leave the tubule and enter the surrounding tissue fluid, or interstitial fluid (IF). They move by several processes previously described in Chapter 3, including:

▶ Diffusion. The movement of substances from an area of higher concentration to an area of lower concentration (following the concentration gradient).
▶ Osmosis. Diffusion of water through a semipermeable membrane.
▶ Active transport. Movement of materials through the plasma membrane against the concentration gradient using energy and transporters.

The substances that leave the nephron and enter the interstitial fluid then enter the peritubular capillaries and return to the circulation. In contrast, most of the urea and other nitrogenous waste materials are kept within the tubule to be eliminated with the urine. Box 19-2 presents additional information on tubular reabsorption in the nephron.

Tubular Secretion Before the filtrate leaves the body as urine, the kidney makes final adjustments in composition by the process of **tubular secretion**. In this process, some substances are actively moved from the blood into the nephron. Potassium ions are moved into the urine by this process. Importantly, the kidneys regulate the acid–base (pH) balance of body fluids by the active secretion of hydrogen ions. Some drugs, such as penicillin, also are actively secreted into the nephron for elimination.

Concentration of the Urine The amount of water that is eliminated with the urine is regulated by a complex mechanism within the nephron that is influenced by **antidiuretic hormone (ADH)**, a hormone released from the posterior pituitary gland (see Table 19-1). The process is called the **countercurrent mechanism** because it involves fluid traveling in opposite directions within the ascending and descending limbs of Henle's loop. The countercurrent mechanism is illustrated in Figure 19-8. Its essentials are as follows:

As the filtrate passes through Henle's loop, electrolytes, especially sodium, are actively pumped out by the nephron's cells, resulting in an increased concentration of the interstitial fluid. Because the ascending limb of Henle's loop is not very permeable to water, the filtrate at this point becomes increasingly dilute (see Fig. 19-8). As the filtrate then passes through the more permeable DCT and collecting duct, the concentrated fluids around the nephron draw water out to be returned to the blood. (Remember, according to the laws of osmosis, water follows salt.) In this manner, the urine becomes more concentrated as it leaves the nephron and its volume is reduced.

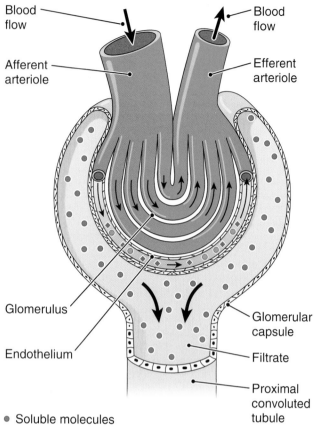

- Blood flow
- Blood flow
- Afferent arteriole
- Efferent arteriole
- Glomerulus
- Glomerular capsule
- Endothelium
- Filtrate
- Proximal convoluted tubule

- ● Soluble molecules
- ◆ Proteins
- ● Blood cells

Figure 19-7 Filtration process in the formation of urine. Blood pressure inside the glomerulus forces water and dissolved substances into the glomerular (Bowman) capsule. Blood cells and proteins remain behind in the blood. The smaller diameter of the efferent arteriole as compared with that of the afferent arteriole maintains the hydrostatic (fluid) pressure. *ZOOMING IN ✦ Which arteriole associated with the glomerulus has the wider diameter?*

The hormone ADH makes the walls of the DCT and collecting tubule more permeable to water, so that more water will be reabsorbed and less will be excreted with the urine. The release of ADH from the posterior pituitary is regulated by a feedback system. As the blood becomes more concentrated, the hypothalamus triggers more ADH release from the posterior pituitary; as the blood becomes more dilute, less ADH is released. In the disease diabetes insipidus, there is inadequate secretion of ADH from the hypothalamus, which results in the elimination of large amounts of dilute urine accompanied by excessive thirst.

Summary of Urine Formation The processes involved in urine formation are summarized below and illustrated in Figure 19-9.

1. Glomerular filtration allows all diffusible materials to pass from the blood into the nephron.
2. Tubular reabsorption moves useful substances back into the blood while keeping waste products in the nephron to be eliminated in the urine.
3. Tubular secretion moves additional substances from the blood into the nephron for elimination. Movement of hydrogen ions is one means by which the pH of body fluids is balanced.
4. The countercurrent mechanism concentrates the urine and reduces the volume excreted. The pituitary hormone ADH allows more water to be reabsorbed from the nephron.

Checkpoint 19-10 What are the four processes involved in the formation of urine?

▶ The Ureters

Each of the two ureters is a long, slender, muscular tube that extends from the kidney down to and through the inferior portion of the urinary bladder (see Fig. 19-1).

Box 19-2   Clinical Perspectives

Transport Maximum

The kidney works efficiently to return valuable substances to the blood after glomerular filtration. However, the carriers that are needed for active transport of these substances can become overloaded, and there is also a limit to the amount of each substance that can be reabsorbed in a given time period. The limit of this rate of reabsorption is called the **transport maximum (Tm)**, or tubular maximum, and it is measured in milligrams (mg) per minute. For example, the Tm for glucose is approximately 375 mg/minute.

If a substance is present in excess in the blood, it may exceed its transport maximum and then, because it cannot be totally reabsorbed, some will be excreted in the urine. Thus, the transport maximum determines the **renal threshold**—the plasma concentration at which a substance will begin to be excreted in the urine, which is measured in mg per deciliter (dL). For example, if the concentration of glucose in the blood exceeds its renal threshold (180 mg/dL), glucose will begin to appear in the urine, a condition called **glycosuria**. The most common cause of glycosuria is uncontrolled diabetes mellitus.

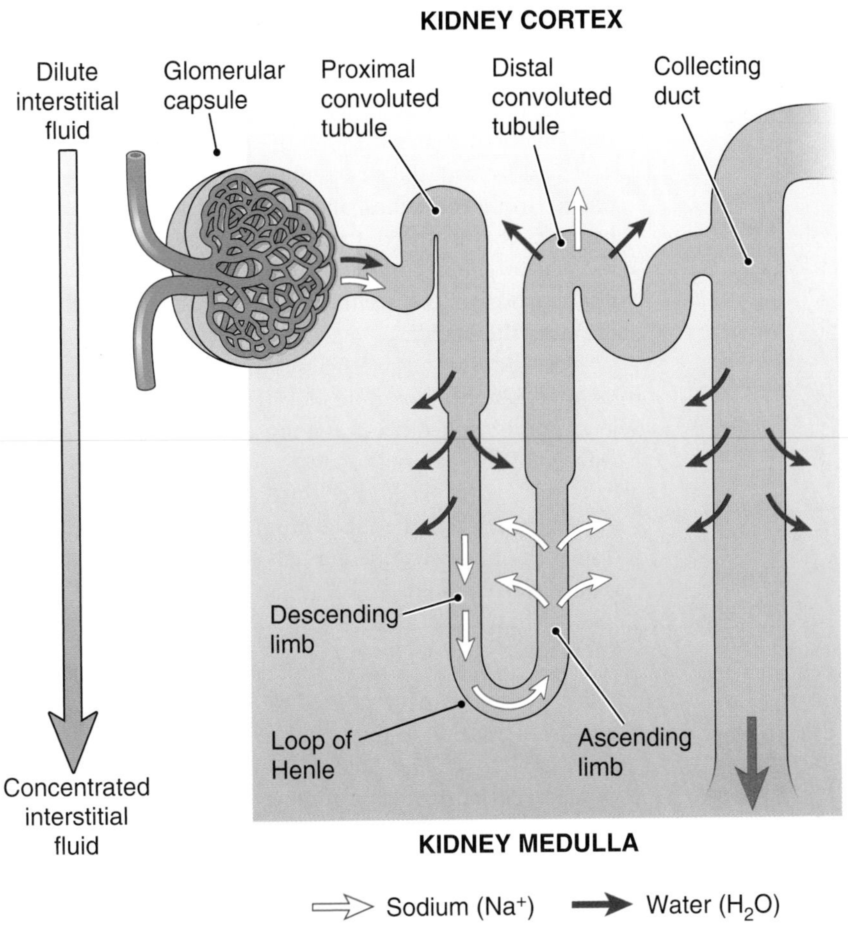

KIDNEY CORTEX

Dilute interstitial fluid

Glomerular capsule

Proximal convoluted tubule

Distal convoluted tubule

Collecting duct

Descending limb

Loop of Henle

Ascending limb

Concentrated interstitial fluid

KIDNEY MEDULLA

⇒ Sodium (Na⁺)   → Water (H_2O)

Figure 19-8 Countercurrent mechanism for concentration of urine. Concentration is regulated by means of intricate exchanges of water and electrolytes, mainly sodium, in the loop of Henle, distal convoluted tubule, and collecting duct. The intensity of color shows changing concentrations of the interstitial fluid and filtrate.

The ureters, which are located posterior to the peritoneum and, at the distal portion, below the peritoneum, are entirely extraperitoneal. Their length naturally varies with the size of the individual, and they may be anywhere from 25 to 32 cm (10–13 inches) long. Nearly 2.5 cm (1 inch) of the ureter's distal portion enters the bladder by passing obliquely (at an angle) through the inferior bladder wall. Because of the oblique direction the ureter takes through the wall, a full bladder compresses the ureter and prevents the backflow of urine.

The wall of the ureter includes a lining of epithelial cells, a relatively thick layer of involuntary muscle, and finally, an outer coat of fibrous connective tissue. The epithelium is the transitional type, which flattens from a cuboidal shape as the tube stretches. This same type of epithelium lines the renal pelvis, the bladder, and the proximal portion of the urethra. The ureteral muscles are capable of the same rhythmic contraction (peristalsis) that occurs in the digestive system. Urine is moved along the ureter from the kidneys to the bladder by gravity and by peristalsis at frequent intervals.

▶ The Urinary Bladder

When it is empty, the urinary bladder (Fig. 19-10) is located below the parietal peritoneum and posterior to the pubic joint. When filled, it pushes the peritoneum upward and may extend well into the abdominal cavity proper. The urinary bladder is a temporary reservoir for urine, just as the gallbladder is a storage sac for bile.

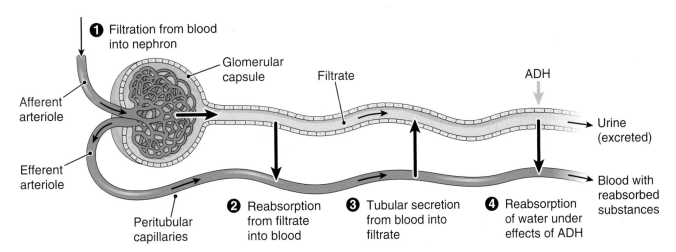

Figure 19-9 **Summary of urine formation in a nephron.**

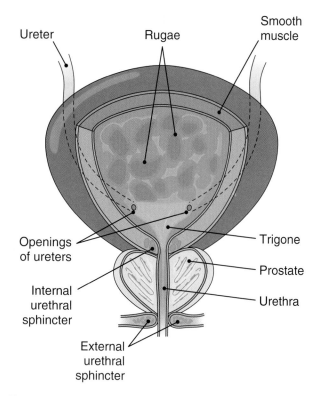

Ureter

Rugae

Smooth muscle

Openings of ureters

Trigone

Prostate

Internal urethral sphincter

Urethra

External urethral sphincter

Figure 19-10 **Interior of the male urinary bladder.** The trigone is a triangular region in the floor of the bladder marked by the openings of the ureters and the urethra. *ZOOMING IN* ✦ *What gland does the urethra pass through in the male?*

The bladder wall has many layers. It is lined with mucous membrane containing transitional epithelium. The bladder's lining, like that of the stomach, is thrown into folds called *rugae* when the organ is empty. Beneath the mucosa is a layer of connective tissue, followed by a three-layered coat of involuntary muscle tissue that can stretch considerably. Finally, there is an incomplete coat of peritoneum that covers only the superior portion of the bladder.

When the bladder is empty, the muscular wall becomes thick, and the entire organ feels firm. As the bladder fills, the muscular wall becomes thinner, and the organ may increase from a length of 5 cm (2 inches) up to as much as 12.5 cm (5 inches) or even more. A moderately full bladder holds about 470 mL (1 pint) of urine.

The **trigone** (TRI-gone) is a triangular-shaped region in the floor of the bladder. It is marked by the openings of the two ureters and the urethra (see Fig. 19-10). As the bladder fills with urine, it expands upward, leaving the trigone at the base stationary. This stability prevents stretching of the ureteral openings and the possible back flow of urine into the ureters.

▶ The Urethra

The **urethra** is the tube that extends from the bladder to the outside (see Fig. 19-1) and is the means by which the bladder is emptied. The urethra differs in men and women; in the male, it is part of both the reproductive system and the urinary system, and it is much longer than is the female urethra.

The male urethra is about 20 cm (8 inches) in length. Proximally, it passes through the prostate gland, where it is joined by two ducts carrying male germ cells (spermatozoa) from the testes and glandular secretions. From here, it leads to the outside through the **penis** (PE-nis), the male organ of copulation. The male urethra serves the dual purpose of conveying semen with the germ cells and draining the bladder.

The urethra in the female is a thin-walled tube about 4 cm (1.5 inches) long. It is located posterior to the pubic joint and is embedded in the muscle of the vagina's anterior wall. The external opening, called the **urinary meatus** (me-A-tus), is located just anterior to the vaginal opening between the labia minora. The female urethra drains the bladder only and is entirely separate from the reproductive system.

Urination

The process of expelling (voiding) urine from the bladder is called **urination** or **micturition** (mik-tu-RISH-un). This process is controlled both voluntarily and involuntarily with the aid of two rings of muscle (sphincters) that surround the urethra (see Fig. 19-10). Near the bladder's outlet is an involuntary **internal urethral sphincter** formed by a continuation of the smooth muscle of the bladder wall. Below this muscle is a voluntary **external urethral** sphincter formed by the muscles of the pelvic floor. By learning to control the voluntary sphincter, one can gain control over emptying of the bladder.

As the bladder fills with urine, stretch receptors in its wall send impulses to a center in the lower part of the spinal cord. Motor impulses from this center stimulate contraction of the bladder wall, forcing urine outward as both the internal and external sphincters are made to relax. In the infant, this emptying occurs automatically as a simple reflex. Early in life, a person learns to control urination from higher centers in the brain until the time is appropriate, a process known as *toilet training.* The impulse to urinate will override conscious controls if the bladder becomes too full.

The bladder can be emptied voluntarily by relaxing the muscles of the pelvic floor and increasing the pressure in the abdomen. The resulting increased pressure in the bladder triggers the spinal reflex that leads to urination.

Checkpoint 19-11 What is the name of the tube that carries urine from the kidney to the bladder?

Checkpoint 19-12 What is the name of the tube that carries urine from the bladder to the outside?

▶ The Urine

Urine is a yellowish liquid that is approximately 95% water and 5% dissolved solids and gases. The pH of freshly collected urine averages 6.0, with a range of 4.5 to 8.0. Diet may cause considerable variation in pH.

The amount of dissolved substances in urine is indicated by its **specific gravity**. The specific gravity of pure water, used as a standard, is 1.000. Because of the dissolved materials it contains, urine has a specific gravity that normally varies from 1.002 (very dilute urine) to 1.040 (very concentrated urine). When the kidneys are diseased, they lose the ability to concentrate urine, and the specific gravity no longer varies as it does when the kidneys function normally.

Normal Constituents

Some of the dissolved substances normally found in the urine are the following:

▶ **Nitrogenous waste products**, including urea, uric acid, and **creatinine** (kre-AT-ih-nin).
▶ **Electrolytes,** including sodium chloride (as in common table salt) and different kinds of sulfates and phosphates. Electrolytes are excreted in appropriate amounts to keep their blood concentration constant.
▶ **Pigment,** mainly yellow pigment derived from certain bile compounds. Pigments from foods and drugs also may appear in the urine.

▶ The Effects of Aging

Even without kidney disease, aging causes the kidneys to lose some of their ability to concentrate urine. With aging, progressively more water is needed to excrete the same amount of waste. Older people find it necessary to drink more water than young people, and they eliminate larger amounts of urine (polyuria), even at night (nocturia).

Beginning at about 40 years of age, there is a decrease in the number and size of the nephrons. Often, more than half of them are lost before the age of 80 years. There may be an increase in blood urea nitrogen (BUN) without serious symptoms. Elderly people are more susceptible than young people to urinary system infections. Childbearing may cause damage to the musculature of the pelvic floor, resulting in urinary tract problems in later years.

Enlargement of the prostate, common in older men, may cause obstruction and back pressure in the ureters and kidneys. If this condition is untreated, it will cause permanent damage to the kidneys. Changes with age, including decreased bladder capacity and decreased muscle tone in the bladder and urinary sphincters, may predispose to incontinence. However, most elderly people (60% in nursing homes, and up to 85% living independently) have no incontinence.

▶ Body Fluids: The Importance of Water in

Water is important to living cells as a solvent, a transport medium, and a participant in metabolic reactions. The normal proportion of body water varies from 50% to 70% of a person's weight. It is highest in the young and in thin, muscular individuals. In infants, water makes up 75% of the total body mass. That's why infants are in greater danger from dehydration than adults. With increase in the amount of fat, the percentage of water in the body decreases, because adipose tissue holds very little water compared with muscle tissue.

Various electrolytes (salts), nutrients, gases, waste, and special substances, such as enzymes and hormones, are dissolved or suspended in body water. The composition of body fluids is an important factor in homeostasis. Whenever the volume or chemical makeup of these fluids deviates even slightly from normal, disease results. The constancy of body fluids is maintained in the following ways:

▶ The thirst mechanism, which maintains the volume of water at a constant level.
▶ Kidney activity, which regulates the volume and composition of body fluids.
▶ Hormones, which serve to regulate fluid volume and electrolytes.
▶ Regulators of pH (acidity and alkalinity), including buffers, respiration, and kidney function.

The maintenance of proper fluid balance involves many of the principles discussed in earlier chapters, such as pH and buffers, the effects of respiration on pH, tonicity of solutions, and forces influencing capillary exchange. Some of these chapters will be referenced in the following sections.

Fluid Compartments

Although body fluids have much in common no matter where they are located, there are some important differences between fluid inside and outside cells. Accordingly, fluids are grouped into two main compartments (Fig. 19-11):

▶ **Intracellular fluid** (ICF) is contained within the cells. About two-thirds to three-fourths of all body fluids are in this category.
▶ **Extracellular fluid** (ECF) includes all body fluids outside of cells. In this group are included the following:
  ▶ **Interstitial** (in-ter-STISH-al) **fluid,** or more simply, tissue fluid. This fluid is located in the spaces between the cells in tissues all over the body. It is estimated that tissue fluid constitutes about 15% of body weight.
  ▶ **Blood plasma,** which constitutes about 4% of a person's body weight.

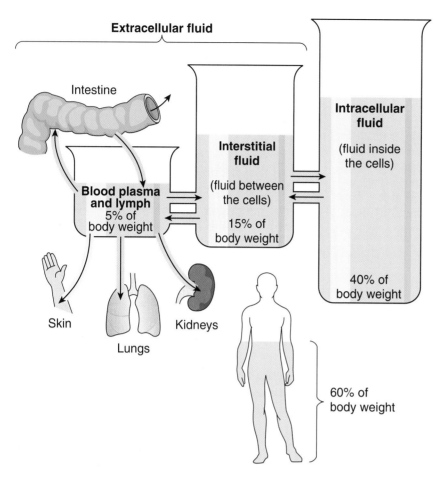

Figure 19-11 Main fluid compartments showing relative percentage by weight of body fluid. Fluid percentages vary but total about 60% of body weight. Fluids are constantly exchanged among compartments, and each day fluids are lost and replaced. *ZOOMING IN* ✦ *What are some avenues through which water is lost?*

▸ **Lymph,** the fluid that drains from the tissues into the lymphatic system. This is about 1% of body weight.

▸ **Fluid in special compartments,** such as cerebrospinal fluid, the aqueous and vitreous humors of the eye, serous fluid, and synovial fluid. Together, these make up about 1% to 3% of total body fluids.

Fluids are not locked into one compartment. There is a constant interchange between compartments as fluids are transferred across semipermeable cell membranes by diffusion and osmosis (see Fig. 19-11). Also, fluids are lost and replaced on a daily basis.

Checkpoint 19-13 What are the two main compartments into which body fluids are grouped?

Water Balance

In a person whose health is normal, the quantity of water gained in a day is approximately equal to the quantity lost (output) (Fig. 19-12). The quantity of water consumed in a day (intake) varies considerably. The average adult in a comfortable environment takes in about 2300 mL of water (about 2½ quarts) daily. About two-thirds of this quantity comes from drinking water and other beverages; about one-third comes from foods—fruits, vegetables, and soups. About 200 mL of water is produced each day as a by-product of cellular respiration. This water, described as *metabolic water*, brings the total average gain to 2500 mL each day.

The same volume of water is constantly being lost from the body by the following routes:

▸ The **kidneys** excrete the largest quantity of water lost each day. About 1 to 1.5 liters of water are eliminated daily in the urine. (Note that beverages containing alcohol or caffeine act as diuretics and increase water loss through the kidneys.)

▸ The **skin.** Although sebum and keratin help prevent dehydration, water is constantly evaporating from the skin's surface. Larger amounts of water are lost from the skin as sweat when it is necessary to cool the body.

▸ The **lungs** expel water along with carbon dioxide.

▸ The **intestinal tract** eliminates water along with the feces.

In many disorders, it is important for the healthcare team to know whether a patient's intake and output are equal; in such a case, a 24-hour intake–output record is kept. The intake record includes *all* the liquid the patient has taken in. This means fluids administered intravenously as well as those consumed by mouth. The healthcare worker must account for water, other beverages, and liquid foods, such as soup and ice cream. The output record includes the quantity of urine excreted in the same 24-hour period as well as an estimation of fluid losses due to fever, vomiting, diarrhea, bleeding, wound discharge, or other causes.

Checkpoint 19-14 What are three routes for water loss from the body?

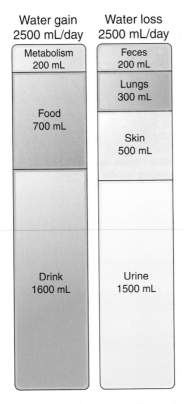

Figure 19-12   **Daily gain and loss of water.**

Sense of Thirst

The control center for the sense of thirst is located in the brain's hypothalamus. This center plays a major role in the regulation of total fluid volume. A decrease in fluid volume or an increase in the concentration of body fluids stimulates the thirst center, causing a person to drink water or other fluids containing large amounts of water. Dryness of the mouth also causes a sensation of thirst. Excessive thirst, such as that caused by excessive urine loss in cases of diabetes, is called **polydipsia** (pol-e-DIP-se-ah).

The thirst center should stimulate enough drinking to balance fluids, but this is not always the case. During vigorous exercise, especially in hot weather, the body can dehydrate rapidly. People may not drink enough to replace needed fluids. In addition, if plain water is consumed, the dilution of body fluids may depress the thirst center. Athletes who are exercising very strenuously may need to drink beverages with some carbohydrates for energy and also some electrolytes to keep fluids in balance. (See Box 19-3, Osmoreceptors: Thinking About Thirst, for more about thirst regulation.)

Checkpoint 19-15 Where is the control center for the sense of thirst located?

▶ Electrolytes and Their Functions

Electrolytes are important constituents of body fluids. These compounds separate into positively and negatively charged ions in solution. Positively charged ions are called *cations;* negatively charged ions are called *anions.* Electrolytes are so-named because they conduct an electrical current in solution. A few of the most important ions are reviewed next:

▶ Positive ions (cations):
  ▶ **Sodium** is chiefly responsible for maintaining osmotic balance and body fluid volume. It is the main positive ion in extracellular fluids. Sodium is required for nerve impulse conduction and is important in maintaining acid–base balance.
  ▶ **Potassium** is also important in the transmission of nerve impulses and is the major positive ion in intracellular fluids. Potassium is involved in cellular enzyme activities, and it helps regulate the chemical reactions by which carbohydrate is converted to energy and amino acids are converted to protein.
  ▶ **Calcium** is required for bone formation, muscle contraction, nerve impulse transmission, and blood clotting.
▶ Negative ions (anions):
  ▶ **Phosphate** is essential in carbohydrate metabolism, bone formation, and acid–base balance. Phosphates are found in plasma membranes, nucleic acids (DNA and RNA) and ATP.
  ▶ **Chloride** is essential for the formation of hydrochloric acid in the stomach. It also helps to regulate fluid balance and pH. It is the most abundant anion in extracellular fluids.

Checkpoint 19-16 What is the main cation in extracellular fluid? In intracellular fluid?

Checkpoint 19-17 What is the main anion in extracellular fluid?

Electrolyte Balance

The body must keep electrolytes in the proper concentration in both intracellular and extracellular fluids. The maintenance of water and electrolyte balance is one of the most difficult problems for health workers in caring for patients. Although some electrolytes are lost in the feces and through the skin as sweat, the job of balancing electrolytes is left mainly to the kidneys, as described earlier in this chapter.

The Role of Hormones Several hormones are involved in balancing electrolytes (see Chapter 11). Aldosterone, produced by the adrenal cortex, promotes the re-

Box 19-3	A Closer Look

Osmoreceptors: Thinking About Thirst

Osmoreceptors are specialized neurons that help to maintain water balances by detecting changes in the concentration of extracellular fluid (ECF). They are located in the hypothalamus of the brain in an area adjacent to the third ventricle, where they monitor the osmotic pressure (concentration) of the circulating blood plasma.

Osmoreceptors respond primarily to small increases in sodium, the most common cation in ECF. As the blood becomes more concentrated, sodium draws water out of the cells, initiating nerve impulses. Traveling to different regions of the hypothalamus, these impulses may have two different but related effects:

▶ They stimulate the hypothalamus to produce antidiuretic hormone (ADH), which is then released from the posterior pituitary. ADH travels to the kidneys and causes these organs to conserve water.

▶ They stimulate the thirst center of the hypothalamus, causing increased consumption of water. Almost as soon as water consumption begins, however, the sensation of thirst disappears. Receptors in the throat and stomach send inhibitory signals to the thirst center, preventing overconsumption of water and allowing time for ADH to affect the kidneys.

Both of these mechanisms serve to dilute the blood and other body fluids. Either mechanism alone can maintain water balance. If both fail, a person soon becomes dehydrated.

---

absorption of sodium (and water) and the elimination of potassium.

When the blood concentration of sodium rises above the normal range, the pituitary secretes more antidiuretic hormone (ADH). This hormone increases water reabsorption in the kidney to dilute the excess sodium.

Hormones from the parathyroid and thyroid glands regulate calcium and phosphate levels. Parathyroid hormone increases blood calcium levels by causing the bones to release calcium and the kidneys to reabsorb calcium. The thyroid hormone calcitonin lowers blood calcium by causing calcium to be deposited in the bones.

Checkpoint 19-18 What are some mechanisms for regulating electrolytes in body fluids?

▶ Acid–Base Balance

The pH scale is a measure of how acidic or basic (alkaline) a solution is. As described in Chapter 2, the pH scale measures the hydrogen ion (H^+) concentration in a solution. Body fluids are slightly alkaline in a pH range of 7.35 to 7.45. These fluids must be kept within a narrow range of pH, or damage, even death, will result. A shift in either direction by three tenths of a point on the pH scale, to 7.0 or 7.7, is fatal.

Regulation of pH

The body constantly produces acids in the course of metabolism. Catabolism of fats yields fatty acids and other acidic byproducts; cellular respiration yields pyruvic acid and, under anaerobic conditions, lactic acid; carbon dioxide dissolves in the blood and yields carbonic acid (see Chapter 16). Conversely, a few abnormal conditions may result in alkaline shifts in pH. Several systems act together to counteract these changes and maintain acid–base balance:

▶ **Buffer systems.** Buffers are substances that prevent sharp changes in hydrogen ion (H^+) concentration and thus maintain a relatively constant pH. Buffers work by accepting or releasing these ions as needed to keep the pH steady. The main buffer systems in the body are bicarbonate buffers, phosphate buffers, and proteins, such as hemoglobin in red blood cells and plasma proteins.

▶ **Respiration.** The role of respiration in controlling pH was described in Chapter 16. Recall that carbon dioxide release from the lungs makes the blood more alkaline by reducing the amount of carbonic acid formed. In contrast, carbon dioxide retention makes the blood more acidic. Respiratory rate can adjust pH for short-term regulation.

▶ **Kidney function.** The kidneys regulate pH by reabsorbing or eliminating hydrogen ions as needed. The kidneys are responsible for long-term pH regulation.

Checkpoint 19-19 What are three mechanisms for maintaining the acid–base balance of body fluids?

Word Anatomy

Medical terms are built from standardized word parts (prefixes, roots, and suffixes). Learning the meanings of these parts can help you remember words and interpret unfamiliar terms.

WORD PART	MEANING	EXAMPLE
The Kidneys		
retro-	backward, behind	The *retroperitoneal* space is posterior to the peritoneal cavity.
ren/o	kidney	The *renal* artery carries blood to the kidney.
nephr/o	kidney	The *nephron* is the functional unit of the kidney.
juxta-	next to	The *juxtaglomerular* apparatus is next to the glomerulus.
The Ureters		
extra-	beyond, outside of	The ureters are *extraperitoneal*.
The Effects of Aging		
noct/i	night	*Nocturia* is excessive urination at night.
Fluid Compartments		
intra-	within	*Intracellular* fluid is within a cell.
extra-	outside of, beyond	*Extracellular* fluid is outside the cells.
semi-	partial, half	A *semipermeable* membrane is partially permeable.
Water Balance		
poly-	many	*Polydipsia* is excessive thirst.
osmo-	osmosis	*Osmoreceptors* detect changes in osmotic concentration of fluids.

Summary

I. Excretion—removal and elimination of metabolic waste

1. Systems that eliminate waste
   a. Urinary- removes waste from blood
      (1) Other functions- regulates blood volume, pH, and electrolytes
   b. Digestive system—eliminates water, salts, bile with digestive residue
   c. Respiratory system—eliminates carbon dioxide, water
   d. Skin—eliminates water, salts, nitrogen waste

II. Organs of the urinary system

1. Kidneys (2)
2. Ureters (2)
3. Urinary bladder (1)
4. Urethra (1)

III. Kidneys

1. In upper abdomen against the back
2. In retroperitoneal space (posterior to the peritoneum)
A. Blood supply
   1. Renal artery—carries blood to kidney from aorta
   2. Renal vein—carries blood from kidney to inferior vena cava
B. Structure of the kidney
   1. Cortex—outer portion
   2. Medulla—inner portion
   3. Pelvis
      a. Upper end of ureter
      b. Calyces—cuplike extensions that receive urine

4. Nephron
   a. Functional unit of kidney
   b. Parts
      (1) Glomerular (Bowman) capsule—around glomerulus
      (2) Proximal convoluted tubule (PCT)
      (3) Loop of Henle- descending and ascending limbs
      (4) Distal convoluted tubule (DCT)
   c. Blood supply to nephron
      (1) Afferent arteriole—enters glomerular capsule
      (2) Glomerulus—coil of capillaries in glomerular capsule
      (3) Efferent arteriole—leaves glomerular capsule
      (4) Peritubular capillaries—surround nephron
      (5) Juxtaglomerular apparatus
         (a) Consists of cells in afferent arteriole and distal convoluted tubule
         (b) Releases renin to regulate blood pressure via angiotensin
C. Functions of the kidney
   1. Excretion of waste, excess salts, toxins
   2. Water balance
   3. Acid–base balance (pH)
   4. Regulation of blood pressure
   5. Releases hormone erythropoietin (EPO)- stimulates red blood cell production
D. Formation of urine
   1. Glomerular filtration—driven by blood pressure in glomerulus
      a. Water and soluble substances forced out of blood and into glomerular capsule

b. Blood cells and proteins remain in blood
c. Glomerular filtrate—material that leaves blood and enters the nephron
2. Tubular reabsorption
a. Most of filtrate leaves nephron by diffusion, osmosis and active transport
b. Returns to blood through peritubular capillaries
3. Tubular secretion—materials moved from blood into nephron for excretion
4. Concentration of urine
a. Countercurrent mechanism—method for concentrating urine based on movement of ions and permeability of tubule
(1) ADH
(a) Hormone from posterior pituitary
(b) Promotes reabsorption of water

IV. The ureters—carry urine from the kidneys to the bladder

V. Urinary bladder
1. Stores urine until it is eliminated
2. Trigone—triangular region in base of bladder; remains stable as bladder fills

VI. Urethra—carries urine out of body
1. Male urethra—20 cm long; carries both urine and semen
2. Female urethra—4 cm long; opening anterior to vagina
A. Urination (micturition)
1. Both voluntary and involuntary
2. Sphincters
a. Internal urethral sphincter—involuntary (smooth muscle)
b. External urethral sphincter—voluntary (skeletal muscle)
3. Stretch receptors in bladder wall signal reflex emptying
4. Can be controlled through higher brain centers

VII. Urine
1. pH averages 6.0
2. Specific gravity—measures dissolved substances
A. Normal constituents—water, nitrogenous waste, electrolytes, pigments

VIII. Effects of aging
1. Polyuria—increased elimination of urine
2. Nocturia—urination at night
3. Incontinence
4. Increased blood urea nitrogen (BUN)
5. Prostate enlargement

IX. Body fluids: the importance of water
1. Functions
a. Solvent
b. Transport medium
c. Participant in metabolic reactions
2. 50% to 70% of body weight
3. Contains electrolytes, nutrients, gases, wastes, hormones, and other substances
4. Important in homeostasis
A. Fluid compartments
1. Intracellular fluid—contained within the cells
2. Extracellular fluid—outside the cells
a. Blood plasma
b. Interstitial (tissue) fluid
c. Lymph
d. Fluid in special compartments
B. Water balance
1. Loss—through kidneys, skin, lungs, intestinal tract,
2. Gain—through beverages, food, metabolic water
3. Sense of thirst
a. Control center in hypothalamus
b. Responds to fluid volume and concentration of body fluids

X. Electrolytes and their functions
1. Electrolytes release ions in solution
a. Positive ions (cations)—e.g., sodium, potassium, calcium
b. Negative ions (anions)—e.g., phosphate, chloride
A. Electrolyte balance
1. Kidneys—main regulators
2. Role of hormones
a. Aldosterone (from adrenal cortex)
(1) Promotes reabsorption of sodium
(2) Promotes excretion of potassium
b. ADH (from pituitary)
(1) Causes kidney to retain water
c. Parathyroid hormone (from parathyroid glands)
(1) Increases blood calcium level
d. Calcitonin (from thyroid)
(1) Decreases blood calcium level

XI. Acid–base balance
1. Normal pH range is 7.35-7.45
A. Regulation of pH
1. Buffers—maintain constant pH
2. Respiration—release of carbon dioxide increases alkalinity; retention of carbon dioxide increases acidity
3. Kidney—regulates amount of hydrogen ion excreted
B. Abnormal pH

Questions for Study and Review

Building Understanding

Fill in the blanks

1. Each kidney is located in a _____ space.
2. The renal artery, vein, and ureter connect to the kidney at the _____.
3. The ureters and urethra open at the _____ of the bladder.
4. The amount of dissolved substances in urine is indicated by its _____.
5. Substances in the blood that prevent sharp changes in hydrogen ion concentration are called _____.

Matching

Match each numbered item with the most closely related lettered item.

___ 6. Produced by the kidney in response to low blood pressure
___ 7. Stimulates vasoconstriction
___ 8. Produced by the kidney in response to hypoxia
___ 9. Stimulates kidneys to produce concentrated urine
___ 10. Produced by the liver during protein catabolism

a. urea
b. erythropoietin
c. antidiuretic hormone
d. renin
e. angiotensin

Multiple choice

___ 11. The functional unit of the renal system is the
    a. renal capsule
    b. kidney
    c. nephron
    d. juxtaglomerular apparatus

___ 12. Fluid moves through the glomerulus by
    a. filtration
    b. diffusion
    c. osmosis
    d. active transport

___ 13. One's ability to delay urination is due to voluntary control of the
    a. trigone
    b. internal urethral sphincter
    c. external urethral sphincter
    d. urinary meatus

___ 14. Body water content is greatest in
    a. infants
    b. children
    c. young adults
    d. elderly adults

___ 15. Fluid located in the spaces between the cells in tissues all over the body is called
    a. cytoplasm
    b. plasma
    c. interstitial fluid
    d. lymph

Understanding Concepts

16. List four organ systems active in excretion. What are the products eliminated by each?

17. Compare and contrast the following terms:
    a. *glomerular capsule* and *glomerulus*
    b. *afferent* and *efferent arteriole*
    c. *proximal* and *distal convoluted tubule*
    d. *ureter* and *urethra*
    e. *intracellular* and *extracellular fluid*
    f. *aldosterone* and *antidiuretic hormone*
    g. *calcitonin* and *parathyroid hormone*

18. Trace the pathway of a molecule of urea from the afferent arteriole to the urinary meatus.

19. Describe the four processes involved in the formation of urine.

20. Compare the male urethra and female urethra in structure and function.

21. List some of the dissolved substances normally found in the urine.

22. Explain the role of the hypothalamus in water balance. In a healthy person, what is the ratio of fluid intake to output?

23. How do the respiratory and renal systems regulate pH?

Conceptual Thinking

24. A class of antihypertensive drugs called loop diuretics prevents sodium reabsorption in the loop of Henle. How could a drug like this lower blood pressure?

25. Lung disease patients who are unable to release carbon dioxide from the lungs often have acidic urine. Why does the the pH of the urine drop?

Perpetuation of Life

*T*he final unit includes two chapters on the structures and functions related to reproduction and heredity. The reproductive system is not necessary for the continuation of the life of the individual but rather is needed for the continuation of the human species. The reproductive cells and their genes have been studied intensively during recent years as part of the rapidly advancing science of genetics.

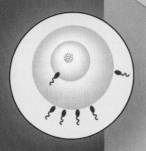

LEARNING OUTCOMES

After careful study of this chapter,
you should be able to:

1. Name the male and female gonads and describe the
   function of each

2. State the purpose of meiosis

3. List the accessory organs of the male and female reproductive
   tracts and cite the function of each

4. Describe the composition and function of semen

5. Draw and label a spermatozoon

6. List in the correct order the hormones produced during the
   menstrual cycle and cite the source of each

7. Describe the functions of the main male and female sex
   hormones

8. Explain how negative feedback regulates reproductive function
   in both males and females

9. Describe the changes that occur during and after menopause

10. Cite the main methods of birth control in use

11. Show how word parts are used to build words related to the
    reproductive systems (see Word Anatomy at the end of the
    chapter)

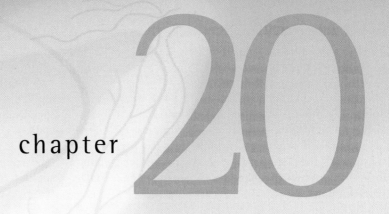

chapter

20

The Male and Female Reproductive Systems

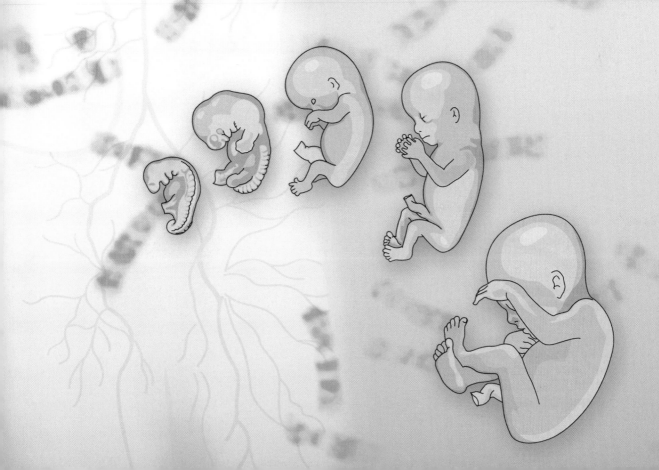

▌ Reproduction

The chapters in this unit deal with what is certainly one of the most interesting and mysterious attributes of life: the ability to reproduce. The simplest forms of life, one-celled organisms, usually need no partner to reproduce; they simply divide by themselves. This form of reproduction is known as **asexual** (nonsexual) reproduction.

In most animals, however, reproduction is **sexual**, meaning that there are two kinds of individuals, males and females, each of which has specialized cells designed specifically for the perpetuation of the species. These specialized sex cells are known as **germ cells**, or **gametes** (GAM-etes). In the male, they are called **spermatozoa** (sper-mah-to-ZO-ah) (sing., spermatozoon), or simply sperm cells, and in the female, they are called **ova** (O-vah) (sing., ovum) or egg cells.

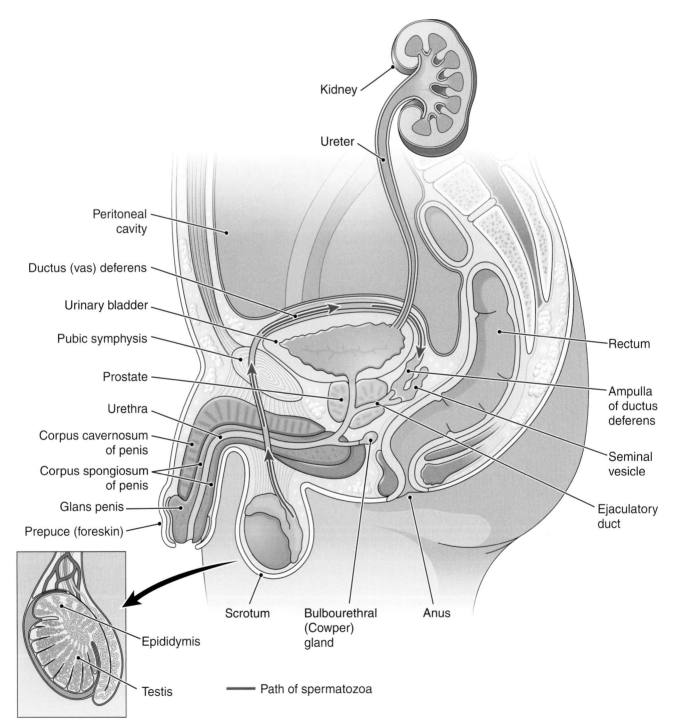

Figure 20-1 Male reproductive system. Organs of the urinary system are also shown. *ZOOMING IN ✦ What four glands empty secretions into the urethra?*

Meiosis

Gametes are characterized by having half as many chromosomes as are found in any other body cell. During their formation, they go through a special process of cell division, called **meiosis** (mi-O-sis), which halves the number of chromosomes. In humans, meiosis reduces the chromosome number in a cell from 46 to 23. The role of meiosis in reproduction is explained in more detail in Chapter 21.

> **Checkpoint 20-1** What is the process of cell division that halves the chromosome number in a cell to produce a gamete?

▶ The Male Reproductive System

The male reproductive system, like that of the female, may be divided into two groups of organs: primary and accessory (see Fig. 20-1).

- ▶ The primary organs are the **gonads** (GO-nads), or sex glands; they produce the germ cells and manufacture hormones. The male gonad is the testis. (In comparison, the female gonad is the ovary, as explained below.)
- ▶ The **accessory organs** include a series of ducts that transport the germ cells as well as various exocrine glands.

The Testes

The male gonads, the **testes** (TES-teze) (sing., testis) are located outside the body proper, suspended between the thighs in a sac called the **scrotum** (SKRO-tum). The testes are oval organs measuring about 4.0 cm (1.5 inches) in length and about 2.5 cm (1 inch) in each of the other two dimensions. During embryonic life, each testis develops from tissue near the kidney.

A month or two before birth, the testis normally descends (moves downward) through the **inguinal** (ING-gwih-nal) **canal** in the abdominal wall into the scrotum. Each testis then remains suspended by a **spermatic cord** (Fig. 20-2) that extends through the inguinal canal. This cord contains blood vessels, lymphatic vessels, nerves, and the tube (ductus deferens) that transports spermatozoa away from the testis. The gland must descend completely if it is to function normally; to produce spermatozoa, the testis must be kept at the temperature of the scrotum, which is several degrees lower than that of the abdominal cavity.

Internal Structure Most of the specialized tissue of the testis consists of tiny coiled **seminiferous** (seh-mih-NIF-er-us) **tubules**. Primitive cells in the walls of these tubules develop into mature spermatozoa, aided by neighboring cells called **sustentacular** (sus-ten-TAK-u-lar) (Sertoli) **cells**. These so-called "nurse" cells nourish and protect the developing spermatozoa. They also se-

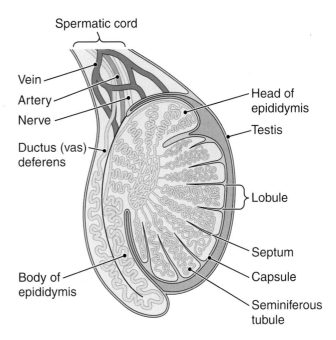

Figure 20-2 Structure of the testis. The epididymis and spermatic cord are also shown. *ZOOMING IN ✦ What duct receives secretions from the epididymis?*

crete a protein that binds testosterone in the seminiferous tubules.

Specialized **interstitial** (in-ter-STISH-al) **cells** that secrete the male sex hormone **testosterone** (*tes-TOS-teh-rone*) are located between the seminiferous tubules. Figure 20-3 is a microscopic view of the testis in cross-section, showing the seminiferous tubules, interstitial cells, and developing spermatozoa.

Testosterone After its secretion, testosterone is absorbed directly into the bloodstream. This hormone has three functions:

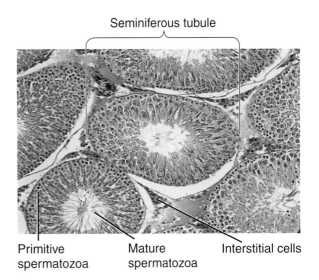

Figure 20-3 Microscopic view of the testis. (Courtesy of Dana Morse Bittus and BJ Cohen.)

▶ Development and maintenance of the reproductive structures.

▶ Development of spermatozoa.

▶ Development of **secondary sex characteristics,** traits that characterize males and females but are not directly concerned with reproduction. In males, these traits include a deeper voice, broader shoulders, narrower hips, a greater percentage of muscle tissue, and more body hair than are found in females.

The Spermatozoa Spermatozoa are tiny individual cells illustrated in Figure 20-4. They are so small that at least 200 million are contained in the average ejaculation (release of semen). After puberty, sperm cells are manufactured continuously in the seminiferous tubules of the testes.

The spermatozoon has an oval head that is largely a nucleus containing chromosomes. The **acrosome** (AK-ro-some), which covers the head like a cap, contains enzymes that help the sperm cell to penetrate the ovum.

Whiplike movements of the tail (flagellum) propel the sperm through the female reproductive system to the ovum. The cell's middle region (midpiece) contains many mitochondria that provide energy for movement.

Checkpoint 20-2 What is the male gonad?

Checkpoint 20-3 What is the main male sex hormone?

Checkpoint 20-4 What is the male sex cell (gamete) called?

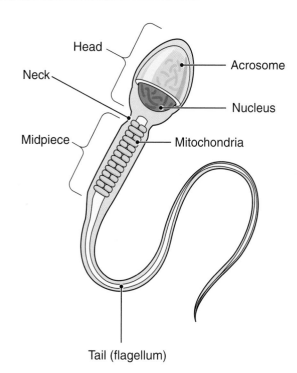

Head

Neck

Acrosome

Nucleus

Midpiece

Mitochondria

Tail (flagellum)

Figure 20-4 **Diagram of a human spermatozoon.** Major structural features are shown. *ZOOMING IN ✦ What organelles provide energy for sperm cell motility?*

Accessory Organs

The system of ducts that transports the spermatozoa begins with tubules inside the testis itself. From these tubules, the cells collect in a greatly coiled tube called the **epididymis** (ep-ih-DID-ih-mis), which is 6 meters (20 feet) long and is located on the surface of the testis inside the scrotal sac (see Fig. 20-2). While they are temporarily stored in the epididymis, the sperm cells mature and become motile, able to move or "swim" by themselves.

The epididymis finally extends upward as the **ductus deferens** (DEF-er-enz), also called the **vas deferens.** This tube, contained in the spermatic cord, continues through the inguinal canal into the abdominal cavity. Here, it separates from the remainder of the spermatic cord and curves behind the urinary bladder. The ductus deferens then joins with the duct of the **seminal vesicle** (VES-ih-kl) on the same side to form the **ejaculatory** (e-JAK-u-lah-to-re) **duct.** The right and left ejaculatory ducts travel through the body of the prostate gland and then empty into the urethra.

Checkpoint 20-5 What is the order in which sperm cells travel through the ducts of the male reproductive system?

Semen

Semen (*SE-men*) (meaning "seed") is the mixture of sperm cells and various secretions that is expelled from the body. It is a sticky fluid with a milky appearance. The pH is in the alkaline range of 7.2 to 7.8. The secretions in semen serve several functions:

▶ Nourish the spermatozoa.

▶ Transport the spermatozoa.

▶ Neutralize the acidity of the male urethra and the female vaginal tract.

▶ Lubricate the reproductive tract during sexual intercourse.

▶ Prevent infection with antibacterial enzymes and antibodies.

The glands discussed next contribute secretions to the semen (see Fig. 20-1).

The Seminal Vesicles The seminal vesicles are twisted muscular tubes with many small outpouchings. They are about 7.5 cm (3 inches) long and are attached to the connective tissue at the posterior of the urinary bladder. The glandular lining produces a thick, yellow, alkaline secretion containing large quantities of simple sugar and other substances that provide nourishment for the sperm. The seminal fluid makes up a large part of the semen's volume.

The Prostate Gland The **prostate gland** lies immediately inferior to the urinary bladder, where it surrounds the first part of the urethra. Ducts from the prostate carry its secretions into the urethra. The thin, alkaline prostatic secretion helps neutralize the acidity of the vaginal tract and enhance the motility of the spermatozoa. The prostate gland is also supplied with muscular tissue, which, upon signals from the nervous system, contracts to aid in the expulsion of the semen from the body.

Bulbourethral Glands The **bulbourethral** (bul-bo-u-RE-thral) **glands**, also called **Cowper glands**, are a pair of pea-sized organs located in the pelvic floor just inferior to the prostate gland. They secrete mucus to lubricate the urethra and tip of the penis during sexual stimulation. The ducts of these glands extend about 2.5 cm (1 inch) from each side and empty into the urethra before it extends into the penis.

Other very small glands secrete mucus into the urethra as it passes through the penis.

> **Checkpoint 20-6** What glands, aside from the testis, contribute secretions to semen?

The Urethra and Penis

The male urethra, as discussed in Chapter 19, serves the dual purpose of conveying urine from the bladder and carrying the reproductive cells with their accompanying secretions to the outside. The ejection of semen into the receiving canal (vagina) of the female is made possible by the **erection,** or stiffening and enlargement, of the penis, through which the longest part of the urethra extends. The penis is made of spongy tissue containing many blood spaces that are relatively empty when the organ is flaccid but fill with blood and distend when the penis is erect. (See Box 20-1 on erectile dysfunction.) This tissue is subdivided into three segments, each called a **corpus** (body) (Fig. 20-5). A single, ventrally located **corpus spongiosum** contains the urethra. On either side is a larger **corpus cavernosum** (pl., corpora cavernosa). At

the distal end of the penis, the corpus spongiosum enlarges to form the **glans** penis, which is covered with a loose fold of skin, the **prepuce** (PRE-puse), commonly called the *foreskin.* It is the end of the foreskin that is removed in a **circumcision** (sir-kum-SIZH-un), a surgery frequently performed on male babies for religious or cultural reasons. Experts disagree on the medical value of circumcision with regard to improved cleanliness and disease prevention.

The penis and scrotum together make up the *external genitalia* of the male.

Ejaculation Ejaculation (e-jak-u-LA-shun) is the forceful expulsion of semen through the urethra to the outside. The process is initiated by reflex centers in the spinal cord that stimulate smooth muscle contraction in the prostate. This is followed by contraction of skeletal muscle in the pelvic floor, which provides the force needed for expulsion. During ejaculation, the involuntary sphincter at the base of the bladder closes to prevent the release of urine.

A male typically ejaculates 2 to 5 mL of semen containing 50 million to 150 million sperm cells per mL. Out of the millions of spermatozoa in an ejaculation, only one, if any, can fertilize an ovum. The remainder of the cells live from only a few hours up to a maximum of 3 days.

> **Checkpoint 20-7** What are the main subdivisions of a spermatozoon?

▶ Hormonal Control of Male Reproduction

The activities of the testes are under the control of two hormones produced by the anterior pituitary. These hormones are named for their activity in female reproduction (described later), although they are chemically the same in both males and females.

▸ **Follicle-stimulating hormone (FSH)** stimulates the sustentacular (Sertoli) cells and promotes the formation of spermatozoa.
▸ **Luteinizing hormone (LH)** stimulates the interstitial cells between the seminiferous tubules to produce testosterone, which is also needed for sperm cell development. An older name for this hormone, which describes its action in males, is *interstitial cell–stimulating hormone* (ICSH).

Starting at puberty, the hypothalamus begins to secrete hormones that trigger the release of FSH and LH. These hormones are secreted continuously in the male.

The activity of the hypothalamus is in turn regulated by a negative feedback mechanism involving testosterone. As the blood level of testosterone increases, the hypothalamus secretes less releasing hormone; as the level of

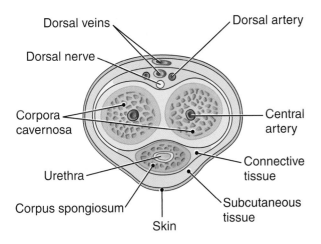

Figure 20-5 Cross-section of the penis. *ZOOMING IN* ✦ *What subdivision of the penis contains the urethra?*

Labels: Dorsal veins; Dorsal artery; Dorsal nerve; Corpora cavernosa; Central artery; Urethra; Connective tissue; Corpus spongiosum; Subcutaneous tissue; Skin

| Box 20-1 | Clinical Perspectives |

Treating Erectile Dysfunction: When NO Means Yes

Approximately 25 million American men and their partners are affected by **erectile dysfunction** (ED), the inability to achieve an erection. Although ED is more common in men over the age of 65, it can occur at any age and can have many causes. Until recently, ED was believed to be caused by psychological factors, such as stress or depression. It is now known that many cases of ED are caused by physical factors, including cardiovascular disease, diabetes, spinal cord injury, and damage to penile nerves during prostate surgery. Antidepressant and antihypertensive medications also can produce erectile dysfunction.

Erection results from interaction between the autonomic nervous system and penile blood vessels. Sexual arousal stimulates parasympathetic nerves in the penis to release a compound called nitric oxide (NO), which activates the vascular smooth muscle enzyme guanylyl cyclase. This enzyme catalyzes production of cyclic GMP (cGMP), a potent vasodilator that increases blood flow into the penis to cause erection.

Physical factors that cause ED prevent these physiologic occurrences.

Until recently, treatment options for ED, such as penile injections, vacuum pumps, and insertion of medications into the penile urethra were inadequate, inconvenient, and painful. Today, drugs that target the physiologic mechanisms that underlie erection are giving men who suffer from ED new hope. The best known of these is sildenafil (Viagra), which works by inhibiting the enzyme that breaks down cGMP, thus prolonging the effects of NO.

Although effective in about 80% of all ED cases, Viagra can cause some relatively minor side effects, including headache, nasal congestion, stomach upset, and blue-tinged vision. Viagra should never be used by men who are taking nitrate drugs to treat angina. Because nitrate drugs elevate NO levels, taking them with Viagra, a drug that prolongs the effects of NO, can cause life-threatening hypotension.

---

testosterone decreases, the hypothalamus secretes more releasing hormone (see Fig. 11-3 in Chapter 11).

Checkpoint 20-8 What two pituitary hormones regulate both male and female reproduction?

The Effects of Aging on Male Reproduction

A gradual decrease in the production of testosterone and spermatozoa begins as early as 20 years of age and continues throughout life. Secretions from the prostate and seminal vesicles decrease in amount and become less viscous. In a few men (less than 10%), sperm cells remain late in life, even to 80 years of age.

▶ The Female Reproductive System

The female gonads are the **ovaries** (O-vah-reze), where the female sex cells, or ova, are formed (Fig. 20-6). The remainder of the female reproductive tract consists of an organ (uterus) to hold and nourish a developing infant, various passageways, and the external genital organs.

The Ovaries

The ovary is a small, somewhat flattened oval body measuring about 4 cm (1.6 inches) in length, 2 cm (0.8 inch) in width, and 1 cm (0.4 inch) in depth. Like the testes, the ovaries descend, but only as far as the pelvic

portion of the abdomen. Here, they are held in place by ligaments, including the broad ligament, the ovarian ligament, and others, that attach them to the uterus and the body wall.

The Ova and Ovulation

The outer layer of the ovary is made of a single layer of epithelium. Beneath this layer, the female gametes, the ova, are produced. The ovaries of a newborn female contain a large number of potential ova. Each month during the reproductive years, several ripen, but usually only one is released.

The complicated process of maturation, or "ripening," of an ovum takes place in a small fluid-filled cluster of cells called the **ovarian follicle** (o-VA-re-an FOL-ih-kl) or **graafian** (GRAF-e-an) **follicle** (Fig. 20-7). As the follicle develops, cells in its wall secrete the hormone estrogen, which stimulates growth of the uterine lining. When an ovum has ripened, the ovarian follicle may rupture and discharge the egg cell from the ovary's surface. The rupture of a follicle allowing the escape of an ovum is called **ovulation** (ov-u-LA-shun). Any developing ova that are not released simply degenerate.

After it is released, the egg cell makes its way to the nearest **oviduct** (O-vih-dukt), a tube that arches over the ovary and leads to the uterus (see Fig. 20-6).

Checkpoint 20-9 What is the female gonad called?

Checkpoint 20-10 What is the female gamete called?

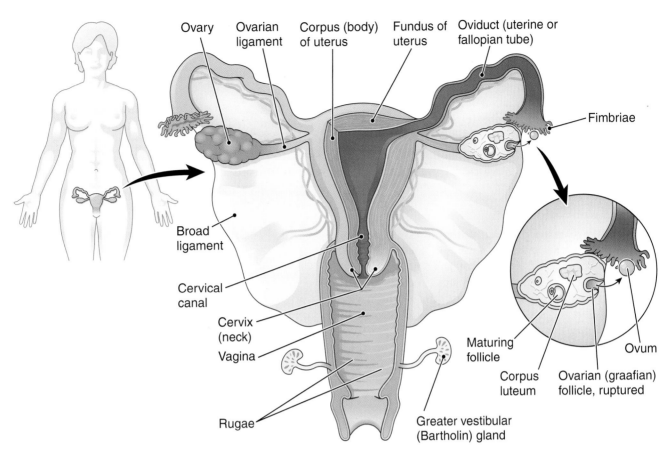

Figure 20-6 **Female reproductive system.** The enlargement (*right*) shows ovulation. *ZOOMING IN ✦ What is the deepest part of the uterus called?*

The Corpus Luteum After the ovum has been expelled, the remaining follicle is transformed into a solid glandular mass called the **corpus luteum** (LU-te-um). This structure secretes estrogen and also progesterone, another hormone needed in the reproductive cycle. Commonly, the corpus luteum shrinks and is replaced by scar tissue. When a pregnancy occurs, however, this structure remains active. Sometimes, as a result of normal ovulation, the corpus luteum persists and forms a small ovarian cyst (fluid-filled sac). This condition usually resolves without treatment.

Checkpoint 20-11 What is the structure that surrounds the egg as it ripens?

Checkpoint 20-12 What is the process of releasing an egg cell from the ovary called?

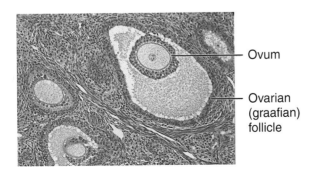

Figure 20-7 **Microscopic view of the ovary.** The photomicrograph shows egg cells (ova) developing within ovarian (graafian) follicles. (Courtesy of Dana Morse Bittus and BJ Cohen.)

Accessory Organs

The accessory organs in the female are the oviducts, the uterus, the vagina, the greater vestibular glands, and the vulva and perineum.

The Oviducts The tubes that transport the ova in the female reproductive system, the oviducts, are also known as **uterine** (U-ter-in) **tubes,** or **fallopian** (fah-LO-pe-an) **tubes.** Each is a small, muscular structure, nearly 12.5 cm (5 inches) long, extending from a point near the ovary to the uterus (womb). There is no direct connection between the ovary and this tube. The ovum is swept into the oviduct by a current in the peritoneal fluid produced by the small, fringelike extensions called **fimbriae** (FIM-bre-e) that are located at the edge of the tube's opening into the abdomen (see Fig. 20-6)

Unlike the sperm cell, the ovum cannot move by itself. Its progress through the oviduct toward the uterus depends on the sweeping action of cilia in the tube's lining and on peristalsis of the tube. It takes about 5 days for an ovum to reach the uterus from the ovary.

Checkpoint 20-13 What does the follicle become after ovulation?

The Uterus The oviducts lead to the **uterus** (U-ter-us), an organ in which a fetus can develop to maturity. The uterus is a pear-shaped, muscular organ about 7.5 cm (3 inches) long, 5 cm (2 inches) wide, and 2.5 cm (1 inch) deep. (The organ is typically larger in women who have borne children and smaller in postmenopausal women.) The superior portion rests on the upper surface of the urinary bladder; the inferior portion is embedded in the pelvic floor between the bladder and the rectum. The wider upper region of the uterus is called the **corpus**, or body; the lower, narrower region is the **cervix** (SER-viks), or neck. The small, rounded region above the level of the tubal entrances is known as the **fundus** (FUN-dus) (see Fig. 20-6).

The broad ligaments support the uterus, extending from each side of the organ to the lateral body wall. Along with the uterus, these two portions of peritoneum form a partition dividing the female pelvis into anterior and posterior areas. The ovaries are suspended from the broad ligaments, and the oviducts lie within the upper borders. Blood vessels that supply these organs are found between the layers of the broad ligament (see Fig. 20-6).

The muscular wall of the uterus is called the **myometrium** (mi-o-ME-tre-um) (Fig. 20-8). The lining of the uterus is a specialized epithelium known as **endometrium** (en-do-ME-tre-um). This inner layer changes during the menstrual cycle, first preparing to nourish a fertilized egg, then breaking down if no fertilization occurs to be released as the menstrual flow. The cavity inside the uterus is shaped somewhat like a capital T, but it is capable of changing shape and dilating as a fetus develops.

Checkpoint 20-14 In what organ does a fetus develop?

The Vagina The cervix leads to the **vagina** (vah-JI-nah), the distal part of the birth canal, which opens to the outside of the body. The vagina is a muscular tube about 7.5 cm (3 inches) long connecting the uterine cavity with the outside. The cervix dips into the superior portion of the vagina forming a circular recess known as the **fornix** (FOR-niks). The deepest area of the fornix, located behind the cervix, is the **posterior fornix** (Fig. 20-9). This recess in the posterior vagina lies adjacent to the most inferior portion of the peritoneal cavity, a narrow passage between the uterus and the rectum named the **cul-de-sac** (from the French meaning "bottom of the sack"). This area is also known as the *rectouterine pouch* or the *pouch of Douglas*. A rather thin layer of tissue separates the posterior fornix from this region, so that abscesses or tumors

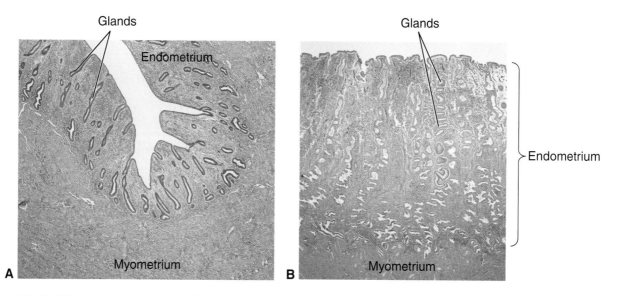

Figure 20-8 **The uterus as seen under the microscope.** The photomicrographs show the myometrium and endometrium and illustrate the changes that occur in the endometrium during the menstrual cycle. (**A**) Proliferative phase (first part of cycle). (**B**) Secretory phase (second part of cycle). (Reprinted with permission from Cormack DH. Essential Histology. 2nd ed. Philadelphia: Lippincott Williams & Wilkins, 2001.) *ZOOMING IN* ✦ *In which part of the menstrual cycle is the endometrium most highly developed?*

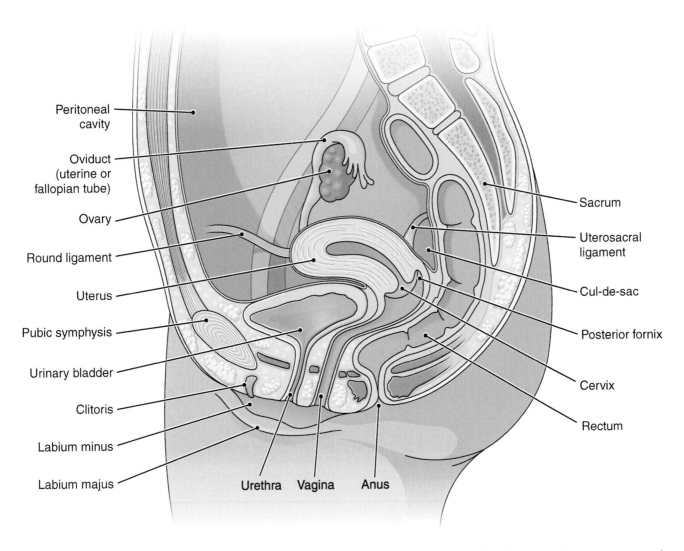

Figure 20-9 Female reproductive system (sagittal section). This view shows the relationship of the reproductive organs to each other and to other structures in the pelvic cavity. *ZOOMING IN* ✦ *Which has the more anterior opening, the vagina or the urethra?*

in the peritoneal cavity can sometimes be detected by vaginal examination.

The lining of the vagina is a wrinkled mucous membrane similar to that found in the stomach. The folds (rugae) permit enlargement so that childbirth usually does not tear the lining. In addition to being a part of the birth canal, the vagina is the organ that receives the penis during sexual intercourse. A fold of membrane called the **hymen** (HI-men) may sometimes be found at or near the vaginal (VAJ-ih-nal) canal opening (see Fig. 20-10).

The Greater Vestibular Glands Just superior and lateral to the vaginal opening are the two mucus-producing **greater vestibular** (ves-TIB-u-lar) **(Bartholin) glands** (see Fig. 20-6). These glands secrete into an area near the vaginal opening known as the **vestibule**. Like the Cowper glands in males, these glands provide lubrication during

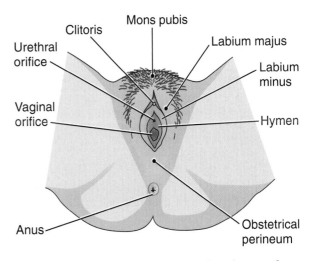

Figure 20-10 External parts of the female reproductive system. Related structures are also shown.

intercourse. If a gland becomes infected, a surgical incision may be needed to reduce swelling and promote drainage.

The Vulva and the Perineum The external parts of the female reproductive system form the **vulva** (VUL-vah), which includes two pairs of lips, or **labia** (LA-be-ah); the **clitoris** (KLIT-o-ris), which is a small organ of great sensitivity; and related structures. Although the entire pelvic floor in both the male and female (see Fig. 7-15 in Chapter 7) is properly called the **perineum** (per-ih-NE-um), those who care for pregnant women usually refer to the limited area between the vaginal opening and the anus as the perineum or obstetrical perineum.

▸ The Menstrual Cycle

In the female, as in the male, reproductive function is controlled by pituitary hormones that are regulated by the hypothalamus. Female activity differs, however, in that it is cyclic; it shows regular patterns of increases and decreases in hormone levels. These changes are regulated by hormonal feedback. The typical length of the menstrual cycle varies between 22 and 45 days, but 28 days is taken as an average, with the first day of menstrual flow being considered the first day of the cycle (Fig. 20-11).

Beginning of the Cycle

At the start of each cycle, under the influence of pituitary FSH, several follicles, each containing an ovum, begin to develop in the ovary. Usually, only one of these follicles will ultimately release an ovum from the ovary in a single month. The follicle produces increasing amounts of **estrogen** as it matures (see Fig. 20-11). (*Estrogen* is the term used for a group of related hormones, the most active of which is estradiol.) The estrogen is carried in the bloodstream to the uterus, where it starts preparing the endometrium for a possible pregnancy. This preparation includes thickening of the endometrium and elongation of the glands that produce the uterine secretion. Estrogen in the blood also acts as a feedback messenger to inhibit the release of FSH and stimulate the release of LH from the pituitary (see Fig. 11-3 in Chapter 11). (Note that there is an unexplained rise in FSH at the time of ovulation, as shown in Fig. 20-11.)

Ovulation

In an average 28-day cycle, ovulation occurs on day 14 and is followed two weeks later by the start of the menstrual flow. However, an ovum can be released any time from day 7 to 21, thus accounting for the variation in the length of normal cycles. About 1 day before ovulation, there is an **LH surge,** a sharp rise of LH in the blood. This hormone causes ovulation and transforms the ruptured follicle into the corpus luteum, which produces some es-

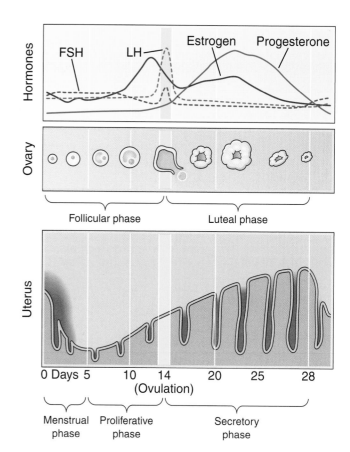

Figure 20-11   The menstrual cycle. Changes in hormones, the ovary, and the uterus are shown during a typical 28-day menstrual cycle with ovulation on day 14. (Pituitary hormones are shown with dashed lines, ovarian hormones with solid lines.) *ZOOMING IN ✦ What hormone peaks closest to ovulation?*

trogen and large amounts of **progesterone.** Under the influence of these hormones, the endometrium continues to thicken, and the glands and blood vessels increase in size. The rising levels of estrogen and progesterone feed back to inhibit the release of FSH and LH from the pituitary. During this time, the ovum makes its journey to the uterus by way of the oviduct. If the ovum is not fertilized while passing through the uterine tube, it dies within 2 to 3 days and then disintegrates.

During each menstrual cycle, changes occur in both the ovary and the uterus (see Fig. 20-11). The time before ovulation is described as the follicular phase in the ovary, because it encompasses development of the ovarian follicle. The uterus during this same time is in a proliferative phase, marked by growth of the endometrium. After ovulation, the ovary is in a luteal phase, with conversion of the follicle to the corpus luteum, and the uterus is described as being in a secretory phase, based on activity of the endometrial glands.

Checkpoint 20-15 What are the two hormones produced in the ovaries?

The Menstrual Phase

If fertilization does not occur, the corpus luteum degenerates, and the levels of estrogen and progesterone decrease. Without the hormones to support growth, the endometrium degenerates. Small hemorrhages appear in this tissue, producing the bloody discharge known as **menstrual flow**, or **menses** (MEN-seze). Bits of endometrium break away and accompany the blood flow during this period of **menstruation** (men-stru-A-shun). The average duration of menstruation is 2 to 6 days.

Even before the menstrual flow ceases, the endometrium begins to repair itself through the growth of new cells. The low levels of estrogen and progesterone allow the release of FSH from the anterior pituitary. FSH causes new follicles to begin to ripen within the ovaries, and the cycle begins anew.

The activity of ovarian hormones as negative feedback messengers is the basis of hormonal methods of contraception (birth control). Estrogen and progesterone inhibit the release of FSH and LH from the pituitary, resulting in a menstrual period but no ovulation.

▶ Menopause

Menopause (MEN-o-pawz) is the period during which menstruation ceases altogether. It ordinarily occurs gradually between the ages of 45 and 55 years and is caused by a normal decline in ovarian function. The ovary becomes chiefly scar tissue and no longer produces ripe follicles or appreciable amounts of estrogen. Eventually, the uterus, oviducts, vagina, and vulva all become somewhat atrophied and the vaginal mucosa becomes thinner, dryer, and more sensitive.

Menopause is an entirely normal condition, but its onset sometimes brings about effects that are temporarily disturbing. The decrease in estrogen levels can cause nervous symptoms, such as anxiety, insomnia, and "hot flashes."

Hormone Replacement Therapy

Physicians may prescribe hormone replacement therapy (HRT) to relieve the discomforts associated with menopause. This medication is usually a combination of estrogen with a synthetic progesterone (progestin), which is included to prevent overgrowth of the endometrium and the risk of endometrial cancer. Early assumptions about the role of estrogen in preventing heart attacks have been disproved by carefully controlled studies, at least with regard to the most commonly prescribed form of HRT. The hormone therapy did lower the incidence of colorectal cancer and hip fractures, a sign of osteoporosis. Studies are continuing with estrogen alone, generally prescribed for women who have undergone a hysterectomy and do not have a uterus.

In addition to an increased risk of breast cancer, HRT also carries a risk of thrombosis and embolism, which is highest among women who smoke. All HRT risks increase with the duration of therapy. Therefore, treatment should be given for a short time and at the lowest effective dose. Women with a history or family history of breast cancer or circulatory problems should not take HRT.

> **Checkpoint 20-16** What is the definition of menopause?

▶ Birth Control

Birth control is most commonly achieved by **contraception**, which is the use of artificial methods to prevent fertilization of the ovum. Birth control measures that prevent implantation of the fertilized ovum are also considered contraceptives, although technically they do not prevent conception and are more accurately called **abortifacients** (ah-bor-tih-FA-shents) (agents that cause abortion). Some of the birth control methods act by both mechanisms. Table 20-1 presents a brief description of the main contraceptive methods currently in use along with some advantages and disadvantages of each. The list is given in rough order of decreasing effectiveness. Unless specifically mentioned as doing so, a given method does *not* prevent the transmission of STIs (see Box 20-2 on lowering risks for STIs).

The various hormonal methods of birth control basically differ in how they administer the hormones. The emergency contraceptive pill (ECP) is a synthetic progesterone (progestin) taken within 72 hours after intercourse, usually in two doses 12 hours apart. It reduces the risk of pregnancy following unprotected intercourse. This so-called "morning after pill" is intended for emergency use and not as a regular birth control method. Birth control hormones can also be implanted as capsules under the skin of the upper arm. This method is highly effective and lasts for 3 to 5 years, but the capsules must be implanted and removed by a health professional, and they have been difficult to remove in some cases. (See Box 20-3 on hormonal contraception for men.)

The female condom is a sheath that fits into the vagina. It does protect against STIs, but is not very convenient to use. Researchers have also done trials with a male contraceptive pill, but none is on the market as yet. Mefipristone (RU 486) is a drug taken after conception to terminate an early pregnancy. It blocks the action of progesterone, causing the uterus to shed its lining and release the fertilized egg. It must be combined with administration of prostaglandins to expel the uterine tissue. Mefipristone is not in widespread use in the U.S., but it has been used in other countries.

> **Checkpoint 20-17** What is the definition of contraception?

Table 20·1 Main Methods of Birth Control Currently in Use

METHOD	DESCRIPTION	ADVANTAGES	DISADVANTAGES
Surgical			
Vasectomy/tubal ligation	Cutting and tying of tubes carrying gametes	Nearly 100% effective; involves no chemical or mechanical devices	Not usually reversible: rare surgical complications
Hormonal			
Birth control pills	Estrogen and progestin or progestin alone taken orally to prevent ovulation	Highly effective; requires no last-minute preparation	Alters physiology; return to fertility may be delayed; risk of cardiovascular disease in older women who smoke or have hypertension
Birth control shot	Injection of synthetic progesterone every 3 months to prevent ovulation	Highly effective; lasts for 3 to 4 months	Alters physiology; same possible side effects as birth control pill; also possible menstrual irregularity, amenorrhea
Birth control patch	Adhesive patch placed on body that administers estrogen and progestin through the skin; left on for 3 weeks and removed for a fourth week	Protects long-term; less chance of incorrect use; no last-minute preparation	Alters physiology; same possible side effects as birth control pill
Birth control ring	Flexible ring inserted into vagina that releases hormones internally; left in place for three weeks and removed for a fourth week	Long-lasting, highly effective; no last minute preparation	Possible infections, irritation; same possible side effects as birth control pill
Barrier			
Male condom	Sheath that fits over erect penis and prevents release of semen	Easily available; does not effect physiology; protects against sexually transmitted disease (STI)	Must be applied just before intercourse; may slip or tear
Diaphragm (with spermicide)	Rubber cap that fits over cervix and prevents entrance of sperm	Does not affect physiology; some protection against STI; no side effects	Must be inserted before intercourse and left in place for 6 hours; requires fitting by physician
Contraceptive sponge (with spermicide)	Soft, disposable foam disk containing spermicide, which is moistened with water and inserted into vagina	Protects against pregnancy for 24 hours; nonhormonal; some STI protection; available without prescription; inexpensive	85%–90% effective depending on proper use; skin irritation
Intrauterine device (IUD)	Metal or plastic device inserted into uterus through vagina; prevents fertilization and implantation by release of copper or birth control hormones	Highly effective for 5–10 years depending on type; reversible; no last-minute preparation	Must be introduced and removed by health professional; heavy menstrual bleeding
Other			
Spermicide	Chemicals used to kill sperm; best when used in combination with a barrier method	Available without prescription; inexpensive; does not affect physiology; some protection against STI	Local irritation; must be used just before intercourse
Fertility awareness	Abstinence during fertile part of cycle as determined by menstrual history, basal body temperature, or quality of cervical mucus	Does not affect physiology; accepted by certain religions	High failure rate; requires careful record keeping

Box 20-2 • Health Maintenance

Sexually Transmitted Infections: Lowering Your Risks

Sexually transmitted infections (STIs) such as chlamydia, gonorrhea, genital herpes, HIV, and syphilis are some of the most common infectious diseases in the United States, affecting more than 13 million men and women each year. These diseases are associated with complications such as pelvic inflammatory disease, epididymitis, infertility, liver failure, neurologic disorders, cancer, and AIDS. Women are more likely to contract STIs than are men. The same mechanisms that transport sperm cells through the female reproductive tract also move infectious organisms. The surest way to prevent STIs is to avoid sexual contact with others. If you are sexually active, the following techniques can lower your risks:

▶ Maintain a monogamous sexual relationship with an uninfected partner.

▶ Correctly and consistently use a condom. While not 100% effective, condoms greatly reduce the risk of contracting an STI.
▶ Avoid having sex during menstruation. Women may be more infectious as well as more susceptible to certain STIs during this time.
▶ Avoid contact with body fluids such as blood, semen, and vaginal fluids, all of which may harbor infectious organisms.
▶ Urinate and wash the genitals after sex. This may help remove infectious organisms before they cause disease.
▶ Have regular checkups for STIs. Most of the time STIs cause no symptoms, particularly in women.

Box 20-3 Hot Topics

Hormonal Contraception: New Options for Men

At present, sexually active men have few effective options for contraception, the most reliable being condoms or vasectomy. While condoms have the additional benefit of preventing sexually transmitted infections, their failure rate for preventing pregnancy is about 10%. With a failure rate of about 1%, vasectomies are much more reliable but are suitable only for couples who do not want children or are finished having children. A new option is on the horizon, however—male hormonal contraception.

Like female contraception, the male version of "the pill" works by suppressing the release of gonadotropin releasing hormone (GnRH) from the hypothalamus. This, in turn, blocks the pituitary's release of luteinizing hormone (LH) and follicle stimulating hormone (FSH), both of which play an important role in spermatogenesis.

Several therapies that decrease LH and FSH production in men are under investigation. One method already in clinical trials uses high levels of testosterone to negatively feed back to the hypothalamus and suppress GnRH secretion. Currently, this method requires regular testosterone injections, which makes it impractical for general use. In addition, doses of testosterone high enough to stop spermatogenesis may be associated with side effects such as acne, weight gain, mood changes, and increased risk of cardiovascular disease. More practical methods of drug delivery, such as pills, transdermal patches, and implants are being developed and may be effective at lower testosterone doses.

Another promising method uses the female hormone progesterone to block GnRH production. While this method suppresses spermatogenesis more effectively than does testosterone alone, it also suppresses normal testosterone production. Thus, the progesterone must be combined with testosterone to prevent the loss of secondary sex characteristics. Investigation is still underway to determine the best way to deliver such combination therapy.

Word Anatomy

Medical terms are built from standardized word parts (prefixes, roots, and suffixes). Learning the meanings of these parts can help you remember words and interpret unfamiliar terms.

WORD PART	MEANING	EXAMPLE
The Male Reproductive System		
semin/o	semen, seed	Sperm cells are produced in the *seminiferous* tubules.
test/o	testis	The hormone *testosterone* is produced in the testis.
acr/o	extreme end	The *acrosome* covers the head of a sperm cell.
fer	to carry	The ductus *deferens* carries spermatozoa away from (de-) the testis.
circum-	around	A cut is made around the glans to remove part of the foreskin in a *circumcision.*
The Female Reproductive System		
ov/o, ov/i	egg	An *ovum* is an egg cell.
ovar, ovari/o	ovary	The *ovarian* follicle encloses a maturing ovum.
metr/o	uterus	The *myometrium* is the muscular (my/o) layer of the uterus.
rect/o	rectum	The *rectouterine* pouch is between the uterus and rectum.

Summary

I. Reproduction
A. Meiosis—reduces chromosome number from 46 to 23
  1. Gametes (sex cells)
      a. Spermatozoa (sperm cells)—male
      b. Ova (egg cells)—female

II. Male reproductive system
  1. Primary organs—gonads
  2. Accessory organs—ducts and exocrine glands
A. Testes
  1. Scrotum—sac that holds the testes
  2. Inguinal canal—channel through which testis descends
  3. Internal structure
      a. Seminiferous tubules—tubes in which sperm cells are produced
          (1) Sustentacular (Sertoli) cells—aid in development of spermatozoa
      b. Interstitial cells (between tubules)—secrete hormones
  4. Testosterone
      a. Maintains reproductive structures
      b. Promotes development of secondary sex characteristics
  5. Spermatozoa
      a. Head—contains chromosomes
      b. Acrosome—covers head; has enzymes to help penetration of ovum
      c. Midpiece—contains mitochondria
      d. Tail (flagellum)—propels sperm
B. Accessory organs
  1. Epididymis—stores spermatozoa until ejaculation
  2. Ductus (vas) deferens—conducts sperm cells through spermatic cord
  3. Ejaculatory duct—empties into urethra
C. Semen
  1. Functions
      a. Nourish spermatozoa
      b. Transport spermatozoa
      c. Neutralize male urethra and vaginal tract

  d. Lubricate reproductive tract during intercourse
  e. Prevent infection
  2. Glands
      a. Seminal vesicles
      b. Prostate—around first portion of urethra
      c. Bulbourethral (Cowper) glands
D. Urethra and penis
  1. Urethra
      a. Conveys urine and semen through penis
  2. Penis
      a. Structure
          (1) Corpus spongiosum—central; contains urethra
          (2) Corpora cavernosa—lateral
          (3) Glans—distal enlargement of corpus spongiosum
          (4) Prepuce—foreskin
      b. Erection—stiffening and enlargement of penis
  3. Ejaculation—forceful expulsion of semen

III. Hormonal control of male reproduction
  1. Pituitary hormones
      a. FSH (follicle stimulating hormone)
          (1) Stimulates Sertoli cells
          (2) Promotes formation of spermatozoa
      b. LH (luteinizing hormone)
          (1) Stimulates interstitial cells to produce testosterone
          (2) Also called ICSH (interstitial cell–stimulating hormone)
A. Effects of aging on male reproduction
  1. Decline in testosterone, spermatozoa, and semen

IV. Female reproductive system
A. Ovaries—gonads in which ova form
B. Ova and ovulation
  1. Egg ripens in graafian follicle
  2. Ovulation—release of ovum from ovary
  3. Corpus luteum
      a. Remainder of follicle in ovary

  b. Continues to function if egg fertilized
  c. Disintegrates if egg not fertilized
C. Accessory organs
 1. Oviducts (uterine tubes, fallopian tubes)
  a. Fimbriae—fringelike extensions that sweep egg into oviduct
 2. Uterus
  a. Holds developing fetus
  b. Supported by broad ligament
  c. Endometrium—lining of uterus
  d. Myometrium—muscle layer
  e. Cervix—narrow, lower part
 3. Vagina
  a. Tube connecting uterus to outside
  b. Hymen—fold of membrane over vaginal opening
  c. Greater vestibular (Bartholin) glands—secrete mucus
 4. Vulva and perineum
  a. Vulva—external genitalia
   (1) Labia—two sets of folds (majora, minora)
   (2) Clitoris—organ of great sensitivity
  b. Perineum—pelvic floor
   (1) In obstetrics—area between vagina and anus

V. Menstrual cycle—average 28 days
A. Beginning of the cycle
 1. FSH stimulates follicle-follicular phase
 2. Follicle secretes estrogen
 3. Estrogen thickens lining of uterus—proliferative phase
B. Ovulation
 1. LH surge 1 day before
 2. Corpus luteum produces progesterone—luteal phase
 3. Progesterone continues growth of endometrium—secretory phase
 4. Ovum disintegrates if not fertilized
C. Menstrual phase (menstruation)
 1. If egg not fertilized, corpus luteum degenerates
 2. Lining of uterus breaks down releasing menses

VI. Menopause—period during which menstruation stops
A. Hormone replacement therapy (HRT)
 1. Reduces adverse symptoms of menopause
 2. Risks of HRT—cardiovascular disorders, breast cancer

VII. Birth control
 1. Contraception—use of artificial methods to prevent fertilization or implantation of fertilized egg
 2. Methods—surgery, hormonal, barrier, IUD, spermicides, fertility awareness

Questions for Study and Review

Building Understanding

Fill in the blanks

1. Gametes go through a special process of cell division called _____.

2. Spermatozoa begin their development in tiny coiled _____.

3. An ovum matures in a small fluid-filled cluster of cells called the _____.

4. The main male sex hormone is _____.

5. The process of releasing an ovum from the ovary is called _____.

Matching

Match each numbered item with the most closely related lettered item.

___ 6. A hormone released by the pituitary that promotes follicular development in the ovary

___ 7. A hormone released by developing follicles that promotes thickening of the endometrium

___ 8. A hormone released by the pituitary that stimulates ovulation

___ 9. A hormone released by the corpus luteum that promotes thickening of the endometrium

 a. follicle stimulating hormone
 b. estrogen
 c. luteinizing hormone
 d. progesterone

Multiple choice

___ 10. A month or two before birth, the testis travels from the abdominal cavity to the scrotum through the
 a. spermatic cord
 b. inguinal canal
 c. seminiferous tubule
 d. vas deferens

___ 11. Enzymes that help the sperm cell to penetrate the ovum are found in the
 a. acrosome
 b. head
 c. midpiece
 d. flagellum

___ 12. The male urethra is contained within the
   a. corpus cavernosum
   b. corpus spongiosum
   c. vas deferens
   d. seminiferous tubules

___ 13. The uterus and ovaries are supported by the
   a. uterine tubes
   b. broad ligaments
   c. fimbriae
   d. fornix

___ 14. The area between the vaginal opening and the anus is referred to as the
   a. vestibule
   b. vulva
   c. hymen
   d. perineum

___ 15. During the menstrual cycle, decreased levels of estrogen and progesterone promote the
   a. luteal phase
   b. menstrual phase
   c. proliferative phase
   d. secretory phase

Understanding Concepts

16. Compare and contrast the following terms:
   a. asexual reproduction and sexual reproduction
   b. spermatozoa and ova

   c. sustentacular cell and interstitial cell
   d. ovarian follicle and corpus luteum
   e. myometrium and endometrium

17. Trace the pathway of sperm from the site of production to the urethra.

18. Describe the components of semen, their sites of production, and their functions.

19. List the hormones that control male reproduction and state their functions.

20. Trace the pathway of an ovum from the site of production to the site of implantation.

21. Beginning with the first day of the menstrual flow, describe the events of one complete cycle, including the role of the hormones involved.

22. Define *contraception*. Describe methods of contraception that involve (1) barriers; (2) chemicals; (3) hormones; (4) prevention of implantation.

Conceptual Thinking

23. Theoretically, it is possible for a brain-dead man to ejaculate. What anatomical and physiological feature makes this possible?

24. Nicole, a middle-aged mother of three, is considering a tubal ligation, a contraceptive procedure that involves cutting the uterine tubes. Nicole is worried that this might cause her to enter early menopause. Should she be worried?

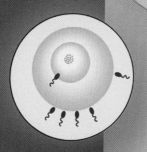

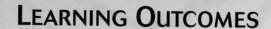

SELECTED KEY TERMS

The following terms and other boldface terms in the chapter are defined in the Glossary

abortion

allele

amniotic sac

autosome

chromosome

dominant

embryo

fertilization

fetus

gene

genotype

gestation

heterozygous

homozygous

implantation

lactation

meiosis

parturition

phenotype

placenta

recessive

sex-linked trait

umbilical cord

zygote

LEARNING OUTCOMES

After careful study of this chapter, you should be able to:

1. Describe fertilization and the early development of the fertilized egg

2. Describe the structure and function of the placenta

3. Briefly describe changes that occur in the fetus and the mother during pregnancy

4. Briefly describe the four stages of labor

5. Compare fraternal and identical twins

6. Cite the advantages of breastfeeding

7. Briefly describe the mechanism of gene function

8. Explain the difference between dominant and recessive genes

9. Compare *phenotype* and *genotype* and give examples of each

10. Describe what is meant by a *carrier* of a genetic trait

11. Define *meiosis* and explain its function in reproduction

12. Explain how sex is determined in humans

13. Describe what is meant by the term *sex-linked* and list several sex-linked traits

14. List several factors that may influence the expression of a gene

15. Define *mutation*

16. Show how word parts are used to build words related to development and heredity (see Word Anatomy at the end of the chapter)

chapter 21

Development and Heredity

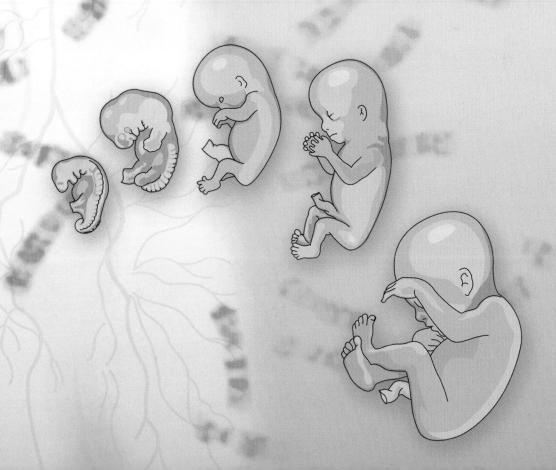

❯ Pregnancy

Pregnancy begins with fertilization of an ovum and ends with delivery of the fetus and afterbirth. During this approximately 38-week period of development, known as **gestation** (jes-TA-shun), all fetal tissues differentiate from a single fertilized egg. Along the way, many changes occur in both the mother and the developing infant.

Fertilization and the Start of Pregnancy

When semen is deposited in the vagina, the many spermatozoa immediately wriggle about in all directions, some traveling into the uterus and oviducts (Fig. 21-1). If an egg cell is present in the oviduct, many spermatozoa cluster around it. Using enzymes, they dissolve the coating around the ovum, so that eventually one sperm cell can penetrate its plasma membrane. The nuclei of the sperm and egg then combine. (See Box 21-1 on artificial methods to assist conception.)

The result of this union is a single cell, called a **zygote** (ZI-gote), with the full human chromosome number of 46. The zygote divides rapidly into two cells and then four cells and soon forms a ball of cells. During this time,

the cell cluster is traveling toward the uterine cavity, pushed along by cilia lining the oviduct and by peristalsis (contractions) of the tube. After reaching the uterus, the little ball of cells burrows into the greatly thickened uterine lining and is soon implanted and completely covered. After **implantation** in the uterus, a group of cells within the dividing cluster becomes an **embryo** (EM-bre-o), the term used for the growing offspring in the early stage of gestation. The other cells within the cluster will differentiate into tissue that will support the developing offspring throughout gestation.

> **Checkpoint 21-1** What structure is formed by the union of an ovum and a spermatozoon?

The Placenta

For a few days after implantation, the embryo gets nourishment from the endometrium. By the end of the second week, however, the outer cells of the embryonic cluster form villi (projections) that invade the uterine wall and maternal blood channels (venous sinuses). Gradually, tissue in the outer embryonic layer and in the uterine lining together form the **placenta** (plah-SEN-tah), a flat, circular organ that consists of a spongy network of blood-filled channels and

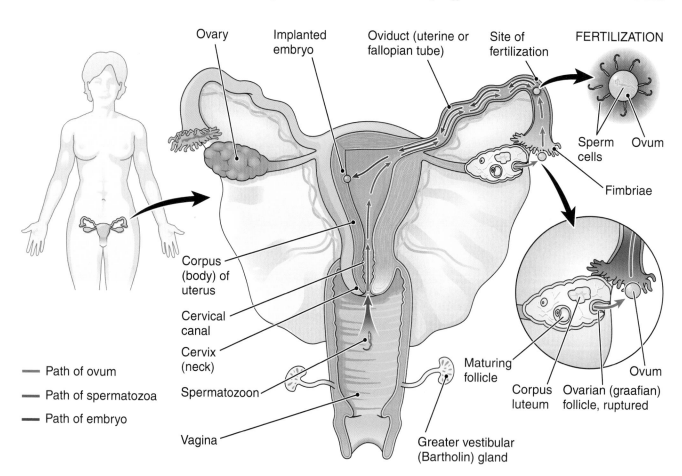

— Path of ovum
— Path of spermatozoa
— Path of embryo

Figure 21-1 The female reproductive system. Arrows show the pathway of the spermatozoa and ovum and also of the fertilization and implantation of the fertilized ovum. *ZOOMING IN ✦ Where is the ovum fertilized?*

Box 21-1 **Clinical Perspectives**

Assisted Reproductive Technology: The "Art" of Conception

At least one in ten American couples is affected by infertility. Assisted reproductive technologies such as in vitro fertilization (IVF), gamete intrafallopian transfer (GIFT), and zygote intrafallopian transfer (ZIFT) can help these couples become pregnant.

In vitro fertilization refers to fertilization of an egg outside the mother's body in a laboratory dish, and it is often used when a woman's fallopian tubes are blocked or when a man has a low sperm count. The woman participating in IVF is given hormones to cause ovulation of several eggs. These are then withdrawn with a needle and fertilized with the father's sperm. After a few divisions, some of the fertilized eggs are placed in the uterus, thus bypassing the fallopian tubes. Additional fertilized eggs can be frozen to repeat the procedure in case of failure or for later pregnancies.

GIFT can be used when the woman has at least one normal fallopian tube and the man has an adequate sperm count. As in IVF, the woman is given hormones to cause ovulation of several eggs, which are collected. Then, the eggs and the father's sperm are placed into the fallopian tube using a catheter. Thus, in GIFT, fertilization occurs inside the woman, not in a laboratory dish.

ZIFT is a combination of both IVF and GIFT. Fertilization takes place in a laboratory dish, and then the zygote is placed into the fallopian tube.

Because of a lack of guidelines or restrictions in the United States in the field of assisted reproductive technology, some problems have arisen. These issues concern the use of stored embryos and gametes, use of embryos without consent, and improper screening for disease among donors. In addition, the implantation of more than one fertilized egg has resulted in a high incidence of multiple births, even up to seven or eight offspring in a single pregnancy, a situation that imperils the survival and health of the babies.

---

capillary-containing villi (Fig. 21-2). (Placenta is from a Latin word meaning "pancake.") The placenta is the organ of nutrition, respiration, and excretion for the developing offspring throughout gestation. Although the blood of the mother and her offspring do not mix—each has its own blood and cardiovascular system—exchanges take place through the capillaries of the placental villi. In this manner, gases (CO_2 and O_2) are exchanged, nutrients are provided to the developing infant, and waste products are released into the maternal blood to be eliminated.

The Umbilical Cord The embryo is connected to the developing placenta by a stalk of tissue that eventually becomes the **umbilical** (um-BIL-ih-kal) **cord**. This structure carries blood to and from the embryo, later called the **fetus** (FE-tus). The cord encloses two arteries that carry deoxygenated blood from the fetus to the placenta, and one vein that carries oxygenated blood from the placenta to the fetus (see Fig. 21-2). (Note that, like the pulmonary vessels, these arteries carry blood low in oxygen and this vein carries blood high in oxygen.) The fetus has special circulatory features used to carry blood to and from the umbilical cord. Several adaptations in the fetal heart allow blood to bypass the lungs, which are not functional in the fetus (see Box 21-2).

Box 21-2 **A Closer Look**

Fetal Circulation: Routing Blood to Miss the Lungs

The developing fetus has several adaptations in the cardiovascular system that change at birth. These adaptations serve to bypass the lungs, which in the fetus are not functional. Fetal blood is oxygenated instead by the placenta (see Fig. 21-2).

Oxygenated blood comes from the placenta to the fetus via the **umbilical vein**, which is contained in the umbilical cord. Most of this blood joins the inferior vena cava by way of a small vessel, the **ductus venosus**, and is carried to the heart. The rest is delivered to the liver. Once in the right atrium, some of the blood flows directly into the left atrium through a hole in the atrial septum called the **foramen ovale**. This blood bypasses the right ventricle and the pulmonary circuit. Blood that does enter the right ventricle is pumped into the pulmonary artery. However, most of this blood shunts directly into the systemic circulation through a small vessel, the **ductus arteriosus**, which connects the pulmonary artery to the aorta. A small portion of blood remains in the pulmonary artery and is delivered to the lungs. Blood returns to the placenta through two **umbilical arteries**.

After birth, when the baby's lungs are functioning, these circulatory adaptations begin to close. The foramen ovale seals to become a depression called the fossa ovalis in the septum between the atria. The various vessels constrict into fibrous cords. Only the proximal parts of the umbilical arteries persist as arteries to the urinary bladder. Except for the foramen ovale, the circulatory adaptations close within 30 minutes after birth. The foramen ovale completely closes within one year. Certain congenital heart defects occur when the foramen ovale or ductus arteriosus fails to close.

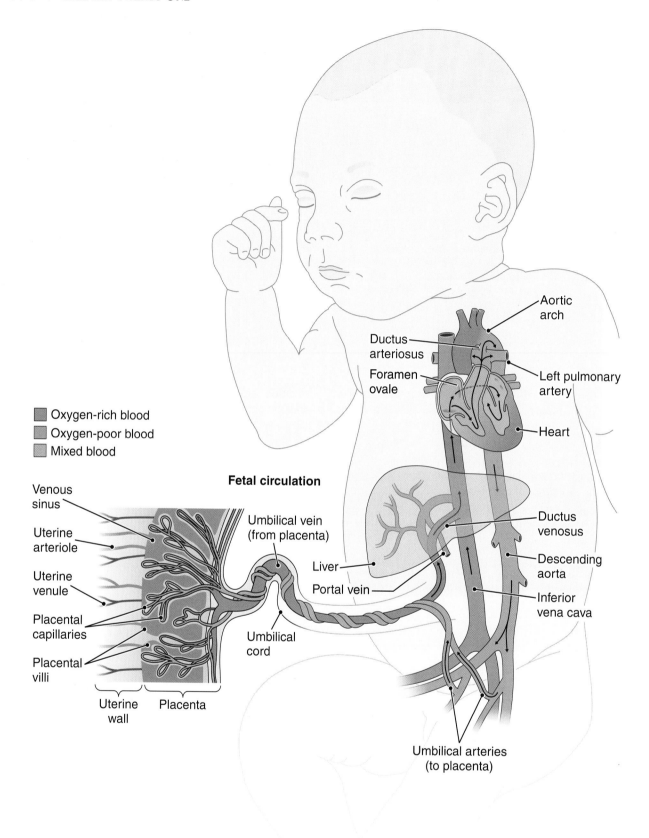

Fetal circulation

Oxygen-rich blood
Oxygen-poor blood
Mixed blood

Venous sinus
Uterine arteriole
Uterine venule
Placental capillaries
Placental villi
Uterine wall
Placenta

Umbilical vein (from placenta)
Liver
Portal vein
Umbilical cord
Umbilical arteries (to placenta)

Aortic arch
Ductus arteriosus
Foramen ovale
Left pulmonary artery
Heart
Ductus venosus
Descending aorta
Inferior vena cava

Figure 21-2 Fetal circulation and section of placenta. Colors show relative oxygen content of blood.   *ZOOMING IN ✦ What is signified by the purple color in this illustration?*

Placental Hormones In addition to maintaining the fetus, the placenta is an endocrine organ. Beginning soon after implantation, some embryonic cells produce the hormone **human chorionic gonadotropin** (ko-re-ON-ik gon-ah-do-TRO-pin) **(hCG)**. This hormone stimulates the ovarian corpus luteum, prolonging its life-span to 11 or 12 weeks and causing it to secrete increasing amounts of progesterone and estrogen. It is hCG that is used in tests as an indicator of pregnancy.

Progesterone is essential for the maintenance of pregnancy. It promotes endometrial secretion to nourish the embryo, maintains the endometrium and decreases the ability of the uterine muscle to contract, thus preventing the embryo from being expelled from the body. During pregnancy, progesterone also helps prepare the breasts for milk secretion.

Estrogen promotes enlargement of the uterus and breasts. By the 11th or 12th week of pregnancy, the corpus luteum is no longer needed; by this time, the placenta itself can secrete adequate amounts of progesterone and estrogen, and the corpus luteum disintegrates. Miscar-

riages (loss of an embryo or fetus) frequently occur during this critical time when hormone secretion is shifting from the corpus luteum to the placenta.

Human placental lactogen (hPL), is a hormone secreted by the placenta during pregnancy, reaching a peak at term, the normal conclusion of pregnancy. HPL stimulates growth of the breasts to prepare the mother for production of milk, or **lactation** (lak-TA-shun). More importantly, it regulates the levels of nutrients in the mother's blood to keep them available for the fetus. This second function leads to an alternate name for this hormone: human chorionic somatomammotropin.

Relaxin is a placental hormone that softens the cervix and relaxes the sacral joints and the pubic symphysis. These changes help to widen the birth canal and aid in delivery.

> **Checkpoint 21-2** What organ nourishes the developing fetus?

> **Checkpoint 21-3** What is the function of the umbilical cord?

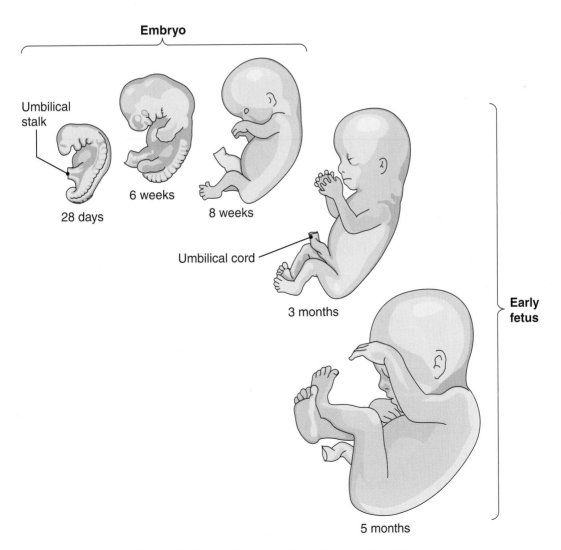

Figure 21-3   Development of an embryo and early fetus.

Development of the Embryo

The developing offspring is referred to as an embryo for the first 8 weeks of life (Fig. 21-3), and the study of growth during this period is called **embryology** (em-bre-OL-o-je). The beginnings of all body systems are established during this time. The heart and the brain are among the first organs to develop. A primitive nervous system begins to form in the third week. The heart and blood vessels originate during the second week, and the first heartbeat appears during week 4, at the same time that other muscles begin to develop.

By the end of the first month, the embryo is approximately 0.62 cm (0.25 inches) long, with four small swellings at the sides called **limb buds**, which will develop into the four extremities. At this time, the heart produces a prominent bulge at the anterior of the embryo.

By the end of the second month, the embryo takes on an appearance that is recognizably human. In male embryos, the primitive testes have formed and have begun to secrete testosterone, which will direct formation of the male reproductive organs as gestation continues. Figure 21-3 shows photographs of embryonic and early fetal development.

Checkpoint 21-4 All body systems originate during the early development of the embryo. At about what time in gestation does the heartbeat first appear?

The Fetus

The term *fetus* is used for the developing offspring from the beginning of the third month until birth. During this period, the organ systems continue to grow and mature. The ovaries form in the female early in this fetal period, and at this stage they contain all the primitive cells (oocytes) that can later develop in mature ova (egg cells).

For study, the entire gestation period may be divided into three equal segments or **trimesters**. The most rapid growth of the fetus occurs during the second trimester (months 4–6). By the end of the fourth month, the fetus is almost 15 cm (6 inches) long, and its external genitalia are sufficiently developed to reveal its sex. By the seventh month, the fetus is usually about 35 cm (14 inches) long and weighs approximately 1.1 kg (2.4 pounds). At the end of pregnancy, the normal length of the fetus is 45 to 56 cm (18–22.5 inches), and the weight varies from 2.7 to 4.5 kg (6–10 pounds).

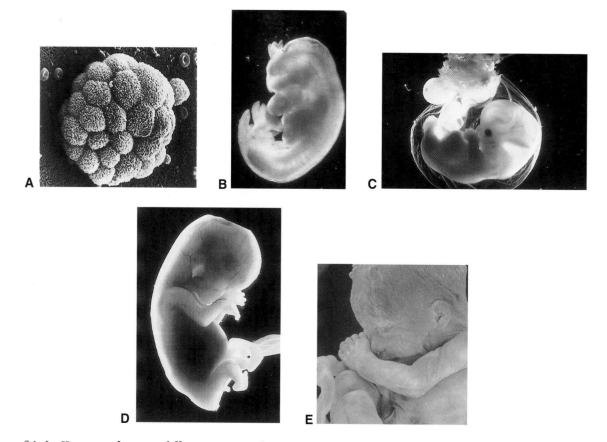

Figure 21-4 **Human embryos at different stages and early fetus.** **(A)** Implantation in uterus 7 to 8 days after conception. **(B)** Embryo at 32 days. **(C)** At 37 days. **(D)** At 41 days. **(E)** Fetus between 12 and 15 weeks. (Reprinted with permission from Pillitteri A. Maternal and Child Health Nursing. 4th ed. Philadelphia: Lippincott Williams & Wilkins, 2003.)

The **amniotic** (am-ne-OT-ik) **sac**, which is filled with a clear liquid known as **amniotic fluid**, surrounds the fetus and serves as a protective cushion for it (Fig. 21-5). The amniotic sac ruptures at birth, an event marked by the common expression that the mother's "water broke."

During development, the fetal skin is protected by a layer of cheeselike material called the **vernix caseosa** (VER-niks ka-se-O-sah) (literally, "cheesy varnish").

Checkpoint 21-5 What is the name of the fluid-filled sac that holds the fetus?

The Mother

The total period of pregnancy, from fertilization of the ovum to birth, is approximately 266 days, also given as 280 days or 40 weeks from the last menstrual period (LMP). During this time, the mother must supply all the food and oxygen for the fetus and eliminate its waste materials. To support the additional demands of the growing fetus, the mother's metabolism changes markedly, and several organ systems increase their output:

▶ The heart pumps more blood to supply the needs of the uterus and the fetus.
▶ The lungs provide more oxygen by increasing the rate and depth of respiration.
▶ The kidneys excrete nitrogenous wastes from both the fetus and the mother.
▶ The digestive system supplies additional nutrients for the growth of maternal organs (uterus and breasts) and growth of the fetus, as well as for subsequent labor and milk secretion.

Nausea and vomiting are common discomforts in early pregnancy. These most often occur upon arising or during periods of fatigue, and are more common in women who smoke cigarettes. The specific cause of these symptoms is not known, but they may be a result of the great changes in hormone levels that occur at this time. The nausea and vomiting usually last for only a few weeks to several months.

Urinary frequency and constipation are often present during the early stages of pregnancy and then usually disappear. They may reappear late in pregnancy as the head of the fetus drops from the abdominal region down into the pelvis, pressing on the rectum and the urinary bladder.

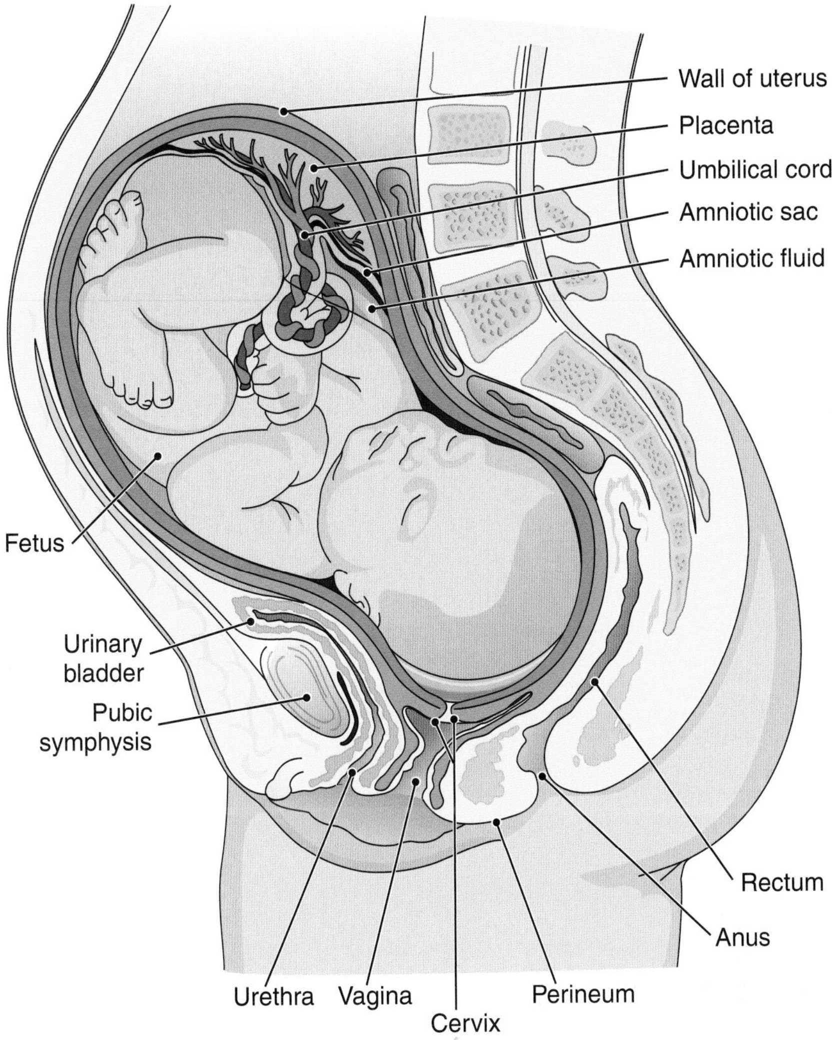

Checkpoint 21-6 What is the approximate duration of pregnancy in days?

The Use of Ultrasound in Obstetrics
Ultrasonography (ul-trah-son-OG-rah-fe) is a safe, painless, and noninvasive method for studying soft tissue. It has proved extremely valuable for monitoring pregnancies and deliveries.

An ultrasound image, called a *sonogram,* is made by sending high-frequency sound waves into the body (Fig. 21-6). Each time a wave meets an interface between two tissues of different densities, an echo is produced. An instrument called a *transducer* converts the reflected sound waves into electrical energy, and a computer is used to generate an image on a viewing screen.

Ultrasound scans can be used in

Figure 21-5 Midsagittal section of a pregnant uterus with intact fetus. *ZOOMING IN ✦ What structure connects the fetus to the placenta?*

Labels in figure: Wall of uterus, Placenta, Umbilical cord, Amniotic sac, Amniotic fluid, Fetus, Urinary bladder, Pubic symphysis, Urethra, Vagina, Cervix, Perineum, Rectum, Anus

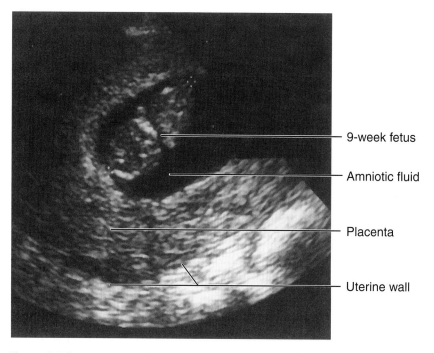

9-week fetus

Amniotic fluid

Placenta

Uterine wall

Figure 21-6 **Sonogram showing a 9-week-old fetus.** (Reprinted with permission from Erkonen WE. Radiology 101: Basics and Fundamentals of Imaging. Philadelphia: Lippincott Williams & Wilkins, 1998.)

obstetrics to diagnose pregnancy, judge fetal age, and determine the location of the placenta. The technique can also show the presence of excess amniotic fluid and fetal abnormalities.

▶ Childbirth

The exact mechanisms that trigger the beginning of uterine contractions for childbirth are still not completely known. Some fetal and maternal factors that probably work in combination to start labor are:

▶ Stretching of the uterine muscle stimulates production of prostaglandin, which promotes uterine contractions.

▶ Pressure on the cervix from the baby stimulates release of **oxytocin** (ok-se-TO-sin) from the posterior pituitary. The uterine muscle becomes increasingly sensitive to this hormone late in pregnancy.

▶ Changes in the placenta that occur with time may contribute to the start of labor.

▶ Cortisol from the fetal adrenal cortex inhibits the mother's progesterone. Increase in the relative amount of estrogen as compared to progesterone stimulates uterine contractions.

After labor begins, stimuli from the cervix and vagina produce reflex secretion of oxytocin, which in turn increases the uterine contractions (an example of positive feedback).

The Four Stages of Labor

The process by which the fetus is expelled from the uterus is known as **labor** and **delivery**; it also may be called **parturition** (par-tu-RISH-un). It is divided into four stages:

1. The **first stage** begins with the onset of regular uterine contractions. With each contraction, the cervix becomes thinner and the opening larger. Rupture of the amniotic sac may occur at any time, with a gush of fluid from the vagina.
2. The **second stage** begins when the cervix is completely dilated and ends with the delivery of the baby. This stage involves the passage of the fetus, usually head first, through the cervical canal and the vagina to the outside.
3. The **third stage** begins after the child is born and ends with the expulsion of the **afterbirth**. The afterbirth includes the placenta, the membranes of the amniotic sac, and the umbilical cord, except for a small portion remaining attached to the baby's **umbilicus** (um-BIL-ih-kus), or navel.
4. The **fourth stage** begins after expulsion of the afterbirth and constitutes a period in which bleeding is controlled. Contraction of the uterine muscle acts to close off the blood vessels leading to the placental site. To prevent tissues of the pelvic floor from being torn during childbirth, as often happens, the obstetrician may cut the mother's perineum just before her infant is born and then repair this clean cut immediately after childbirth; such an operation is called an **episiotomy** (eh-piz-e-OT-o-me). The area between the vagina and the anus that is cut in an episiotomy is referred to as the *surgical* or *obstetrical perineum* (see Fig. 20-10 in Chapter 20).

Checkpoint 21-7 What is parturition?

Cesarean Section

A **cesarean** (se-ZAR-re-an) **section** (C section) is an incision made in the abdominal wall and in the uterine wall for delivery of a fetus. A cesarean section may be required for a variety of reasons, including placental abnormalities, abnormal fetal position, disproportion between the head of the fetus and the mother's pelvis that makes vaginal delivery difficult or dangerous, and other problems that may arise during pregnancy and delivery.

> **Checkpoint 21-8** What is a cesarean section?

Multiple Births

Until recently, statistics indicated that twins occurred in about 1 of every 80 to 90 births, varying somewhat in different countries. Triplets occurred much less frequently, usually once in several thousand births, whereas quadruplets occurred very rarely. The birth of quintuplets represented a historic event unless the mother had taken fertility drugs. Now these fertility drugs, usually gonadotropins, are given more commonly, and the number of multiple births has increased significantly. Multiple fetuses tend to be born prematurely and therefore have a high death rate. However, better care of infants and newer treatments have resulted in more living multiple births than ever.

Twins originate in two different ways, and on this basis are divided into two types:

▶ **Fraternal twins** are formed as a result of the fertilization of two different ova by two spermatozoa. Two completely different individuals, as distinct from each other as brothers and sisters of different ages, are produced. Each fetus has its own placenta and surrounding sac.
▶ **Identical twins** develop from a single zygote formed from a single ovum fertilized by a single spermatozoon. Sometime during the early stages of development, the embryonic cells separate into two units. Usually, there is a single placenta, although there must be a separate umbilical cord for each fetus. Identical twins are always the same sex and carry the same inherited traits.

Other multiple births may be fraternal, identical, or combinations of these. The tendency to multiple births seems to be hereditary.

Termination of Pregnancy

A pregnancy may end before its full term has been completed. The term **live birth** is used if the baby breathes or shows any evidence of life such as heartbeat, pulsation of the umbilical cord, or movement of voluntary muscles. An **immature** or **premature** infant is one born before the organ systems are mature. Infants born before the 37th week of gestation or weighing less than 2500 grams (5.5 pounds) are considered **preterm**.

Loss of the fetus is classified according to the duration of the pregnancy:

▶ The term **abortion** refers to loss of the embryo or fetus before the 20th week or weight of about 500 grams (1.1 pound). This loss can be either spontaneous or induced.

▷ **Spontaneous abortion** occurs naturally with no interference. The most common causes are related to an abnormality of the embryo or fetus. Other causes include abnormality of the mother's reproductive organs, infections, or chronic disorders, such as kidney disease or hypertension. **Miscarriage** is the lay term for spontaneous abortion.
▷ **Induced abortion** occurs as a result of artificial or mechanical interruption of pregnancy. A **therapeutic abortion** is an abortion performed by a physician as a treatment for a variety of reasons. More liberal access to this type of abortion has dramatically reduced the incidence of death related to illegal abortion.
▶ The term **fetal death** refers to loss of the fetus after the eighth week of pregnancy. **Stillbirth** refers to the delivery of an infant who is lifeless.

Immaturity is a leading cause of death in the newborn. After the 20th week of pregnancy, the fetus is considered **viable,** that is, able to live outside the uterus. A fetus expelled before the 24th week or before reaching a weight of 1000 grams (2.2 pounds) has little more than a 50% chance of survival. One born at a point closer to the full 40 weeks stands a much better chance of living. Increasing numbers of immature infants are being saved because of advances in neonatal intensive care.

> **Checkpoint 21-9** What does the term *viable* mean with reference to a fetus?

▶ The Mammary Glands and Lactation

The **mammary glands,** or breasts, of the female are accessories of the reproductive system. They provide nourishment for the baby after its birth. The mammary glands are similar in construction to the sweat glands. Each gland is divided into a number of lobes composed of glandular tissue and fat, and each lobe is further subdivided. Secretions from the lobes are conveyed through **lactiferous** (lak-TIF-er-us) **ducts,** all of which converge at the papilla (nipple) (Fig. 21-7).

The mammary glands begin developing during puberty, but they do not become functional until the end of a pregnancy. Placental lactogen (hPL) helps to prepare the breasts for lactation, and the hormone **prolactin (PRL),** produced by the anterior pituitary gland, stimulates the secretory cells of the mammary glands. The first mammary gland secretion is a thin liquid called **colostrum** (ko-LOS-trum). It is nutritious but has a somewhat different composition from milk. Milk secretion begins within a few days following birth and can continue for several years as long as milk is frequently removed by the suckling baby or by pumping. Stimulation

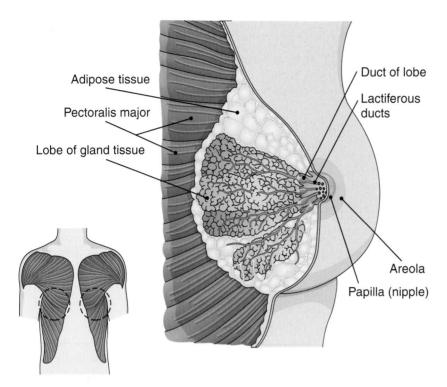

Figure 21-7 Section of the breast (mammary gland). *ZOOMING IN* ✦ *What muscle underlies the breast?*

Labels in figure:
- Adipose tissue
- Pectoralis major
- Lobe of gland tissue
- Duct of lobe
- Lactiferous ducts
- Areola
- Papilla (nipple)

of the breast by the suckling infant causes oxytocin release from the posterior pituitary. This hormone causes the milk ducts to contract, resulting in the ejection, or *letdown*, of milk.

The digestive tract of the newborn baby is not ready for the usual adult mixed diet. Mother's milk is more desirable for the young infant than milk from other animals for several reasons, some of which are listed below:

▶ Infections that may be transmitted by foods exposed to the outside air are avoided by nursing.

▶ Both breast milk and colostrum contain maternal antibodies that help protect the baby against pathogens.

▶ The proportions of various nutrients and other substances in human milk are perfectly suited to the human infant. Substitutes are not exact imitations of human milk. Nutrients are present in more desirable amounts if the mother's diet is well balanced.

▶ The psychological and emotional benefits of nursing are of infinite value to both the mother and the infant.

Checkpoint 21-10 What is lactation?

▶ Heredity

We are often struck by the resemblance of a baby to one or both of its parents, yet rarely do we stop to consider *how* various traits are transmitted from parents to offspring. This subject—heredity—has fascinated humans

for thousands of years. The *Old Testament* contains numerous references to heredity (although, of course, the word was unknown in biblical times). It was not until the 19th century, however, that methodical investigation into heredity was begun. At that time, an Austrian monk, Gregor Mendel, discovered through his experiments with garden peas that there was a precise pattern in the appearance of differences among parents and their **progeny** (PROJ-eh-ne), their offspring or descendents. Mendel's most important contribution to the understanding of heredity was the demonstration that there are independent units of heredity in the cells. Later, these independent units were given the name **genes**.

Genes and Chromosomes

Genes are actually segments of DNA (deoxyribonucleic acid) contained in the threadlike chromosomes within the nucleus of each cell. Genes govern the cell by controlling the manufacture of proteins, especially enzymes, which are necessary for all the chemical reactions that occur within the cell. Other proteins regulated by genes are those used for structural materials, hormones and growth factors.

When body cells divide by the process of mitosis, the DNA that makes up the chromosomes is duplicated and distributed to the daughter cells, so that each daughter cell gets exactly the same kind and number of chromosomes as were in the original cell. Each chromosome (aside from the Y chromosome, which determines sex) may carry thousands of genes, and each gene carries the code for a specific trait (characteristic). These traits constitute the physical, biochemical, and physiologic makeup of every cell in the body. (See Box 21-3 to learn about the Human Genome Project.)

In humans, every cell except the gametes (sex cells) contains 46 chromosomes. The chromosomes exist in pairs. One member of each pair was received at the time of fertilization from the offspring's father, and one was received from the mother. The paired chromosomes, except for the pair that determines sex, are alike in size and appearance. Thus, each body cell has one pair of sex chromosomes and 22 pairs (44 chromosomes) that are not involved in sex determination and are known as **autosomes** (AW-to-somes).

The paired autosomes carry genes for the same traits at exactly the same sites on each. The genes for each trait thus exist in pairs; each member of the gene pair that controls a given trait is known as an **allele** (al-LELE).

Box 21-3	Hot Topics

The Human Genome Project: Reading the Book of Life

Packed tightly in nearly every one of your body cells (except the red blood cells) is a complete copy of your genome—the genetic instructions that direct all of your cellular activities. Written in the language of DNA, these instructions consist of genes parceled into 46 chromosomes that code for proteins. In 1990, a consortium of scientists from around the world set out to crack the genetic code and read the human genome, our "book of life." This monumental task, called the Human Genome Project, was completed in 2003 and succeeded in mapping the entire human genome—3 billion DNA base pairs arranged into about 30,000 genes. Now, scientists can pinpoint the exact location and chemical code of every gene in the body.

The human genome was decoded using a technique called sequencing. Samples of human DNA were fragmented into smaller pieces and then inserted into bacteria. As the bacteria multiplied, they produced more and more copies of the human DNA fragments, which the scientists extracted. The DNA copies were loaded into a sequencing machine capable of "reading" the string of DNA nucleotides that composed each fragment. Then, using computers, the scientists put all of the sequences from the fragments back together to get the entire human genome.

Now, scientists hope to use all these pages of the book of life to revolutionize the treatment of human disease. The information obtained from the Human Genome Project may lead to improved disease diagnosis, new drug treatments, and even gene therapy.

Checkpoint 21-11 What is a gene and what is a gene made of?

Dominant and Recessive Genes

Another of Mendel's discoveries was that genes can be either dominant or recessive. A **dominant** gene is one that expresses its effect in the cell regardless of whether its allele on the matching chromosome is the same as or different from the dominant gene. The gene must be received from only one parent to be expressed in the offspring. When the matching genes for a trait are different, the alleles are described as **heterozygous** (het-er-o-ZI-gus), or hybrid.

The effect of a **recessive** gene is not evident unless its paired allele on the matching chromosome is also recessive. Thus, a recessive trait appears only if the recessive genes for that trait are received from both parents. For example, the gene for brown eyes is dominant over the gene for blue eyes, which is recessive. Blue eyes appear in the offspring only if genes for blue eyes are received from both parents. When both the genes for a trait are the same, that is, both dominant or both recessive, the alleles are said to be **homozygous** (ho-mo-ZI-gus), or pure-bred. A recessive trait only appears if a person's genes are homozygous for that trait.

Any characteristic that can be observed or can be tested for is part of a person's **phenotype** (FE-no-tipe). Eye color, for example, can be seen when looking at a person. Blood type is not visible but can be determined by testing and is also a part of a person's phenotype. When someone has the recessive phenotype, his or her genetic make-up, or **genotype** (JEN-o-tipe), is obviously homozygous recessive. When a dominant phenotype appears, the person's genotype can be either homozygous dominant or heterozygous. Only genetic studies or family studies can reveal which it is.

A recessive gene is not expressed if it is present in the cell together with a dominant allele. However, the recessive gene can be passed on to offspring and may thus appear in future generations. An individual who shows no evidence of a trait but has a recessive gene for that trait is described as a **carrier** of the gene. Using genetic terminology, that person shows the dominant phenotype but has a heterozygous genotype for that trait.

Checkpoint 21-12 What is the difference between a dominant and a recessive gene?

Distribution of Chromosomes to Offspring

The reproductive cells (ova and spermatozoa) are produced by a special process of cell division called **meiosis** (mi-O-sis). This process divides the chromosome number in half, so that each reproductive cell has 23 chromosomes. Moreover, the division occurs in such a way that each cell receives one member of each chromosome pair that was present in the original cell. The separation occurs at random, meaning that either member of the original pair may be included in a given germ cell. Thus, the maternal and paternal sets of chromosomes get mixed up and redistributed at this time, leading to increased variety within the population. Children in a family resemble each other, but no two look exactly alike (unless they are identical twins), because they receive different combinations of maternal and paternal chromosomes.

Geneticists use a grid called a **Punnett square** to show all the combinations of genes that can result from a given parental cross (Fig. 21-8). In these calculations, a capital letter is used for the dominant gene and the recessive gene is represented by the lower case of the same letter.

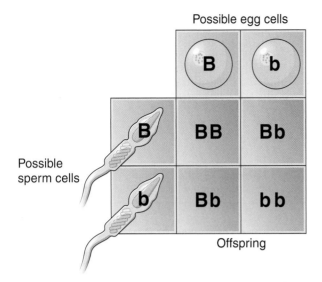

Possible egg cells

Possible sperm cells

Offspring

Figure 21-8 A Punnett square. Geneticists use this grid to show all the possible combinations of a given cross. *ZOOMING IN ✦ What percentage of children will show the recessive phenotype blond hair?*

For example, if *B* is the gene for the dominant trait brown eyes, then *b* would be the recessive gene for blue eyes. In the offspring, the genotype BB is homozygous dominant and the genotype Bb is heterozygous, both of which will show the dominant phenotype brown eyes. The homozygous recessive genotype bb will show the recessive phenotype blue eyes.

A Punnett square shows all the possible gene combinations of a given cross and the theoretical ratios of all the genotypes produced. Actual ratios may differ if the number of offspring is small. For example, the chances of having a male or female baby are 50-50 with each birth, but a family might have several girls before having a boy, and vice versa. The chances of seeing the theoretical ratios improve as the number of offspring increases.

Checkpoint 21-13 What is the process of cell division that forms the gametes?

Sex Determination

The two chromosomes that determine the offspring's sex, unlike the autosomes (the other 22 pairs of chromosomes), are not matched in size and appearance. The female X chromosome is larger than most other chromosomes and carries genes for other characteristics in addition to that for sex. The male Y chromosome is smaller than other chromosomes and mainly determines sex. A female has two X chromosomes in each body cell; a male has one X and one Y.

By the process of meiosis, each male sperm cell receives either an X or a Y chromosome, whereas every egg cell receives only an X chromosome (Fig. 21-9). If a sperm cell with an X chromosome fertilizes an ovum, the

resulting infant will be female; if a sperm with a Y chromosome fertilizes an ovum, the resulting infant will be male (see Fig. 21-9).

Sex-Linked Traits

Any trait that is carried on a sex chromosome is said to be **sex-linked.** Because the Y chromosome carries few traits aside from sex determination, most sex-linked traits are carried on the X chromosome and are best described as *X-linked.* Examples are hemophilia, certain forms of baldness, and red-green color blindness.

Sex-linked traits appear almost exclusively in males. The reason for this is that most of these traits are recessive, and if a recessive gene is located on the X chromosome in a male it cannot be masked by a matching dominant gene. (Remember that the Y chromosome with which the X chromosome pairs is very small and carries few genes.) Thus, a male who has only one recessive gene for a trait will exhibit that characteristic, whereas a female must have

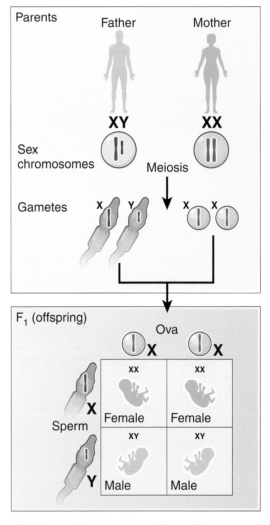

Figure 21-9 Sex determination. If an X chromosome from a male unites with an X chromosome from a female, the child is female (XX); if a Y chromosome from a male unites with an X chromosome from a female, the child is male (XY).

two recessive genes to show the trait. The female must inherit a recessive gene for that trait from each parent and be homozygous recessive in order for the trait to appear.

> **Checkpoint 21-14** What sex chromosome combination determines a female? A male?

> **Checkpoint 21-15** What term is used to describe a trait carried on a sex chromosome?

▶ Hereditary Traits

Some observable hereditary traits are skin, eye, and hair color and facial features. Also influenced by genetics are less clearly defined traits, such as weight, body build, life span, and susceptibility to disease.

Some human traits, including the traits involved in many genetic diseases, are determined by a single pair of genes; most, however, are the result of two or more gene pairs acting together in what is termed **multifactorial inheritance**. This type of inheritance accounts for the wide range of variations within populations in such characteristics as coloration, height, and weight, all of which are determined by more than one pair of genes.

Gene Expression

The effect of a gene on a person's phenotype may be influenced by a variety of factors, including the individual's sex and the presence of other genes. For example, the genes for certain types of baldness and certain types of color blindness may be inherited by either males or females, but the traits appear mostly in males under the effects of male sex hormone.

Environment also plays a part in gene expression. One inherits a potential for a given size, for example, but one's actual size is additionally influenced by such factors as nutrition, development, and general state of health. The same is true of life span and susceptibility to diseases.

Genetic Mutation

As a rule, chromosomes replicate exactly during cell division. Occasionally, however, for reasons not yet totally understood, the genes or chromosomes change. This change may involve a single gene or whole chromosomes. Alternatively, it may consist of chromosomal breakage, in which there is loss or rearrangement of gene fragments. Often these changes occur during cell division (mitosis or meiosis) as chromosomes come together, re-assort, and get distributed to two new cells. Such changes are termed genetic **mutations**. Mutations may occur spontaneously or may be induced by some agent, such as ionizing radiation or chemicals, described as a **mutagen** (MU-tah-jen) or mutagenic agent.

If a mutation occurs in an ovum or a sperm cell, the altered trait will be inherited by the offspring. The vast majority of harmful mutations never are expressed because the affected fetus dies and is spontaneously aborted. Most remaining mutations are so inconsequential that they have no visible effect. Beneficial mutations, on the other hand, tend to survive and increase as a population evolves.

> **Checkpoint 21-16** What is a mutation?

Word Anatomy

Medical terms are built from standardized word parts (prefixes, roots, and suffixes). Learning the meanings of these parts can help you remember words and interpret unfamiliar terms.

WORD PART	MEANING	EXAMPLE
Pregnancy		
zyg/o	joined	An ovum and spermatozoon join to form a *zygote*.
chori/o	membrane, chorion	Human *chorionic* gonadotropin is produced by the outermost cells (chorion) of the embryo and acts on the corpus luteum in the ovary.
somat/o	body	Human chorionic *somatomammotropin* controls nutrients for the body and acts on the mammary glands (mamm/o).
Childbirth		
ox/y	sharp, acute	*Oxytocin* is a hormone that stimulates labor.
toc/o	labor	See preceding example.
Genes and Chromosomes		
chrom/o	color	*Chromosomes* color darkly with stains.
aut/o-	self	*Autosomes* are all the chromosomes aside from the two that determine sex.

WORD PART	MEANING	EXAMPLE
heter/o	other, different	*Heterozygous* paired genes (alleles) are different from each other.
homo-	same	*Homozygous* paired genes (alleles) are the same.
phen/o	to show	Traits that can be observed or tested for make a up a person's *phenotype*.

Hereditary Traits

multi-	many	*Multifactorial* traits are determined by multiple pairs of genes.

Summary

I. Pregnancy (gestation)—lasts about 38 weeks

A. Fertilization and the start of pregnancy
   1. Fertilization occurs in oviduct
   2. Zygote (fertilized egg)—formed by fusion of egg and sperm nuclei
      a. Divides rapidly
      b. Travels to uterus
      c. Implants in lining and becomes embryo
B. The placenta
   1. Formed by tissue around embryo and in lining of uterus
   2. Functions
      a. Nourishment
      b. Gas exchange
      c. Removal of waste
      d. Production of hormones
         (1) Human chorionic gonadotropin (hCG)—maintains corpus luteum for 11–12 weeks
         (2) Human placental lactogen (hPL)
         (3) Relaxin—relaxes birth canal
   3. Umbilical cord—connects fetus to placenta
C. Development of the embryo
   1. First 8 weeks
   2. All body systems begin to develop
D. The fetus
   1. Third month to birth
   2. Amniotic sac
      a. Surrounds fetus
      b. Contains fluid to cushion and protect fetus
E. The mother
   1. Increased demands on heart, lungs, kidneys
   2. Increased nutritional needs
   3. Ultrasound used to monitor pregnancy and delivery

II. Childbirth—initiated by changes in uterus, placenta, fetus

A. Four stages of labor
   1. Contractions
   2. Delivery of baby
   3. Expulsion of afterbirth
   4. Contraction of uterus
B. Cesarean section
   1. Incision to remove fetus
C. Multiple births
   1. Fraternal twins formed from two different ova
   2. Identical twins develop from a single zygote

   3. Larger multiples follow either pattern or a combination
   4. Increased by fertility drugs
D. Termination of pregnancy
   1. Immature (premature) infant—born before organ system mature
   2. Preterm—born before 37th week or weighing less than 2500 grams
   3. Abortion—loss of fetus before 20th week or weighing less than 500 grams
   4. Fetal death—loss of fetus after 8 weeks of pregnancy

III. Mammary glands and lactation

   1. Lactation—secretion of milk
      a. Colostrum—first mammary secretion
   2. Hormones
      a. HPL—prepares prepares breasts for lactation
      b. Prolactin—stimulates secretory cells
      c. Oxytocin—promotes letdown (ejection) of milk
   3. Advantages of breastfeeding
      a. Reduces infections
      b. Transfers antibodies
      c. Provides best form of nutrition
      d. Emotional satisfaction

IV. Heredity

A. Genes and chromosomes
   1. Genes
      a. Hereditary units
      b. Segments of DNA
      c. Control manufacture of proteins (*e.g.*, enzymes, hormones)
   2. Chromosomes
      a. Threadlike bodies in nucleus; 46 in humans
      b. Composed of genes
      c. 22 pairs autosomes (non-sex chromosomes)
      d. 1 pair sex chromosomes
B. Dominant and recessive genes
   1. Dominant gene—always expressed
      a. May be heterozygous (two genes different)
      b. May be homozygous dominant (two genes the same)
   2. Recessive gene—expressed only if homozygous recessive (received from both parents)
      a. Carrier—person with recessive gene that is not apparent but can be passed to offspring
      b. Phenotype—characteristic that can be seen or tested for
      c. Genotype—genetic make-up
C. Distribution of chromosomes to offspring

1. Meiosis
   a. Cell division that forms sex cells with 23 chromosomes
   b. Each cell receives one of each chromosome pair
   c. Punnett square shows results of crosses
D. Sex determination
   1. X chromosome larger and carries other traits
   2. Y smaller and carries mainly gene for sex determination
   3. Female cells have XX; male cells have XY
E. Sex-linked traits
   1. Traits carried on sex chromosome (usually X)
   2. Sex-linked traits appear mostly in males
      a. Passed from mother to son on X chromosome
      b. If recessive, not masked by dominant gene on Y
      c. Examples—hemophilia, baldness, red-green color blindness

V. Hereditary traits
   1. Genes determine physical, biochemical, and physiologic characteristics of every cell

2. Some traits determined by single gene pairs
3. Most determined by multifactorial inheritance
   a. Involves multiple gene pairs
   b. Produces a range of variations in a population
   c. Examples—height, weight, coloration, susceptibility to disease
A. Gene expression
   1. Factors
      a. Sex
      b. Presence of other genes
      c. Environment
B. Genetic mutation
   1. Change in genes or chromosomes
   2. May be passed to offspring if occurs in germ cells
   3. Mutagenic agents
      a. Factors causing mutation
      b. Examples—ionizing radiation, chemicals

Questions for Study and Review

Building Understanding

Fill in the blanks

1. Fetal skin is protected by a cheeselike material called_____.
2. The first mammary secretion is called _____.
3. Sound waves can be used to safely monitor pregnancy with a technique called _____.
4. The basic unit of heredity is a(n) _____.
5. Chromosomes not involved in sex determination are known as _____.

Matching

Match each numbered item with the most closely related lettered item.

___ 6. A placental hormone that stimulates the ovaries to secrete progesterone and estrogen
___ 7. A placental hormone that regulates maternal blood nutrient levels
___ 8. A placental hormone that softens the cervix, which widens the birth canal
___ 9. A pituitary hormone that stimulates uterine contractions
___ 10. A pituitary hormone that stimulates maternal milk production

a. human placental lactogen
b. prolactin
c. oxytocin
d. relaxin
e. human chorionic gonadotropin

Multiple choice

___ 11. For a few days after implantation, the embryo is nourished by the
   a. endometrium
   b. placenta
   c. yolk sac
   d. umbilical cord
___ 12. The total period of pregnancy, from fertilization to birth, is about
   a. 240 days
   b. 260 days
   c. 280 days
   d. 300 days
___ 13. With regard to identical twins, which of the following statements is incorrect?
   a. they develop from a single zygote
   b. they each have their own placenta
   c. they are always the same sex

   d. they carry the same inherited traits
___ 14. Genes govern the cell by controlling the manufacture of
   a. carbohydrates
   b. lipids
   c. proteins
   d. electrolytes
___ 15. Paired genes for a given trait are known as
   a. chromosomes
   b. ribosomes
   c. nucleotides
   d. alleles

Understanding Concepts

16. Distinguish among the following: *zygote, embryo,* and *fetus*:
17. Explain the role of the placenta in fetal development.

18. Is blood in the umbilical arteries relatively high or low in oxygen? In the umbilical vein?

19. What is the major event of each of the four stages of parturition?

20. List several reasons why breast milk is best for baby.

21. How many chromosomes are there in a human body cell? In a human gamete?

22. Dana has one dominant allele for brown eyes (B) and one recessive allele for blue eyes. What is Dana's genotype? What is her phenotype?

23. Describe the process of meiosis and explain how it results in genetic variation.

Conceptual Thinking

24. If mitosis were used to produce gametes, what consequences would this have on the offspring's genotype, phenotype, and chromosome number?

25. Jason and Nicole are expecting their first child and are wondering what their child's eye color might be. Jason has blue eyes (a recessive trait) and Nicole has brown eyes (a dominant trait). Both of Jason's parents have blue eyes. One of Nicole's parents has brown eyes, the other has blue eyes. What are Jason's and Nicole's genotype and phenotype? What are the possible genotypes and phenotypes of their children?

Glossary

abdominopelvic (ab-dom-ih-no-PEL-vik) Pertaining to the abdomen and pelvis

abduction (ab-DUK-shun) Movement away from the midline

abortion (ah-BOR-shun) Loss of an embryo or fetus before the 20th week of pregnancy

absorption (ab-SORP-shun) Transfer of digested nutrients from the digestive tract into the circulation

accommodation (ah-kom-o-DA-shun) Coordinated changes in the lens of the eye that enable one to focus on near and far objects

acetylcholine (as-e-til-KO-lene) (**ACh**) Neurotransmitter; released at synapses within the nervous system and at the neuromuscular junction

acid (AH-sid) Substance that can donate a hydrogen ion to another substance

acidosis (as-ih-DO-sis) Condition that results from a decrease in the pH of body fluids

acquired immunodeficiency syndrome (AIDS) Viral disease that attacks the immune system, specifically the T-helper lymphocytes with CD4 receptors

acrosome (AK-ro-some) Caplike structure over the head of the sperm cell that helps the sperm to penetrate the ovum

ACTH See adrenocorticotropic hormone

actin (AK-tin) One of the two contractile proteins in muscle cells, the other being myosin

action potential Sudden change in the electrical charge on a cell membrane, which then spreads along the membrane; nerve impulse

active transport Movement of a substance into or out of a cell in an opposite direction to the way in which it would normally flow by diffusion; active transport requires energy and transporters

adduction (ad-DUK-shun) Movement toward the midline

adenosine triphosphate (ah-DEN-o-sene tri-FOS-fate) (**ATP**) Energy-storing compound found in all cells

ADH See antidiuretic hormone

adipose (AD-ih-pose) Referring to a type of connective tissue that stores fat or to fats

adrenal (ah-DRE-nal) **gland** Endocrine gland located above the kidney; suprarenal gland

adrenaline (ah-DREN-ah-lin) See epinephrine

adrenergic (ad-ren-ER-jik) An activity or structure that responds to epinephrine (adrenaline)

adrenocorticotropic (ah-dre-no-kor-tih-ko-TRO-pik) **hormone (ACTH)** Hormone produced by the pituitary that stimulates the adrenal cortex

aerobic (air-O-bik) Requiring oxygen

afferent (AF-fer-ent) Carrying toward a given point, such as a sensory neuron that carries nerve impulses toward the central nervous system

agglutination (ah-glu-tih-NA-shun) Clumping of cells due to an antigen–antibody reaction

agranulocyte (a-GRAN-u-lo-site) Leukocyte without visible granules in the cytoplasm when stained; lymphocyte or monocyte

AIDS See acquired immunodeficiency syndrome

albumin (al-BU-min) Protein in blood plasma and other body fluids; helps maintain the osmotic pressure of the blood

aldosterone (al-DOS-ter-one) Hormone released by the adrenal cortex that promotes the reabsorption of sodium and water in the kidneys

alkali (AL-kah-li) Substance that can accept a hydrogen ion (H^+); substance that donates a hydroxide ion (OH^-); a base

alkalosis (al-kah-LO-sis) Condition that results from an increase in the pH of body fluids

allele (al-LELE) One member of the pair of genes that controls a given trait

alveolus (al-VE-o-lus) Small sac or pouch; usually a tiny air sac in the lungs through which gases are exchanged between the outside air and the blood; tooth socket; pl., alveoli

amino (ah-ME-no) **acid** Building block of protein

amniotic (am-ne-OT-ik) Pertaining to the sac that surrounds and cushions the developing fetus or to the fluid that fills that sac

amphiarthrosis (am-fe-ar-THRO-sis) Slightly movable joint

anabolism (ah-NAB-o-lizm) Metabolic building of simple compounds into more complex substances needed by the body

anaerobic (an-air-O-bik) Not requiring oxygen

anaphase (AN-ah-faze) The third stage of mitosis in which chromosomes separate to opposite sides of the cell

anastomosis (ah-nas-to-MO-sis) Communication between two structures, such as blood vessels

anatomy (ah-NAT-o-me) Study of body structure

androgen (AN-dro-jen) Any male sex hormone

angiotensin (an-je-o-TEN-sin) Substance formed in the blood by the action of the enzyme renin from the kidneys. It increases blood pressure by causing constriction of the blood vessels and

stimulating the release of aldosterone from the adrenal cortex

anion (AN-i-on) Negatively charged particle (ion)

anoxia (ah-NOK-se-ah) See hypoxia

ANP See atrial natriuretic peptide

ANS See autonomic nervous system

antagonist (an-TAG-o-nist) Muscle that has an action opposite that of a given movement; substance that opposes the action of another substance

anterior (an-TE-re-or) Toward the front or belly surface; ventral

antibody (AN-te-bod-e) (**Ab**) Substance produced in response to a specific antigen; immunoglobulin

antidiuretic (an-ti-di-u-RET-ik) **hormone (ADH)** Hormone released from the posterior pituitary gland that increases the reabsorption of water in the kidneys, thus decreasing the volume of urine excreted

antigen (AN-te-jen) (**Ag**) Foreign substance that produces an immune response

antioxidant (an-te-OX-ih-dant) Substances in the diet that protect against harmful free radicals

antiserum (an-te-SE-rum) Serum containing antibodies that may be given to provide passive immunity; immune serum

anus (A-nus) Distal opening of the digestive tract

aorta (a-OR-tah) The largest artery; carries blood out of the left ventricle of the heart

apex (A-peks) The pointed region of a cone-shaped structure

apnea (AP-ne-ah) Temporary cessation of breathing

apocrine (AP-o-krin) Referring to a gland the releases some cellular material along with its secretions

aponeurosis (ap-o-nu-RO-sis) Broad sheet of fibrous connective tissue that attaches muscle to bone or to other muscle

appendicular (ap-en-DIK-u-lar) **skeleton** Part of the skeleton that includes the bones of the upper extremities, lower extremities, shoulder girdle, and hips

appendix (ah-PEN-diks) Fingerlike tube of lymphatic tissue attached to the first portion of the large intestine; vermiform (wormlike) appendix

aqueous (A-kwe-us) Pertaining to water; an aqueous solution is one in which water is the solvent

aqueous (A-kwe-us) **humor** Watery fluid that fills much of the eyeball anterior to the lens

arachnoid (ah-RAK-noyd) Middle layer of the meninges

areolar (ah-RE-o-lar) Referring to loose connective tissue, any small spaces or to an areola, a circular area of marked color

arrector pili (ah-REK-tor PI-li) Muscle attached to a hair follicle that raises the hair

arteriole (ar-TE-re-ole) Vessel between a small artery and a capillary

artery (AR-ter-e) Vessel that carries blood away from the heart

articular (ar-TIK-u-lar) Pertaining to a joint

atom (AT-om) Smallest subunit of a chemical element

atomic number The number of protons in the nucleus of an element's atoms; a number characteristic of each element

ATP See adenosine triphosphate

atrial natriuretic (*na-tre-u-RET-ik*) **peptide (ANP)** Hormone produced by the atria of the heart which lowers blood pressure

atrioventricular (a-tre-o-ven-TRIK-u-lar) **(AV) node** Part of the conduction system of the heart

atrium (A-tre-um) One of the two upper chambers of the heart; adj., atrial

attenuated (ah-TEN-u-a-ted) Weakened

autonomic (aw-to-NOM-ik) **nervous system (ANS)** The part of the nervous system that controls smooth muscle, cardiac muscle, and glands; the visceral or involuntary nervous system

autosome (AW-to-some) One of the 44 chromosomes not involved in sex determination

AV node See atrioventricular node

axial (AK-se-al) **skeleton** The part of the skeleton that includes the skull, spinal column, ribs, and sternum

axilla (ak-SIL-ah) Hollow beneath the arm where it joins the body; armpit

axon (AK-son) Fiber of a neuron that conducts impulses away from the cell body

basal ganglia (BA-sal GANG-le-ah) Gray masses in the lower part of the forebrain that aid in muscle coordination

base Substance that can accept a hydrogen ion (H$^+$); substance that donates a hydroxide ion (OH$^-$) an alkali

basophil (BA-so-fil) Granular white blood cell that shows large, dark blue cytoplasmic granules when stained with basic stain

B cell Agranular white blood cell that gives rise to antibody-producing plasma cells in response to an antigen; B lymphocyte

bile Substance produced in the liver that emulsifies fats

bilirubin (BIL-ih-ru-bin) Pigment derived from the breakdown of hemoglobin and found in bile

blood urea nitrogen (BUN) Amount of nitrogen from urea in the blood; test to evaluate kidney function

bolus (BO-lus) A concentrated mass; the portion of food that is moved to the back of the mouth and swallowed

Bowman capsule Enlarged portion of the nephron that contains the glomerulus; glomerular capsule

bone Hard connective tissue that makes up most of the skeleton, or any structure composed of this type of tissue

bradycardia (brad-e-KAR-de-ah) Heart rate of less than 60 beats per minute

brain The controlling area of the central nervous system (CNS)

brain stem Portion of the brain that connects the cerebrum with the spinal cord; contains the midbrain, pons, and medulla oblongata

Broca (bro-KAH) **area** Area of the cerebral cortex concerned with motor control of speech

bronchiole (BRONG-ke-ole) Microscopic terminal branch of a bronchus

bronchus (BRONG-kus) Large air passageway in the lung; pl., bronchi (BRONG-ki)

buffer (BUF-er) Substance that prevents sharp changes in the pH of a solution

bulbourethral (bul-bo-u-RE-thral) **gland** Gland that secretes mucus to lubricate the urethra and tip of penis during sexual stimulation; Cowper gland

bulk transport Movement of large amounts of material through the plasma membrane of a cell

BUN See blood urea nitrogen

bursa (BER-sah) Small, fluid-filled sac found in an area subject to stress around bones and joints; pl., bursae (BER-se)

calcitonin (kal-sih-TO-nin) Hormone from the thyroid gland that lowers blood calcium levels and promotes deposit of calcium in bones; thyrocalcitonin

calcitriol (kal-sih-TRI-ol) The active form of vitamin D; dihydroxycholecalciferol (di-hi-drok-se-ko-le-kal-SIF-eh-rol)

calyx (KA-liks) Cuplike extension of the renal pelvis that collects urine; pl., calyces (KA-lih-seze)

cancellous (KAN-sel-us) Referring to spongy bone tissue

capillary (CAP-ih-lar-e) Microscopic vessel through which exchanges take place between the blood and the tissues

carbohydrate (kar-bo-HI-drate) Simple sugar or compound made from simple sugars linked together, such as starch or glycogen

carbon Element that is the basis of organic chemistry

carbon dioxide (di-OX-ide) **(CO$_2$)** The gaseous waste product of cellular metabolism

cardiac (KAR-de-ak) Pertaining to the heart

cardiovascular system (kar-do-o-VAS-ku-lar) The system consisting of the heart and blood vessels that transports blood throughout the body

carrier Individual who has a gene that is not expressed but that can be passed to offspring

cartilage (KAR-tih-lij) Type of hard connective tissue found at the ends of bones, the tip of the nose, larynx, trachea and the embryonic skeleton

CAT See computed tomography

catabolism (kah-TAB-o-lizm) Metabolic breakdown of substances into simpler substances; includes the digestion of food and the oxidation of nutrient molecules for energy

catalyst (KAT-ah-list) Substance that speeds the rate of a chemical reaction

cation (KAT-i-on) Positively charged particle (ion)

caudal (KAWD-al) Toward or nearer to the sacral region of the spinal column

cecum (SE-kum) Small pouch at the beginning of the large intestine

cell Basic unit of life

cell membrane Outer covering of a cell; regulates what enters and leaves cell; plasma membrane

cellular respiration Series of reactions by which nutrients are oxidized for energy within the cell

central nervous system (CNS) Part of the nervous system that includes the brain and spinal cord

centrifuge (SEN-trih-fuje) An instrument that separates materials in a mixture based on density

centriole (SEN-tre-ole) Rod-shaped body near the nucleus of a cell; functions in cell division

cerebellum (ser-eh-BEL-um) Small section of the brain located under the cerebral hemispheres; functions in coordination, balance, and muscle tone

cerebral (SER-e-bral) **cortex** The very thin outer layer of gray matter on the surface of the cerebral hemispheres

cerebrospinal (ser-e-bro-SPI-nal) **fluid (CSF)** Fluid that circulates in and around the brain and spinal cord

cerebrum (SER-e-brum) Largest part of the brain; composed of two cerebral hemispheres

cerumen (seh-RU-men) Earwax; adj., ceruminous (seh-RU-min-us)

cervix (SER-vix) Constricted portion of an organ or part, such as the lower portion of the uterus; neck.; adj., cervical

chemistry (KEM-is-tre) Study of the composition and properties of matter

chemoreceptor (ke-mo-re-SEP-tor) Receptor that responds to chemicals in body fluids

cholecystokinin (ko-le-sis-to-KI-nin) **(CCK)** Hormone from the duodenum that stimulates release of pancreatic enzymes and bile from the gallbladder

cholesterol (ko-LES-ter-ol) An organic fatlike compound found in animal fat, bile, blood, myelin, liver, and other parts of the body

cholinergic (ko-lin-ER-jik) An activity or structure that responds to acetylcholine

chondrocyte (KON-dro-site) Cell that produces cartilage

chordae tendineae (KOR-de ten-DIN-e-e) Fibrous threads that stabilize the AV valve flaps in the heart

choroid (KO-royd) Pigmented middle layer of the eye

choroid plexus (KO-royd PLEKS-us) Vascular network in the ventricles of the brain that forms cerebrospinal fluid

creatinine (kre-AT-in-in) A nitrogenous waste product in the blood

chromosome (KRO-mo-some) Dark-staining, threadlike body in the nucleus of a cell; contains genes that determine hereditary traits

chyle (kile) Milky-appearing fluid absorbed into the lymphatic system from the small intestine; consists of lymph and droplets of digested fat

chyme (kime) Mixture of partially digested food, water, and digestive juices that forms in the stomach

cilia (SIL-e-ah) Hairs or hairlike processes, such as eyelashes or microscopic extensions from the surface of a cell; sing., cilium

ciliary (SIL-e-ar-e) **muscle** Muscle of the eye that controls the shape of the lens

circumduction (ser-kum-DUK-shun) Circular movement at a joint

cisterna chyli (sis-TER-nah KI-li) First part of the thoracic lymph duct, which is enlarged to form a temporary storage area

clitoris (KLIT-o-ris) Small organ of great sensitivity in the external genitalia of the female

CNS See central nervous system

coagulation (ko-ag-u-LA-shun) Clotting, as of blood

cochlea (KOK-le-ah) Coiled portion of the inner ear that contains the organ of hearing

collagen (KOL-ah-jen) Flexible white protein that gives strength and resilience to connective tissue, such as bone and cartilage

colloid (kol-OYD) Mixture in which suspended particles do not dissolve but remain distributed in the solvent because of their small size (*e.g.*, cytoplasm); colloidal suspension

colon (KO-lon) Main portion of the large intestine

colostrum (ko-LOS-trum) Secretion of the mammary glands released prior to secretion of milk

complement (KOM-ple-ment) Group of blood proteins that helps antibodies to destroy foreign cells

compliance (kom-PLI-ans) The ease with which the lungs and thorax can be expanded

compound Substance composed of two or more chemical elements

computed tomography (to-MOG-rah-fe) **(CT)** Imaging method in which multiple radiographic views taken from different angles are analyzed by computer to show a cross-section of an area; used to detect tumors and other abnormalities; also called computed axial tomography (CAT)

concha (KON-ka) Shell-like bone in the nasal cavity; pl., conchae (KON-ke)

condyle (KON-dile) Rounded projection, as on a bone

cone Receptor cell in the retina of the eye; used for vision in bright light

conjunctiva (kon-junk-TI-vah) Membrane that lines the eyelid and covers the anterior part of the sclera (white of the eye)

contraception (con-trah-SEP-shun) Prevention of fertilization of an ovum or implantation of a fertilized ovum; birth control

convergence (kon-VER-jens) The centering of both eyes on the same visual field

cornea (KOR-ne-ah) Clear portion of the sclera that covers the front of the eye

coronary (KOR-on-ar-e) Referring to the heart or to the arteries supplying blood to the heart

corpus callosum (kal-O-sum) Thick bundle of myelinated nerve cell fibers, deep within the brain, that carries nerve impulses from one cerebral hemisphere to the other

corpus luteum (LU-te-um) Yellow body formed from ovarian follicle after ovulation; produces estrogen and progesterone

cortex (KOR-tex) Outer layer of an organ, such as the brain, kidney, or adrenal gland

countercurrent mechanism Mechanism for concentrating urine as it flows through the distal portions of the nephron

covalent (KO-va-lent) **bond** Chemical bond formed by the sharing of electrons between atoms

cranial (KRA-ne-al) Pertaining to the cranium, the part of the skull that encloses the brain; toward the head or nearer to the head

creatine (KRE-ah-tin) **phosphate** Compound in muscle tissue that stores energy in high energy bonds

creatinine (kre-AT-ih-nin) Nitrogenous waste product eliminated in urine

crenation (kre-NA-shun) Shrinking of a cell, as when placed in a hypertonic solution

crista (KRIS-tah) Receptor for the sense of dynamic equilibrium; pl., cristae

CSF See cerebrospinal fluid

CT See computed tomography

cutaneous (ku-TA-ne-us) Referring to the skin

cuticle (KU-tih-kl) Extension of the stratum corneum that seals the space between the nail plate and the skin above the root of the nail

cystic (SIS-tik) **duct** Duct that carries bile into and out of the gallbladder

cytology (si-TOL-o-je) Study of cells

cytoplasm (SI-to-plazm) Substance that fills the cell, consisting of a liquid cytosol and organelles

cytosol (SI-to-sol) Liquid portion of the cytoplasm, consisting of nutrients, minerals, enzymes, and other materials in water

deamination (de-am-ih-NA-shun) Removal of amino groups from proteins in metabolism

defecation (def-e-KA-shun) Act of eliminating undigested waste from the digestive tract

deglutition (deg-lu-TISH-un) Act of swallowing

dehydration (de-hi-DRA-shun) Excessive loss of body fluid

denaturation (de-nah-tu-RA-shun) Change in structure of a protein, such as an enzyme, so that it can no longer function

dendrite (DEN-drite) Fiber of a neuron that conducts impulses toward the cell body

deoxyribonucleic (de-OK-se-ri-bo-nu-kle-ik) **acid (DNA)** Genetic material of the cell; makes up the chromosomes in the nucleus of the cell

depolarization (de-po-lar-ih-ZA-shun) A sudden reversal of the charge on a cell membrane

dermal papillae (pah-PIL-le) Extensions of the dermis that project up into the epidermis; they contain blood vessels that supply the epidermis

dermatome (DER-mah-tome) A region of the skin supplied by a single spinal nerve

dermis (DER-mis) True skin; deeper part of the skin

dextrose (DEK-strose) Glucose; simple sugar

dialysis (di-AL-ih-sis) Method for separating molecules in solution based on differences in their ability to pass through a semipermeable membrane; method for removing nitrogenous waste products from the body, as by hemodialysis or peritoneal dialysis

diaphragm (DI-ah-fram) Dome-shaped muscle under the lungs that flattens during inhalation; separating membrane or structure

diaphysis (di-AF-ih-sis) Shaft of a long bone

diarthrosis (di-ar-THRO-sis) Freely movable joint; synovial joint

diastole (di-AS-to-le) Relaxation phase of the cardiac cycle; adj., diastolic (di-as-TOL-ik)

diencephalon (di-en-SEF-ah-lon) Region of the brain between the cerebral hemispheres and the midbrain; contains the thalamus, hypothalamus, and pituitary gland

diffusion (dih-FU-zhun) Movement of molecules from a region where they are in higher concentration to a region where they are in lower concentration

digestion (di-JEST-yun) Process of breaking down food into absorbable particles

digestive system (di-JES-tiv) The system involved in taking in nutrients, converting them to a form the body can use and absorbing them into the circulation

dihydroxycholecalciferol (di-hi-drok-se-ko-le-kal-SIF-eh-rol) The active form of vitamin D

dilation (di-LA-shun) Widening of a part, such as the pupil of the eye, a blood vessel, or the uterine cervix; dilatation

disaccharide (di-SAK-ah-ride) Compound formed of two simple sugars linked together, such as sucrose and lactose

dissect (dis-sekt) To cut apart or separate tissues for study

distal (DIS-tal) Farther from the origin of a structure or from a given reference point

DNA See deoxyribonucleic acid

dominant (DOM-ih-nant) Referring to a gene that is always expressed if present

dopamine (DO-pah-mene) A neurotransmitter

dorsal (DOR-sal) Toward the back; posterior

dorsiflexion (dor-sih-FLEK-shun) Bending the foot upward at the ankle

duct Tube or vessel

ductus deferens (DEF-er-enz) Tube that carries sperm cells from the testis to the urethra; vas deferens

duodenum (du-o-DE-num) First portion of the small intestine

dura mater (DU-rah MA-ter) Outermost layer of the meninges

dyspnea (disp-NE-ah) Difficult or labored breathing

eccrine (EK-rin) Referring to sweat glands that regulate body temperature and vent directly to the surface of the skin through a pore

ECG See electrocardiograph

echocardiograph (ek-o-KAR-de-o-graf) Instrument to study the heart by means of ultrasound; the record produced is an echocardiogram

EEG See electroencephalograph

effector (ef-FEK-tor) Muscle or gland that responds to a stimulus; effector organ

efferent (EF-fer-ent) Carrying away from a given point, such as a motor neuron that carries nerve impulses away from the central nervous system

ejaculation (e-jak-u-LA-shun) Expulsion of semen through the urethra

EKG See electrocardiograph

electrocardiograph (e-lek-tro-KAR-de-o-graf) **(ECG, EKG)** Instrument to study the electrical activity of the heart; record made is an electrocardiogram

electroencephalograph (e-lek-tro-en-SEF-ah-lo-graf) **(EEG)** Instrument used to study electrical activity of the brain; record made is an electroencephalogram

electrolyte (e-LEK-tro-lite) Compound that separates into ions in solution; substance that conducts an electric current in solution

electron (e-LEK-tron) Negatively charged particle located in an energy level outside the nucleus of an atom

element (EL-eh-ment) One of the substances from which all matter is made; substance that cannot be decomposed into a simpler substance

embryo (EM-bre-o) Developing offspring during the first 2 months of pregnancy

emulsify (e-MUL-sih-fi) To break up fats into small particles; n., emulsification

endocardium (en-do-KAR-de-um) Membrane that lines the heart chambers and covers the valves

endocrine (EN-do-krin) Referring to a gland that secretes directly into the bloodstream

endocrine system The system composed of glands that secrete hormones

endocytosis (en-do-si-TO-sis) Movement of large amounts of material into a cell (*e.g.,* phagocytosis and pinocytosis)

endolymph (EN-do-limf) Fluid that fills the membranous labyrinth of the inner ear

endomysium (en-do-MIS-e-um) Connective tissue around an individual muscle fiber

endometrium (en-do-ME-tre-um) Lining of the uterus

endoplasmic reticulum (en-do-PLAS-mik re-TIK-u-lum) **(ER)** Network of membranes in the cytoplasm of a cell; may be smooth or rough based on absence or presence of ribosomes

end-organ Modified ending on a dendrite that functions as a sensory receptor

endorphin (en-DOR-fin) Pain-relieving substance released naturally from the brain

endosteum (en-DOS-te-um) Thin membrane that lines the marrow cavity of a bone

endothelium (en-do-THE-le-um) Epithelium that lines the heart, blood vessels, and lymphatic vessels

enzyme (EN-zime) Organic catalyst; speeds the rate of a reaction but is not changed in the reaction

eosinophil (e-o-SIN-o-fil) Granular white blood cell that shows beadlike, bright pink cytoplasmic granules when stained with acid stain; acidophil

epicardium (ep-ih-KAR-de-um) Membrane that forms the outermost layer of the heart wall and is continuous with the lining of the pericardium; visceral pericardium

epicondyle (ep-ih-KON-dile) Small projection on a bone above a condyle

epidermis (ep-ih-DER-mis) Outermost layer of the skin

epididymis (ep-ih-DID-ih-mis) Coiled tube on the surface of the testis in which sperm cells are stored and in which they mature

epigastric (ep-ih-GAS-trik) Pertaining to the region just inferior to the sternum (breastbone)

epiglottis (ep-e-GLOT-is) Leaf-shaped cartilage that covers the larynx during swallowing

epimysium (ep-ih-MIS-e-um) Sheath of fibrous connective tissue that encloses a muscle

epinephrine (ep-ih-NEF-rin) Neurotransmitter and hormone; released from neurons of the sympathetic nervous system and from the adrenal medulla; adrenaline

epiphysis (eh-PIF-ih-sis) End of a long bone; adj epiphyseal (ep-ih-FIZ-e-al)

episiotomy (eh-piz-e-OT-o-me) Cutting of the perineum between the vaginal opening and the anus to reduce the tearing of tissue in childbirth

epithelium (ep-ih-THE-le-um) One of the four main types of tissue; forms glands, covers surfaces, and lines cavities; adj., epithelial

EPO See erythropoietin

equilibrium (e-kwih-LIB-re-um) Sense of balance

ER See endoplasmic reticulum

erythrocyte (eh-RITH-ro-site) Red blood cell

erythropoietin **(EPO)** (eh-rith-ro-POY-eh-tin) Hormone released from the kidney that stimulates the production of red blood cells in the red bone marrow

esophagus (eh-SOF-ah-gus) Tube that carries food from the throat to the stomach

estrogen (ES-tro-jen) Group of female sex hormones that promotes development of the uterine lining and maintains secondary sex characteristics

eustachian (u-STA-shun) tube Tube that connects the middle ear cavity to the throat; auditory tube

eversion (e-VER-zhun) Turning outward, with reference to movement of the foot

excitability In cells, the ability to transmit an electrical current along the plasma membrane

excretion (eks-KRE-shun) Removal and elimination of metabolic waste products from the blood

exhalation (eks-hah-LA-shun) Expulsion of air from the lungs; expiration

exocrine (EK-so-krin) Referring to a gland that secretes through a duct

exocytosis (eks-o-si-TO-sis) Movement of large amounts of material out of the cell using vesicles

extension (eks-TEN-shun) Motion that increases the angle at a joint

extracellular (EK-strah-sel-u-lar) Outside the cell

extremity (ek-STREM-ih-te) Limb; an arm or leg

facilitated diffusion Movement of materials across the plasma membrane as they would normally flow by diffusion but using transporters to speed movement

fallopian (fah-LO-pe-an) tube See oviduct

fascia (FASH-e-ah) Band or sheet of fibrous connective tissue

fascicle (FAS-ih-kl) Small bundle, as of muscle cells or nerve cell fibers

fat Type of lipid composed of glycerol and fatty acids

feces (FE-seze) Waste material discharged from the large intestine; excrement; stool

feedback Return of information into a system, so that it can be used to regulate that system

fertilization (fer-til-ih-ZA-shun) Union of an ovum and a spermatozoon

fetus (FE-tus) Developing offspring from the third month of pregnancy until birth

fever (FE-ver) Abnormally high body temperature

fibrin (FI-brin) Blood protein that forms a blood clot

fibrinogen (fi-BRIN-o-jen) Plasma protein that is converted to fibrin in blood clotting

filtration (fil-TRA-shun) Movement of material through a semipermeable membrane under mechanical force

fimbriae (FIM-bre-e) Fringelike extensions of the oviducts that sweep a released ovum into the oviduct

fissure (FISH-ure) Deep groove

flagellum (flah-JEL-lum) Long whiplike extension from a cell used for locomotion; pl., flagella

flexion (FLEK-shun) Bending motion that decreases the angle between bones at a joint

follicle (FOL-lih-kl) Sac or cavity, such as the ovarian follicle or hair follicle

follicle-stimulating hormone (FSH) Hormone produced by the anterior pituitary that stimulates development of ova in the ovary and spermatozoa in the testes

fontanel (fon-tah-NEL) Area in the infant skull where bone formation has not yet occurred; also spelled fontanelle; "soft spot"

foramen (fo-RA-men) Opening or passageway, as into or through a bone; pl., foramina (fo-RAM-in-ah)

foramen magnum Large opening in the occipital bone of the skull through which the spinal cord passes to join the brain

formed elements Cells and cell fragments in the blood

fornix (FOR-niks) A recess or archlike structure

fossa (FOS-sah) Hollow or depression, as in a bone; pl., fossae (FOS-se)

fovea (FO-ve-ah) Small pit or cup-shaped depression in a surface; the fovea centralis near the center of the retina is the point of sharpest vision

frontal (FRONT-al) Describing a plane that divides a structure into anterior and posterior parts

FSH See follicle-stimulating hormone

fulcrum (FUL-krum) Pivot point in a lever system; joint in the skeletal system

fundus (FUN-dus) The deepest portion of an organ, such as the eye or the uterus

gamete (GAM-ete) Reproductive cell; ovum or spermatozoon

gamma globulin (GLOB-u-lin) Protein fraction in the blood plasma that contains antibodies

ganglion (GANG-le-on) Collection of nerve cell bodies located outside the central nervous system

gastric-inhibitory peptide (GIP) Hormone from the duodenum that inhibits release of gastric juice and stimulates release of insulin from the pancreas

gastrin (GAS-trin) Hormone released from the stomach that stimulates stomach activity

gastrointestinal (gas-tro-in-TES-tih-nal) (GI) Pertaining to the stomach and intestine or the digestive tract as a whole

gene Hereditary factor; portion of the DNA on a chromosome

genetic (jeh-NET-ik) Pertaining to the genes or heredity

genotype (JEN-o-tipe) Genetic make-up of an organism

gestation (jes-TA-shun) Period of development from conception to birth

GH See growth hormone

GI See gastrointestinal

gingiva (JIN-jih-vah) Tissue around the teeth; gum

glans The enlarged distal portion of the penis

glial cells (GLI-al) The connective tissue cells of the nervous system; neuroglia

glomerular (glo-MER-u-lar) filtrate Fluid and dissolved materials that leave the blood and enter the kidney nephron through Bowman capsule

glomerulus (glo-MER-u-lus) Cluster of capillaries in the glomerular (Bowman) capsule of the nephron

glottis (GLOT-is) Space between the vocal cords

glucagon (GLU-kah-gon) Hormone from the pancreatic islets that raises blood glucose level

glucocorticoid (glu-ko-KOR-tih-koyd) Steroid hormone from the adrenal cortex that raises nutrients in the blood during times of stress, e.g., cortisol

glucose (GLU-kose) Simple sugar; main energy source for the cells; dextrose

glycemic (gli-SE-mik) effect Measure of how rapidly a food raises the blood glucose level and stimulates release of insulin

glycogen (GLI-ko-jen) Compound built from glucose molecules that is stored for energy in liver and muscles

glycolysis (gli-KOL-ih-sis) First, anaerobic phase of the metabolic breakdown of glucose for energy

goblet cell A single-celled gland that secretes mucus

Golgi (GOL-je) apparatus System of membranes in the cell that formulates special substances; also called Golgi complex

gonad (GO-nad) Sex gland; ovary or testis

gonadotropin (gon-ah-do-TRO-pin) Hormone that acts on a reproductive gland (ovary or testis), e.g., FSH, LH

Graafian (GRAF-e-an) follicle See ovarian follicle

gram (g) Basic unit of weight in the metric system

granulocyte (GRAN-u-lo-site) Leukocyte with visible granules in the cytoplasm when stained

gray matter Nervous tissue composed of unmyelinated fibers and cell bodies

greater vestibular (ves-TIB-u-lar) gland Gland that secretes mucus into the vagina; Bartholin gland

growth hormone (GH) Hormone produced by anterior pituitary that promotes growth of tissues; somatotropin

gustatory (GUS-tah-to-re) Pertaining to the sense of taste (gustation)

gyrus (JI-rus) Raised area of the cerebral cortex; pl., gyri (JI-ri)

Haversian (ha-VER-shan) canal Channel in the center of an osteon (haversian system), a subunit of compact bone

Haversian system See osteon

heart (hart) The organ that pumps blood through the cardiovascular system

hemapheresis (hem-ah-fer-E-sis) Return of blood components to a donor following separation and removal of desired components

hematocrit (he-MAT-o-krit) (Hct) Volume percentage of red blood cells in whole blood; packed cell volume

hemocytometer (he-mo-si-TOM-eh-ter) Device used to count blood cells under the microscope

hemodialysis (he-mo-di-AL-ih-sis) Removal of impurities from the blood by their passage through a semipermeable membrane in a fluid bath

hemoglobin (he-mo-GLO-bin) (Hb) Iron-containing protein in red blood cells that binds oxygen

hemolysis (he-MOL-ih-sis) Rupture of red blood cells; v., hemolyze (HE-mo-lize)

hemopoiesis (he-mo-poy-E-sis) Production of blood cells; hematopoiesis

hemostasis (he-mo-STA-sis) Stoppage of bleeding

heparin (HEP-ah-rin) Substance that prevents blood clotting; anticoagulant

heredity (he-RED-ih-te) Transmission of characteristics from parent to offspring by means of the genes; the genetic makeup of the individual

hereditary (he-RED-ih-tar-e) Transmitted or transmissible through the genes; familial

heterozygous (het-er-o-ZI-gus) Having unmatched alleles for a given trait; hybrid

hilum (HI-lum) Indented region of an organ where vessels and nerves enter or leave

hippocampus (hip-o-KAM-pus) Sea horse-shaped region of the limbic system that functions in learning and formation of long-term memory

histamine (HIS-tah-mene) Substance released from tissues during an antigen–antibody reaction

histology (his-TOL-o-je) Study of tissues

HIV See human immunodeficiency virus

homeostasis (ho-me-o-STA-sis) State of balance within the body; maintenance of body conditions within set limits

homozygous (ho-mo-ZI-gus) Having identical alleles for a given trait; purebred

hormone Secretion of an endocrine gland; chemical messenger that has specific regulatory effects on certain other cells

human chorionic gonadotropin (ko-re-ON-ik gon-ah-do-TRO-pin) (hCG) Hormone produced by embryonic cells soon after implantation that maintains the corpus luteum

human immunodeficiency virus (HIV) The virus that causes AIDS

human placental lactogen (hPL) Hormone produced by the placenta that prepares the breasts for lactation and maintains nutrient levels in maternal blood

humoral (HU-mor-al) Pertaining to body fluids, such as immunity based on antibodies circulating in the blood

hyaline (HI-ah-lin) Clear, glasslike; referring to a type of cartilage

hydrolysis (hi-DROL-ih-sis) Splitting of large molecules by the addition of water, as in digestion

hydrophilic (hi-dro-FIL-ik) Mixing with or dissolving in water, such as salts; literally "water-loving"

hydrophobic (hi-dro-FO-bik) Repelling and not dissolving in water, such as fats; literally "water-fearing"

hymen Fold of membrane near the opening of the vaginal canal

hypercapnia (hi-per-KAP-ne-ah) Increased level of carbon dioxide in the blood

hyperglycemia (hi-per-gli-SE-me-ah) Abnormal increase in the amount of glucose in the blood

hyperpnea (hi-PERP-ne-ah) Abnormal increase in the depth and rate of respiration

hypertonic (hi-per-TON-ik) Describing a solution that is more concentrated than the fluids within a cell

hyperventilation (hi-per-ven-tih-LA-shun) Increased amount of air entering the alveoli of the lungs due to deep and rapid respiration

hypocapnia (hi-po-KAP-ne-ah) Decreased level of carbon dioxide in the blood

hypochondriac (hi-po-KON-dre-ak) Pertaining to a region just inferior to the ribs

hypogastric (hi-po-GAS-trik) Pertaining to an area inferior to the stomach or the most inferior midline region of the abdomen

hypoglycemia (hi-po-gli-SE-me-ah) Abnormal decrease in the amount of glucose in the blood

hypophysis (hi-POF-ih-sis) Pituitary gland

hypopnea (hi-POP-ne-ah) Decrease in the rate and depth of breathing

hypothalamus (hi-po-THAL-ah-mus) Region of the brain that controls the pituitary and maintains homeostasis

hypotonic (hi-po-TON-ik) Describing a solution that is less concentrated than the fluids within a cell

hypoventilation (hi-po-ven-tih-LA-shun) Insufficient amount of air entering the alveoli

hypoxemia (hi-pok-SE-me-ah) Lower than normal concentration of oxygen in arterial blood

hypoxia (hi-POK-se-ah) Lower than normal level of oxygen in the tissues

ileum (IL-e-um) The last portion of the small intestine

iliac (IL-e-ak) Pertaining to the ilium, the upper portion of the hipbone

immunity (ih-MU-nih-te) Power of an individual to resist or overcome the effects of a particular disease or other harmful agent

immunization (ih-mu-nih-ZA-shun) Use of a vaccine to produce immunity; vaccination

immunoglobulin (im-mu-no-GLOB-u-lin) (Ig) See antibody

implantation (im-plan-TA-shun) The embedding of the fertilized egg into the lining of the uterus

inferior (in-FE-re-or) Below or lower

inferior vena cava (VE-nah KA-vah) Large vein that drains the lower part of the body and empties into the right atrium of the heart

inflammation (in-flah-MA-shun) Response of tissues to injury; characterized by heat, redness, swelling, and pain

infundibulum (in-fun-DIB-u-lum) Stalk that connects the pituitary gland to the hypothalamus of the brain

ingestion (in-JES-chun) The intake of food

inguinal (IN-gwih-nal) Pertaining to the groin region or the region of the inguinal canal

inhalation (in-hah-LA-shun) Drawing of air into the lungs; inspiration

insertion (in-SER-shun) Muscle attachment connected to a movable part

insulin (IN-su-lin) Hormone from the pancreatic islets that lowers blood glucose level

integument (in-TEG-u-ment) Skin; adj., integumentary

integumentary system The skin and all its associated structures

intercalated (in-TER-cah-la-ted) disk A modified plasma membrane in cardiac tissue that allows rapid transfer of electrical impulses between cells

intercellular (in-ter-SEL-u-lar) Between cells

intercostal (in-ter-KOS-tal) Between the ribs

interferon (in-ter-FERE-on) (IFN) Group of substances released from virus-infected cells that prevent spread of infection to other cells; also nonspecifically boost the immune system

interleukin (in-ter-LU-kin) A substance released by a T cell or macrophage that stimulates other cells of the immune system

interneuron (in-ter-NU-ron) A nerve cell that transmits impulses within the central nervous system

interphase (IN-ter-faze) Stage in the life of a cell between one mitosis and the next when a cell is not dividing

interstitial (in-ter-STISH-al) Between; pertaining to spaces or structures in an organ between active tissues

interstitial cell–stimulating hormone (ICSH) see Luteinizing hormone

intestine (in-TES-tin) Organ of the digestive tract between the stomach and the anus, consisting of the small and large intestine

intracellular (in-trah-SEL-u-lar) Within a cell

inversion (in-VER-zhun) Turning inward, with reference to movement of the foot

ion (I-on) Charged particle formed when an electrolyte goes into solution

ionic bond Chemical bond formed by the exchange of electrons between atoms

iris (I-ris) Circular colored region of the eye around the pupil

islets (I-lets) Groups of cells in the pancreas that produce hormones; islets of Langerhans (LAHNG-er-hanz)

isometric (i-so-MET-rik) **contraction** Muscle contraction in which there is no change in muscle length but an increase in muscle tension, as in pushing against an immovable force

isotonic (i-so-TON-ik) Describing a solution that has the same concentration as the fluid within a cell

isotonic contraction Muscle contraction in which the tone within the muscle remains the same but the muscle shortens to produce movement

isotope (I-so-tope) Form of an element that has the same atomic number as another form of that element but a different atomic weight; isotopes differ in their numbers of neutrons

isthmus (IS-mus) Narrow band, such as the band that connects the two lobes of the thyroid gland

jejunum (je-JU-num) Second portion of the small intestine

joint Area of junction between two or more bones; articulation

juxtaglomerular (juks-tah-glo-MER-u-lar) **(JG) apparatus** Structure in the kidney composed of cells of the afferent arteriole and distal convoluted tubule that secretes the enzyme renin when blood pressure decreases below a certain level

karyotype (KAR-e-o-tipe) Picture of the chromosomes arranged according to size and form

keratin (KER-ah-tin) Protein that thickens and protects the skin; makes up hair and nails

kidney (KID-ne) Organ of excretion

kilocalorie (kil-o-KAL-o-re) A measure of the energy content of food; technically, the amount of heat needed to raise 1 kg of water 1° centigrade

kinesthesia (kin-es-THE-ze-ah) Sense of body movement

Kupffer (KOOP-fer) **cells** Macrophages in the liver that help to fight infection

labium (LA-be-um) Lip; pl., labia (LA-be-ah)

labyrinth (LAB-ih-rinth) Inner ear, named for its complex shape

lacrimal (LAK-rih-mal) Referring to tears or the tear glands

lactation (lak-TA-shun) Secretion of milk

lacteal (LAK-te-al) Capillary of the lymphatic system; drains digested fats from the villi of the small intestine

lactic (LAK-tik) **acid** Organic acid that accumulates in muscle cells functioning without oxygen

laryngeal (lah-RIN-je-al) **pharynx** Lowest portion of the pharynx, opening into the larynx and esophpagus

larynx (LAR-inks) Structure between the pharynx and trachea that contains the vocal cords; voice box

lateral (LAT-er-al) Farther from the midline; toward the side

lens Biconvex structure of the eye that changes in thickness to accommodate for near and far vision; crystalline lens

lesion (LE-zhun) Wound or local injury

leukocyte (LU-ko-site) White blood cell

leukocytosis (lu-ko-si-TO-sis) Increase in the number of white cells in the blood, such as during infection

LH See luteinizing hormone

ligament (LIG-ah-ment) Band of connective tissue that connects a bone to another bone; thickened portion or fold of the peritoneum that supports an organ or attaches it to another organ

limbic system Area between the cerebrum and diencephalon of the brain that is involved in emotional states and behavior

lipid (LIP-id) Type of organic compound, one example of which is a fat

liter (LE-ter) **(L)** Basic unit of volume in the metric system

loop of Henle Hairpin shaped segment of the renal tubule between the proximal and distal convoluted tubules

lumbar (LUM-bar) Pertaining to the region of the spine between the thoracic vertebrae and the sacrum

lumen (LU-men) Central opening of an organ or vessel

lung Organ of respiration

lunula (LU-nu-la) The pale half-moon shaped area at the proximal end of the nail

luteinizing (LU-te-in-i-zing) **hormone** Hormone produced by the anterior pituitary that induces ovulation and formation of the corpus luteum in females; in males, it stimulates cells in the testes to produce testosterone and may be called *interstitial cell–stimulating hormone (ICSH)*

lymph (limf) Fluid in the lymphatic system

lymphatic duct (lim-FAH-tic) Vessel of the lymphatic system

lymphatic system System consisting of the lymphatic vessels and lymphoid tissue; invovled in immunity, digestion, and fluid balance

lymph node Mass of lymphoid tissue along the path of a lymphatic vessel that filters lymph and harbors white blood cells active in immunity

lymphocyte (LIM-fo-site) Agranular white blood cell that functions in immunity

lysosome (LI-so-some) Cell organelle that contains digestive enzymes

macrophage (MAK-ro-faj) Large phagocytic cell that develops from a monocyte; presents antigen to lymphocytes in immune response

macula (MAK-u-lah) Spot; flat, discolored spot on the skin, such as a freckle or measles lesion; also called macule; small yellow spot in the retina of the eye that contains the fovea, the point of sharpest vision; receptor for the sense of static equilibrium

magnetic resonance imaging (MRI) Method for studying tissue based on nuclear movement after exposure to radio waves in a powerful magnetic field

major histocompatibility complex Group of genes that codes for specific proteins (antigens) on the surface of cells; these antigens are important in cross-matching for tissue transplantation, in immune reactions

MALT Mucosal-associated lymphoid tissue; tissue in the mucous membranes that helps fight infection

mammary (MAM-er-e) **gland** Breast

mastication (mas-tih-KA-shun) Act of chewing

matrix (MA-triks) The nonliving background material in a tissue; the intercellular material

meatus (me-A-tus) Short channel or passageway, as in a bone

medial (ME-de-al) Nearer the midline of the body

mediastinum (me-de-as-TI-num) Region between the lungs and the organs and vessels it contains

medulla (meh-DUL-lah) Inner region of an organ; marrow

medullary (MED-u-lar-e) **cavity** Channel at the center of a long bone that contains bone marrow

medulla oblongata (ob-long-GAH-tah) Part of the brain stem that connects the brain to the spinal cord

megakaryocyte (meg-ah-KAR-e-o-site) Very large cell that gives rise to blood platelets

meibomian (mi-BO-me-an) **gland** Gland that produces a secretion that lubricates the eyelashes

meiosis (mi-O-sis) Process of cell division that halves the chromosome number in the formation of the reproductive cells

melanin (MEL-ah-nin) Dark pigment found in skin, hair, parts of the eye, and certain parts of the brain

melanocyte (MEL-ah-no-site) Cell that produces melanin

melatonin (mel-ah-TO-nin) Hormone produced by the pineal gland

membrane Thin sheet of tissue

Mendelian (men-DE-le-en) **laws** Principles of heredity discovered by an Austrian monk named Gregor Mendel

meninges (men-IN-jeze) Three layers of fibrous membranes that cover the brain and spinal cord

menopause (MEN-o-pawz) Time during which menstruation ceases

menses (MEN-seze) Monthly flow of blood from the female reproductive tract

menstruation (men-stru-A-shun) The period of menstrual flow

mesentery (MES-en-ter-e) Membranous peritoneal ligament that attaches the small intestine to the dorsal abdominal wall

mesocolon (mes-o-KO-lon) Peritoneal ligament that attaches the colon to the dorsal abdominal wall

mesothelium (mes-o-THE-le-um) Epithelial tissue found in serous membranes

metabolic rate Rate at which energy is released from nutrients in the cells

metabolism (meh-TAB-o-lizm) All the physical and chemical processes by which an organism is maintained

metaphase (MET-ah-faze) Second stage of mitosis, during which the chromsomes line up across the equator of the cell

metarteriole (met-ar-TE-re-ole) Small vessel that connects the arterial system directly with the venous system in a blood shunt; thoroughfare channel

meter (ME-ter) **(m)** Basic unit of length in the metric system

MHC See major histocompatibility complex

micrometer (MI-kro-me-ter) (μm) 1/1000th of a millimeter; micron; also an instrument for measuring through a microscope (pronounced mi-KROM-eh-ter)

microscope (MI-kro-skope) Magnifying instrument used to examine cells and other structures not visible with the naked eye; examples are the compound light microscope, transmission electron microscope (TEM) and scanning electron microscope (SEM)

microvilli (mi-kro-VIL-li) Small projections of the plasma membrane that increase surface area; sing., microvillus

micturition (mik-tu-RISH-un) Act of urination; voiding of the urinary bladder

midbrain Upper portion of the brainstem

mineral (MIN-er-al) Inorganic substance; in the diet, an element needed in small amounts for health

mineralocorticoid (min-er-al-o-KOR-tih-koyd) Steroid hormone from the adrenal cortex that regulates electrolyte balance, *e.g.*, aldosterone

mitochondria (mi-to-KON-dre-ah) Cell organelles that manufacture ATP with the energy released from the oxidation of nutrients; sing., mitochondrion

mitosis (mi-TO-sis) Type of cell division that produces two daughter cells exactly like the parent cell

mitral (MI-tral) **valve** Valve between the left atrium and left ventricle of the heart; bicuspid valve

mixture Blend of two or more substances

molecule (MOL-eh-kule) Particle formed by chemical bonding of two or more atoms; smallest subunit of a compound

monocyte (MON-o-site) Phagocytic agranular white blood cell

monosaccharide Simple sugar; basic unit of carbohydrates

motor (MO-tor) Describing structures or activities involved in transmitting impulses away from the central nervous system; efferent

motor end plate Region of a muscle cell membrane that receives nervous stimulation

motor unit Group consisting of a single neuron and all the muscle fibers it stimulates

mouth Proximal opening of the digestive tract where food is ingested, chewed, mixed with saliva, and swallowed

MRI See magnetic resonance imaging

mucosa (mu-KO-sah) Lining membrane that produces mucus; mucous membrane

mucus (MU-kus) Thick protective fluid secreted by mucous membranes and glands; adj., mucous

murmur Abnormal heart sound

muscle (MUS-l) Tissue that contracts to produce movement; includes skeletal, smooth and cardiac types; adj., muscular

muscular (MUS-ku-lar) **system** The system of skeletal muscles that moves the skeleton, supports and protects the organs and maintains posture

mutation (mu-TA-shun) Change in a gene or a chromosome

myelin (MI-el-in) Fatty material that covers and insulates the axons of some neurons

myocardium (mi-o-KAR-de-um) Middle layer of the heart wall; heart muscle

myoglobin (MI-o-glo-bin) Compound that stores oxygen in muscle cells

myometrium (mi-o-ME-tre-um) The muscular layer of the uterus

myosin (MI-o-sin) One of the two contractile proteins in muscle cells, the other being actin

narcotic (nar-KOT-ik) Drug that acts on the CNS to alter perception and response to pain

nasopharynx (na-zo-FAR-inks) Upper portion of the pharynx located behind the nasal cavity

natural killer (NK) cell Type of lymphocyte that can nonspecifically destroy abnormal cells

negative feedback Self-regulating system in which the result of an action is the control over that action; a method for keeping body conditions within a normal range and maintaining homeostasis

nephron (NEF-ron) Microscopic functional unit of the kidney

nerve Bundle of neuron fibers outside the central nervous system

nerve impulse Electrical charge that spreads along the membrane of a neuron; action potential

nervous (NER-vus) **system** The system that transports information in the body by means of electrical impulses

neurilemma (nu-rih-LEM-mah) Thin sheath that covers certain peripheral axons; aids in regeneration of the axon

neuroglia (nu-ROG-le-ah) Supporting and protective cells of the central nervous system; glial cells

neuromuscular junction Point at which a nerve fiber contacts a muscle cell

neuron (NU-ron) Conducting cell of the nervous system

neurotransmitter (nu-ro-TRANS-mit-er) Chemical released from the ending of an axon that enables a nerve impulse to cross a synapse

neutron (NU-tron) Noncharged particle in the nucleus of an atom

neutrophil (NU-tro-fil) Phagocytic granular white blood cell; polymorph; poly; PMN; seg

nitrogen Chemical element found in all proteins

node Small mass of tissue, such as a lymph node; space between cells in the myelin sheath

norepinephrine (nor-epi-ih-NEF-rin) Neurotransmitter similar to epinephrine; noradrenaline

normal saline Isotonic or physiologic salt solution

nucleic acid (nu-KLE-ik) Complex organic substance composed of nucleotides that makes up DNA and RNA

nucleolus (nu-KLE-o-lus) Small unit within the nucleus that assembles ribosomes

nucleotide (NU-kle-o-tide) Building block of DNA and RNA

nucleus (NU-kle-us) Largest organelle in the cell, containing the DNA, which directs all cell activities; group of neurons in the central nervous system; in chemistry, the central part of an atom

olfactory (ol-FAK-to-re) Pertaining to the sense of smell (olfaction)

omentum (o-MEN-tum) Portion of the peritoneum; greater omentum extends over the anterior abdomen; lesser omentum extends between the stomach and liver

ophthalmic (of-THAL-mik) Pertaining to the eye

ophthalmoscope (of-THAL-mo-skope) Instrument for examining the posterior (fundus) of the eye

organ (OR-gan) Body part containing two or more tissues functioning together for specific purposes

organelle (or-gan-EL) Specialized subdivision within a cell

organic (or-GAN-ik) Referring to the complex compounds found in living things that contain carbon, and usually hydrogen, and oxygen

organism (OR-gan-izm) Individual plant or animal; any organized living thing

organ of Corti (KOR-te) Receptor for hearing located in the cochlea of the inner ear

origin (OR-ih-jin) Source; beginning; muscle attachment connected to a non-moving part

oropharynx (o-ro-FAR-inks) Middle portion of the pharynx, located behind the mouth

orthopnea (or-THOP-ne-ah) Difficulty in breathing that is relieved by sitting in an upright position

osmosis (os-MO-sis) Movement of water through a semipermeable membrane

osmotic (os-MOT-ik) **pressure** Tendency of a solution to draw water into it; is directly related to the concentration of the solution

osseus (OS-e-us) Pertaining to bone tissue

ossicle (OS-ih-kl) One of three small bones of the middle ear: malleus, incus, or stapes

ossification (os-ih-fih-KA-shun) Process of bone formation

osteoblast (OS-te-o-blast) Bone-forming cell

osteoclast (OS-te-o-clast) Cell that breaks down bone

osteocyte (OS-te-o-site) Mature bone cell; maintains bone but does not produce new bone tissue

osteon (OS-te-on) Subunit of compact bone, consisting of concentric rings of bone tissue around a central channel; haversian system

otoliths (O-to-liths) Crystals that add weight to fluids in the inner ear and function in the sense of static equilibrium

ovarian follicle (o-VA-re-an FOL-ih-kl) Cluster of cells in which the ovum develops within the ovary; Graafian follicle

ovary (O-vah-re) Female reproductive gland

oviduct (O-vih-dukt) Tube that carries ova from the ovaries to the uterus; fallopian tube, uterine tube

ovulation (ov-u-LA-shun) Release of a mature ovum from a follicle in the ovary

ovum (O-vum) Female reproductive cell or gamete; pl., ova

oxidation (ok-sih-DA-shun) Chemical breakdown of nutrients for energy

oxygen (OK-sih-jen) (O_2) The gas needed to break down nutrients completely for energy within the cell

oxygen debt Amount of oxygen needed to reverse the effects produced in muscles functioning without oxygen

oxytocin (*ok-se-TO-sin*) Hormone from the posterior pituitary that causes uterine contraction and milk ejection ("letdown") from the breasts

pacemaker Sinoatrial (SA) node of the heart; group of cells or artificial device that sets the rate of heart contractions

palate (PAL-at) Roof of the oral cavity; anterior portion is hard palate, posterior portion is soft palate

pancreas (PAN-kre-as) Large, elongated gland behind the stomach; produces digestive enzymes and hormones (*e.g.*, insulin)

papilla (pah-PIL-ah) Small nipplelike projection or elevation

parasympathetic nervous system Craniosacral division of the autonomic nervous system; generally reverses the fight-or-flight (stress) response

parathyroid (par-ah-THI-royd) **gland** Any of four to six small glands embedded in the capsule enclosing the thyroid gland; produces parathyroid hormone, which raises the blood calcium level by causing release of calcium from bones

parietal (pah-RI-eh-tal) Pertaining to the wall of a space or cavity

parturition (par-tu-RISH-un) Childbirth; labor

pedigree (PED-ih-gre) Family history; used in the study of heredity; family tree

pelvis (PEL-vis) Basinlike structure, such as the lower portion of the abdomen or the upper flared portion of the ureter (renal pelvis)

penis (PE-nis) Male organ of urination and sexual intercourse

perforating canal Channel across a long bone that contains blood vessels and nerves; Volkmann canal

pericardium (per-ih-KAR-de-um) Fibrous sac lined with serous membrane that encloses the heart

perichondrium (per-ih-KON-dre-um) Layer of connective tissue that covers cartilage

perilymph (PER-e-limf) Fluid that fills the bony labyrinth of the inner ear

perimysium (per-ih-MIS-e-um) Connective tissue around a fascicle of muscle tissue

perineum (per-ih-NE-um) Pelvic floor; external region between the anus and genital organs

periosteum (per-e-OS-te-um) Connective tissue membrane covering a bone

peripheral (peh-RIF-er-al) Located away from a center or central structure

peripheral nervous system (PNS) All the nerves and nervous tissue outside the central nervous system

peristalsis (per-ih-STAL-sis) Wavelike movements in the wall of an organ or duct that propel its contents forward

peritoneum (per-ih-to-NE-um) Serous membrane that lines the abdominal cavity and forms outer layer of abdominal organs; forms supporting ligaments for some organs

peroxisome (per-OK-sih-some) Cell organelle that enzymatically destroys harmful substances produced in metabolism

Peyer (PI-er) **patches** Clusters of lymphatic nodules in the mucous membranes lining the distal portion of the small intestine

pH Symbol indicating hydrogen ion (H^+) concentration; scale that measures the relative acidity and alkalinity (basicity) of a solution

phagocyte (FAG-o-site) Cell capable of engulfing large particles, such as foreign matter or cellular debris, through the plasma membrane

phagocytosis (fag-o-si-TO-sis) Engulfing of large particles through the plasma membrane

pharynx (FAR-inks) Throat; passageway between the mouth and esophagus

phenotype (FE-no-tipe) All the characteristics of an organism that can be seen or tested for

phospholipid (fos-fo-LIP-id) Complex lipid containing phosphorus

phrenic (FREN-ik) Pertaining to the diaphragm

physiology (fiz-e-OL-o-je) Study of the function of living organisms pia mater (PI-ah MA-ter) Innermost layer of the meninges

pineal (PIN-e-al) gland Gland in the brain that is regulated by light; involved in sleep–wake cycles

pinna (PIN-nah) Outer projecting portion of the ear; auricle

pinocytosis (pi-no-si-TO-sis) Intake of small particles and droplets by the plasma membrane of a cell

pituitary (pih-TU-ih-tar-e) gland Endocrine gland located under and controlled by the hypothalamus; releases hormones that control other glands; hypophysis

placenta (plah-SEN-tah) Structure that nourishes and maintains the developing fetus during pregnancy

plasma (PLAZ-mah) Liquid portion of the blood

plasma cell Cell derived from a B cell that produces antibodies

plasma membrane Outer covering of a cell; regulates what enters and leaves cell; cell membrane

plasmapheresis (plas-mah-fer-E-sis) Separation and removal of plasma from a blood donation and return of the formed elements to the donor

platelet (PLATE-let) Cell fragment that forms a plug to stop bleeding and acts in blood clotting; thrombocyte

pleura (PLU-rah) Serous membrane that lines the chest cavity and covers the lungs

plexus (PLEK-sus) Network of vessels or nerves

PNS See peripheral nervous system

polycythemia (pol-e-si-THE-me-ah) Increase in the number of red cells in the blood

polydipsia (pol-e-DIP-se-ah) Excessive thirst

polysaccharide Compound formed from many simple sugars linked together, such as starch and glycogen

pons (ponz) Area of the brain between the midbrain and medulla; connects the cerebellum with the rest of the central nervous system

portal system Venous system that carries blood to a second capillary bed through which it circulates before returning to the heart

positive feedback A substance or condition that acts within a system to promote more of the same activity

positron emission tomography (to-MOG-rah-fe) (PET) Imaging method that uses a radioactive substance to show activity in an organ

posterior (pos-TE-re-or) Toward the back; dorsal

potential (po-TEN-shal) An electrical charge, as on the neuron plasma membrane

precipitation (pre-sip-ih-TA-shun) Clumping of small particles as a result of an antigen-antibody reaction; seen as a cloudiness

pregnancy (PREG-nan-se) The period during which an embryo or fetus is developing in the body

prepuce (PRE-puse) Loose fold of skin that covers the glans penis; foreskin

presbyopia (pres-be-O-pe-ah) Loss of visual accommodation that occurs with age, leading to farsightedness

prime mover Muscle that performs a given movement; agonist

PRL see prolactin

progeny (PROJ-eh-ne) Offspring, descendent

progesterone (pro-JES-ter-one) Hormone produced by the corpus luteum and placenta; maintains the lining of the uterus for pregnancy

prolactin (pro-LAK-tin) Hormone from the anterior pituitary that stimulates milk production in the breasts; PRL

prone Face down or palm down

prophase (PRO-faze) First stage of mitosis, during which the chromosomes become visible and the organelles disappear

proprioceptor (pro-pre-o-SEP-tor) Sensory receptor that aids in judging body position and changes in position; located in muscles, tendons, and joints

prostaglandin (pros-tah-GLAN-din) Any of a group of hormones produced by many cells; these hormones have a variety of effects

prostate (PROS-tate) gland Gland that surrounds the urethra below the bladder and contributes secretions to the semen

protein (PRO-tene) Organic compound made of amino acids; contains nitrogen in addition to carbon, hydrogen, and oxygen (some contain sulfur or phosphorus)

prothrombin (pro-THROM-bin) Clotting factor; converted to thrombin during blood clotting

prothrombinase (pro-THROM-bih-nase) Blood clotting factor that converts prothrombin to thrombin

proton (PRO-ton) Positively charged particle in the nucleus of an atom

proximal (PROK-sih-mal) Nearer to point of origin or to a reference point

puerperal (pu-ER-per-al) Related to childbirth

pulmonary circuit Pathway that carries blood from the heart to the lungs for oxygenation and then returns the blood to the heart

pulse Wave of increased pressure in the vessels produced by contraction of the heart

pupil (PU-pil) Opening in the center of the eye through which light enters

Purkinje (pur-KIN-je) fibers Part of the conduction system of the heart; conduction myofibers

pylorus (pi-LOR-us) Distal region of the stomach that leads to the pyloric sphincter

pyruvic (pi-RU-vik) acid Intermediate product in the breakdown of glucose for energy

radioactivity (ra-de-o-ak-TIV-ih-te) Emission of rays of atomic particles from an element

radiography (RA-de-o-graf-e) Production of an image by passage of x-rays through the body onto sensitized film; record produced is a radiograph

receptor (re-SEP-tor) Specialized cell or ending of a sensory neuron that can be excited by a stimulus; also, a site in the cell membrane to which a special substance (e.g., hormone, antibody) may attach

recessive (re-SES-iv) Referring to a gene that is not expressed if a dominant gene for the same trait is present

reflex (RE-flex) Simple, rapid, automatic response involving few neurons

reflex arc (ark) A pathway through the nervous system from stimulus to response; commonly involves a receptor, sensory neuron, central neuron(s), motor neuron, and effector

refraction (re-FRAK-shun) Bending of light rays as they pass from one medium to another of a different density

relaxin (re-LAKS-in) Placental hormone that softens the cervix and relaxes the pelvic joints

renin (RE-nin) Enzyme released from the juxtaglomerular apparatus of the kidneys that indirectly increases blood pressure by activating angiotensin

repolarization (re-po-lar-ih-ZA-shun) A sudden return to the original charge on a cell membrane following depolarizaiton

resorption (re-SORP-shun) Loss of substance, such as that of bone or a tooth

respiration (res-pih-RA-shun) Process by which oxygen is obtained from the environment and delivered to the cells

respiratory system The system consisting of the lungs and breathing passages involved in exchange of oxygen and carbon dioxide between the outside air and the blood

reticular (reh-TIK-u-lar) formation Network in the limbic system that governs wakefulness and sleep

reticuloendothelial (reh-tik-u-lo-en-do-THE-le-al) system Protective system consisting of highly phagocytic cells in body fluids and tissues, such as the spleen, lymph nodes, bone marrow, and liver

retina (RET-ih-nah) Innermost layer of the eye; contains light-sensitive cells (rods and cones)

retroperitoneal (ret-ro-per-ih-to-NE-al) Behind the peritoneum, as are the kidneys, pancreas, and abdominal aorta

Rh factor Red cell antigen; D antigen

rhodopsin (ro-DOP-sin) Light-sensitive pigment in the rods of the eye; visual purple

rib One of the slender curved bones that make up most of the thorax; costa; adj., costal

ribonucleic (RI-bo-nu-kle-ik) **acid (RNA)** Substance needed for protein manufacture in the cell

ribosome (RI-bo-some) Small body in the cytoplasm of a cell that is a site of protein manufacture

RNA See ribonucleic acid

rod Receptor cell in the retina of the eye; used for vision in dim light

roentgenogram (rent-GEN-o-gram) Image produced by means of x-rays; radiograph

rotation (ro-TA-shun) Twisting or turning of a bone on its own axis

rugae (RU-je) Folds in the lining of an organ, such as the stomach or urinary bladder; sing., ruga (RU-gah)

SA node See sinoatrial node

saliva (sah-LI-vah) Secretion of the salivary glands; moistens food and contains an enzyme that digests starch

salt Compound formed by reaction between an acid and a base (*e.g.,* NaCl, table salt)

sagittal (SAJ-ih-tal) Describing a plane that divides a structure into right and left portions

saturated fat Fat that has more hydrogen atoms and fewer double bonds between carbons than do unsaturated fats

Schwann cell (shvahn) Cell in the nervous system that produces the myelin sheath around peripheral axons

sclera (SKLE-rah) Outermost layer of the eye; made of tough connective tissue; "white" of the eye

scrotum (SKRO-tum) Sac in which testes are suspended

sebum (SE-bum) Oily secretion that lubricates the skin; adj., sebaceous (se-BA-shus)

secretin (se-KRE-tin) Hormone from the duodenum that stimulates pancreatic release of water and bicarbonate

selectively permeable Describing a membrane that regulates what can pass through (*e.g.,* the plasma membrane of a cell)

sella turcica (SEL-ah TUR-sih-ka) Saddlelike depression in the floor of the skull that holds the pituitary gland

semen (SE-men) Mixture of sperm cells and secretions from several glands of the male reproductive tract

semicircular canal Bony canal in the inner ear that contains receptors for the sense of dynamic equilibrium; there are three semicircular canals in each ear

semilunar (sem-e-LU-nar) Shaped like a half-moon, such as the flaps of the pulmonary and aortic valves

seminal vesicle (VES-ih-kl) Gland that contributes secretions to the semen

seminiferous (seh-mih-NIF-er-us) **tubules** Tubules in which sperm cells develop in the testis

semipermeable (sem-e-PER-me-ah-bl) Capable of being penetrated by some substances and not others

sensory (SEN-so-re) Describing cells or activities involved in transmitting impulses toward the central nervous system; afferent

sensory adaptation Gradual loss of sensation when sensory receptors are exposed to continuous stimulation

septum (SEP-tum) Dividing wall, as between the chambers of the heart or the nasal cavities

serosa (se-RO-sah) Serous membrane; epithelial membrane that secretes a thin, watery fluid

Sertoli cells See sustentacular cells

serum (SE-rum) Liquid portion of blood without clotting factors; thin, watery fluid; adj., serous (SE-rus)

sex-linked Referring to a gene carried on a sex chromosome, usually the X chromosome

sinoatrial (si-no-A-tre-al) **(SA) node** Tissue in the upper wall of the right atrium that sets the rate of heart contractions; pacemaker of the heart

sinus (SI-nus) Cavity or channel, such as the paranasal sinuses in the skull bones

sinus rhythm A normal heart rhythm originating at the SA node

sinusoid (SI-nus-oyd) Enlarged capillary that serves as a blood channel

skeletal (SKEL-eh-tal) **system** The body system that includes the bones and joint

skeleton (SKEL-eh-ton) The complete bony framework of the body; adj., skeletal

skull Bony framework of the head

solute (SOL-ute) Substance that is dissolved in another substance (the solvent)

solution (so-LU-shun) Homogeneous mixture of one substance dissolved in another; the components in a mixture are evenly distributed and cannot be distinguished from each other

solvent (SOL-vent) Substance in which another substance (the solute) is dissolved

somatic (so-MAT-ik) **nervous system** The division of the nervous system that controls voluntary activities and stimulates skeletal muscle

somatotropin (so-mah-to-TRO-pin) Growth hormone

specific gravity The weight of a substance as compared to the weight of an equal volume of pure water

spermatic (sper-MAT-ik) **cord** Cord that extends through the inguinal canal and suspends the testis; contains blood vessels nerves and ductus deferens

spermatozoon (sper-mah-to-ZO-on) Male reproductive cell or gamete; pl., spermatozoa

sphincter (SFINK-ter) Muscular ring that regulates the size of an opening

sphygmomanometer (sfig-mo-mah-NOM-eh-ter) Device used to measure blood pressure; blood pressure apparatus or cuff

spinal cord Nervous tissue contained in the spinal column; major relay area between the brain and the peripheral nervous system

spirometer (spi-ROM-eh-ter) Instrument for recording lung volumes; tracing is a spirogram

spleen Lymphoid organ in the upper left region of the abdomen

squamous (SKWA-mus) Flat and irregular, as in squamous epithelium

stasis (STA-sis) Stoppage in the normal flow of fluids, such as blood, lymph, urine, or contents of the digestive tract

stem cell Cell that has the potential to develop into different types of cells

steroid (STE-royd) Category of lipids that includes the hormones of the sex glands and the adrenal cortex

stethoscope (STETH-o-skope) Instrument for conveying sounds from the patient's body to the examiner's ears

stimulus (STIM-u-lus) Change in the external or internal environment that produces a response

stomach (STUM-ak) Organ of the digestive tract that stores food, mixes it with digestive juices and moves it into the small intestine

stratified (STRAT-ih-fide) In multiple layers (strata)

stratum (STRA-tum) A layer; pl., strata

stratum basale (bas-A-le) Deepest layer of the epidermis; layer that produces new epidermal cells; stratum germinativum

stratum corneum (KOR-ne-um) The thick uppermost layer of the epidermis

striations (stri-A-shuns) Stripes or bands, as seen in skeletal muscle and cardiac muscle

subcutaneous (sub-ku-TA-ne-us) Under the skin

submucosa (sub-mu-KO-sah) Layer of connective tissue beneath the mucosa

substrate Substance on which an enzyme works

sudoriferous (su-do-RIF-er-us) Producing sweat; referring to the sweat glands

sulcus (SUL-kus) Shallow groove, as between convolutions of the cerebral cortex; pl., sulci (SUL-si)

superior (su-PE-re-or) Above; in a higher position

superior vena cava (VE-nah KA-vah) Large vein that drains the upper part of the body and empties into the right atrium of the heart

supine (SU-pine) Face up or palm up

surfactant (sur-FAK-tant) Substance in the alveoli that prevents their collapse by reducing surface tension of the contained fluids

suspension (sus-PEN-shun) Heterogeneous mixture that will separate unless shaken

suspensory ligaments Filaments attached to the ciliary muscle of the eye that hold the lens in place

sustentacular (sus-ten-TAK-u-lar) **cells** Cells in the seminiferous tubules that aid in development of spermatozoa; Sertoli cells

suture (SU-chur) Type of joint in which bone surfaces are closely united, as in the skull

sympathetic nervous system Thoracolumbar division of the autonomic nervous system; stimulates a fight-or-flight (stress) response

synapse (SIN-aps) Junction between two neurons or between a neuron and an effector

synarthrosis (sin-ar-THRO-sis) Immovable joint

synergist (SIN-er-jist) A substance or structure that enhances the work of another; a muscle that works with a prime mover to produce a given movement

synovial (sin-O-ve-al) Pertaining to a thick lubricating fluid found in joints, bursae, and tendon sheaths; pertaining to a freely movable (diarthrotic) joint

system (SIS-tem) Group of organs functioning together for the same general purposes

systemic circuit Pathway that carries blood to all tissues of the body except the lungs

systole (SIS-to-le) Contraction phase of the cardiac cycle; adj., systolic (sis-TOL-ik)

tachycardia (tak-e-KAR-de-ah) Heart rate more than 100 beats per minute

tachypnea (tak-IP-ne-ah) Excessive rate of respiration

tactile (TAK-til) Pertaining to the sense of touch

target tissue Tissue that is capable of responding to a specific hormone

T cell Lymphocyte active in immunity that matures in the thymus gland; destroys foreign cells directly; T lymphocyte

tectorial (tek-TO-re-al) **membrane** Part of the hearing apparatus; generates nerve impulses as cilia move against it in response to sound waves

telophase (TEL-o-faze) Final stage of mitosis, during which new nuclei form and the cell contents usually divide

tendon (TEN-don) Cord of fibrous connective tissue that attaches a muscle to a bone

teniae (TEN-e-e) **coli** Bands of smooth muscle in the wall of the large intestine

testis (TES-tis) Male reproductive gland; pl., testes (TES-teze)

testosterone (tes-TOS-ter-one) Male sex hormone produced in the testes; promotes the development of sperm cells and maintains secondary sex characteristics

tetanus (TET-an-us) Constant contraction of a muscle

thalamus (THAL-ah-mus) Region of the brain located in the diencephalon; chief relay center for sensory impulses traveling to the cerebral cortex

thorax (THO-raks) Chest; adj., thoracic (tho-RAS-ik)

thrombocyte (THROM-bo-site) Blood platelet; cell fragment that participates in clotting

thymosin (THI-mo-sin) Hormone produced by the thymus gland

thymus (THI-mus) Endocrine gland in the upper portion of the chest; stimulates development of T cells

thyroid (THI-royd) Endocrine gland in the neck

thyroid-stimulating hormone (TSH) Hormone produced by the anterior pituitary that stimulates the thyroid gland; thyrotropin

thyroxine (thi-ROK-sin) Hormone produced by the thyroid gland; increases metabolic rate and needed for normal growth; T_4

tinea (TIN-e-ah) Common term for fungal infection of the skin

tissue Group of similar cells that performs a specialized function

tonicity (to-NIS-ih-te) The osmotic concentration or osmotic pressure of a solution; the effect that a solution will have on osmosis

tonsil (TON-sil) Mass of lymphoid tissue in the region of the pharynx

tonus (TO-nus) Partially contracted state of muscle; also, tone

toxoid (TOK-soyd) Altered toxin used to produce active immunity

trachea (TRA-ke-ah) Tube that extends from the larynx to the bronchi; windpipe

tract Bundle of neuron fibers within the central nervous system

trait Characteristic

transverse Describing a plane that divides a structure into superior and inferior parts

tricuspid (tri-KUS-pid) **valve** Valve between the right atrium and right ventricle of the heart

triglyceride (tri-GLIS-er-ide) Simple fat composed of glycerol and three fatty acids

trigone (TRI-gone) Triangular shaped region in the floor of the bladder that remains stable as the bladder fills

triiodothyronine (tri-i-o-do-THI-ro-nin) Thyroid hormone that functions with thyroxine to raise cellular metabolism; T_3

tropomyosin (tro-po-MI-o-sin) A protein that works with troponin to regulate contraction in skeletal muscle

troponin (tro-PO-nin) A protein that works with tropomyosin to regulate contraction in skeletal muscle

TSH See thyroid-stimulating hormone

tympanic (tim-PAN-ik) **membrane** Membrane between the external and middle ear that transmits sound waves to the bones of the middle ear; eardrum

ultrasound (UL-trah-sound) Very high frequency sound waves

umbilical (um-BIL-ih-kal) **cord** Structure that connects the fetus with the placenta; contains vessels that carry blood between the fetus and placenta

umbilicus (um-BIL-ih-kus) Small scar on the abdomen that marks the former attachment of the umbilical cord to the fetus; navel

universal solvent Term used for water because it dissolves more substances than any other solvent

unsaturated fat Fat that has fewer hydrogen atoms and more double bonds between carbons than do saturated fats

urea (u-RE-ah) Nitrogenous waste product excreted in the urine; end product of protein metabolism

ureter (U-re-ter) Tube that carries urine from the kidney to the urinary bladder

urethra (u-RE-thrah) Tube that carries urine from the urinary bladder to the outside of the body

urinary bladder Hollow organ that stores urine until it is eliminated

urinary system (U-rin-ar-e) The system involved in elimination of soluble waste, water balance, and regulation of body fluids

urination (u-rin-A-shun) Voiding of urine; micturition

urine (U-rin) Liquid waste excreted by the kidneys

uterus (U-ter-us) Muscular, pear-shaped organ in the female pelvis within which the fetus develops during pregnancy

uvea (U-ve-ah) Middle coat of the eye, including the choroid, iris, and ciliary body; vascular and pigmented structures of the eye

uvula (U-vu-lah) Soft, fleshy, V-shaped mass that hangs from the soft palate

vaccination (vak-sin-A-shun) Administration of a vaccine to protect against a specific disease; immunization

vaccine (vak-SENE) Substance used to produce active immunity; usually, a suspension of attenuated or killed pathogens or some component of a pathogen given by inoculation to prevent a specific disease

vagina (vah-JI-nah) Lower part of the birth canal that opens to the outside of the body; female organ of sexual intercourse

valence (VA-lens) The combining power of an atom; the number of electrons lost or gained by atoms of an element in chemical reactions

valve Structure that prevents fluid from flowing backward, as in the heart, veins, and lymphatic vessels

vas deferens (DEF-er-enz) Tube that carries sperm cells from the testis to the urethra; ductus deferens

vasectomy (vah-SEK-to-me) Surgical removal of part or all of the ductus (vas) deferens; usually done on both sides to produce sterility

vasoconstriction (vas-o-kon-STRIK-shun) Decrease in the diameter of a blood vessel

vasodilation (vas-o-di-LA-shun) Increase in the diameter of a blood vessel

vein (vane) Vessel that carries blood toward the heart

vena cava (VE-nah KA-vah) A large vein that carries blood into the right atrium of the heart; superior vena cava or inferior vena cava

venous sinus (VE-nus SI-nus) Large channel that drains deoxygenated blood

ventilation (ven-tih-LA-shun) Movement of air into and out of the lungs

ventral (VEN-tral) Toward the front or belly surface; anterior

ventricle (VEN-trih-kl) Cavity or chamber; one of the two lower chambers of the heart; one of the four chambers in the brain in which cerebrospinal fluid is produced; adj., ventricular (ven-TRIK-u-lar)

venule (VEN-ule) Vessel between a capillary and a vein

vernix caseosa (VER-niks ka-se-O-sah) Cheeselike sebaceous secretion that covers a newborn

vertebra (VER-teh-brah) A bone of the spinal column; pl., vertebrae (VER-teh-bre)

vesicle (VES-ih-kl) Small sac filled with fluid

vesicular transport Use of vesicles to move large amounts of material through the plasma membrane of a cell

vestibule (VES-tih-bule) Part of the inner ear that contains receptors for the sense of static equilibrium; any space at the entrance to a canal or organ

villi (VIL-li) Small fingerlike projections from the surface of a membrane; projections in the lining of the small intestine through which digested food is absorbed; sing., villus

viscera (VIS-er-ah) Organs in the ventral body cavities, especially the abdominal organs; adj., visceral

viscosity (vis-KOS-ih-te) Thickness, as of the blood or other fluid

vitamin (VI-tah-min) Organic compound needed in small amounts for health

vitreous (VIT-re-us) **body** Soft, jellylike substance that fills the eyeball and holds the shape of the eye; vitreous humor

vocal cords Folds of mucous membrane in the larynx used in producing speech

Volkmann canal See perforating canal

Wernicke (VER-nih-ke) **area** Portion of the cerebral cortex concerned with speech recognition and the meaning of words

white matter Nervous tissue composed of myelinated fibers

x-ray Ray or radiation of extremely short wavelength that can penetrate opaque substances and affect photographic plates and fluorescent screens

zygote (ZI-gote) Fertilized ovum; cell formed by the union of a sperm and an egg

Glossary of Word Parts

▶ Use of Word Parts in Medical Terminology

Medical terminology is based on an understanding of a relatively few basic elements. These elements—roots, prefixes, and suffixes—form the foundation of almost all medical terms. A useful way to familiarize yourself with each term is to learn to pronounce it correctly and say it aloud several times. Soon it will become an integral part of your vocabulary.

The foundation of a word is the word root. Examples of word roots are *abdomin-*, referring to the belly region; and *aden-*, pertaining to a gland. A word root is often followed by a vowel to facilitate pronunciation, as in *abdomino-* and *adeno-*. We then refer to it as a "combining form." The hyphen appended to a combining form indicates that it is not a complete word; if the hyphen precedes the combining form, then it commonly appears as the word ending, as in *-cyte*, meaning "cell."

A prefix is a part of a word that precedes the word root and changes its meaning. For example, the prefix *-sub* in *subcutaneous* means "below." A suffix, or word ending, is a part that follows the word root and adds to or changes its meaning. The suffix *-ase* means "enzyme," as in lipase, an enzyme that digests fat.

Many medical words are compound words; that is, they are made up of more than one root or combining form. Examples of such compound words are *erythrocyte* (red blood cell) and *histology* (study of tissue), and many more difficult words, such as *sternoclavicular* (indicating relations to both the sternum and the clavicle).

A general knowledge of language structure and spelling rules is also helpful in mastering medical terminology. For example, adjectives describe something and include, among others, words that end in *-al*, as in *sternal* (the noun is *sternum*), and words that end in *-ous*, as in *mucous* (the noun is *mucus*).

The following list includes some of the most commonly used word roots, combining forms, prefixes, and suffixes, as well as examples of their use. Prefixes are followed by a hyphen; suffixes are preceded by a hyphen; and word roots have no hyphen. Commonly used combining vowels are added following a slash.

▶ Word Parts

a-, an- absent, deficient, lack of: *atrophy, amorphous, anaerobic*

ab- away from: *abduction, aboral*

abdomin/o belly or abdominal area: *abdominal, abdominopelus*

acous, acus hearing, sound: *acoustic*

acr/o- extreme end of a part, especially of the extremities: *acromion*

ad- (sometimes converted to *ac-, af-, ag-, ap-, as-, at-,*) toward, added to, near: *adrenal, accretion, agglomerated, afferent*

aden/o gland: *adenoid, adenocyte*

aer/o air, gas: *aerobic, aerate*

-agogue inducing, leading, stimulating: *cholagogue, galactagogue*

-al pertaining to, resembling: *skeletal, surgical, ileal*

amb/i- both, on two sides: *ambidexterity, ambivalent*

amphi on both sides, around, double: *amphiarthrosis, amphibian*

amyl/o starch: *amylase, amyloid*

an- absent, deficient, lack of: *anaerobic, anoxia*

ana- upward, back, again, excessive: *anatomy, anastomosis, anabolism*

andr/o male: *androgen, androgenous*

angi/o vessel: *angiogram, angiotensin*

ant/i- against; to prevent, suppress, or destroy: *antarthritic, antibiotic, anticoagulant*

ante- before, ahead of: *antenatal, antepartum*

anter/o- position ahead of or in front of (i.e., anterior to) another part: *anterolateral, anteroventral*

ap/o- separation, derivation from: *apocrine, apoptosis, apophysis*

aqu/e water: *aqueous, aquatic, aqueduct*

-ar pertaining to, resembling: *muscular, nuclear*

arthr/o joint or articulation: *arthritis, arthrosis*

-ary pertaining to, resembling: *salivary, dietary, urinary*

-ase enzyme: *lipase, protease*

-asis see *–sis*

audi/o sound, hearing: *audiogenic, audiometry, audiovisual*

aut/o- self: *autodigestion, autoimmune, autonomic*

bas/o- alkaline: *basic, basophilic*

bi- two, twice: *bifurcate, bisexual*

bil/i bile: *biliary, bilirubin*

bio- life, living organism: *antibiotic, biology, biochemistry*

blast/o, -blast early stage of a cell, immature cell: *blastula, blastophore, erythroblast*

brachi, brachi/o arm: *brachial, brachiocephalic, brachiotomy*

brady- slow: *bradycardia*

bronch/o-, bronch/i windpipe or other air tubes: *bronchiol, bronchoscope*

bucc cheek: *buccal*

capn/o carbon dioxide: *hypocapnia, hypercapnia*

cardi/o, cardi/a heart: *carditis, cardiac, cardiologist, cardiovascular*

cata- down: *catabolism, catalyst*

celi/o abdomen: *celiac*

centi- relating to 100 (used in naming units of measurements): *centigrade, centimeter*

cephal/o head: *cephalic, cephalopelvic*

cerebro brain: *cerobrospinal, cerebrum*

cervi neck: *cervical, cervix*

chem/o, chem/i chemistry, chemical: *chemotherapy, chemoreceptor*

chir/o, cheir/o hand: *cheiromegaly, chiropractic*

chol/e, chol/o bile, gall: *chologogue, cholecyst, cholecystokinin*

chondr/o, chondri/o cartilage: *chondrocyte, perichondrium*

chori/o membrane: *chorion, choroid*

chrom/o, chromat/o color: *chromosome, chromatin, chromophilic*

circum- around, surrounding: *circumorbital, circumrenal, circumduction*

-clast break: *osteoclast*

clav/o, cleid/o clavicle: *cleidomastoid, subclavian*

co- with, together: *cofactor, cohesion*

colp/o vagina: *colposcope, colpotomy*
con- with: *concentric, concentrate, conduct*
contra- opposed, against: *contraindication, contralateral*
corne/o horny: *corneum, cornified, cornea*
cortic/o cortex: *cortical, corticotropic, cortisone*
cost/a, cost/o- ribs: *intercostal, costosternal*
counter- against, opposite to: *counteract, counterirritation, countertraction*
crani/o skull: *cranium, craniosacral*
cry/o- cold: *cryalgesia, cryogenic, cryotherapy*
crypt/o- hidden, concealed: *cryptic, cryptogenic, cryptorchidism*
-cusis hearing: *acusis, presbyacusis*
cut- skin: *subcutaneous, cuticle*
cyt/o, -cyte cell: *cytology, cytoplasm, osteocyte*

dactyl/o digits (usually fingers, but sometimes toes): *dactylitis, polydactyly*
de- remove: *detoxify, dehydration*
dendr tree: *dendrite*
dent/o, dent/i tooth: *dentition, dentin, dentifrice*
derm/o, dermat/o skin: *dermatitis, dermatology, dermis*
di- twice, double: *dimorphism, dibasic, dihybrid*
dipl/o- double: *diploid*
dia- through, between, across, apart: *diaphragm, diaphysis*
dis- apart, away from: *dissect, dissolve, distal*
dors/i, dors/o- back (in the human, this combining form is the same as poster/o-): *dorsal, dorsiflexion, dorsonuchal*

e- out: *erection, ejection*
-ectasis expansion, dilation, stretching: *angiectasis, bronchiectasis*
ecto- outside, external: *ectoderm, ectogenous*
-ectomy surgical removal or destruction by other means: *appendectomy, thyroidectomy*
edem swelling: *edema*
-emia condition of blood: *glycemia, hyperemia*
encephal/o brain: *dienecephalor, encephalogram*
end/o- in, within, innermost: *endarterial, endocardium, endothelium*
enter/o intestine: *enteric, mesentery*
epi- on, upon: *epicardium, epidermis*
equi- equal: *equidistant, equivalent, equilibrium*
erg/o work: *ergonomic, energy, synergy*
eryth-, erythr/o red: *erythrocyte, erythropoiesis*
-esthesia sensation: *anesthesia, paresthesia*
eu- well, normal, good: *euphoria, eupnea*
ex/o- outside, out of, away from: *excretion, exocrine, exophthalmic*
extra- beyond, outside of, in addition to: *extracellular, extrasystole, extravascular*

fasci fibrous connective tissue layers: *fascia, fascicle*
fer, -ferent to bear, to carry: *afferent, efferent, transfer*
fibr/o threadlike structures, fibers: *fibrillation, fibroblast, myofibril*

gastr/o stomach: *gastric, gastrointestinal*
-gen an agent that produces or originates: *allergen, fibrinogen, pepsinogen*
-genic produced from, producing: *neurogenic, psychogenic*
genit/o organs of reproduction: *genitoplasty, genitourinary*
gen/o- a relationship to reproduction or sex: *genealogy, generate, genetic, genotype*
-geny manner of origin, development or production: *ontogeny, progeny*
gest/o gestation, pregnancy: *progesterone, gestagen*
glio, -glia gluey material; specifically, the connective tissue of the central nervous system: *neuroglia*
gloss/o tongue: *glossal, glossopharyngeal*
glyc/o- relating to sugar, glucose, sweet: *glycogen, glycemia*
gnath/o related to the jaw: *prognathic, gnathoplasty*
gnos to perceive, recognize: *agnostic, prognosis, diagnosis*
gon seed, knee: *gonad, gonarthritis*
-gram record, that which is recorded: *electrocardiogram, electroencephalogram*
graph/o, -graph instrument for recording, record, writing: *electrocardiograph, electroencephalograph, micrograph*
-graphy process of recording data: *photography, radiography*
gyn/o, gyne, gynec/o female, woman: *gynecology, gynecomastia, gynoplasty*
gyr/o circle: *gyroscope, gyrus, gyration*

hem/a, hem/o, hemat/o blood: *hematoma, hematuria, hemorrhage*
hemi- one half: *hemisphere, heminephrectomy, hemiplegia*
hepat/o liver: *hepatitis, hepatogenous*
heter/o- other, different: *heterogenous, heterosexual, heterochromia*
hist/o, histi/o tissue: *histology, histiocyte*
homeo-, homo- unchanging, the same: *hemeostasis, homosexual*
hydr/o water: *hydrolysis, hydrocephalus*
hyper- above, over, excessive: *hyperglycemia, hypertrophy*
hypo- deficient, below, beneath: *hypochondrium, hypodermic, hypogastrium*
hyster/o uterus: *hysterectomy*

-ia state of, condition of: *myopia, hypochondria, ischemia*
-iatrics, -trics medical specialty: *pediatrics, obstetrics*
iatr/o physician, medicine: *iatrogenic*

-ic pertaining to, resembling: *metric, psychiatric, geriatric*
idio- self, one's own, separate, distinct: *idiopathic, idiosyncrasy*
-ile pertaining to, resembling: *febrile, virile*
im-, in- in, into, lacking: *implantation, inanimate, infiltration*
infra- below, inferior: *infraspinous, infracortical*
insul/o pancreatic islet, island: *insulin, insulation, insuloma*
inter- between: *intercostal, interstitial*
intra- within a part or structure: *intracranial, intracellular, intraocular*
isch suppression: *ischemia*
-ism state of: *alcoholism, hyperthyroidism*
iso- same, equal: *isotonic, isometric*
-ist one who specializes in a field of study: *cardiologist, gastroenterologist*
-itis inflammation: *dermatitis, keratitis, neuritis*

juxta- next to: *juxtaglomerular, juxtaposition*

kary/o nucleus: *karyotype, karyoplasm*
kerat/o cornea of the eye, certain horny tissues: *keratin, keratoplasty*
kine movement: *kinetic, kinesiology, kinesthesia*

lacri- tear: *lacrimal*
lact/o milk: *lactation, lactogenic*
laryng/o larynx: *laryngeal, laryngectomy*
later/o- side: *lateral*
-lemma sheath: *neurilemma, sarcolemma*
leuk/o- (also written as *leuc-, leuco-*) white, colorless: *leukocyte, leukoplakia*
lip/o lipid, fat: *lipase, lipid*
lig- bind: *ligament, ligature*
lingu/o tongue: *lingual, linguodental*
-logy study of: *physiology, gynecology*
lute/o yellow: *macula lutea, corpus luteum*
lymph/o lymph, lymphatic system, lymphocyte: *lymphoid, lymphedema*
lyso-, -lysis, -lytic loosening, dissolving, separating: *hemolysis, paralysis, lysosome*

macr/o- large, abnormal length: *macrophage, macroblast.* See also -mega, mega/o-
mamm/o breast, mammary gland: *mammogram, mammoplasty, mammal*
man/o pressure: *manometer, sphygmomanometer*
mast/o breast: *mastectomy, mastitis*
meg/a-, megal/o, -megaly unusually or excessively large: *megacolon, megaloblast, splenomegaly, megakaryocyte*
melan/o dark, black: *melanin, melanocyte*
men/o physiologic uterine bleeding, menses: *menses, menopause*
mening/o membranes covering the brain and spinal cord: *meninges, meningitis*
mes/a, mes/o- middle, midline: *mesencephalon, mesoderm*

meta- change, beyond, after, over, near: *metabolism, metacarpal, metaplasia*

-meter, metr/o measure: *hemocytometer, sphygmomanometer, spirometer, isometric*

metr/o uterus: *endometrium*

micro- very small: *microscope, microbiology, microsurgery, micrometer*

mon/o- single, one: *monocyte, mononucleosis*

morph/o shape, form: *morphogenesis, morphology*

multi- many: *multiple, multifactorial, multipara*

my/o muscle: *myocardium, myometrium, myoglobin*

myc/o, mycet fungi: *mycid, mycete, mycology, mycosis, mycelium*

myel/o marrow (often used in reference to the spinal cord): *myeloid, myeloblast*

nas/o nose: *nasopharynx, paranasal*

natri sodium: *hyponatremia, natriuretic*

necr/o death, corpse: *necrosis*

neo- new: *neoplasm, neonatal*

neph, nephr/o kidney: *nephrectomy, nephron*

neur/o, neur/i nerve, nervous tissue: *neuron, neuralgia*

neutr/o neutral: *neutrophil, neutron*

ocul/o eye: *oculist, oculomotor, oculomycosis*

odont/o tooth, teeth: *odontogenesis, orthodontics*

-oid like, resembling: *lymphoid, myeloid*

olig/o- few, a deficiency: *oligospermia, oligodendrocyte*

-one ending for steroid hormone: *testosterone, progesterone*

oo, ov/i, ov/o ovum, egg: *oocyte, oviduct, ovoplasm* (do not confuse with **oophor-**)

oophor/o ovary: *oophorectomy, oophoritis, oophorocystectomy.* See also **ovar-**

ophthalm/o eye: *ophthalmia, ophthalmologist, ophthalmoscope*

-opia disorder of the eye or vision: *heterotropia, myopia, hyperopia*

or/o mouth: *oropharynx, oral*

orchi/o, orchid/o testis: *orchitis, cryptorchidism*

orth/o- straight, normal: *orthopedics, orthopnea, orthosis*

-ory pertaining to, resembling: *respiratory, circulatory*

oscill/o to swing to and fro: *oscilloscope*

osmo- osmosis: *osmoreceptor; osmotic*

oss/i, osse/o, oste/o bone, bone tissue: *osseous, ossicle, osteocyte*

ot/o ear: *otolith, otoscope*

-ous pertaining to, resembling: *fibrous, venous, androgynous*

ov/o egg, ovum: *oviduct, ovulation*

ovar, ovari/o ovary: *ovariectomy.* See also **oophor**

ox-, -oxia pertaining to oxygen: *hypoxemia, hypoxia, anoxia*

oxy sharp, acute: *oxygen, oxytocia*

papill/o nipple: *papilloma, papillary*

para- near, beyond, apart from, beside: *paramedical, parametrium, parathyroid, parasagittal*

pariet/o wall: *parietal*

ped/o, pedia child, foot: *pedal, pedicel, pediatrician*

-penia lack of: *leukopenia, thrombocytopenia*

per- through, excessively: *percutaneous, perfusion*

peri- around: *pericardium, perichondrium*

phag/o to eat, to ingest: *phage, phagocyte*

-phagia, -phagy eating, swallowing: *aphagia, dysphagia*

-phasia speech, ability to talk: *aphasia, dysphasia*

phen/o to show: *phenotype*

-phil, -philic to like, have an affinity for: *eosinophilic, hemophilia, hydrophilic*

phot/o light: *photoreceptor*

phren/o diaphragm: *phrenic, phrenicotomy*

physi/o natural, physical: *physiology, physician*

pil/e, pil/i, pil/o hair, resembling hair: *pileous, piliation*

pin/o to drink: *pinocytosis*

pleur/o side, rib, pleura: *pleural*

-pnea air, breathing: *dyspnea, eupnea*

pneum/o, pneumat/o air, gas, respiration: *pneumatic, pneumonia*

pod/o foot: *podiatry, pododynia*

-poiesis making, forming: *erythropoiesis, hematopoiesis*

poly- many: *monopoly, polysaccharide*

post- behind, after, following: *postnatal, postocular, postpartum*

pre- before, ahead of: *precancerous, preclinical, prenatal*

presby- old age: *presbycusis, presbyopia*

pro- before, in front of, in favor of: *prodromal, prosencephalon, prolapse, prothrombin*

proct/o rectum: *proctitis, proctocele, proctologist*

propri/o own: *proprioception*

pseud/o false: *pseudoarthrosis, pseudostratified, pseudopod*

psych/o mind: *psychosomatic, psychotherapy*

pulm/o, pulmon/o lung: *pulmonic, pulmonology*

pyel/o renal pelvis: *pyelitis, pyelogram, pyelonephrosis*

pyr/o fire, fever: *pyrogen, antipyretic, pyromania*

quadr/i- four: *quadriceps, quadriplegic*

rachi/o spine: *rachicentesis, rachischisis*

radio- emission of rays or radiation: *radioactive, radiography, radiology*

re- again, back: *reabsorption, reaction, regenerate*

rect/o rectum: *rectal, rectouterine*

ren/o kidney: *renal, renopathy*

reticul/o network: *reticulum, reticular*

retro- backward, located behind: *retrocecal, retroperitoneal*

rhin/o nose: *rhinitis, rhinoplasty*

-rhage, -rhagia* bursting forth, excessive flow: *hemorrhage, menorrhagia*

-rhea* flow, discharge: *diarrhea, gonorrhea, seborrhea*

sacchar/o sugar: *monosaccharide, polysaccharide*

salping/o tube: *salpingitis, salpingoscopy*

sarc/o flesh: *sarcolemma, sarcoplasm, sarcomere*

scler/o hard, hardness; *scleroderma, sclerosis*

-scope instrument used to look into or examine a part: *bronchoscope, endoscope, arthroscope*

semi- partial, half: *semipermeable, semicoma*

semin/o semen, seed: *seminiferous, seminal*

sin/o sinus: *sinusoid, sinoatrial*

-sis condition or process, usually abnormal: *dermatosis, osteoporosis*

soma-, somat/o, -some body: *somatic, somatotype, somatotropin*

son/o sound: *sonogram, sonography*

sphygm/o pulse: *sphygmomanometer*

spir/o breathing: *spirometer, inspiration, expiration*

splanchn-, splanchno- internal organs: *splanchnic, splanchnoptosis*

splen/o spleen: *splenectomy, splenic*

stat, -stasis stand, stoppage, remain at rest: *hemostasis, static, homeostasis*

sthen/o, -sthenia, -sthenic strength: *asthenic, calisthenics, neurasthenia*

steth/o chest: *stethoscope*

stoma, stomat/o mouth: *stomatitis*

-stomy surgical creation of an opening into a hollow organ or an opening between two organs: *colostomy, tracheostomy, gastroenterostomy*

sub- under, below, near, almost: *subclavian, subcutaneous, subluxation*

super- over, above, excessive: *superego, supernatant, superficial*

supra- above, over, superior: *supranasal, suprarenal*

sym-, syn- with, together: *symphysis, synapse*

tach/o-, tachy- rapid: *tachycardia, tachypnea*

tars/o eyelid, foot: *metatarsal, tarsoplasty*

-taxia, -taxis order, arrangement: *chemotaxis, taxonomy*

tel/o end: *telophase, telomere*

tens- stretch, pull: *extension, tensor*

test/o testis: *testosterone, testicular*

tetr/a four: *tetralogy, tetraplegia*

therm/o-, -thermy heat: *thermalgesia, thermocautery, diathermy, thermometer*

*When a suffix beginning with *rh* is added to a word root, the *r* is doubled.

thromb/o blood clot: *thrombosis, thrombocyte*

toc/o labor: *oxytocin*

tom/o, -tomy incision of, cutting: *anatomy, phlebotomy, laparotomy*

ton/o tone, tension: *tonicity, tonic*

tox, toxic/o poison: *toxin, cytotoxic, toxemia, toxicology*

trache/o trachea, windpipe: *tracheal, tracheotomy*

trans- across, through, beyond: *transorbital, transpiration, transplant, transport*

tri- three: *triad, triceps*

troph/o, -trophic, -trophy nutrition, nurture: *atrophic, hypertrophy*

trop/o, -tropin, -tropic turning toward, acting on, influencing, changing: *thyrotropin, adrenocorticotropic, gonadotropic*

tympan/o drum: *tympanic, tympanum*

ultra- beyond or excessive: *ultrasound, ultraviolent, ultrastructure*

uni- one: *unilateral, uniovular, unicellular*

-uria urine: *glycosuria, hematuria, pyuria*

ur/o urine, urinary tract: *urology, urogenital*

vas/o vessel, duct: *vascular, vasectomy, vasodilation*

viscer/o internal organs, viscera: *visceral, visceroptosis*

vitre/o glasslike: *vitreous*

xer/o dryness: *xeroderma, xerophthalmia, xerosis*

-y condition of: *tetany, atony, dysentery*

zyg/o joined: *zygote, heterozygous, monozygotic*

Appendices

Appendix 1   Metric Measurements

UNIT	ABBREVIATION	METRIC EQUIVALENT	U.S. EQUIVALENT
Units of length			
Kilometer	km	1000 meters	0.62 miles; 1.6 km/mile
Meter*	m	100 cm; 1000 mm	39.4 inches; 1.1 yards
Centimeter	cm	1/100 m; 0.01 m	0.39 inches; 2.5 cm/inch
Millimeter	mm	1/1000 m; 0.001 m	0.039 inches; 25 mm/inch
Micrometer	μm	1/1000 mm; 0.001 mm	
Units of Weight			
Kilogram	kg	1000 g	2.2 lb
Gram*	g	1000 mg	0.035 oz.; 28.5 g/oz
Milligram	mg	1/1000 g; 0.001 g	
Microgram	μg	1/1000 mg; 0.001 mg	
Units of volume			
Liter*	L	1000 mL	1.06 qt
Deciliter	dL	1/10 L; 0.1 L	
Milliliter	mL	1/1000 L; 0.001 L	0.034 oz.; 29.4 mL/oz
Microliter	μL	1/1000 mL; 0.001 mL	

*Basic unit.

Appendix 2 Celsius–Fahrenheit Temperature Conversion Scale

CELSIUS TO FAHRENHEIT

Use the following formula to convert Celsius readings to Fahrenheit readings:
°F= 9/5°C + 32
For example, if the Celsius reading is 37°
°F= (9/5 × 37) + 32
  =6.6 + 32
  =98.6°F (normal body temperature)

FAHRENHEIT TO CELSIUS

Use the following formula to convert Fahrenheit readings to Celsius readings:
°C= 5/9 (°F − 32)
For example, if the Fahrenheit reading is 68°:
°C =5/9 (68 − 32)
  =5/9 × 36
  =20°C (a nice spring day)

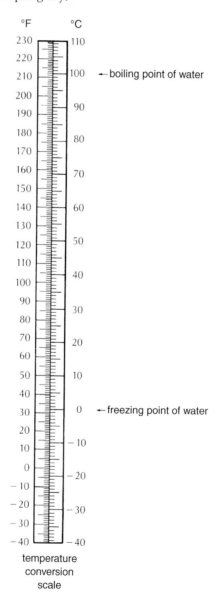

temperature
conversion
scale

Appendix 3 — Periodic Table of Elements

The periodic table lists the chemical elements according to their atomic numbers. The boxes in the table have information about the elements, as shown by the example at the top of the table. The upper number in each box is the atomic number, which represents the number of protons in the nucleus of the atom. Under the name of the element is its chemical symbol, an abbreviation of its modern or Latin name. The Latin names of four common elements are shown under the chart. The bottom number gives the atomic weight (mass) of each atom of that element as compared to the weight of carbon. Atomic weight is the sum of the weights of the protons and neutrons in the nucleus of an atom.

All the elements in a column share similar chemical properties based on the number of electrons in their outermost energy levels. Those in column VIII are nonreactive (inert) and are referred to as the *noble gases*. The 26 elements found in the body are color coded according to quantity (see legend above chart). Carbon, hydrogen, oxygen, and nitrogen make up 96% of body weight. The first three of these are present in all carbohydrates, lipids, proteins, and nucleic acids. Nitrogen is an additional component of all proteins. Nine other elements make up almost all the rest of body weight. The remaining 13 elements are present in very small amounts and are referred to as *trace elements*. Although needed in very small quantities, they are essential for good health, as they are parts of enzymes and other compounds used in metabolism.

PERIODIC TABLE OF THE ELEMENTS

Legend:
- 96% of body weight
- 3.9% of body weight
- 0.1% of body weight

Notation:
- 6 — Atomic number
- Carbon — Name
- C — Symbol
- 12.01 — Atomic weight

I	II											III	IV	V	VI	VII	VIII
1 Hydrogen **H** 1.01																	2 Helium **He** 4.00
3 Lithium **Li** 6.94	4 Beryllium **Be** 9.01											5 Boron **B** 10.81	6 Carbon **C** 12.01	7 Nitrogen **N** 14.01	8 Oxygen **O** 16.00	9 Fluorine **F** 19.00	10 Neon **Ne** 20.18
11 Sodium **Na** 22.99	12 Magnesium **Mg** 24.31											13 Aluminum **Al** 26.98	14 Silicon **Si** 28.09	15 Phosphorus **P** 30.97	16 Sulfur **S** 32.07	17 Chlorine **Cl** 35.45	18 Argon **Ar** 39.95
19 Potassium **K** 39.10	20 Calcium **Ca** 40.08	21 Scandium **Sc** 44.96	22 Titanium **Ti** 47.88	23 Vanadium **V** 50.94	24 Chromium **Cr** 52.00	25 Manganese **Mn** 54.94	26 Iron **Fe** 55.85	27 Cobalt **Co** 58.93	28 Nickel **Ni** 58.69	29 Copper **Cu** 63.55	30 Zinc **Zn** 65.39	31 Gallium **Ga** 69.72	32 Germanium **Ge** 72.59	33 Arsenic **As** 74.92	34 Selenium **Se** 78.96	35 Bromine **Br** 79.90	36 Krypton **Kr** 83.80
37 Rubidium **Rb** 85.47	38 Strontium **Sr** 87.62	39 Yttrium **Y** 88.91	40 Zirconium **Zr** 91.22	41 Niobium **Nb** 92.91	42 Molybdenum **Mo** 95.94	43 Technetium **Tc** (98)	44 Ruthenium **Ru** 101.1	45 Rhodium **Rh** 102.9	46 Palladium **Pd** 106.4	47 Silver **Ag** 107.9	48 Cadmium **Cd** 112.4	49 Indium **In** 114.8	50 Tin **Sn** 118.7	51 Antimony **Sb** 121.8	52 Tellurium **Te** 127.6	53 Iodine **I** 126.9	54 Xenon **Xe** 131.3
55 Cesium **Cs** 132.91	56 Barium **Ba** 137.34		72 Hafnium **Hf** 178.5	73 Tantalum **Ta** 180.9	74 Tungsten **W** 183.9	75 Rhenium **Re** 186.2	76 Osmium **Os** 190.2	77 Iridium **Ir** 192.2	78 Platinum **Pt** 195.1	79 Gold **Au** 196.9	80 Mercury **Hg** 200.6	81 Thallium **Tl** 204.4	82 Lead **Pb** 207.2	83 Bismuth **Bi** 209.0	84 Polonium **Po** (210)	85 Astatine **At** (210)	86 Radon **Rn** (222)
87 Francium **Fr** (223)	88 Radium **Ra** (226)		104 Rutherfordium **Rf** (257)	105 Dubnium **Db** (260)	106 Seaborgium **Sg** (263)	107 Bohrium **Bh** (262)	108 Hassium **Hs** (265)	109 Meitnerium **Mt** (267)	110 Darmstadtium **Ds** (271)	111 Unnamed (272)	112 Unnamed (277)						

57-71 Lanthanides

57 Lanthanum **La** 138.9	58 Cerium **Ce** 140.1	59 Praseodymium **Pr** 140.9	60 Neodymium **Nd** 144.2	61 Promethium **Pm** (145)	62 Samarium **Sm** (150.4)	63 Europium **Eu** 152.0	64 Gadolinium **Gd** 157.3	65 Terbium **Tb** 158.9	66 Dysprosium **Dy** 162.5	67 Holmium **Ho** 164.9	68 Erbium **Er** 167.3	69 Thulium **Tm** 168.9	70 Ytterbium **Yb** 173.0	71 Lutetium **Lu** 175.0

89-103 Actinides

89 Actinium **Ac** (227)	90 Thorium **Th** 232.0	91 Protactinium **Pa** (231)	92 Uranium **U** (238)	93 Neptunium **Np** (237)	94 Plutonium **Pu** (244)	95 Americium **Am** (243)	96 Curium **Cm** (247)	97 Berkelium **Bk** (247)	98 Californium **Cf** (251)	99 Einsteinium **Es** (254)	100 Fermium **Fm** (257)	101 Mendelevium **Md** (256)	102 Nobelium **No** (259)	103 Lawrencium **Lr** (257)

Name	Latin name	Symbol
Copper	*cuprium*	Cu
Iron	*ferrum*	Fe
Potassium	*kalium*	K
Sodium	*natrium*	Na

Appendix 4 Answers to Chapter Checkpoint and Zooming In Questions

CHAPTER 1

Answers to Checkpoint Questions

1-1 Study of body structure is anatomy; study of body function is physiology.

1-2 The breakdown phase of metabolism is catabolism; the building phase of metabolism is anabolism.

1-3 Negative feedback systems are primarily used to maintain homeostasis.

1-4 The three planes in which the body can be cut are sagittal, frontal (coronal), and transverse (horizontal). The midsagittal plane divides the body into two equal halves.

1-5 The posterior cavity is the dorsal cavity; the anterior cavity is the ventral cavity.

1-6 The three central regions of the abdomen are the epigastric, umbilical, and hypogastric regions; the three left and right lateral regions of the abdomen are the hypochondriac, lumbar, and iliac (inguinal) regions.

1-7 The basic unit of length in the metric system is the meter; of weight, the gram; of volume, the liter.

Answers to Zooming In Questions

1-7 The small figure is standing in the anatomical position.

1-8 The transverse (horizontal) plane divides the body into superior and inferior parts. The frontal (coronal) plane divides the body into anterior and posterior parts.

1-11 The ventral cavity contains the diaphragm.

CHAPTER 2

Answers to Checkpoint Questions

2-1 Atoms are subunits of elements.

2-2 Three types of particles found in atoms are protons, neutrons, and electrons.

2-3 Molecules are units composed of two or more atoms. They are the subunits of compounds.

2-4 Water is the most abundant compound in the body.

2-5 In a solution, the components dissolve and remain evenly distributed (the mixture is homogeneous); in a suspension, the particles settle out unless the mixture is shaken (the mixture is heterogeneous).

2-6 When an electrolyte goes into solution, it separates into charged particles called ions (cations and anions).

2-7 A covalent bond is formed by the sharing of electrons.

2-8 A value of 7.0 is neutral on the pH scale. An acid measures lower than 7.0; a base measures higher than 7.0.

2-9 A buffer is a substance that maintains a steady pH of a solution.

2-10 Isotopes that break down to give off radiation are termed radioactive.

2-11 Organic compounds are found in living things.

2-12 The element carbon is the basis of organic chemistry.

2-13 The three main categories of organic compounds are carbohydrates, lipids, and proteins.

2-14 A catalyst is a compound that speeds up the rate of a chemical reaction.

Answers to Zooming In Questions

2-1 The number of protons is equal to the number of electrons. There are eight protons and eight electrons.

2-2 Two hydrogen atoms bond with an oxygen atom to form water.

2-4 Two electrons are needed to complete the energy level of each hydrogen atom.

2-5 The amount of hydroxide ion (OH^-) in a solution decreases when the amount of hydrogen ion (H^+) increases.

2-7 Monosaccharides are the building blocks of disaccharides and polysaccharides.

2-8 There are three carbon atoms in glycerol.

2-9 The amino group of an amino acid contains nitrogen.

2-10 The shape of the enzyme after the reaction is the same as it was before the reaction.

CHAPTER 3

Answers to Checkpoint Questions

3-1 The cell shows organization, metabolism, responsiveness, homeostasis, growth, and reproduction.

3-2 Three types of microscopes are the compound light microscope, transmission electron microscope (TEM), and scanning electron microscope (SEM).

3-3 The main substance of the plasma membrane is a bilayer of phospholipids. Three types of materials found within the membrane are cholesterol, proteins, and carbohydrates (glycoproteins and glycolipids).

3-4 The cell organelles are specialized structures that perform different tasks.

3-5 The nucleus is called the control center of the cell because it contains the chromosomes, hereditary units that control all cellular activities.

3-6 The two types of organelles used for movement are the cilia, which are small and hairlike, and the flagellum, which is long and whiplike.

3-7 Nucleotides are the building blocks of nucleic acids.

3-8 DNA codes for proteins in the cell.

3-9 The three types of RNA are messenger RNA (mRNA), ribosomal RNA (rRNA) and transfer RNA (tRNA).

3-10 Before mitosis can occur, the DNA must double (duplicate). The doubling occurs during interphase.

3-11 The four stages of mitosis are prophase, metaphase, anaphase, and telophase

12-8 Neutrophils, eosinophils, and basophils are the granular leukocytes. Lymphocytes and monocytes are the agranular leukocytes.

12-9 The main function of leukocytes is to destroy pathogens.

12-10 The blood platelets are essential to blood coagulation (clotting).

12-11 When fibrinogen converts to fibrin a blood clot forms.

12-12 A, B, AB, and O are the four ABO blood type groups.

12-13 The blood antigens most often involved in incompatibility reactions are the A antigen, the B antigen, and the Rh antigen.

12-14 Blood is commonly separated into its component parts by a centrifuge.

12-15 The hematocrit is the percentage of red cell volume in whole blood.

Answers to Zooming In Questions

12-2 Erythrocytes (red blood cells) are the most numerous cells in the blood.

12-3 Erythrocytes are described as biconcave because they have an inward depression on both sides.

12-4 The granulocytes have segmented nuclei. Monocytes are the largest in size. Lymphocytes are the smallest in size.

12-6 Simple squamous epithelium makes up the capillary wall.

12-8 Fibrin in the blood forms a clot.

12-9 No. To test for Rh antigen, you have to use anti-Rh serum. The two types of antigens are independent.

CHAPTER 13

Answers to Checkpoint Questions

13-1 The innermost layer of the heart is the endocardium, the middle is the myocardium, and the outermost is the epicardium.

13-2 The pericardium is the sac that encloses the heart.

13-3 The upper chamber on each side of the heart is the atrium; each lower chamber is the ventricle.

13-4 Valves direct the flow of blood through the heart.

13-5 The coronary circulation is the blood supply to the myocardium.

13-6 The contraction phase of the cardiac cycle is systole; the relaxation phase is diastole.

13-7 Cardiac output is determined by the stroke volume, the volume of blood ejected from the ventricle with each beat, and by the heart rate, the number of times the heart beats per minute.

13-8 The small mass of tissue that starts the heartbeat is the sinoatrial (SA) node.

13-9 The autonomic nervous system is the main influence on the rate and strength of heart contractions.

13-10 A heart murmur is an abnormal heart sound.

13-11 ECG and EKG stand for electrocardiography.

Answers to Zooming In Questions

13-1 The left lung is smaller than the right lung because the heart is located more toward the left of the thorax.

13-2 The left ventricle has the thickest wall.

13-4 The aorta carries blood into the systemic circuit.

13-5 The myocardium is the thickest layer of the heart wall.

13-6 The right AV valve has three cusps; the left AV valve has two.

13-10 The AV (tricuspid and mitral) valves close when the ventricles contract, and the semilunar (pulmonary and aortic) valves open.

13-11 The internodal pathways connect the SA and AV nodes.

13-12 The SA and AV nodes are affected by the autonomic nervous system.

13-16 The cardiac cycle shown in the diagram is 0.8 seconds.

CHAPTER 14

Answers to Checkpoint Questions

14-1 The five types of blood vessels are arteries, arterioles, capillaries, venules, and veins.

14-2 The pulmonary circuit carries blood from the heart to the lungs and back to the heart; the systemic circuit carries blood to and from all remaining tissues in the body.

14-3 Smooth muscle makes up the middle layer of arteries and veins. Smooth muscle is involuntary muscle controlled by the autonomic nervous system.

14-4 There is one cell layer in the wall of a capillary.

14-5 The aorta is divided into the ascending aorta, aortic arch, thoracic aorta, and abdominal aorta.

14-6 The common iliac arteries are formed by the final division of the abdominal aorta.

14-7 The brachiocephalic trunk supplies the arm and head on the right side.

14-8 An anastomosis is a communication between two vessels.

14-9 Superficial means near the surface.

14-10 The superior vena cava and inferior vena cava drain the systemic circuit and empty into the right atrium.

14-11 A venous sinus is a large channel that drains deoxygenated blood.

14-12 The hepatic portal system takes blood from the abdominal organs to the liver.

14-13 As materials diffuse across the capillary wall, blood pressure helps to push materials out of the capillaries, and osmotic pressure of the blood helps to draw materials into the capillaries.

14-14 Vasodilation and vasoconstriction are the two type of vasomotor changes.

14-15 Vasomotor activities are regulated in the medulla of the brain stem.

14-16 The pulse is the wave of pressure that begins at the heart and travels along the arteries.

14-17 Blood pressure is the force exerted by blood against the walls of the vessels.

14-18 Systolic and diastolic blood pressure are measured.

Answers to Zooming In Questions

14-1 Pulmonary capillaries pick up oxygen. Systemic capillaries release oxygen.

14-2 Veins have valves to control the flow of blood.

14-3 The artery has a thicker wall than the vein.

14-4 There is one brachiocephalic artery.

14-8 There are two brachiocephalic veins.

14-10 The hepatic veins drain into the inferior vena cava.

14-12 The proximal valve is closer to the heart.

CHAPTER 15

Answers to Checkpoint Questions

15-1 The lymphatic system drains excess fluid and proteins from the tissues, protects against pathogens, absorbs fats from the small intestine.

15-2 The lymphatic capillaries are more permeable than blood capillaries and begin blindly. They are closed at one end and do not bridge two vessels.

15-3 The two main lymphatic vessels are the right lymphatic duct and the thoracic duct.

15-4 The lymph nodes filter lymph. They also have lymphocytes and monocytes to fight infection.

15-5 The spleen filters blood.

15-6 T cells of the immune system develop in the thymus.

15-7 Tonsils are located in the vicinity of the pharynx (throat).

15-8 The unbroken skin and mucous membranes constitute the first line of defense against the invasion of pathogens.

15-9 Some nonspecific factors that help to control infection are chemical and mechanical barriers, phagocytosis, natural killer cells, inflammation, fever, and interferon.

15-10 Inborn immunity is inherited in a person's genetic material; acquired immunity develops during an individual's lifetime.

15-11 An antigen is any foreign substance, usually a protein, that induces an immune response.

15-12 Four types of T cells are cytotoxic, helper, regulatory, and memory.

15-13 An antibody is a substance produced in response to an antigen.

15-14 Plasma cells, derived from B cells, produce antibodies.

15-15 Complement is a group of proteins in the blood that sometimes is required for the destruction of foreign cells.

15-16 The active form of naturally acquired immunity comes from contact with a disease organism; the passive form comes from the passage of antibodies from a mother to her fetus through the placenta or breast milk.

Answers to Zooming In Questions

15-1 A vein receives lymph collected from the body.

15-5 An afferent vessel carries lymph into a node. An efferent vessel carries lymph out of a node.

15-9 The phagocytic vesicle in step 2 contains fragments of foreign antigen

15-10 Plasma cells and memory cells develop from activated B cells.

CHAPTER 16

Answers to Checkpoint Questions

16-1 The three phases of respiration are pulmonary ventilation, external exchange of gases, and internal exchange of gases.

16-2 As air passes over the nasal mucosa, it is filtered, warmed, and moistened.

16-3 The scientific name for the throat is pharynx, for the voice box is larynx, and for the windpipe is trachea.

16-4 The three regions of the pharynx are the nasopharynx, the oropharynx, and the laryngeal pharynx.

16-5 The cells that line the respiratory passageways have cilia to filter impurities and to move fluids.

16-6 Gas exchange in the lungs occurs in the alveoli.

16-7 The pleura is the membrane that encloses the lung.

16-8 The two phases of breathing are inhalation, which is active, and exhalation, which is passive.

16-9 Diffusion is the movement of molecules from an area in which they are in higher concentration to an area where they are in lower concentration.

16-10 The substance in red blood cells that carries almost all of the oxygen in the blood is hemoglobin.

16-11 The main form in which carbon dioxide is carried in the blood is as bicarbonate ion.

16-12 The medulla of the brain stem sets the basic pattern of respiration.

16-13 The phrenic nerve is the motor nerve that controls the diaphragm.

16-14 Carbon dioxide is the main chemical controller of respiration.

Answers to Zooming In Questions

16-2 The heart is located in the medial depression of the left lung.

16-4 The epiglottis is named for its position above the glottis.

16-7 The external and internal intercostals are the muscles between the ribs.

16-8 Gas pressure decreases as the volume of its container increases.

16-9 Residual volume can not be measured with a spirometer.

CHAPTER 17

Answers to Checkpoint Questions

17-1 Food must be broken down by digestion into particles small enough to pass through the plasma membrane.

17-2 The digestive tract has a wall composed of a mucous membrane (mucosa), a submucosa, smooth muscle, and a serous membrane (serosa).

17-3 The peritoneum is the large serous membrane that lines the abdominopelvic cavity and covers the organs it contains.

17-4 There are 20 baby teeth, which are also called deciduous teeth.

17-5 Proteins are digested in the stomach.

17-6 The three divisions of the small intestine are the duodenum, jejunum, and ileum.

17-7 Most digestion takes place in the small intestine under the effects of digestive juices from the small intestine and the accessory organs. Most absorption of digested food and water also occurs in the small intestine.

17-8 The divisions of the large intestine are the cecum, ascending colon, transverse colon, descending colon, sigmoid colon, and rectum.

17-9 The large intestine reabsorbs some water and stores, forms, and eliminates the stool. It also houses bacteria that provide some vitamins.

17-10 The salivary glands are the parotid, submandibular (submaxillary), and sublingual.

17-11 The gallbladder stores bile.

17-12 Bile emulsifies fats.

17-13 The pancreas produces the most complete digestive secretions.

17-14 Absorption is the movement of digested nutrients into the circulation.

17-15 The two types of control over the digestive process are nervous control and hormonal control.

Answers to Zooming In Questions

17-1 Smooth muscle (circular and longitudinal) is between the submucosa and the serous membrane in the digestive tract wall.

17-3 The mesentery is the part of the peritoneum around the small intestine.

17-4 The salivary glands are the accessory organs that secrete into the mouth.

17-7 The oblique muscle layer is an additional muscle layer in the stomach as compared to the rest of the digestive tract.

17-8 The ileum of the small intestine joins the cecum.

17-10 The accessory organs shown secrete into the duodenum.

CHAPTER 18

Answers to Checkpoint Questions

18-1 The two phases of metabolism are catabolism, the breakdown phase of metabolism, and anabolism, the building phase of metabolism.

18-2 Cellular respiration is the series of reactions that releases energy from nutrients in the cell.

18-3 Glucose is the main energy source for the cells.

18-4 An essential amino acid or fatty acid cannot be made metabolically and must be taken in as part of the diet.

18-5 Minerals are chemical elements, and vitamins are complex organic substances.

18-6 The normal range of blood glucose is 85 to 125 mg/dL.

18-7 Typical recommendations are 55% to 60% carbohydrate; 30% or less fat; 15% to 20% protein.

18-8 Some factors that affect heat production are exercise, hormone production, food intake, and age.

18-9 The hypothalamus of the brain is responsible for regulating body temperature.

18-10 Normal body temperature is 36.2°C to 37.6°C (97°F to 100°F).

Answers to Zooming In Questions

18-1 Pyruvic acid produces lactic acid under anaerobic conditions; it produces CO_2 and H_2O under aerobic conditions.

CHAPTER 19

Answers to Checkpoint Questions

19-1 Systems other than the urinary system that eliminate waste include the digestive, respiratory, and integumentary systems.

19-2 The urinary system consists of two kidneys, two ureters, the bladder, and the urethra.

19-3 The retroperitoneal space is posterior to the peritoneum.

19-4 The renal artery supplies blood to the kidney, and the renal vein drains blood from the kidney.

19-5 The outer region of the kidney is the renal cortex; the inner region is the renal medulla.

19-6 The nephron is the functional unit of the kidney.

19-7 The glomerulus is the coil of capillaries in the glomerular (Bowman) capsule.

19-8 The JG apparatus produces renin when blood pressure falls too low for the kidneys to function effectively.

19-9 Glomerular filtration is the movement of materials under pressure from the blood into glomerular capsule of the nephron.

19-10 The four processes involved in the formation of urine are glomerular filtration, tubular reabsorption, tubular secretion, and the countercurrent mechanism for concentrating the urine.

19-11 The ureter carries urine from the kidney to the bladder.

19-12 The urethra carries urine from the bladder to the outside.

19-13 Body fluids are grouped into intracellular fluid and extracellular fluid.

19-14 Water is lost from the body through the kidneys, the skin, the lungs, and the intestinal tract.

19-15 The control center for the sense of thirst is located in the hypothalamus of the brain.

19-16 Sodium is the main cation in extracellular fluid. Potassium is the main cation in intracellular fluid.

19-17 Chloride is the main anion in extracellular fluid

19-18 Some electrolytes are lost through the feces and through sweat. The kidneys have the main job of balancing electrolytes. Several hormones, such as aldosterone, parathyroid hormone, and calcitonin, are also involved.

19-19 The acid–base balance of body fluids is maintained by buffer systems, respiration, and kidney function.

Answers to Zooming In Questions

19-1 The renal artery supplies blood to the kidney. The renal vein drains blood from the kidney.

19-2 The aorta supplies blood to the renal artery. The inferior vena cava receives blood from the renal vein.

19-3 The outer region of the kidney is the renal cortex. The inner region of the kidney is the renal medulla

19-4 The proximal convoluted tubule is closer to the glomerular capsule. The distal convoluted tubule is farther away from the glomerular capsule.

19-6 The juxtaglomerular apparatus is made up of cells from the afferent arteriole and the distal convoluted tubule.

19-7 The afferent arteriole has a wider diameter than the efferent arteriole.

19-10 The urethra passes through the prostate gland in the male.

19-11 Water is lost through the skin, the lungs, the kidneys and the intestine.

CHAPTER 20

Answers to Checkpoint Questions

20-1 Meiosis is the process of cell division that halves the chromosome number in a cell to produce a gamete.

20-2 The testis is the male gonad.

20-3 Testosterone is the main male sex hormone.

20-4 The spermatozoon, or sperm cell, is the male sex cell (gamete).

20-5 Sperm cells leave the seminiferous tubules within the testis and then travel through the epididymis, ductus (vas) deferens, ejaculatory duct, and urethra.

20-6 Glands that contribute secretions to the semen, aside from the testes, are the seminal vesicles, prostate, and bulbourethral glands.

20-7 The main subdivisions of the sperm cell are the head, midpiece, and tail (flagellum).

20-8 Follicle-stimulating hormone (FSH) and luteinizing hormone (LH), also called ICSH, are the pituitary hormones that regulate male and female reproduction.

20-9 The ovary is the female gonad.

20-10 The ovum (egg cell) is the female gamete.

20-11 The ovarian (graafian) follicle surrounds the egg as it ripens.

20-12 Ovulation is the process of releasing an egg cell from the ovary.

20-13 The follicle becomes the corpus luteum after ovulation.

20-14 The fetus develops in the uterus.

20-15 The two hormones produced in the ovaries are estrogen and progesterone.

20-16 Menopause is the period during which menstruation ceases.

20-17 Contraception is the use of artificial methods to prevent fertilization of the ovum or implantation of the fertilized ovum.

Answers to Zooming In Questions

20-1 The four glands that empty secretions into the urethra are the testes, seminal vesicles, prostate, and bulbourethral glands.

20-2 The ductus (vas) deferens receives secretions from the epididymis.

20-4 Mitochondria are the organelles that provide energy for sperm cell motility.

20-5 The corpus spongiosum of the penis contains the urethra.

20-6 The fundus of the uterus is the deepest part.

20-8 The endometrium is most highly developed in the second part of the menstrual cycle.

20-9 The opening of the urethra is anterior to the opening of the vagina.

20-11 LH shows the greatest increase at the time of ovulation.

CHAPTER 21

Answers to Checkpoint Questions

21-1 A zygote is formed by the union of an ovum and a spermatozoon.

21-2 The placenta nourishes the developing fetus.

21-3 The umbilical cord carries blood between the fetus and the placenta.

21-4 The heartbeat first appears during the fourth week of embryonic development.

21-5 The amniotic sac is the fluid-filled sac that holds the fetus.

21-6 The approximate length of pregnancy in days is 266.

21-7 Parturition is the process of labor and delivery.

21-8 A cesarean section is an incision made in the abdominal wall and the wall of the uterus for delivery of a fetus.

21-9 The term viable with reference to a fetus means able to live outside the uterus.

21-10 Lactation is the secretion of milk from the mammary glands.

21-11 A gene is an independent unit of heredity. Each is a segment of DNA contained in a chromosome.

21-12 A dominant gene is always expressed, regardless of the gene on the matching chromosome. A recessive gene is only expressed if the gene on the matching chromosome is also recessive.

21-13 Meiosis is the process of cell division that forms the gametes.

21-14 The sex chromosome combination that determines a female is XX; a male is XY.

21-15 A trait carried on a sex chromosome is described as sex-linked.

21-16 A mutation is a change in the genetic material (a gene or chromosome) of a cell.

Answers to Zooming In Questions

21-1 The ovum is fertilized in the oviduct (fallopian, uterine) tube.

21-2 The purple color signifies a mixture of oxygenated and unoxygenated blood.

21-5 The umbilical cord connects the fetus to the placenta.

21-7 The pectoralis major underlies the breast.

21-8 25% of children will show the recessive phenotype blond hair. 50% of children will be heterozygous.

Index

Page numbers in *italics* indicate figures. Those followed by "t" indicate tables. Page numbers followed by *B* indicate boxed material.